Meeting the Physical Therapy Needs of Children

Meeting the Physical Therapy Needs of Children

Susan K. Effgen, PT, PhD
Joseph Hamburg Professorship in Rehabilitation Sciences and Director
Rehabilitation Sciences Doctoral Program
College of Health Sciences
University of Kentucky
Lexington, Kentucky

F. A. Davis Company • Philadelphia

F. A. Davis Company
1915 Arch Street
Philadelphia, PA 19103
www.fadavis.com

Printed in the United States of America

Last digit indicates print number: 10 9 8 7 6 5

Acquisitions Editor: Margaret Biblis
Developmental Editor: Jennifer Pine
Production Editor: Jessica Howie Martin
Design Manager: Joan Wendt

As new scientific information becomes available through basic and clinical research, recommended treatments and drug therapies undergo changes. The author and publisher have done everything possible to make this book accurate, up to date, and in accord with accepted standards at the time of publication. The author, editors, and publisher are not responsible for errors or omissions or for consequences from application of the book, and make no warranty, expressed or implied, in regard to the contents of the book. Any practice described in this book should be applied by the reader in accordance with professional standards of care used in regard to the unique circumstances that may apply in each situation. The reader is advised always to check product information (package inserts) for changes and new information regarding dose and contraindications before administering any drug. Caution is especially urged when using new or infrequently ordered drugs.

Library of Congress Cataloging-in-Publication Data

Meeting the physical therapy needs of children / [edited by] Susan K. Effgen.
   p. ; cm.
  Includes bibliographical references and index.
  ISBN 10: 0-8036-0250-2 (alk. paper)   ISBN 13: 978-0-8036-0250-2
  1. Physical therapy for children.
[DNLM: 1. Physical Therapy Techniques—Adolescent. 2. Physical Therapy Techniques—Child. 3. Physical Therapy Techniques—Infant. 4. Health Facility Environment. 5. Needs Assessment—Adolescent. 6. Needs Assessment—Child. 7. Needs Assessment—Infant. 8. Patient Participation. WB 460 M495 2005] I. Effgen, Susan K., 1949-
  RJ53 . P5M446 2005
  615.8′2′083—dc22

                                  2004018944

To those wonderful men in my life:
Arthur, Michael, Brenton, Patrick, and Jonathan

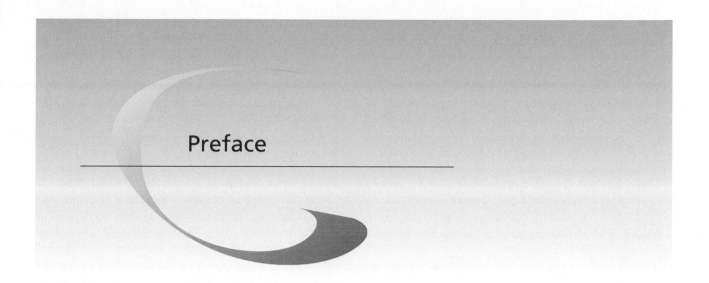

Preface

What a challenging and exciting time to work in pediatric physical therapy! Children with disabilities and special health-care needs are now active participants in their community. They are being educated and served in their local schools and local health care agencies. Services are being provided in functional, natural environments where generalization or transfer of skills is most likely to occur. Managed care has challenged therapists to be creative in dealing with the restricted provision of services, and the importance of families and others as therapy extenders has been acknowledged. The clinical decision making that drives our practice is becoming increasingly supported by research evidence. In the next decade, we expect to have almost all of our interventions supported by research so that we can provide evidence-based practice.

This rapid period of change in pediatric physical therapy service delivery and the major advances in the theoretical foundations of intervention are the impetus for writing this book. These factors require a fresh perspective from the historical disease-based or treatment approach-based texts of the past. The authors want to share their expertise in these new arenas so that future generations of therapists are best prepared to enter the fast-paced and changing world of practice in the twenty-first century.

Since the II STEP Conference, physical therapists have embraced contemporary management models of motor control problems. The central nervous system is no longer viewed as the predominant controller of movement, and there is recognition of the importance of all systems in the dynamic emergence of a coordinated movement activity. In addition, there is an understanding that the biomechanical,

psychological, and social environments also influence motor learning and motor control. No one system dominates, and the interplay of all systems is critical for learning to perform a motor skill.

Another factor in the evolution in practice is the movement from deficit-based models to ability-based models of service delivery. In the past, therapists would look for impairments in body structure and function, and limitations in activities. They would then plan their interventions. In 1991, Dr. Philippa Campbell, a noted early childhood educator and occupational therapist, published her classic article outlining a top-down approach to evaluation, which was later embraced by physical therapists. In this model, the child and family determine the desired goals and objectives that are important to them before the evaluation of the child. Then the examination, evaluation, and intervention are completed with a focus on those family goals and objectives. Pediatric physical therapists have come to accept this family-centered model. Throughout this text, the importance of the child and family in the decision-making process is emphasized, and an entire chapter is devoted to family-centered care. Recognizing the importance of the family in the decision-making process and being able to work effectively with children and families from diverse cultural backgrounds are critical for therapists who are being educated for service delivery in the future.

The *Guide to Physical Therapist Practice, Second Edition* (2001), published by the American Physical Therapy Association, has reshaped physical therapy practice and the terminology we use. The *Guide* language of *Examination, Evaluation, Diagnosis, Prognosis, Intervention,* and *Outcomes* is fully integrated throughout this text. In addition, the chapters are organized around the practice patterns of the four categories of conditions provided in the *Guide:* Musculoskeletal (Chapters 4 and 5), Neuromuscular (Chapters 6 and 7), Cardiopulmonary (Chapter 8), and Integumentary (Chapter 9). This was done not just because of the *Guide* but because a systems approach to intervention is far more comprehensive, dynamic, and problem based than the disease-based and deficit-based models of the past. Readers must understand that the problems many children face involve multiple systems and are referred frequently to chapters on other systems throughout the text. A dynamic systems perspective requires an understanding of all systems to fully comprehend problems in movement and health in general.

In this preface and throughout the text, the phrases "impairments of body functions and structures" and "limitations in activities and participation" are used. These are not new words to therapy, but what is new is that they are part of the organizational structure of a classification system developed by the World Health Organization, first called *International Classification of Impairments, Disabilities, and Handicaps* (ICIDH) (1980 and 1999) and now referred to as the *International Classification of Functioning, Disability and Health* (ICF) (2001). The aim of the "classification is to provide a unified and standard language and framework for the description of human functioning and disability as an important component of health." This model of disablement is somewhat similar to the Nagi Model (1991) and the National Center for Medical Rehabilitation Research (NCMRR) (1992) classification. However, because ICF is international in scope, it will most likely become the accepted disablement model used across the nation. Some members of the Tri-Alliance have already embraced ICF. Having a unified language is critical as we join the international community in our research and service delivery efforts.

The ICF model has been used throughout this text, although terms from the Nagi model are also sometimes used because they are so much a part of our common professional language. This can lead to some confusion, and we have tried to provide clarification as necessary. Use of the term "impairment" is common, but it is certainly not always used as part of the Nagi model of *pathology, impairment, functional limitation,* and *disability.* These models are discussed in Chapter 1.

The first chapter of this text provides a foundation of physical therapy service delivery for children with disabilities and special health care needs. This is followed by a review of child development with a focus on motor devel-

opment. Of course, reading about development does not compare with observing development, and readers are encouraged to go to playgrounds, churches, and preschools to observe the motor skills and interactions of children of a variety of ages. The best environment would be where there are children with disabilities included with children who are developing typically. That allows for comparisons of development and will expose the observer to the benefits of full participation of those with disabilities in the community. These experiences will bring to life the written discussion of the development of movement. Also included in Chapter 2 is a review of the developmental and functional examination and evaluation measurement tools used in pediatric physical therapy. The chapters on specific systems in Section 2 provide information on the measurement tools used to examine each specific system. Section 1 ends with a chapter on family-centered care. This is a critical area of practice and is intentionally placed early in the text to provide an understanding of family-centered care, which is discussed throughout the text.

The major portion of this text is contained in Section 2: Systems. The *examination, evaluation, prognosis including plan of care,* and *intervention* for each of the systems are reviewed. The theoretical foundations and a framework for examination, evaluation, and intervention, along with evidence to support our interventions, are discussed in detail. Unfortunately, as noted by Dr. Valvano in Chapter 7, "at this time, most research on the effectiveness of intervention techniques is limited, sometimes equivocal and sometimes based on studies with small numbers of children…each therapist is encouraged to problem solve for each child, monitor motor function to determine effectiveness…and keep current with research findings." A text can only summarize the research evidence to date, and it is the professional obligation of therapists to keep abreast of the recent literature.

The unique environments and requirements of several service delivery settings are presented in Section 3. Practice today is very much influenced by the setting. Federal and state laws govern service delivery in early intervention and school-based settings; insurance companies and reimbursement issues govern outpatient services; and the financial limitations of prospective payment affect hospital and rehabilitation services. The infants, toddlers, children, and adolescents seen in each of these environments also differ. Therapists must understand the unique elements of working in each of these settings and how they can provide quality services.

The past 10 years have brought about a revolution in assistive technology and the supports available to aid all individuals with disabilities. Therapists play a vital role in the selection, utilization, and modification of these technologies. Section 4 provides foundational information on this evolving aspect of intervention.

The final section of this text is case studies. Although we want to emphasize a systems approach to service delivery, the entry-level physical therapist tends to focus on medical diagnoses. Therefore, we have selected common medical diagnoses seen by pediatric therapists and have presented a life-span approach to the intervention of infants, toddlers, children, and adolescents with these diagnoses. The case studies follow the model of the *Guide* and provide an overall perspective of the role of the therapist in examination, evaluation, and intervention throughout the life of the child with a specific diagnosis in a variety of service delivery settings.

Meeting the physical therapy needs of children in the 21st century will involve a continuous process of change and refinement. This text is one of the first of the new millennium to include many of the new aspects of serving children with disabilities and special health-care needs. The therapist must be prepared for direct access, especially in school settings, where the need was first recognized. They must discard deficit models of evaluation and focus on the goals and objectives of the child and family in a culturally sensitive manner. Intervention must be based on evidence supporting its effectiveness or, at the very least, on sound clinical judgment and experience. Interventions must be discarded if there is no evidence to support continued use.

The *Guide's* emphasis on *coordination, communication,* and *documentation* as part of the intervention process must be embraced. Hands-on intervention is of little value if there is no carryover throughout the child's day and if services are not coordinated and communicated. These processes assist in making certain the child receives the "appropriate, comprehensive, efficient, and effective quality of care" (APTA, 2001, p. 47/S39) from initial examination through to graduation from services.

Susan K. Effgen

REFERENCES

American Physical Therapy Association (2001). Guide to physical therapist practice (2nd ed.). *Physical Therapy, 81,* 9–744.

Campbell, P.H. (1991). Evaluation and assessment in early intervention for infants and toddlers. *Journal of Early Intervention, 15,* 42.

Nagi, S.Z. (1991). Disability concepts revisited: Implications for prevention. In A.N. Pope and A.R. Tarlow (Eds.). *Disability in America: Toward a national agenda for prevention* (pp 309–327). Washington, D.C.: National Academy Press.

National Institutes of Health (1993). *Research plan for the National Center for Medical Rehabilitation Research.* NIH Publication No. 93–3509, Bethesda, MD: Author.

World Health Organization (1980). *International classification of impairments, disabilities, and handicaps.* Geneva: Author.

World Health Organization (2001). *International classification of functioning, disability and health.* Geneva: Author.

Acknowledgments

Where does one begin to thank all of the individuals responsible for assisting in moving a project from merely an idea through production into a useful product? The delightful individuals at F. A. Davis Company are certainly a good place to start. Jean-François Vilain convinced me that a pediatrics textbook that was systems based and not "disease of the week" was an important project. Margaret Biblis and Susan Rhyner inherited the project and supported it through completion. Along the way there were a number of developmental editors, with Jennifer Pine finally taking charge and setting deadlines for everyone and actually getting the project done!

Over the years there have been numerous graduate students who provided valuable assistance and, I hope, learned through the process. They include, but are certainly not limited to, Jonathan Averdick, Lori Bolgla, Laurie Chan, and Rachel Unanue Rose. Linda Pax Lowes enthusiastically stepped forward to develop the Instructor's Resource Disk. A special thanks is also offered to the numerous administrative support staff who helped in so many important ways across two continents. The time, effort, and expertise of the many reviewers are greatly appreciated, especially their ability to engage us in the invigorating process of revision! There are certainly more people to thank, but with yet another deadline, I must send apologies to those inadvertently left out.

Contributors

Donna Bernhardt Bainbridge, PT, EdD, ATC
Special Olympics Global Advisor for FUNfitness and
    Fitness Programming and Project Director
The University of Montana
Missoula, Montana

Katie Bergeron, PT, MS
President and COO
Adaptivemall.com, LLC
Dolgeville, New York

Heather Lever Brossman, MS, DPT, CCS
The Children's Hospital *of* Philadelphia
Philadelphia, Pennsylvania

Donna J. Cech, PT, MS, PCS
Program Director and Associate Professor
Physical Therapy Program
Midwestern University
Downers Grove, Illinois

Lisa Ann Chiarello, PT, PhD, PCS
Associate Professor
Drexel University
Hahnemann Programs in Rehabilitation Sciences
Philadelphia, Pennsylvania

Shirley Albinson Daniels, PT, MS
Physical Therapist
Gloucester County Special Services School District
Sewell, New Jersey

Carol Gildenberg Dichter, PT, PhD, PCS
Deceased, formerly Consultant
Office of Education
New Jersey Department of Human Services
Trenton, New Jersey

Caroline Goulet, PT, PhD
Associate Professor
Director of the Transitional DPT Program
Department of Physical Therapy
Creighton University
Omaha, Nebraska

Sylvia Gray, MS, ATP
Assistive Technology Consultant
Andrews, Texas

Pamela Girvin Hackett, MPT
Vice President, Pediatric Therapeutic Services, Inc.
Philadelphia, Pennsylvania

Maria A. Jones, PT, PhD, ATP
Clinic Manager/Clinical Physical Therapist
Oklahoma Assistive Technology Center
Department of Rehabilitation Sciences
College of Allied Health
University of Oklahoma Health Sciences Center
Oklahoma City, Oklahoma

Jane O'Regan Kleinert, MSPA, CCC-SLP
Rehabilitation Sciences Doctoral Program
College of Health Sciences
University of Kentucky
Lexington, Kentucky

Linda Pax Lowes, PT, PhD, PCS
Private Practice and Adjunct Faculty
Program in Physical Therapy
The Ohio State University
Columbus, Ohio

Victoria Gocha Marchese, PT, PhD
Rehabilitation Services
St. Jude Children's Research Hospital
Memphis, Tennessee

Suzanne F. Migliore, PT, MS, PCS
Physical Therapy Supervisor
The Children's Seashore House of The Children's Hospital
    of Philadelphia
Philadelphia, Pennsylvania

Margo N. Orlin, PT, PhD, PCS
Director, Entry-Level Doctor of Physical Therapy
    Program
Programs in Rehabilitation Sciences
Drexel University
Philadelphia, Pennsylvania

Shree Devi Pandya, PT, MS
Assistant Professor
Neurology and Physical Medicine and Rehabilitation
University of Rochester
Rochester, New York

Coleen Schrepfer, PT, MS
Former Staff Physical Therapist
The Children's Hospital of Philadelphia
Philadelphia, Pennsylvania

Julie Ann Starr, PT, MS, CCS
Clinical Associate Professor
Department of Rehabilitation Sciences
Sargent College of Health and Rehabilitation Sciences
Boston University and Physical Therapist
Beth Israel Deaconess Medical Center
Boston, Massachusetts

Carole A. Tucker, PT, PhD, PCS
Research Department
Shriners' Hospital
Philadelphia, Pennsylvania

Joanne Valvano, PT, PhD
Assistant Professor
Program in Physical Therapy
University of Colorado Health Sciences Center
Denver, Colorado

Sarah L. Westcott, PT, PhD
Adjunct Associate Professor
Programs in Rehabilitation Sciences
Drexel University and Associate Professor
University of Puget Sound
Tacoma, Washington

Sharon T. White, PT, MS
Chief Pediatric Therapist
California Children Services
Contra Costa County, California

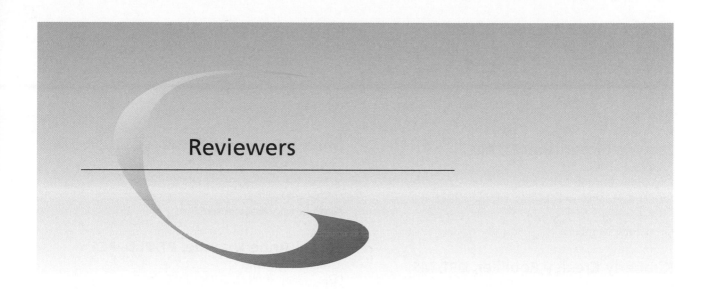

Reviewers

Wendy D. Bircher, PT, MS
Director
Physical Therapist Assistant Program
San Juan College
Farmington, New Mexico

Jill Bloss, PT, MPH
Former Chairperson and Associate Professor
Department of Physical Therapy
Nazareth College
Rochester, New York

Heather Carling-Smith, PT, MA, PCS
Former Academic Coordinator of Clinical Education
Department of Physical Therapy
California State University
Sacramento, California

Lynn A. Colby, PT, MS
Faculty Emeritus
Physical Therapy Division
College of Medicine and Public Health
School of Allied Medical Professions
Ohio State University
Columbus, Ohio

Claudia B. Fenderson, PT, EdD, PCS
Associate Professor
Department of Physical Therapy
Division of Health Sciences
Mercy College
Dobbs Ferry, New York

Carrie Gajdosik, PT, MS
Associate Professor
Department of Physical Therapy
University of Montana
Missoula, Montana

Caroline Goulet, PT, PhD
Associate Professor
Department of Physical Therapy
Creighton University
Omaha, Nebraska

Patricia Stavrakas Hodson, PT, MS, PCS
Clinical Associate Professor and ACCE
Department of Physical Therapy
East Carolina University
Greenville, North Carolina

Toby Long, PT, PhD
Associate Director for Training
Center for Child and Human Development
Georgetown University
Washington, DC

Janet Audrey Macdonald, BPT, MSEd, MSc
Assistant Professor
Department of Physical Therapy
University of Manitoba
Winnipeg, Manitoba, Canada

Jamyne Richardson, PT, ACCE
Adjunct Faculty
Department of Physical Therapy
Montana State University–Great Falls College of
    Technology
Great Falls, Montana

Kimberly Crealey Rouillier, DPT, MS
Chairperson and Associate Professor
Rehabilitative Health Programs
Community College of Rhode Island
Warwick, Rhode Island

Marjane B. Selleck, PT, MS, PCS
Chairperson and Associate Professor
Physical Therapy Department
School of Nursing and Health Sciences
The Sage Colleges
Troy, New York

Joyce Whitaker Sparling, PT, PhD, OT
Associate Professor (Retired)
Division of Human Movement Sciences
University of North Carolina at Chapel Hill
Chapel Hill, North Carolina

MaryAnn Delaney Tuttle, PT, MS
Formerly Academic Coordinator of Clinical Education
    and Assistant Professor
Physical Therapy Program
University of Hartford
West Hartford, Connecticut

Linda J. Tsoumas, PT, MS
Chairperson and Associate Professor
Department of Physical Therapy
Springfield College
Belchertown, Massachusetts

Rachel Anne Unanue, PT, PhD, PCS
Assistant Professor
Department of Physical Therapy
The University of Alabama at Birmingham
Birmingham, Alabama

Judith C. Vestal, PhD, LOTR
Program Director and Associate Professor
Program in Occupational Therapy
Department of Rehabilitation Sciences
Louisiana State University Health Sciences
    Center–Shreveport
Shreveport, Louisiana

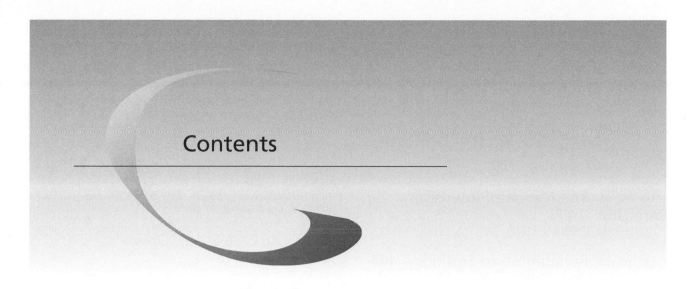

Contents

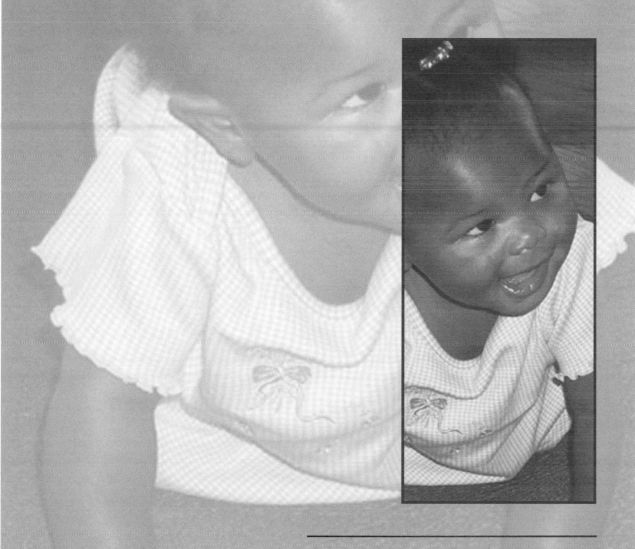

Foundations of Service Delivery

Chapter *1*

Serving the Needs of Children and Their Families

— Susan K. Effgen, PT, PhD

The loving mother teaches her child to walk alone. She is far enough from him so that she cannot actually support him, but she holds out her arms to him. She imitates his movements, and if he totters, she swiftly bends as if to seize him, so that the child might believe that he is not walking alone.... And yet, she does more. Her face beckons like a reward, an encouragement. Thus, the child walks alone with his eyes fixed on his mother's face, not on the difficulties in his way. He supports himself by the arms that do not hold him and constantly strives towards the refuge in his mother's embrace, little suspecting that in the very same moment that he is emphasizing his need of her, he is proving that he can do without her, because he is walking alone.
(Kierkegaard, 1846)

Little did Kierkegaard realize over a century and a half ago that he was describing not only the responsibilities of a mother to nurture her child and then allow the child to go alone but also the role of the physical therapist in serving children. Our responsibility is to provide support, guidance, and specific interventions and also to prepare the child and family for the time when our services are no longer needed. Competent therapists work themselves out of a job. This is not to say that all children achieve their desired goals and objectives, but rather that we help them to achieve their greatest potential and then recognize when we can no longer contribute to the advancement of their goals and objectives. It is often difficult for therapists to discharge a child from services, especially when the child has not achieved the desired goals,

just as it is sometimes difficult for a mother to let her new walker walk alone, or her teenager drive the family car. Our direct role is episodic, although we may provide periodic services over many years.

Throughout this text we will describe the role of the physical therapist in meeting the physical therapy needs of children and their families in a culturally appropriate context. Each body system will be discussed in terms of examination, evaluation, diagnosis, prognosis, and intervention for children with a wide range of diagnoses, impairments in body structure and function, limitations in activities, and restrictions in participation in the community. In some areas there is evidence to support the frequency, intensity, and specifics of our interventions; however, more commonly there is a dearth of empirical support, and therapists rely on experience and consensus decision making. As we move through the 21st century, physical therapists must strive to obtain the scientific data that will support our interventions because those who pay for our services are appropriately requiring evidence of the effectiveness of our interventions. Now therapists must not only provide intervention but also collect data that will support our continued efforts.

This chapter covers a number of diverse topics that set the stage for meeting the physical therapy needs of children and their families. The history of pediatric physical therapy is reviewed so that the reader can understand the evolution of the profession. Pioneering approaches to intervention are reviewed briefly and elaborated in later chapters as appropriate. The World Health Organization (WHO)'s International Classification of Functioning, Disability and Health (ICF) (2001) is presented and serves as a framework for the terminology and classification used in this text, as is the American Physical Therapy Association's (APTA's) *Guide to Physical Therapist Practice* (2001). Health care and educational services for children with disabilities require the collaboration of a number of professionals. The models of team interaction are presented, along with models of service delivery. Service delivery has changed over the past decade in all areas of physical therapy practice, but especially in pediatric physical therapy, in which federal laws play a significant role. Additional issues that influence practice conclude the chapter.

Background of Pediatric Physical Therapy

The history of physical therapy is usually traced to the "reconstruction aides" of World War I. However, the significance of poliomyelitis (polio), an inflammation of the gray matter of the spinal cord, in the history of physical therapy cannot be understated. Children and young adults were most likely to contract polio. This disease became a major health-care issue in the United States in 1917, when 27,363 cases were reported with 7,179 deaths (Murphy, 1995, p. 35). It was then that physical therapists began to work with people recovering from polio as well as with those with war injuries.

There were many treatments for polio, and one of the more successful approaches was implemented by Robert W. Lovett, a Boston orthopedist. Assisting Dr. Lovett was Wilhelmine Wright, who ran a "gymnasium" clinic at the Boston Children's Hospital. She developed and published a testing procedure called *manual muscle testing*. The procedures of Lovett and Wright remained among the primary treatments of polio until the 1940s, when an Australian nurse known as Sister Elizabeth Kenny arrived in the United States. The standard polio treatment at that time was bed rest and immobilization. Sister Kenny, however, believed in a more aggressive, active treatment that included exercise (Murphy, 1995, p. 123).

Numerous schools, institutions, and clinics for children with polio and other physical disabilities were established by charitable organizations early in the 20th century. Many children lived at these special schools or hospitals for extended periods of time because of the limitations of the transportation and health-care systems and the belief that experts, including physical and occupational therapists, could better meet the children's needs than their families.

Unfortunately, children with mental retardation or serious physical limitations had a more difficult time obtaining services, and all too often they were placed in institutions where they were "taken care of" but did not receive the services necessary to reach their potential. The growth of these institutions during the early part of the 20th century was tremendous. This growth was stimulated by the misguided beliefs that families could not "handle" children with these conditions and that both the child and the family would be better off if the child were "put away." The widespread public health policy promoting the use of the polio vaccine in the 1950s ended the need for physical therapists to serve children with polio. At the same time, however, the potential for physical therapists to contribute to the treatment of children with cerebral palsy (CP) was beginning to be recognized. CP is a nonprogressive neurological disorder occurring early in life. Children with milder degrees of CP could receive services at special clinics and schools. Those with more serious disabilities that prevented ambulation or included mental retardation were often "sent" to institutions.

Early physical therapists were guided by two enlightened physicians who combined orthopedics and neurology in serving children with CP. Bronson Crothers, a pediatric neurologist at the Boston Children's Hospital, worked with Mary Trainor, a physical therapist. Ms. Trainor is the apparent source of the once-famous technique of singing songs to accompany exercises for children with CP. She would sing "… a little descriptive song to the child… the child is taught by imitation to go through certain actions" (Mary McMillan, Massage and Therapeutic Exercise, as cited in Murphy, 1995, p. 164). Dr. Crothers also trained Dr. Winthrop Phelps, who in 1932 published an important, and now classic, paper on CP that emphasized that children with CP were not necessarily mentally retarded, which was a prevailing thought at the time (American Academy for Cerebral Palsy and Developmental Medicine, 1996, p. 9). Drs. Crothers and Phelps and four other physicians founded the American Academy of Cerebral Palsy in 1946. In 1957, this medical association established an associate category that allowed nonphysicians with doctoral degrees, including physical therapists, to join. Today this organization, called the American Academy of Cerebral Palsy and Developmental Medicine (AACPDM), is truly multidisciplinary, and all members, with or without doctoral degrees, have full voting privileges. Many therapists are active members who support education and research efforts to find effective interventions for CP and other developmental disabilities.

In the 1940s a group of parents got together to see if there was anything more they could do at home to help meet the needs of their children with CP. In 1947, the national United Cerebral Palsy Association (UCPA) was founded to help people become more aware of the needs of children with CP. Many schools that had once served children with polio now extended their services to children with CP and other disabilities. Physical therapists were already on staff at these schools.

The APTA has always supported the work of pediatric physical therapists, as evidenced by numerous journal articles and conference proceedings. Bud DeHaven, a leader in the advancement of the pediatric physical therapy profession, was instrumental in establishing the APTA Section on Pediatrics in 1973. This was one of the first components of the APTA to address the needs of therapists serving a specific clinical population. The APTA Section on Pediatrics continues to support the work of physical therapists in meeting the needs of children and their families, and is responsible for the publication of the journal *Pediatric Physical Therapy*.

Approaches to Intervention

The work of the early pioneers clearly demonstrated that children with CP and other developmental disabilities could benefit from physical therapy intervention. The contributions of these pioneers and those of contemporary leaders are discussed throughout this text. An overview of significant intervention methods developed during the 20th century is presented in this section.

Throughout the 1940s, 1950s, and 1960s, therapists sought a neurophysiological foundation to support their clinical interventions. However, the words of Sedwich Mead, in his 1967 presidential address to the American Academy of Cerebral Palsy, were prophetic: "Neurophysiologic doctrine is a most perishable commodity and it is a mistake to pin one's hopes on a current interpretation" (Mead, 1968). Therapists did, however, place their hopes for a scientific rationale for treatment in the rapidly evolving science of neurophysiology. Unfortunately, many of the theoretic foundations of those treatments have not withstood the test of time in light of recent findings in neuroscience. Some techniques have gained a scientific foundation and are presented in this text. Others continue to be accepted because of assumed clinical effectiveness, good salesmanship, and the search by parents to find a cure for their child with a disability.

Proprioceptive Neuromuscular Facilitation

One of the early neurophysiological approaches, and the one that still has a partly scientific basis for its continued use, is **proprioceptive neuromuscular facilitation (PNF)**, which was developed by Herman Kabot, a physician, and physical therapists Maggie Knott and Dorothy Voss (Knott & Voss, 1968; Voss, Ionta, & Myers, 1985). PNF is a developmental approach that uses normal motor developmental patterns and includes specific procedures to promote motor learning, strengthening, and function. PNF treatment is "based upon the idea that all human beings respond in accordance with demand: that movements must be specific and directed toward a goal; that the activity is necessary to the best development of coordination, strength, and endurance; and that the stronger cooperation leads toward a goal of optimum function"(Knott & Voss, 1968). Spiral and diagonal patterns of movement and exercise are used for strengthening, combining flexion, extension, abduction, adduction, and internal or external rotation instead of the traditional straight planes of motion. Coordination is encouraged through the timed sequence of muscle contraction in a distal-to-proximal sequence. The child's cooperation is necessary if he or she is to benefit fully from this approach. It is interesting that the same Dr. Mead who questioned pinning our hopes on neurophysiological doctrine wrote in the foreword to the third edition of *Proprioceptive Neuromuscular Facilitation* that "Our attempts to rationalize it [PNF] using neurophysiology currently in our grasp may be drastically modified by future discoveries, but PNF does work..." (Voss, Ionta, & Myers, 1985, p. vi).

Sensorimotor Approach

Margaret Rood, a physical and occupational therapist, developed an approach frequently referred to as the **sensorimotor approach** to treatment. She was concerned with the interaction of somatic, autonomic, and psychic factors and how they regulated motor behavior. She outlined a four-stage sequence for the development of movement: (1) mobility, also called reciprocal innervation; (2) stability, also called coinnervation; (3) mobility superimposed on stability, also called heavy work; and (4) skill, which combined mobility and stability in non–weight-bearing activities. Mobility is characterized by antigravity movement such as supine flexion and rolling. Stability involves the development of muscle cocontraction at the proximal joints. This stability allows the child to maintain antigravity weight-bearing postures such as prone on elbows, sitting, and standing. Once the child has stability, mobility is superimposed on the stability. This involves proximal movement on a fixed distal limb, such as when an infant rocks on all fours. When that rocking progresses to forward movement and reaching on all fours, it is termed **skill.** Skilled movement involves the ability to combine mobility and stability in non–weight-bearing postures (Stockmeyer, 1967).

Rood is credited with attempting to ground her theory in the latest scientific research and encouraging others to do the same (Stockmeyer, 1967). Unfortunately, the scientific foundation of many of her techniques has not withstood the evolution of scientific knowledge. However, the implications of the four stages of development, consideration of the differences in the role of tonic and phasic muscles, and the use of various sensory stimulation techniques remain a part of clinical practice today.

Neurodevelopmental Treatment

During the 1960s and 1970s, the most widely used approaches for the treatment of CP and other developmental disabilities were those developed by Karl Bobath, a physician, and his wife Berta, a physical therapist. Berta Bobath developed the technique named **neurodevelopmental treatment (NDT)** and Karl Bobath explained the scientific rationale of the intervention (Bly, 1991; Bobath, 1971; Bobath & Bobath, 1972; Seamans, 1967). This approach, as originally presented, was based on the now-questioned, hierarchical model of motor control and the clinical results of Mrs. Bobath's skilled interventions with children and adults with neurologic dysfunction.

The Bobaths believed that normal child development is characterized by "the increase of inhibition of the maturing brain leading to a gradual breaking up and resynthesis of the early total synergies of muscular coordination" (Bobath & Bobath, 1972, p. 44); "the inhibition or suppression of the abnormal tonic reflex activity which is responsible for the patterns of hypertonus"; and the "facilitation of the normal, higher integrated righting and equilibrium reactions in their proper developmental sequence, with a progression towards skilled activities" (Bobath, 1980, p. 77).

In NDT, the therapist uses a "hands-on" approach to facilitate normal movement patterns and to inhibit abnormal reflex mechanisms. The normal movement patterns are expected to carry over into daily functional activities. Although the hierarchical model of motor control and the inhibition of abnormal tone on which this theory is based have not been supported with subsequent research, a number of the tenets of the Bobath approach are still widely accepted and merit serious continued consideration. The Bobaths said that *treatment* is a misleading term. They preferred *management* as "a better term as it indicates not only dealing with the motor handicap, but also with the totality of the child's needs and especially with the establishment of a good mother-child relationship. The main argument for the early recognition and management…is the combination of therapy with a programme of thorough parent training" (Bobath, 1980, p. 3). A colleague of the Bobaths, physical therapist Nancie Finnie, elaborated on the issue of family involvement and authored one of the first books for parents, *Handling the Young Child with Cerebral Palsy at Home.* The book is in its third edition (1997) and is still a valuable resource. Its concepts of family involvement are now widely embraced in family-centered early intervention. A discussion of the importance of developing good parent-child relationships appears in Chapter 3.

Bobath notes that knowledge of motor milestones is "largely statistical, with great variations due to culture, nutrition and other factors. It is necessary, however, to understand **why** a baby can do certain things at certain times" (Bobath, 1980, p. 4). The Bobaths provide extensive descriptions of the characteristics of children with CP, emphasizing the importance of early identification and treatment, and encouraging the team approach. "A united team must, therefore, have the same fundamental approach and the same concept of treatment in order to plan and execute an integrated and well-coordinated treatment program" (Bobath & Bobath, 1972, p. 173). In their training programs, they required the participation of physical, occupational, and speech therapists and frequently teachers. Many of the characteristics of the multidisciplinary and transdisciplinary teams used today were developed and encouraged by the Bobaths. Elements of NDT are still used widely in clinical practice today and are summarized in the published works of Bly (1999), Bly and Whiteside (1997), and Howle (2002). Contemporary implementation of NDT is discussed in more detail in Chapter 7.

Conductive Education

Another approach to serving children with CP and similar disabilities is **conductive education.** This educational approach was developed by a Hungarian neurologist, Andras Peto, beginning in the 1940s (Kozma & Balogh, 1995; Spivack, 1995). Conductive education combines elements of education and rehabilitation into a "multidisciplinary system of education focusing on the child's emotional and cognitive growth as well as motor function. Children are taught to see themselves as active and self-reliant participants in the world. Motor skills are taught in a comprehensive way integrating the skills needed for everyday tasks with songs and games. The children learn to move their bodies, constantly transitioning from one position to the next" (Capital Association for Conductive Education, 1997). The constant practice of each task may be one of the keys to the suggested success of conductive education. A recent study of movement activity in Philadelphia preschool programs suggests that there is very little active movement by children with disabilities in both integrated and segregated preschools (Ott & Effgen, 2000). Research also suggests that there is little difference in child outcomes when participating in a "traditional" therapy program or conductive education when the intensity of the intervention is controlled (Reddihough, King, Coleman, & Catanese, 1998).

A "conductor," trained in Hungary to meet the educational and rehabilitation needs of children with CP, provides all the services. Conductive education in Hungary and many European countries does not include the participation of occupational or physical therapists and relies solely on the expertise of the conductor. In other areas of the world, such as Hong Kong, Australia, and the United States, therapists often participate in service delivery or consultation (Effgen, 2000a; O'Shea, 2000). The role of the therapist in conductive education is very similar to the role of the therapist in any transdisciplinary team model. The therapist works with all team members to achieve the goals and objectives determined for each individual child.

This is a very integrated, functional model of service delivery, consistent with contemporary practice in which all appropriate professionals are involved and not just a conductor.

Sensory Integration

During the 1960s and 1970s, an occupational therapist, A. Jean Ayres, conceptualized a different way to view the neural organization of sensory information for functional behavior. She developed a clinical framework for the assessment and treatment of children who had disorders in sensory processing. Her approach, termed **sensory integration**, related to the "organization of sensation for use" (Ayres, 1979, p. 5). Dr. Ayres's work focused on sensory processing in children, specifically their vestibular, tactile, and proprioceptive systems, at a time when few people were considering these systems. Her work continues to have applications for children with developmental coordination disorders and other sensory-processing problems, and is an important area of practice for occupational therapists.

Mobility Opportunities Via Education (MOVE)

The MOVE curriculum was developed by Linda Bidabe, an educator, and John Lollar, a physical therapist, to help children to systematically acquire motor skills (Bidabe & Lollar, 1990). The selection of motor skill goals is based on a top-down model in which the specific targeted skills are determined first and then activities to acquire those skills are determined. The program provides naturally occurring practice of functional motor skills while the child is engaged in educational or leisure activities. It consists of 16 categories of functional motor skills and 74 individual skills within these categories. The child is tested to determine his or her skill level, and then a task analysis is performed to target the skills needed to achieve the desired result. Prompting is used to help perform the task, as are various mechanical devices or adaptive equipment. The prompts are systematically reduced as soon as the child gains independence. There are few studies to support the effectiveness of the MOVE curriculum; however, this structured, focused approach to functional movement has its advocates, especially among those servicing children with severe physical disabilities when other approaches have not been effective in achieving mobility goals.

Systems Approach/ Task-Oriented Model

In 1968, a conference titled "An Exploratory and Analytical Survey of Therapeutic Exercise," referred to as NUSTEP, was held to study the evolving neurodevelopmental and facilitation techniques in physical therapy. For the next decade, the proceedings of that conference served as the foundation for most therapeutic exercise. Despite the widespread use of these approaches, there was little empirical evidence to support their continued use (Gordon, 1987; Harris, 1997; Horak, 1991). As a new body of literature supporting different motor-learning and motor-control methods developed, leaders in the field held a new conference, "II STEP," in 1990. The presenters recommended a task-oriented model of neurological rehabilitation using a systems model of motor control. "The **task-oriented model** does not assume that therapeutic influence on motor control should be aimed only peripherally at the musculoskeletal system and environment, or only centrally at the nervous system. It targets both peripheral and central systems. From the systems model of motor control, the task-oriented model assumes that control of movement is organized around goal-directed, functional behaviors rather than on muscles or movement patterns" (Horak, 1991, p. 20). The proceedings of this conference are published in *Contemporary Management of Motor Control Problems* (Lister, 1991). During the summer of 2005, yet another major conference will address contemporary management of motor-control problems. These newer approaches to the intervention of children with neurological disabilities are presented in Chapter 7.

Models That Influence Practice

Nagi and NCMRR Disablement Models

Systems that classify an individual's findings into patterns provide a foundation for examination, evaluation, intervention, and analysis of outcomes of intervention. A number of models have been proposed to study the consequences of diseases. Widely adopted models in physical therapy include the Nagi model, the five-dimension National Center for Medical Rehabilitation Research (NCMRR) model (National Institutes of Health, 1993), and the WHO ICF model. The **Nagi model** serves as the organiza-

tional framework for the APTA's *Guide to Physical Therapist Practice* (2001).

The first dimension of the Nagi model is *pathophysiology*. This refers to the underlying medical or injury process at the cellular and tissue levels. Rarely does a physical therapist contribute to this level of intervention. The second dimension is *impairment*, which involves tissue, organ, and system disorders that might impair functioning at the organ or person level. Physical therapists frequently focus their interventions on strategies to reduce the primary and secondary impairments associated with the disease process. In a child with a motor delay, impairments might include decreased muscle power, range of motion (ROM), balance, coordination, and endurance. These impairments might, though not necessarily, limit the child's ability to optimally perform some tasks or activities.

One or more impairments may lead to the third dimension within the Nagi model, *functional limitations*. Functional limitations involve the inability to perform the usual activities of daily living such as walking, climbing stairs, or getting in and out of a car. Physical therapists play an active role in trying to decrease or eliminate functional limitations. Collectively, children may have similar functional limitations, but the pathophysiology and impairments causing the functional limitations may differ from child to child. Conversely, similar pathophysiology and impairments may lead to different degrees of functional limitations in different children. Many individuals can overcome significant pathophysiology and have few functional limitations. On the other hand, some individuals have serious functional limitations but relatively minor pathophysiology. An individual's response to the disease process and demands of society can vary greatly, and we must be cautious in our prognostications regarding the capabilities of individuals.

According to the Nagi model, when functional limitations are not corrected or overcome, *disabilities* may result. Disabilities are limitations "in performance of socially defined roles and tasks within a sociocultural and physical environment" (APTA, 2001, p. 28). Children who are unable to participate fully in school and the community because of functional limitations are said to be disabled. Their quality of life may be seriously affected. The amount of impairment and functional limitation may not be directly proportional to the degree of disability. Many factors are involved. Low self-esteem and lack of confidence may also impair social interaction and decrease participation in community activities, leading to further disability.

The NCMRR model adds another dimension of *societal limitations*. Societal limitations result when society imposes barriers that prevent individuals from functioning at their highest level. Societal barriers include, for example, the stairs to enter the U.S. Supreme Court Building, the lack of curb cuts on city streets, and inaccessible public transportation. Therapists usually do not work directly on the issues of societal limitations; however, our active advocacy and modeling in the community with individuals with disabilities do help society recognize and reduce societal barriers.

World Health Organization International Classification of Functioning, Disability, and Health

The WHO has developed the most widely known models of disablement. In the 1980s, they published the *International Classification of Impairments, Disabilities and Handicaps* (ICIDH), which was later revised and referred to as ICIDH-2. In 2001, after extensive international review, the WHO approved a revised system called the *International Classification of Functioning, Disability and Health* (ICF). ICF provides a unified and standard language and framework to describe and measure health

and health-related states. Traditional classification systems focus on mortality; ICF focuses on "life." Determining how people can live with their health conditions and how people can be helped to achieve a productive, fulfilling life is more important than noting their inabilities. ICF strives to place all disease and health conditions on an equal footing. An adolescent might miss school because of a cold or a broken leg but also because of depression. ICF takes a neutral approach and places mental disorders on a par with physical illness.

The ICF has two parts, and each part has two components. Part 1, Functioning and Disability, includes (a) Body Functions and Structures and (b) Activities and Participation. Part 2, Contextual Factors, includes (a) Environmental Factors and (b) Personal Factors (Table 1.1). "Each component consists of various domains and, within each domain, categories, which are the units of classification. Health and health-related states of an individual may be recorded by selecting the appropriate category code, or codes, and then adding qualifiers" (WHO, 2001, p. 10–11). The qualifiers are a numeric coding system that indicates the degree of the problem ranging from *No problem* to *Complete problem* (Table 1.2). The ICF codes and

Table 1.1 An Overview of the *International Classification of Functioning, Disability and Health*

	Part 1: Functioning and Disability		Part 2: Contextual Factors	
Components	Body Functions and Structures	Activities and Participation	Environmental Factors	Personal Factors
Domains	Body functions Body structures	Life areas (tasks, actions)	External influences on functioning and disability	Internal influences on functioning and disability
Constructs	Change in body functions (physiological) Change in body structures (anatomical)	Capacity: Executing tasks in a standard environment Performance: Executing tasks in the current environment	Facilitating or hindering impact of features of the physical, social, and attitudinal world	Impact of attributes of the person
Positive aspect	Functional and structural integrity	Activities: Participation	Facilitators	Not applicable
	Functioning			
Negative aspect	Impairment	Activity limitation Participation Restriction	Barriers/hindrances	Not applicable
	Disability			

Source: World Health Organization (2001). *International Classification of Functioning, Disability and Health* (p. 11). Geneva: Author. Copyright by the World Health Organization. Reprinted with permission of the author.

Table 1.2 International Classification of Functioning, Disability, and Health Scoring System

If an impairment in body functions or body structure, limitation in activity, or restriction in participation is present, the following generic performance qualifiers may be used to indicate degree of difficulty in accomplishing an activity.

	Impairment, Limitation or Restriction Level		Magnitude of Impairment
0	NO problem	Functioning is within expected norms (none, absent, negligible…)	0–4%
1	MILD problem	Slight deviation from expected norm and functioning (slight, low…)	5–24%
2	MODERATE problem	Significant impairment of functioning and person likely to need assistance (medium, fair…)	25–49%
3	SEVERE problem	Seriously compromised functioning and person may be unable to perform functions, even with assistance (high, extreme…)	50–95%
4	COMPLETE problem	Total loss of function (total…)	96–100%
8	Not specified	Insufficient data	
9	Not applicable	Qualifier not applicable in this instance	

This performance qualifier can be used in conjunction with another qualifier that implies the level of difficulty, such as using an assistive device or personal help. Additional qualifiers can be used to describe the individual's ability to perform the task.

Source: Adapted from World Health Organization (2001). *International Classification of Functioning, Disability and Health* (p. 222). Geneva: Author. Copyright by the World Health Organization. Reprinted with permission of the author. Adapted from American Psychological Association (APA) & World Health Organization (2003). *International classification of functioning, disability and health procedural manual and guide for a standardized application of the ICF: A manual for health professionals.* Washington, DC: Author.

qualifiers provide a "condensed version" of the information found in clinical records.

The terminology used in ICF is relatively straightforward; however, the different meanings of similar words among ICF, the NCMRR model, and the *Guide* (APTA, 2001) can lead to some confusion. The WHO (2001, p. 10) defines the ICF components as follows:

- **Body functions** are the physiological functions of body systems (including psychological functions).
- **Body structures** are anatomical parts of the body, such as organs, limbs, and their components.
- **Impairments** are problems in body function or structure such as a significant deviation or loss.
- **Activity** is the execution of a task or an action by an individual.

- **Participation** is involvement in a life situation.
- **Activity limitations** are difficulties an individual may have in executing activities.
- **Participation restrictions** are problems an individual may experience in involvement in life situations.
- **Environmental factors** make up the physical, social, and attitudinal environment in which people live and conduct their lives.

Under ICF, function relates to body organ or system function, *not* functional activities. In the ICF model, functional activities, as therapists have used the term in the past, are activities and participation. Impairments are of the body, not of the activity. We would discuss *limitations* in the activity of walking, not impairments, because there might be an impairment of the anatomical structure of the limb influencing the activity of walking. Throughout this text we attempt to use the ICF terminology. This has been a difficult task because traditionally we refer to "functional" activities and "impairments" in balance and gait. Occasionally in this text, we use two sets of terminology so that the reader, who may not be familiar with ICF, will understand the concepts being presented.

To provide a comprehensive understanding of the individual's life, ICF includes the Contextual Factors, which consist of the components of environmental and personal factors. These factors can be expressed in positive or negative terms. Environmental factors include *individual influences,* such as the immediate environment and the people in that environment, and *societal influences,* such as formal and informal social structures. Environmental factors interact with body functions and structures, activities, and participation. Personal factors include the part of the child's background that is not related to a health condition or health status, as well as demographics and past and current life experiences. There is no classification of personal factors in ICF (WHO, 2001, p. 17–18). A procedure manual is being developed for the standardized application of the ICF for adults, which will be followed by a manual for use with children (APA, 2003).

Management of Children With Disabilities

Physical therapy practice for children with disabilities previously followed the medical model of determining the symptoms; establishing a diagnosis, usually provided by the physician; determining the child's weaknesses and, it is hoped, strengths; therapist determination of goals and objectives; and treatment based on the therapist's experience. Over the past decade, practice has changed substantially. The child and family are primary in determining goals and objectives; the child and family's strengths are vital in developing appropriate interventions; interventions are increasingly evidence based; and service settings have shifted from hospital- or center-based environments to the community and home.

Management of children with disabilities is based on clinical decision making and evidence-based practice. Unfortunately, it has been noted that a therapist's decision making is usually based only on expert opinion, advice from a colleague, textbooks, continuing education courses, and personal experience, all of which are subject to bias (Thomson-O'Brien & Moreland, 1998). A stronger foundation for decision making is provided by evidence-based practice. Evidence-based practice or

> … *evidence-based medicine movement is the conscientious, explicit, and judicious use of current evidence in making decisions about the care of individual patients. The practice of evidence-based medicine means integrating individual clinical expertise with the best available external clinical evidence from systematic research (Sackett, Rosenberg, Gray, Haynes, & Richardson, 1996).*

Evidence-based practice emphasizes findings from sound clinical research and de-emphasizes intuition, unsystematic clinical experience, and explanations based on pathophysiology (Evidence-based Medical Working Group, 1992). However, it includes a fine balance between "clinical expertise" and "external clinical evidence" (Law, 2002). Clinical knowledge is not ignored, but it means critically evaluating what we do. "Health care is an imperfect science that requires both overarching clinical guidelines and individual judgment in equal parts. Evidence-based practice works with the interplay of these two factors, making it a powerful tool that practitioners can use to guide their clinical decisions" (Law, 2002, p. 5). Evidence-based practice strongly supports a client-centered approach; clinical experience is critical because knowledgeable therapists must implement the findings based on the evidence, and it makes use of the best methods of intervention currently available (Law, 2002).

Mary Law, a well-known pediatric occupational therapist, in her recent text *Evidence-based Rehabilitation: A Guide to Practice* (2002) notes four elements of good evidence-based practice in rehabilitation. The first is *awareness.* The therapist must be aware of the evidence that is available. Unless one is aware of it, evidence cannot be used in clinical decision making. Second is *consultation.* The child and family must be consulted as part of the decision-making process. We must communicate our knowledge so that they can make informed decisions about various options. *Judgment,* the third element, is important in deciding how and when to apply the recommendations of evidence-based practice. Information must be analyzed as it applies to a particular child at a particular time. It takes sound professional judgment to avoid blindly embracing evidence. Finally, *creativity* is necessary because even when there is evidence, it must be applied creatively and not in a "cookie-cutter" fashion.

In 1997, APTA published the *Guide to Physical Therapist Practice* to describe, standardize, and delineate preferred physical therapist practice. The *Guide*, as it is referred to in this text, was revised in 2001 and describes patient management and preferred practice patterns for physical therapists. The practice patterns are divided into musculoskeletal, neuromuscular, cardiovascular/pulmonary, and integumentary systems, as is the organizational structure used in this text. The *Guide*, although not geared to the pediatric population, provides the preferred standards of care and professional terminology to be used by all physical therapists. The *Guide* terminology and practice patterns are used throughout this text, with the exception that new ICF language is used to describe health and health-related issues. Now that the ICF has been finalized, this WHO system is gaining popularity worldwide and will probably influence future editions of the *Guide*.

According to the *Guide* (APTA, 2001), there are six elements of management of the individual with a disability or illness: *examination, evaluation, diagnosis, prognosis, intervention,* and *outcomes*. They are discussed in this section and outlined in Figure 1–1.

Examination

The *Guide* (APTA, 2001) divides **examination** into three components: *History, Systems Review,* and *Tests and Measures*. The examination starts with a review of the child's *History* and a *Systems Review*, as outlined in Display 1.1 and Figure 1–2. After analyzing the information gained from the history and systems review, specific *Tests and Measurements* are administered by the physical therapist. Specific tests and measures of development, sensory integration, function, and quality of life are discussed in Chapter 2 and described in Appendix 2-B. Tests and measures used to examine each body system are presented in the chapters on the systems. These must be performed before intervention. How and by whom the examination data are collected in pediatric settings will vary significantly by the type of service delivery setting (see Chapters 10 through 15).

Management of children with disabilities and complex medical problems usually requires a team approach. Collaboration by team members is critical for a comprehensive examination and evaluation and for the provision of coordinated, integrated services. To facilitate this collaboration, team members frequently perform the examination together. Any member of the team might collect the history data and perform portions of the examination. Duplication of examination procedures is avoided by a coordinated plan. For example, blood pressure, pulse, and respiration

should be collected only once unless there is a need to collect this information under different conditions, such as after stair climbing. Many professionals from different disciplines can collect this data.

Careful consideration must be given to the setting and conditions under which the examination will be performed. One of the first issues to consider is the time of day of the examination. This is especially important for an infant or a young child. Testing near nap time or just before feeding will not encourage optimal results. Taking school-aged children out of their favorite class is also not a good way of establishing rapport! One must also consider the effects of long commutes to the examination and multiple examinations by several professionals. When possible, both parents should be present, so nontraditional work hours should be considered. Although evenings may be best for parents, it is generally not best for children. Saturdays may be the best day to get all of the participants together.

The setting of the examination is important because it influences the child's performance. If the child is fearful in a strange clinical environment, he or she may not participate at all; even when comfortable, the child may not be able to generalize skills to a new environment. As a result, the findings might be inaccurate. When possible, the best place to conduct an examination is in the child's **natural environment**. This will vary depending on the age, medical status, and disability of the child. If the child is not a hospital inpatient, the home, day care center, or educational setting is frequently the natural environment of choice. Familiarity with the physical environment and people helps the child and family to be more comfortable and to obtain the child's best performance.

The examination should first include **naturalistic observation**. During naturalistic observation, you observe the child functioning in the regular environment—be it home, day care center, or school—doing whatever is normally done in that environment. Naturalistic observation has a number of advantages. How and when the child typically moves under normal circumstances are observed. Information is learned regarding the child's behavior, interaction with adults and children if available, mobility, preferred positions and movement patterns, use of verbal and nonverbal language, indications of cognitive ability based on play behaviors and communication, manipulation of objects, and indications of endurance. The more comfortable and enriched the environment, the more likely it is that typical behaviors will be observed. Very "clinical" settings do not promote observation of optimal, typical behaviors. Observation of the child in the waiting room might provide a more realistic view of the child's behavior

DIAGNOSIS

Both the process and the end result of evaluating examination data, which the physical therapist organizes into defined clusters, syndromes, or categories to help determine the prognosis (including the plan of care) and the most appropriate intervention strategies.

PROGNOSIS
(Including Plan of Care)

Determination of the level of optimal improvement that may be attained through intervention and the amount of time required to reach that level. The plan of care specifies the interventions to be used and their timing and frequency.

EVALUATION

A dynamic process in which the physical therapist makes clinical judgments based on data gathered during the examination. This process also may identify possible problems that require consultation with or referral to another provider.

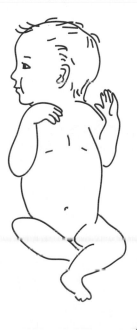

INTERVENTION

Purposeful and skilled interaction of the physical therapist with the patient/client and, if appropriate, with other individuals involved in care of patient/client, using various physical therapy methods and techniques to produce changes in the condition that are consistent with the diagnosis and prognosis. The physical therapist conducts a re-examination to determine changes in patient/client status and to modify or redirect intervention. The decision to re-examine may be based on new clinical findings or on lack of patient/client progress. The process of re-examination also may identify the need for consultation with or referral to another provider.

EXAMINATION

The process of obtaining a history, performing a systems review, and selecting and administering tests and measures to gather data about the patient/client. The initial examination is a comprehensive screening and specific testing process that leads to a diagnostic classification. The examination process also may identify possible problems that require consultation with or referral to another provider.

OUTCOMES

Result of patient/client management, which includes the impact of physical therapy interventions in the following domains: pathology/pathophysiology (disease, disorder, or condition); impairments, functional limitations, and disabilities; risk reduction/prevention; health, wellness, and fitness; societal resources; and patient/client satisfaction.

Figure 1–1   Elements of child management leading to optimal outcomes. (From American Physical Therapy Association [2001]. *Guide to physical therapist practice* [2nd ed.]. *Physical Therapy, 81*[1], 43. Copyright 2001 by the American Physical Therapy Association. Reprinted with permission of the author.)

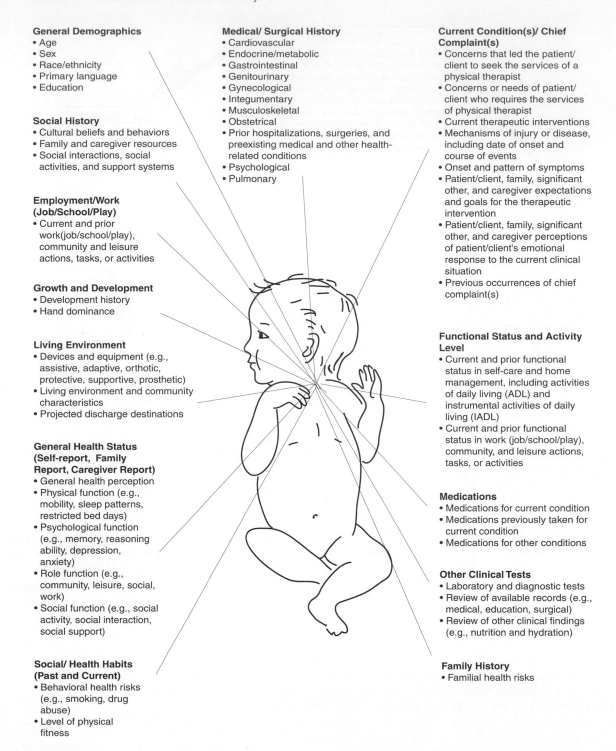

General Demographics
• Age
• Sex
• Race/ethnicity
• Primary language
• Education

Social History
• Cultural beliefs and behaviors
• Family and caregiver resources
• Social interactions, social activities, and support systems

Employment/Work (Job/School/Play)
• Current and prior work(job/school/play), community and leisure actions, tasks, or activities

Growth and Development
• Development history
• Hand dominance

Living Environment
• Devices and equipment (e.g., assistive, adaptive, orthotic, protective, supportive, prosthetic)
• Living environment and community characteristics
• Projected discharge destinations

General Health Status (Self-report, Family Report, Caregiver Report)
• General health perception
• Physical function (e.g., mobility, sleep patterns, restricted bed days)
• Psychological function (e.g., memory, reasoning ability, depression, anxiety)
• Role function (e.g., community, leisure, social, work)
• Social function (e.g., social activity, social interaction, social support)

Social/ Health Habits (Past and Current)
• Behavioral health risks (e.g., smoking, drug abuse)
• Level of physical fitness

Medical/ Surgical History
• Cardiovascular
• Endocrine/metabolic
• Gastrointestinal
• Genitourinary
• Gynecological
• Integumentary
• Musculoskeletal
• Obstetrical
• Prior hospitalizations, surgeries, and preexisting medical and other health-related conditions
• Psychological
• Pulmonary

Current Condition(s)/ Chief Complaint(s)
• Concerns that led the patient/client to seek the services of a physical therapist
• Concerns or needs of patient/client who requires the services of physical therapist
• Current therapeutic interventions
• Mechanisms of injury or disease, including date of onset and course of events
• Onset and pattern of symptoms
• Patient/client, family, significant other, and caregiver expectations and goals for the therapeutic intervention
• Patient/client, family, significant other, and caregiver perceptions of patient/client's emotional response to the current clinical situation
• Previous occurrences of chief complaint(s)

Functional Status and Activity Level
• Current and prior functional status in self-care and home management, including activities of daily living (ADL) and instrumental activities of daily living (IADL)
• Current and prior functional status in work (job/school/play), community, and leisure actions, tasks, or activities

Medications
• Medications for current condition
• Medications previously taken for current condition
• Medications for other conditions

Other Clinical Tests
• Laboratory and diagnostic tests
• Review of available records (e.g., medical, education, surgical)
• Review of other clinical findings (e.g., nutrition and hydration)

Family History
• Familial health risks

Figure 1–2 Types of data generated from history. (From American Physical Therapy Association [2001]. *Guide to physical therapist practice* [2nd ed.]. *Physical Therapy, 81*[1], 44. Copyright 2001 by the American Physical Therapy Association. Reprinted with permission of the author.)

Display 1.1 Pediatric Physical Therapy Evaluation and Plan of Care

Child's name:	Child's date of birth:
Physical therapist's name:	Date of examination:

I. Parents' and Child's Concerns
What are the major concerns of the child and family?
What is the child trying to do?
What do the child and parents want the child to be able to do?

II. Child's History (APTA, 2001, p. 44) See Figure 1–2 for items to include under each heading.
General Demographics
Social History
Employment/Work (Job/School/Play)
Growth and Development
Living Environment
General Health Status
Social/Health Habits
Medical/Surgical History
Current Conditions(s)/Chief Complaints(s)
Functional Status and Activity Level
Medications
Other Clinical Tests
Family History

III. Systems Review
The systems review is a brief or limited examination of each of the systems that will assist in determining what tests and measures to use and in formulating a diagnosis, prognosis, plan of care, and interventions.

IV. Present Function
Description of present function, preferably in natural environment.

V. Tests and Measures (APTA, 2001, p. 52)
Based on the history and systems review, specific tests and measures are selected to be administered. These tests and measures, given in alphabetical order, not by level of significance, might include:
Aerobic Capacity/Endurance
Anthropometric Characteristics
Arousal, Attention, and Cognition
Assistive and Adaptive Devices
Circulation
Cranial and Peripheral Nerve Integrity
Environmental, Home, and Work (Job/School/Play) Barriers
Ergonomics and Body Mechanics
Gait, Location, and Balance
Integumentary Integrity
Joint Integrity and Mobility
Motor Function (Motor Control and Motor Learning)
Muscle Performance (including Strength, Power, and Endurance)
Neuromotor Development and Sensory Integration
Orthotic, Protective, and Supportive Devices
Pain
Posture
Prosthetic Requirements
Range of Motion (including Muscle Length)
Reflex Integrity
Self-Care and Home Management (including Activities of Daily Living [ADL] and Instrumental Activities of Daily Living [IADL])
Sensory Integrity
Ventilation, Respiration, and Circulation
Work (Job/School/Play), Community, and Leisure Integration or Reintegration (including IADL)

(Continued)

Display 1.1 Pediatric Physical Therapy Evaluation and Plan of Care (Continued)

Standardized Tests and Measures of neuromotor development, sensory integration, function, and quality of life are commonly used in a pediatric examination and are listed in Appendix 2.B. Tests and Measures of body functions and structures and additional activities are provided in the chapters on body systems.

VI. **Summary of Findings**
A concise evaluation and summary of the findings, this is a critical section because it is the area most commonly read by others.

VII. **Factors Affecting Function**

Factors Affecting Function	Objective Examination Findings Regarding Factors	Factor Aids or Hinders Function (+/−)
Internal factors	*Include as many findings as appropriate.*	*Indicate if factor in column to the left aids or hinders function.*
External factors	*Include as many findings as appropriate.*	*Indicate if factor in column to the left aids or hinders function.*

VIII. **Measurable Goals, Outcomes, and Objectives**
List goals, outcomes, and objectives to address the problems noted above.

IX. **Intervention Plan (APTA, 2001), as appropriate, might include:**
   1. Coordination, Communication, and Documentation
   2. Child- and Family-Related Instruction
   3. Procedural Interventions:
   Therapeutic Exercise
   Functional Training in Self-Care and Home Management (including ADL and IADL)
   Functional Training in Work (Job/School/Play), Community and Leisure Integration or Reintegration (including IADL, Work Hardening, and Work Conditioning)
   Manual Therapy Techniques (including Mobilization/Manipulation)
   Prescription, Application, and Fabrication of Devices and Equipment
   Airway Clearance Techniques
   Integumentary Repair and Protective Techniques
   Electrotherapeutic Modalities
   Physical Agents and Mechanical Modalities

   For Procedural Interventions the following need to be considered (see Chapter 7):
   1. Setting Goals
   2. Practice
   3. Intrinsic Meaning of the Task
   4. Content of Practice
   5. Adaptation to Practice
   6. Structure and Schedule of Practice
   7. Physical Environment
   8. Natural Environment vs. the Practice Environment
   9. Psychosocial Environment
   10. Performance Environment: Augmented Information
   11. Attributes That Support Learning
   12. Strategies to Address

X. **Re-examination**
What is the planned frequency of reexamination?

XI. **Criteria for Discharge**
Critical part of the plan of care because proper discharge planning improves and maintains outcomes and reduces potential of later problems regarding continued intervention.

than other clinic rooms. During the observation, the therapist does *not* handle the child, a very difficult task for some experienced therapists! As the child becomes comfortable with the setting, the therapist slowly starts to interact with the child, providing objects to play with to encourage natural movement. With older, cooperative children, the therapist can ask the child to perform tasks while the therapist observes. Therapists have a number of systematic techniques available for observation and recording of movement (Bailey & Wolery, 1992, p. 104–110; Effgen, 1991; Ott & Effgen, 2000). Naturalistic, classroom observation is required in school settings as part of the federal Individuals with Disabilities Education Act (IDEA) Amendments of 1997.

Observation of the child's best performance in the natural environment allows accurate determination of environmental obstacles, needed supports, and the child's strengths. This encourages realistic remediation. For example, suggesting that a child practice stair climbing in a home without stairs is not realistic, nor is cruising along a sofa if there is no sofa. In a clinical setting, parents are frequently reluctant to admit that they do not have certain items. Knowing the resources in the home allows the therapist to best determine what realistic and practical activities can be done in the home. If specialized examination equipment is necessary, a portion of the examination can be done in a setting that has the equipment; however, one should first consider selecting portable equipment and alternative means of measurement. Instead of using a computerized isokinetic system, a portable, handheld dynamometer is a reliable tool to measure muscle force production (Effgen & Brown, 1992) and is easily carried into homes and schools.

During the observation, the therapist determines areas of development and functioning that warrant further examination. In addition, the observation provides rich information that may be included in the tests-and-measures portion of the examination. When working with children, especially young children, their schedule and desires must be followed, not the predetermined examination plans of the therapist. The examination data are frequently obtained in a random order based on the child's activity and cooperation, unless a specific sequence must be followed for a standardized test. With infants, toddlers, and children with severe disabilities, it is generally best to perform an examination in one position at a time and to not request frequent position changes.

Play-based assessment is a form of naturalistic observation of young children popular in early childhood education (Linder, 1993). Professionals watch as the child interacts with selected play materials and with other children. Materials are carefully arranged to encourage the child's participation in activities that will provide the observers with information needed to evaluate the child's strengths and weaknesses based on their profession's frame of reference. An occupational therapist might evaluate the play behaviors, including sensorimotor, imaginary, constructional, and gross and fine motor game play (Olson, 1999). An educator might focus on creativity, social skills, and spontaneous language; the speech-language pathologist would note articulation and word usage. The physical therapist would focus on spontaneity and ease of movement during functional skills, gross motor activities, and transitions between play activities. The strength of this form of examination is that it is very functional and activity based; however, it provides limited information about impairment of body structures or functions, such as ROM and muscle strength. In addition, numerical scores have not been developed for this assessment, which might be required to determine eligibility for services for young children.

Arena assessments are commonly used in examination of infants in early intervention and for children with severe disabilities. This involves team members, including the parents, observing the child at the same time. One team member usually does the majority of the handling, and others provide direction, take notes, and talk with the parents.

When an examination is to be done in the child's home, generally the full team will not participate, and a decision must be made regarding what professionals will participate in the examination. If all team members are necessary, the examination might initially be done in the home with a few professionals present, with a follow-up by members of other disciplines at the home or in a center. Center-based assessment, however, is artificial and does not provide an accurate picture of the child's abilities (Rainforth & York-Barr, 1997).

History

Obtaining an acute **history** is a vital part of the examination process. Data are collected from various sources including medical and educational records, parent and child interviews, and interviews with significant others.

The types of data generated are outlined in Figure 1–2. After the history has been obtained and analyzed and the setting and structure of the examination determined, the examination can be started.

Systems Review

According to the *Guide* (APTA, 2001), the **systems review** is a *brief* or *limited* examination of the status of the cardiovascular/pulmonary, integumentary, musculoskeletal, and neuromuscular systems, based on pertinent information obtained from the history. In addition, the communication ability, social maturity, cognition, and learning style of the child may be determined.

The *Guide* (APTA, 2001, p. 42–43) suggests that the systems review include the following:

- For the cardiovascular/pulmonary system, assessment of heart rate, respiratory rate, blood pressure, and edema

- For the integumentary system, assessment of skin integrity, skin color, and presence of scar formation

- For the musculoskeletal system, assessment of gross symmetry, gross ROM, gross strength, height, and weight

- For the neuromuscular system, a general assessment of gross coordinated movement (e.g., balance, locomotion, transfers, and transitions)

- For communication ability, affect, cognition, language, and learning style; the assessment of the ability to make needs known; consciousness; orientation (person, place, and time); expected emotional/behavioral responses; and learning preferences (e.g., learning barriers, education needs)

The extent of the systems review will depend on the child's age and cognitive ability, the requirements of the setting, and reimbursement issues. The systems review helps determine what specific tests and measures would be appropriate to administer and whether consultation with another provider is necessary.

Tests and Measures

The history and systems review help determine what specific **tests** and **measures** should be performed to confirm or rule out the causes of impairment in body functions and structures, limitations in activities, and restrictions in participation. They also assist in establishing a diagnosis, prognosis, and plan of care. If a medical diagnosis is available, that will frequently guide the examination. For example, a child with cystic fibrosis will definitely require a comprehensive examination of the cardiopulmonary system, and the brief systems review would probably determine that further examination of the integumentary system is not warranted. A child with burns will require a thorough examination of the integumentary system, and the systems review would indicate which other systems might require more extensive examination.

Tests and measures help confirm or reject a hypothesis regarding what factors are contributing to the child's current level of performance and "support the physical therapist's clinical judgments about appropriate interventions, anticipated goals, and expected outcomes" (APTA, 2001, p. 43). Measurement is the "numeral assigned to an object, event, or person or the class (category) to which an object, event, or person is assigned according to rules" (APTA, 1991). We collect measurements by many methods, including interviewing, observing, and conducting performance-based assessments; taking photographs or videographic recordings; and using scales, indexes, inventories, self-assessments, and logs (APTA, 2001).

The tests and measurements that therapists use should be **reliable** (produce consistent, repeatable results) and **valid** (measure what they are supposed to measure). The test or measurement should have the **sensitivity** to detect dysfunction and the **specificity** to detect normality. If the test has high sensitivity, there should be few false-negative results, and if it has high specificity, there should be few false positives. Tests and measures must be administered as directed in test manuals or standardized protocols if they are to be reliable. Results of standardized tests and measures are reported in several ways, depending on how the test was developed. The **raw score** indicates the total number of items passed on a test. When providing raw scores, usually the basal and ceiling levels are indicated. The basal level is the item preceding the earliest failed item, and the ceiling level is the item representing the most difficult success. A score that is easy to understand for the family and caregivers is the **age-equivalent score**. The performance of a child is compared with the mean age when 50% of children would have mastered those skills. For example, an infant of 12 months' chronological age (CA) may be described as having an age-equivalent score of 6 months because the infant has just learned to sit and has other skills common to most 6-month-olds as noted on a developmental test. The age equivalent score is not a truly accurate appraisal of the child's ability, but most families easily understand it.

Another useful score is the **developmental quotient.** This is the ratio between the child's actual score based on the developmental age achieved on a test and the child's CA.

The developmental quotient in the previous example would be 6 months/12 months = 0.50, or 50%. This would indicate a significant delay in development. If the child had scored at the 12-month level and was 12 months old, the developmental quotient would be 12 months/12 months = 1, or 100%, indicating no delay at all.

Descriptive statistics are used to compare an individual to other individuals based on a normal distribution called the normal, or bell-shaped, curve (Figure 1–3). **Standard scores** are used to express deviation or variations from the mean score of a group and include Z-scores, T-scores, IQ scores, developmental index scores, percentile scores, and age-equivalent scores (Richardson, 2001). Percentile scores are used to indicate the number of children of the same age expected to score lower than the subject child. A child scoring in the 75th percentile on a norm-referenced test would be scoring *above* 75% of the children in the normative sample of the test. The Z-score and T-score are computed using standard deviation scores. The Z-score is determined by subtracting the mean for a test from the child's score and then dividing it by the published standard deviation for the test. The equation would be

$$Z = \frac{child's\ score\ -\ test\ mean\ score}{test\ standard\ deviation}$$

The T-score is derived from the Z-score; however, the mean is always 50 and the standard deviation is always 10. The equation would be:

$$T = 10(Z\ score) + 50$$

The T-score is always a positive value, and any result below 50 indicates a score below the mean.

Frequently in clinical practice, a test is used that is within the performance level of the child, but the test's norms were determined on a younger population of children. In this situation, the standard norms are invalid because the child's age is outside the test's age norms, even though the child scores within the test's range. The test is not valid, but the results can provide a standardized indication of performance and an indication of developmental level.

Most tests are either **criterion referenced** or **norm referenced**. Criterion-referenced tests have become common in physical therapy practice and early intervention. Cut-off scores are used to compare individual performance against a defined standard (description of desired performance) and not against group performance. Criterion-referred tests, such as the Functional Independence Measure for Children (WEEFIM), are used frequently in ongoing examination and for program planning because they are sensitive to the effects of intervention. Norm-referenced tests compare

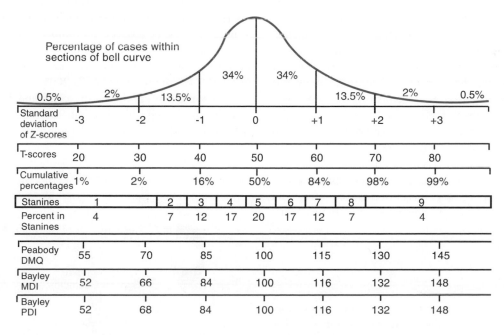

Figure 1–3 Normal curve and associated standard scores. (From Richardson, P.K. (2001). Use of standardized tests in pediatric practice. In J. Case-Smith (Ed.): *Occupational therapy for children,* 4th ed., p. 336. St Louis: Mosby. Reprinted with permission of the author.)

individual performance against a known group performance, and deviations from the normal distribution are determined. IQ and SATs are common norm-referenced tests. Other norm-referenced tests, such as the Bayley Scales of Infant Development and Peabody Developmental Motor Scales, are frequently used to determine the program eligibility of young children. They are not sensitive to the effects of intervention but have all too frequently been used inappropriately to evaluate intervention outcomes.

Selecting the right test for the right purpose is critical. You must consider what the test measures, the age group of children for which the test was developed, the reliability and validity of the test, how well the test correlates with other "gold standard" tests, the time and cost involved in administering the test, and why the test is being given. The purpose of the examination is critical in determining what measurement tools to use. When the purpose is **screening**, the test should generally be brief and cost effective, with minimal false-negative results. Children who screen positive then receive a more comprehensive test as part of the examination. A **diagnostic** examination should determine if a child has a specific disability or is at risk of the development of one. A common purpose of examinations in pediatrics, especially in early intervention and school-based services, is to determine eligibility for services. Standardized tests are frequently administered to determine eligibility for services. Once the child is determined to be eligible for services, the **prescriptive** examination can be completed to assist in determining the most appropriate intervention and plan of care. Frequently, there is overlap in the purposes of the examination, and many tests and measures serve multiple functions. Selecting the correct test or measure can be critical for determining services, documenting outcomes, and receiving reimbursement for services.

Section 2 of this text discusses appropriate tests and measures for each of the body systems. In addition to the examination of specific systems, it is important when working with children to determine their developmental and functional status, sensory integration functioning, and quality of life and health. These tests and measures are discussed in Chapter 2.

Evaluation

After the physical process of performing the examination, the intellectual process of the **evaluation** is completed. The *Guide* (APTA, 2001, p. 43) states that evaluation is a "dynamic process in which the physical therapist makes clinical judgments based on data gathered during the exam-ination." The evaluation involves the synthesis of findings from the history, systems review, and tests and measures of impairments of body structures and functions, limitations in activities, and restrictions in participation. In pediatrics, the terms *evaluation, examination,* and *assessment* are frequently used interchangeably or have different meanings than indicated in the *Guide*, as discussed in Chapter 2.

There are many approaches to the evaluation of children with disabilities. The theoretical model that serves as the foundation for the process varies based on the setting, diagnoses, resources, payer, and provider. P. H. Campbell (1991) has described both top-down and bottom-up approaches to examination and evaluation. In the top-down approach (Figure 1–4), the desired outcomes (goals or objectives) are determined first, with extensive input from the child and family. Then the strengths and obstacles to achieving the goals are determined through the examination and evaluation process. A plan of care with appropriate interventions is then developed and implemented with ongoing re-examination. This family-centered, top-down approach is commonly used for children with known problems or diagnoses, those with severe limitations in activities, and those in early intervention programs. The bottom-up approach is the more traditional approach in which the child's strengths and weaknesses are identified through the examination process and then the professionals usually determine the goals and objectives. This approach is more common in medical settings. The evaluation process is influenced by the severity and complexity of the findings, extent of loss of function, family and home situation, school situation, functional level, and activities and participation in the community (APTA, 2001).

In a top-down approach, the child and family might identify that being able to climb the stairs at the high-school football stadium is very important to them. It is

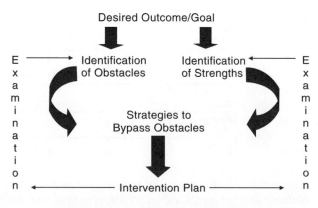

Figure 1–4   Top-down approach.

unlikely that the therapist would have thought about stadium stairs without family input, but with the family's assistance, the therapist can develop a plan of care to achieve this goal. The therapist would determine what skills and abilities the child has that would assist in performing this task. Strengths might include the ability to walk with crutches on level ground and climb stairs using a railing in an empty stairwell. Possible obstacles might include lacking the balance required for stair climbing without a railing, distractibility in crowded places, and lacking the cardiopulmonary endurance required for the task. The plan of care to achieve this goal would then be developed and provided for the child.

Diagnosis

Diagnosis is a term used to describe a cluster of signs and symptoms, arranged in syndromes or categories. The diagnosis is based on the results of the examination and evaluation process. Physicians usually use a medical diagnosis to identify a disease, disorder, or condition at the cell, tissue, organ, or system level. A physical therapist, when determining a diagnosis, will use "labels that identify the *impact of a condition on function at the level of the system (especially the movement system) and at the level of the whole person*" (APTA, 2001, p. 45). A physical therapist, after a comprehensive examination and evaluation, will assign a diagnostic label based on the specific practice patterns outlined in the *Guide*. If this process does not yield an appropriate practice pattern, as is frequently the case in pediatrics, "the physical therapist may administer interventions for the alleviation of symptoms and remediation of impairments" (APTA, 2001, p. 45) guided by the child's responses. Each practice pattern represents a diagnostic classification and "indicates the primary dysfunctions toward which the physical therapist directs intervention" (APTA, 2001, p. 45). The preferred practice patterns can thereby serve as a guide to direct the management and intervention of individuals who are grouped together by clusters of impairments.

The diagnostic process is complex and should be systematically addressed. At the moment, few diagnostic tests are available "with adequate sensitivity and specificity for identifying and defining impairments and functional limitations" (Palisano, Campbell, & Harris, 2000, p. 204). In addition, the *Guide* (APTA, 2001) has mainly focused on adult practice patterns, and it is only in the most recent edition that a major area of practice in pediatric physical therapy was represented by the practice pattern: Impaired Neuromotor Development. The diagnostic process may reveal that the findings are outside the scope of physical therapy practice and that referral to another, more appropriate practitioner is indicated.

Prognosis (Including Plan of Care)

Prognosis involves determining the "predicted optimal level of improvement in function and the amount of time needed to reach that level, and may also include a prediction of levels of improvement that may be reached at various intervals during the course of therapy" (APTA, 2001, p. 46). Determining a prognosis can be very difficult and usually requires a great deal of experience in working with children with a specific diagnosis at a specific age. There is insufficient information regarding prognosis, and even less information on time to achieve goals in the pediatric literature. A few studies have tried to determine ambulation prognosis in children with developmental delay or CP based on the presence of primitive reflexes (Bleck, 1975; Effgen, 1982; Montgomery, 1998). Parents and others need an estimate of their child's potential functional abilities and realistic expectations of what intervention can offer. Some parents wrongly believe that "more is better," and unfortunately, we do not have the data to support ideal frequencies and intensities of intervention. This is an area requiring intensive investigation.

The culmination of the examination, evaluation, diagnosis, and prognosis is development of the **plan of care**. The plan is developed in full collaboration with the child, family, and other service providers. Various formats are used across the nation for documenting examination, evaluation findings, and the plan of care. Some of this variation is a result of the purpose of the examination and the setting. Hospital- and clinic-based therapists must provide daily documentation to reflect the changing status of an ill child, or as required by insurance companies. This documentation is generally concise and frequently is in the form of the "SOAP" notes (S = subjective, O = objective, A = assessment, P = plan) (Kettenbach, 2001). Early intervention and school-based therapists must provide documentation that meets the legal requirements of IDEA and state regulations.

Display 1.1 is a comprehensive sample template for a **Pediatric Physical Therapy Evaluation and Plan of Care** based on the areas suggested in the *Guide* (APTA, 2001) and common pediatric physical therapy practice. The documentation templates provided in the *Guide* are not generally appropriate to pediatric practice. The document presented starts with the *Parent and Child's Concerns,* as advocated in a family-centered, top-down approach to evaluation. The *History* and *Systems Review* follow this, as outlined in the *Guide*. *Present Function*, when possible, is observed during naturalistic observation and then reported. The findings of the *Tests and Measures* are then given. The tests and measures administered to a child depend on the findings of the *History* and *Systems Review* and observation of *Present Function*. All of these results are then analyzed, synthesized, and reported under *Summary of Findings*. *Factors Affecting Function* are then listed based on the examination results. Internal factors, those within the individual, include impairments of body structures and functions, limitations in activities, and cognitive ability, emotional stability, motivation, and language ability. *External Factors* are personal and environmental factors such as family support, access to health care, financial resources, accessible schools, and so on. Factors that both aid and hinder function should be included because they can affect intervention. The negative *Factors Affecting Function* are really a list of problems similar to those used in many physical therapy reporting systems (Kettenbach, 2001). *Measurable Goals, Outcomes and /or Objectives* are then listed. The *Intervention Plan* comes next, with the major categories of Coordination, Communication, Documentation; Child and Family Instruction; and Procedural Interventions. The plan for *Re-examination* and the *Criteria for Discharge* follow.

The plan of care includes the anticipated goals and predicted outcomes that are the intended results of the intervention. The plan of care indicates the expected changes in impairments of body structures and functions, limitations in activities, and restrictions in participation. The plan might "also address risk reduction, prevention, impact on societal resources and … satisfaction" (APTA, 2001, p. 46). "The anticipated goals and expected outcomes may be expressed as short-term and long-term goals" (APTA, 2001, p. 46). Several goals and objectives may be developed within a plan of care to achieve an outcome.

Goals, Outcomes, and Objectives

As in other areas of physical therapy practice, there have been changes in the terminology and definitions used to describe goals, outcomes, and objectives. Goals and objectives might best be considered *expectations* of the intervention, whereas the outcomes are the *results*. This becomes complicated, because in the *Guide* (APTA, 2001, p. 46) the word "expected" is placed before outcomes, which would lead one to wonder what the difference is between "antici-

pated goals" and "expected outcomes." Differences were provided in the first edition of the *Guide* (APTA, 1997) but not in the second edition. Goals should precede objectives (Alberto & Troutman, 2002). In the past, goals and outcomes were global statements that were usually not measurable (APTA, 1997; Montgomery, 1987). However, in the second edition of the *Guide* (APTA, 2001), it is noted that "anticipated goals and expected outcomes … should be measurable and time limited" (p. 48). The term "objective" is not defined in the *Guide,* although it is used in the *Guide* and is standard terminology in physical therapy practice, especially in pediatrics. **Objectives** are measurable statements regarding desired (anticipated/expected) results (goals/outcomes). There appears to be an agreement that **outcomes** are "factors that identify the results of interventions (e.g., functional health status, morbidity, mortality, quality of life, satisfaction, and cost)" (Nicholson, 2002, p. 214). Montgomery and Connolly (2003) now note that two-part outcomes may be indicated: one at the impairment of body structure and function level, and one at the limitations in activities and participation level. These outcomes should both be measurable. For the sake of consistency, we have tried to use the term *objective* when referring to measurable expectations, recognizing that goals and outcomes may also, but not necessarily, be stated in measurable terms.

Determining a desired goal, outcome, or objective can be as simple as asking the child what activity he or she wants to perform, or so complex that it requires several interdisciplinary team meetings. The goals, outcomes, and objectives are developed based on the child's and family's desires and the findings of the evaluation.

The ability to measure whether or not a child has achieved a desired outcome is critical in determining the success of the intervention and the need for continued intervention and program evaluation. Nebulous statements such as "The child will achieve normal motor development" or "The child's tone will normalize" say very little, and it is impossible to know when and if the child attained normal motor development or normal tone. Use of nonmeasurable goal statements hinders the profession's efforts to acquire the data necessary to support the effectiveness of our interventions.

Writing measurable objectives (Table 1.3) is not difficult, but it does require thoughtful consideration of numerous variables. An objective (Effgen, 1991; Mager, 1962) must contain a statement of the behavior that the child is expected to perform, the conditions under which the behavior is performed, and the criteria expected for ultimate performance.

Table 1.3 Considerations for Objectives

Behavior Examples
- Maintaining sitting position
- Transferring oneself while lying
- Carrying an object from place to place
- Walking on different surfaces

Conditions (might include more than one condition)
- *Equipment*: such as using an assistive device or wearing an orthosis
- *Physical environment*: such as at home or in the school cafeteria
- *Social environment*: such as with the parents or therapist
- *Antecedent stimuli*: such as verbal requests or demonstration

Criteria (might include more than one criterion)
- *Frequency*: number of correct behaviors in a specific number of trials (e.g., 2 of 5 trials) or percentage correct (75% of the time)
- *Duration*: how long a behavior will last (e.g., 3 seconds, 30 seconds, 5 minutes, 6 repetitions)
- *Amount of assistance provided*: independent; with supervision; standby assistance; minimal, moderate, or maximum assistance

Examples of Objectives*
- Patrick will sit independently on the floor at home for 5 minutes.
- Kathy will transfer from lying on her bed to sitting at the side of her bed with moderate assistance in 3 of 5 trials.
- Julie will carry her books to class from the bus without dropping them 75% of the time.
- Jonathan will walk across his lawn with his walker with standby assistance.

*Examples selected from World Health Organization (2001). International classification of functioning, disability and health. Geneva: Author, Mobility Chapter of Activities and Participation.

Changes in the behavior may reflect maturation of the behavior itself, progressing from basic skills to more complex skills or increasing levels of completing the activity. Changes in conditions may be from simple to complex, such as walking at home to walking in a mall filled with people, or transferring with assistance to transferring independently. Progression of criteria may be increased frequency or duration of an activity, or changes in the amount of assistance required. Using criteria such as three of four trials, or 80% of the time, should be considered carefully. Successfully transferring into a car 80% of the time could mean that 20% of the time the child

ends up on the street! That is not an acceptable outcome or criterion. Selection of the behavior, conditions, and criteria for each objective for each individual child must be based on sound professional judgment. "Cookbooks" of objectives should not replace the judgment of the professional.

Commonly, a long-term objective or goal is determined first and then broken down into several short-term objectives. Short-term objectives are based on a task analysis of the major or long-term objective. In some settings, the word *goal* refers only to the long-term goal, and *objective* refers to the short-term objective (Richardson & Shultz-Krohn, 2001). When possible, each short-term objective should be a desired activity the child wants to perform. There are situations when some short-term objectives relate to impairment of body functions and structures, and when these objectives are attained, they will assist the child in achieving an activity objective. For example, sitting is an important activity; however, without the prerequisite trunk muscle strength and hip ROM, independent sitting is impossible. In such a case, the therapist might write objectives regarding the ability to sit independently and also write objectives about increasing trunk strength and hip ROM. In educational environments, the activity of sitting and manipulating an object might be an objective placed in the child's Individualized Education Plan (IEP), but the impairment level objectives of muscle strengthening and ROM would be part of the plan of care that the therapist writes. Documentation of the achievement of each goal/objective is important and should be reported to both the child and the family. Many small gains should be recognized and rewarded instead of waiting, perhaps forever, for the achievement of the major, long-term objective.

A task analysis should be completed to determine the short-term objectives. In a task analysis, the therapist determines the component parts of the task, including both activity requirements and prerequisites. For example, a standing transfer from a wheelchair to a car requires the ability to lock the wheel chair, come to a standing position, pivot, and lower one's self to sitting. To perform this activity, the child requires the cognitive ability to understand the activity, the motivation to perform the activity, the motor planning ability to execute the activity, the muscle strength to stand and pivot, the flexion and extension ROM required to stand and sit, and the balance to sit, stand, and pivot. These are only a few of the components required to perform this complex task. The therapist must select the most important elements for an individual child and systematically develop the objectives.

Consideration of the level of learning of the activity is also important and is referred to as the Hierarchy of Response Competence (Figure 1–5) (Alberto & Troutman, 2002). Skill must first be **acquired**. This might be the initial behavior of propped sitting of an infant, the first few steps with a walker, or a roll from prone to supine. This is followed by **fluency** or proficiency, in which the quality and level of learning and performance move beyond merely performance of the task as in acquisition. Fluency occurs when the infant then learns to sit without propping, the child can walk around the room with the walker, and the child can roll around from place to place. Fluency may be reflected under conditions or criteria of the objective. After fluency there must be **maintenance** of the ability to perform the activities/skills/behaviors over time. The child should be able to perform the activity several days, weeks, or months later. Maintenance is followed by **generalization.** The child must be able to perform the activity in multiple environments, with different individuals (usually referred to as **trainers**), and with different types of equipment. In the motor learning literature, generalization is referred to as **transfer**. The condition statement may be written to reflect generalization of environments, equipment, and individuals. *Acquisition, fluency, maintenance,* and *generalization of behaviors* are terms used by educators and others. Using this terminology is very helpful when we need to convey the

ACQUISITION
Initial learning of a new activity

FLUENCY
Developing proficiency at the activity

MAINTENANCE
Performing the activity over time

GENERALIZATION
Performing the activity in numerous environments,
with new people and different equipment

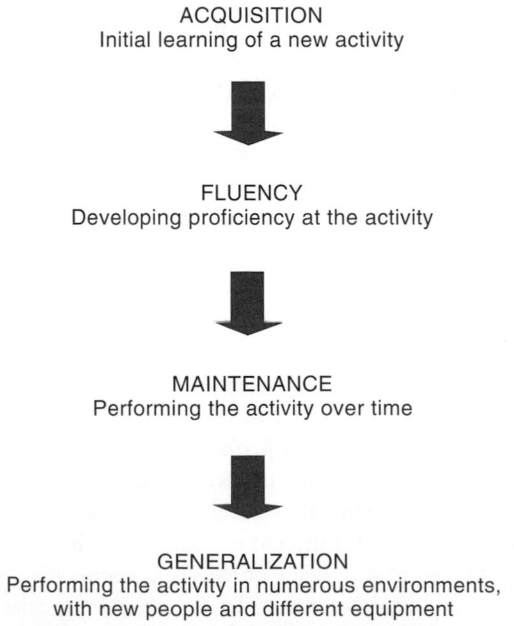

Figure 1–5   Hierarchy of response competence.

rationale for providing services past the initial phase of acquisition of a behavior.

For children, the time stipulated to achieve the long-term objective is setting specific. In educational settings, the long-term objectives are for 1 year; in early intervention programs, they are generally for 6 months; and in acute-care settings, they might be for 1 week or less. The ability to write realistic objectives that can be achieved in the specified time frame is based, in no small part, on the skill and experience of the therapist writing the objectives. How to develop appropriate goals and objectives for specific limitations and restrictions is discussed in later chapters.

The plan of care must also include plans for discharge or "graduation" from services. The primary criterion for discharge should be achievement of the objectives, not an arbitrary criterion based on number of intervention sessions determined by an insurance company or school administrator, and physical therapy should not be an ongoing continuous activity with no discharge plan. Although discharging children from physical therapy services can be difficult, therapists who discuss discharge planning when initiating intervention in school settings do not report problems in "graduating" children from therapy (Effgen, 2000b).

Intervention

Intervention is the term used throughout the *Guide* to describe "the purposeful and skilled interaction of the physical therapist with the patient/client and, if appropriate, with other individuals involved in the care of the patient/client, using various physical therapy methods and techniques to produce changes in the condition that are consistent with the diagnosis and prognosis" (APTA, 2001, p. 43). Judgments regarding intervention are made based on the timely monitoring of the child's responses and progress in achieving the anticipated goals, objectives, and outcomes. The concept of intervention is far more encompassing than just the term treatment and, according to the *Guide,* intervention should be composed of three important components: coordination, communication, and documentation; child- and family-related instruction; and procedural intervention.

Coordination

Coordination involves the organization and management of services with all parties working together to ensure that the child and family "receive appropriate, comprehensive, efficient, and effective quality of care" (APTA, 2001, p. 47) from the initiation of services to the end of services. The therapist, or a designated case manager, might provide coordination of services. Coordination may involve arranging for durable medical equipment; working with an orthotist or a prosthetist in determining the most appropriate orthotic or prosthesis; arranging transportation; arranging with teachers about the best time and place to observe a child's classroom performance; and scheduling parent and teacher meetings.

Communication

Communication includes written and verbal correspondence to convey information to the child, family, and other approved parties. Therapists must make certain that private health information is released to only those authorized to receive that information as required under the federal Health Insurance Portability and Accountability Act of 1996 (HIPAA). This act limits the nonconsensual use and release of private health information, provides individuals access to their medical records, and restricts disclosure. In school settings, the Family Education Right to Privacy Act (FERPA) also applies. No matter what the setting, professionals must be very careful that information about a child is shared with only those individuals who have a documented need for that information.

Documentation

Documentation is written information that may include the evaluation report, plan of care, request for approval for services, summary letters to physicians and other service providers, referrals, home and school programs, discharge planning, and information provided to those who pay for the services. Comprehensive documentation is mandatory for reimbursement for services. Although reimbursement may not be an issue in school-based settings, the therapist must still maintain appropriate documentation and meet the state standards for physical therapy documentation. HIPAA regulations must be complied with regarding the distribution of these records.

Child- and Family-Related Instruction

Child- and family-related instruction, along with instruction to other team members, is a critical area of pediatric practice. The family and other professionals and paraprofessionals are frequently largely responsible for assisting the child in carrying out or practicing many intervention activities. This instruction is to promote and maximize the physical therapy services and expedite achievement of the goals. Physical therapy intervention done once a week for perhaps gait training will be of little benefit if the family and others are not able to assist the child in practicing this activity throughout the week. Positioning devices are of little value if the child is improperly positioned in the device in the classroom or intensive care unit. Instruction given to physical therapist assistants, teachers, aides, and day care workers is vital if the child is to function on a daily basis by relying on the assistance of others.

Procedural Interventions

Procedural interventions occur when the physical therapist "selects, applies, or modifies ... interventions ... based on examination data, the evaluation, the diagnosis and the prognosis, and the anticipated goals and expected outcomes" (APTA, 2001, p. 47). The type, frequency, and duration of the interventions are based on many factors, including the following:

- Child's age
- Anatomical and physiological changes related to growth and development
- Chronicity or severity of the condition
- Comorbidities
- Degree of limitations and restrictions
- Accessibility and availability of resources
- Concurrent services
- Family desires and degree of participation
- Caregiver ability and expertise
- Community support
- Psychosocial and socioeconomic factors
- Child's level of cognitive ability and cooperation

The specific interventions selected depend on these numerous variables. There are different models and rationales for providing physical therapy procedural interventions. Interventions that are provided based on impairments of body structures and functions and limitations in activities are discussed in the chapters on body systems in Section 2 of this text. Section 3, Service Delivery Settings, discusses the most common environments for pediatric physical therapy service delivery. Interventions are determined based not only on the needs of the child but also on the requirements of the settings. For example, physical therapy in an educational environment for school-aged children must be "educationally relevant." If a needed intervention does not relate to an educationally relevant goal, then that intervention, which is also needed by the child, must be provided in a different setting such as an outpatient clinic. Some settings will only serve a child with a specific diagnosis, and if the child has an additional diagnosis, services for that secondary diagnosis must be received elsewhere. Some insurance companies limit the number of treatment visits for which they will pay, which influences the plan of care.

There has been an increasing trend in health care to use algorithms, clinical practice guidelines, and clinical pathways to increase efficiency and improve quality of care. **Algorithms** are "written guidelines to stepwise evaluation and management strategies that require observations to be made, decisions to be considered, and actions to be taken" (Nicholson, 2002, p. 214). They assist in decision making and make it easier to list essential clinical steps that might later be used to develop clinical practice guidelines. **Clinical practice guidelines** are systematically developed plans to assist in health-care decision making for specific clinical circumstances (Nicholson, 2002). They may be based on expert opinion, consensus, or evidence-based practice. They help the service provider determine the most effective and appropriate interventions. The *Guide* (APTA, 2001) is a global clinical practice guideline. More explicit than an algorithm or a clinical practice guideline is the critical or clinical pathway. **Clinical, critical,** or **care pathways,** as they are frequently named, are predetermined protocols that define the critical steps in examining, evaluating, and providing intervention for a clinical problem to improve quality of care, reduce variability of care, and enhance efficiency (Fleischman et al., 2002). These pathways were initially developed for nurses and physicians; however, there is a trend toward multidisciplinary pathways that will facilitate achievement of expected outcomes in a defined length of time for individuals who require a team approach to intervention. The clinical pathway sets locally agreed-on standards of care for individuals with similar conditions. The APTA Section on Pediatrics is developing a clinical pathway for providing services for children with spastic diplegia. Clinical pathways will become more common as efforts continue to make services more cost efficient and consistent. Therapists should recognize the value of these pathways in guiding practice but recognize that they have a professional obligation to evaluate the appropriateness of a particular pathway or intervention for every child.

Re-examination

The process of re-examination and re-evaluation or reappraisal of a child is an ongoing, continual process. Throughout the intervention process, the therapist should constantly be re-examining and re-evaluating the child's impairments in body structures and functions, limitations in activities, and restrictions in participation. The child's progress toward achieving the agreed-on goals/outcomes/objectives should be discussed with the parents and other team members. There may also be a need for formal periodic re-examinations. The frequency of re-examination depends on whether the child has an acute or a chronic disability, the requirements of the setting and payor, and the rate of progress. In an acute-care hospital, re-examination might be daily, and in a rehabilitation setting, weekly; in early intervention programs, re-examination occurs at least every 6 months, and in school settings, annually.

Outcomes

The final element of the *Guide* (APTA, 2001) is outcomes. **Outcomes** are the result of the intervention process. Outcomes are usually measured in terms of achievement of the goals and objectives resulting in reduced limitations in body structures or functions, improved performance in activities, child and family satisfaction, and prevention of secondary problems. Outcomes are measured near the end of the episode of care or during care through re-examination.

According to Guralnick (1997), a leader in early intervention research, outcomes must be measured along three dimensions: child and family characteristics, program/intervention features, and goals and objectives. Outcome measures in pediatrics need to expand beyond domains of development and must consider quality of life issues (McLaughlin & Bjornson, 1998). The interventions done by physical therapists may be successful in terms of achieving the goals and objectives; however, if the goals and objectives are not meaningful to the child and family, it is unlikely that the child's quality of life will improve, or that the child and family will experience satisfaction. Measurement of quality of life issues is becoming a standard part of practice in many settings.

Models of Team Interaction

Understanding models of team interaction and the role of the therapist in each model is important for effective and efficient team functioning in health-care and educational settings. The complex needs of the children we serve require the expertise of several disciplines, and there are different opinions about the best ways to function together. The preferred model of team interaction can vary based on the setting.

The landmark work of Deming (2000) in the manufacturing sector has slowly brought changes in all service delivery, including health-care delivery, over the past several decades. The autocratic, hierarchical model of the "captain of the ship" and the isolated uniprofessional models have evolved into more democratic models. Models of team interaction are presented in Table 1.4 and Figure 1–6. The **unidisciplinary model** is not really a "team" model because it generally involves an individual discipline providing services in isolation from all other disciplines. This is the approach described in the APTA *Guide* (2001) (McEwen, 2000, p. 89). In pediatrics, this might be the only model possible in rural areas where there are no other team members. The **multidisciplinary model** is the oldest form of teaming and involves the least active interaction among team members. Several professions will perform independent evaluations and then meet to discuss their examination and evaluation findings and determine goals, outcomes, and a plan of care. Usually the interventions are provided individually by each discipline, although communication among providers is maintained. In the **interdisciplinary model,** the team works together and there is extensive interaction among the team members from the initial examination through the intervention phase. Formal channels of communication are established and all information is shared. Confusion in terminology occurred when the meaning of multidisciplinary changed because of its use in Public Law (PL) 99-457, Education of the Handicapped Act Amendments of 1986. According to the law, "Multidisciplinary means the involvement of two or more disciplines or professions in the provision of integrated and coordinated services, including evaluation and assessment activities" (Federal Register, June 22, 1989, 303.17, pp. 26, 313). This is consistent with the definition of an interdisciplinary model presented here; however, there is often confusion when using these terms.

Another model of team interaction is the **transdisciplinary model.** This is the model most commonly used in early intervention programs. The definition and application of the transdisciplinary model also vary greatly. In a transdisciplinary model there should be continuous sharing of information, skills, and programming across disciplines. There is usually joint examination, evaluation, and intervention, coupled with professional role release. Role release

Table 1.4 Models of Team Interaction

Unidisciplinary	Professional works independently of all others.
Intradisciplinary	Members of the same profession work together without significant communication with members of other professions.
Multidisciplinary	Professionals work independently but recognize and value the contributions of other professions. There may be little interaction or ongoing communication among professionals. However, the Rules and Regulations (Federal Register, June 22, 1989, p. 26313) for PL 99-457 redefines multidisciplinary to mean "the involvement of two or more disciplines or professions in the provision of integrated and coordinated services, including evaluation and assessment."
Interdisciplinary	Individuals from different disciplines work together cooperatively to evaluate and develop programs. Emphasis is on teamwork. Role definitions are relaxed.
Transdisciplinary	There is teaching and ongoing work among professionals across traditional disciplinary boundaries. Role release occurs when a team member assumes the responsibilities of other disciplines for service delivery.
Collaborative	All team members work together in equal participation and consensus decision making. The team interaction of the transdisciplinary model is combined with the integrated service delivery model.

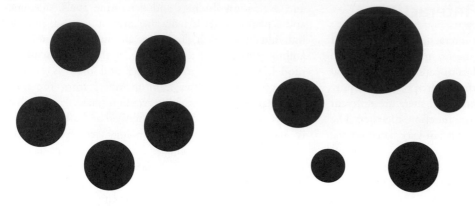

Equal team members   **Unequal team members**

Figure 1–6   Representation of equal and unequal teams.

involves not merely the sharing of information but also sharing performance competencies and cross-training. Team members teach each other specific interventions to meet the child's needs. This model developed out of the need for consistent services for children with severe disabilities and for infants who would not tolerate being handled by multiple individuals. The transdisciplinary model should lead to more effective interventions because the interventions are provided at increased frequencies throughout the day during functional activities. Some professionals are concerned about the liability involved in teaching others to provide interventions, the legal restrictions, the inability of some to properly carry out the interventions, and the watering down of professional involvement in service delivery. However, in 1997, Rainforth examined role release in relation to the legally defined scope of physical therapy practice and found that the roles of evaluation, intervention, planning, and supervision may not be delegated, but intervention could be done by others who are trained and supervised by a physical therapist.

As the team process has developed, the use of the terms **collaboration** and **collaborative teamwork** has evolved. A summary of the defining characteristics of collaborative teamwork, as conceptualized by Rainforth and York-Barr (1997), is presented in Box 1.1. Collaborative teamwork involves equal participation in the process by the family and service providers, consensus decision making regarding goals and interventions, skills that are embedded in the intervention program, infusion of knowledge across disciplines, and role release.

Older hierarchical medical or educational models of team interaction dictated the team leaders, but in

newer models, the needs of the child determine who is the team leader, if indeed there is a team leader. Dormans and Pellegrino (1998), two leading pediatric orthopedic surgeons, note in *Caring for Children With Cerebral Palsy: A Team Approach* that an effective team requires effective leadership, but that the "specific person and discipline that provide that leadership are usually determined by the primary mission of the team and by the setting" (p. 59).

BOX 1.1 Collaborative Teamwork

Collaborative team includes:

- Equal participation on the team by family members and service providers
- Consensus decision making in determining priorities for goals and objectives
- Consensus decision making about the type and amount of intervention
- Motor and communication skills embedded throughout the intervention program
- Design and implementation of the intervention that include infusion of knowledge and skills from different disciplines
- Role release so team members develop confidence and competence necessary to encourage the child's learning

Source: Adapted from Rainforth, B., & York-Barr, J. (1997). *Collaborative teams for students with severe disabilities* (2nd ed.). Baltimore, MD: Paul H. Brookes.

Children with severe disabilities (Hunt, Soto, Maier, & Doering, 2003) or complex medical problems generally require the services of an extensive team of professionals. For that team to prevent duplication of services and conflicting services and to maximize resources to provide efficient and effective intervention, the members must collaborate. The different discipline members on teams provide support for each other and enhance each other's problem-solving capabilities. The hopes are that each member of the team will be equally valued and that no member of the team will have inappropriate authority based on personality or self-perceived importance (see Figure 1–6).

When working in a new setting or joining a team, you should ask for a clarification and definition of terms regarding models or expectations of team interaction. All individuals involved should have the same understanding to avoid miscommunication and conflict.

Models of Service Delivery

The models of physical therapy service delivery are often closely connected with models of team interaction. There is also an array of confusing and conflicting terms used to describe the various models. The framework for these models of service delivery is outlined in Table 1.5 and presented here.

Direct Model

In the **direct model**, the therapist is usually the primary service provider to the child. This is the traditional model used to provide physical therapy. Direct intervention may be given when *specific therapeutic techniques cannot be safely delegated and when there is emphasis on acquisition of new motor skills*. Direct therapy should, when possible, be done in the natural environment. Only when it is in the best interests of the child should the therapy session be in a restrictive environment, such as a treatment room or clinic setting. A restrictive treatment environment might be necessary if extensive equipment is required, if the child is highly distractible, or when it is the safest environment for either the therapist or child. Rarely, if ever, should direct intervention be given without instructing and working with the child's parents and other service providers. It is not unusual for a child to receive direct intervention for a specific objective and receive other models of service deliv-

ery to achieve other goals. Direct intervention is common in acute-care hospital settings because of the seriousness and complexity of the problems and the usually very short length of stay.

Integrated Model

A number of different definitions of the **integrated model** have been described. They vary by the setting in which they are implemented. The integrated model in educational settings is one in which the therapist's contact is not only the child but also the teacher, aide/associate, and family. The service is generally delivered in the learning environment and the method of intervention is educationally related—activities with an emphasis on practice of newly acquired motor skills during the child's daily routine. The *implementer of the activities may be the teacher, aide/associate, other professionals, parent, and/or physical therapist or physical therapist assistant* (Iowa Department of Education, 2001).

The integrated model of service delivery can, and frequently does, include direct physical therapy intervention and consultative services. The physical therapist collaborates with all other key individuals serving the child such as the occupational therapist, speech-language pathologist, and teachers. Goals and objectives are jointly developed, and all individuals serving the child are instructed in how to achieve these objectives within their capability. Direct services, when necessary, are provided in the most natural environment; natural environments include the child's home, preschool classroom, regular classroom, and community at large.

Dunn (1991) states that the integrated model also consists of peer integration, functional integration, practice integration, and comprehensive integration. Peer integration occurs when a child with a disability functions in a classroom or at a social event with children without disabilities. The child functions in multiple settings with other peers. Functional integration involves the child's use of a therapeutic strategy or newly acquired skill in the natural environment. Functional integration is one rationale behind providing therapy in natural environments, especially when the objectives involve fluency (refinement of skills) and generalization of skills (ability to perform skills in multiple environments with different individuals and equipment). Practice integration involves the collaboration of professionals to meet a child's individual needs. Comprehensive integration combines all the areas of integration and is the level to which we must strive.

Table 1.5 Physical Therapy Service Delivery Models

	Direct	Integrated	Consultative	Monitoring	Collaborative
Therapist's Primary Contact	Child	Child, team, and family	Family and team	Child	Child, team, and family
Environment for Service Delivery	Usually hospital or outpatient setting Distraction-free environment Specialized equipment might be needed	Usually early intervention or school-based setting Natural environment Therapy area if necessary for a specific child	Can occur in all intervention settings Natural environment	Usually school-based setting Natural environment Therapy area if necessary for a specific child	Can occur in all intervention settings Natural environment
Methods of Intervention	Functional activities and intervention for impairments limiting function Specific therapeutic techniques that cannot safely be delegated Emphasis on acquisition of new motor skills	Functional activities Positioning Emphasis on practice of newly acquired motor skills in the daily routine	Functional activities Positioning Adaptive materials Emphasis on adapting to natural environment and generalization of acquired skills	Emphasis on making certain child maintains functional status	Functional activities
Amount of Service Time	Regularly scheduled sessions	Routinely scheduled Flexible amount of time depending on needs of staff or child	Intermittent, depending on needs of staff or child	Intermittent, depending on needs of child, may be as infrequent as once in 6 months	Ongoing intervention Discipline-referenced knowledge shared among team members so relevant activities occur throughout day

Source:: Adapted from Effgen, S.K. (2000c). The educational environment. In S.K. Campbell, D.W. Vander Linden, & R.J. Palisano (Eds.), *Physical therapy for children* (2nd ed., p. 920). Philadelphia: W.B. Saunders; and Iowa Department of Education (2001). *Iowa guidelines for educationally related physical therapy services*. Des Moines: Author.

Consultative Model

In the **consultative model**, the therapist's contact is other health professionals, the teacher, aide, parent, and child. All personnel, *except the therapist,* implement the activities and interventions. The therapist meets with and demonstrates activities to all appropriate staff so that they can carry out the interventions to help the child achieve the determined goals and objectives. The *responsibility for the outcome lies with the consultee,* the individual receiving the consultation (Dunn, 1991; Iowa Department of Education, 2001). The service is generally provided in the natural environment.

Consultation is usually thought of in terms of a specific child, as outlined in Table 1.5. However, there is also a need for more global, programmatic consultation. Programmatic consultation includes issues related to safety, transportation, architectural barriers, equipment, documentation, continuing education, and quality improvement (Lindsey, O'Neal, Haas, & Tewey, 1980). These are all very important issues that ultimately relate to successful service provision. In many settings, but especially a school setting, the therapist must consult with the administration regarding overall safety issues, proper positioning during transportation, and the removal of architectural barriers. In programmatic consultation, the therapist makes recommendations but does not necessarily perform the activity, such as removing architectural barriers.

Monitoring Model

Another model of indirect service delivery is **monitoring**. Monitoring is an important element of transition from direct or integrated services to no services. In the **monitoring model** the *therapist remains responsible* for the outcome of the intervention. The therapist, although not providing direct intervention, maintains regular contact with the child to check on the child's status and to instruct others. Monitoring is important for the follow-up of children who have impairments that might deteriorate over time or limitations that might require direct, integrated, or consultative intervention at a later date. Monitoring allows the therapist to check on the need for modifications in equipment and to make recommendations quickly. Monitoring provides the family, child, and therapist with a sense that the child is being watched. If the child should then require a change in the model of physical therapy intervention, monitoring generally allows a more rapid transition of services because the child is known to the physical therapist and justification for services can be expedited to meet the child's immediate needs.

Collaborative Model

The **collaborative model** of service delivery is defined as a combination of transdisciplinary team interaction and an integrated service delivery model. Some would say that it is not a model of service delivery at all and is just the preferred model of professional and family interaction. As noted in Table 1.5 and Box 1.1, many team members, as in an integrated model, provide services in a collaborative model but with a greater degree of role release and crossing of disciplinary boundaries than in the integrated model. The team assumes responsibility for consensus decision making on the goals and objectives, and implementation of the program activities. Any member of the team, including the family, implements the activities in the natural routine of the home, school, and community. The amount of service delivery or therapeutic practice of an activity should be greater than in other models because the entire team is carrying out the activities. In practice, this might not be the case because of the varied levels of skill of the implementers, insufficient "natural" opportunities to practice an activity, competing activities, and the difficulty of some activities (Ott & Effgen, 2000; Prieto, 1992; Soccio, 1991). Teams must strive for collaboration and consensus, even if in some situations there is little actual crossing of discipline boundaries with regard to service delivery.

Issues Influencing Practice

Advocacy and Public Policy

In 1961, President John F. Kennedy established a President's Panel on Mental Retardation. On this panel were major proponents for normalization and deinstitutionalization of persons with disabilities, advocating models that were already successful in Scandinavia. The excellent work of this panel, along with later television documentaries such as the one done on the Willowbrook State Institution by Geraldo Rivera, and Blatt and Kaplan's book, *Christmas in Purgatory: A Photographic Essay on Mental Retardation* (1966), raised national concern for the care and treatment of all people with disabilities, especially those in institutions. This public awareness and interest, the decisions by state and federal judicial systems, and the work by special masters appointed by the courts to oversee compliance with litigation led to the federal Developmental Disabilities Assistance and Bill of Rights Act of 1975 (PL 94-103). This law included a provision that required states to develop and incorporate a "deinstitutionalization and institutional reform" plan (Braddock, 1987, p. 71). Advocacy groups gained power, and the location, extent, and type of all service delivery, including physical therapy and rehabilitation services, would see major changes.

Since the 1960s, important federal legislation has provided rights and services to individuals with disabilities. This legislation includes provisions for early intervention services, the right to a free and appropriate public education, the right to health care for those with disabilities, reduction in discrimination, and access to society. These federal laws are summarized in Table 1.6. A review of each of these important pieces of legislation is beyond the scope

Table 1.6 Federal Legislation Affecting Children With Disabilities

Year Enacted	Public Law (PL) Number	Name of Legislation	Impact on Children With Disabilities
1963	PL 88-164	Mental Retardation Facilities and Community Mental Health Centers Construction Act	Provided financial aid for building community-based facilities for people with developmental disabilities and mental illness, and authorized research centers and university-affiliated facilities (UAFs).
1963	PL 88-156	The Maternal and Child Health and Mental Retardation Planning Act	Expanded the Maternal and Child Health Program to improve prenatal care to high-risk women from low-income families to prevent mental retardation.
1963	PL 88-210	Vocation Education Act of 1963	Recognized that individuals with special needs required assistance to achieve success in regular vocational programs.
1964	PL 88-452	Economic Opportunity Act of 1963	Established Project Head Start, offering health, education, nutritional, and social services to economically deprived preschool children. In 1972, PL 92-424 set aside a minimum of 10% of Head Start enrollment for children with disabilities. Now includes an Early Head Start Program for infants.
1965	PL 89-97	Social Security Amendments	Authorized Medicare/Medicaid to provide public funding for the poor, aged, and disabled. This was one of the reforms recommended by President Kennedy's Panel on Mental Retardation.
1967	PL 90-248	Early and Periodic Screening, Diagnosis, and Treatment (EPSDT) Program, part of the Social Security Act of 1967	Provided early and periodic screening, diagnosis, and treatment for all Medicaid-eligible children. Became mandatory as part of Medicaid in 1972.
1970	PL 91-230	ESEA Amendments of 1970 creates the Education of the Handicapped Act (EHA)	Several special education statutes consolidated into Title VI, referred to as the "Education of the Handicapped Act."
1970	PL 91-517	The Developmental Disabilities Services and Facilities Construction Amendments	Expands PL 88-164 into a comprehensive statute that required states to establish a governor's council on developmental disabilities. Term "developmental disabilities" replaced "mental retardation." Children with cerebral palsy and epilepsy were now eligible for services under this definition.
1972	PL 92-223	Social Security Amendments	"Intermediate care facilities" (ICF) to be reimbursed if states ensured that residents received "active treatment."
1972	PL 92-603	Social Security Amendments	Supplemental Security Income (SSI) provided to people in need, including those with developmental disabilities.
1973	PL 93-112	Rehabilitation Act, Section 504	Extended basic civil rights protections to individuals with disabilities. The rules applied to all institutions, agencies, schools, and organizations that received federal assistance.

Year Enacted	Public Law (PL) Number	Name of Legislation	Impact on Children With Disabilities
1974	PL 93-247	Child Abuse and Prevention and Treatment Act and its later amendments (1992, 1996, & 1997)	Provided protection and treatment for children who were abused or neglected. Included a reporting system.
1975	PL 94-142	Education of All Handicapped Children Act and its later amendments (1986, 1991, 1997, & 2004)	Provided the right to a free and appropriate public education and related services for all children ages 5 (6) to 21 years, regardless of their degree of disability.
1978	PL 95-602	Rehabilitation Comprehensive Services and Developmental Disability Act	"Developmental disabilities" defined in functional terms.
1981	PL 97-35 Section 2176	Omnibus Reconciliation Act, "Home-Based Waiver"	Allowed states to finance a variety of community-based services for those with developmental disabilities instead of institutional settings.
1982	PL 97-248	Social Security Amendments ("Katie Beckett" Amendments)	Permitted states to use Medicaid for certain children with disabilities to stay home rather than be institutionalized.
1984	PL 98-248	Carl Perkins Vocational Technical Education Act	Authorized development of vocational education programs with 10% of the funds used to train individuals with disabilities.
1984	PL 98-527	Developmental Disabilities Act Amendments and later amendments of 1987, PL 100-146	Amended the purpose of the Developmental Disabilities Act to ensure that individuals receive necessary services and to establish a coordination and monitoring system. Later added family support.
1986	PL 99-372	The Handicapped Children's Protection Act	Allowed for reasonable attorney's fees incurred by parents who prevailed in hearings related to the child's right to an education under IDEA.
1986	PL 99-401	Temporary Child Care for Handicapped Children and Crisis Nurseries Act and Amendment PL 101-127	Provided funding for temporary respite care for children with disabilities or chronic illness who are at risk of abuse or neglect.
1986	PL 99-457	Education of the Handicapped Act amendments later reauthorized as PL 102-119 Individuals with Disabilities Education Act amendments of 1991	Expanded PL 94-142 to provide special education and related services to preschool children with disabilities, age 3–5 years. Also established early intervention state grant program for infants and toddlers with disabilities age 0 to 36 months and their families.
1986	PL 101-336	The Americans with Disabilities Act (ADA)	Ensured full civil rights to individuals with disabilities. Guaranteed equal opportunity in employment, public and private accommodations, transportation, government services, and telecommunications.
1988	PL 100-407	Technology-Related Assistance for Individuals	Provided state funding to develop technology-related assistance programs and to offer assistive technology to individuals with disabilities.

(Continued)

Table 1.6 Federal Legislation Affecting Children With Disabilities (Continued)

Year Enacted	Public Law (PL) Number	Name of Legislation	Impact on Children With Disabilities
1988	PL 100-360	Medicare Catastrophic Coverage Act	Clarified that Medicaid funds can pay for the cost of "related services" in a school-age child's IEP or IFSP, if the services would have been paid for if PL 94-142 was not in effect.
1997	PL 105-17	Individuals with Disabilities Education Act Amendments (IDEA), 1997)	Refined comprehensive right to education law. Expanded purpose to prepare students for life after school.
1997	PL 105-33	Title XXI of the Social Security Act; State Child Health Insurance Program (SCHIP)	Provided funding for states to initiate and expand health insurance coverage for uninsured, low-income children
2002	PL 107-110	No Child Left Behind (NCLB) Act of 2001	Education reform for all children, designed to close achievement gap through accountability, increased flexibility, parents, options, and evidence-based instruction.
2004	PL 108-446	Amendments to IDEA	Reauthorization of IDEA. Provides more flexibility for IEP content and meetings. Removed requirements for short-term objectives and benchmarks.

Source: Adapted in part from Hanft, B.E. (1991). Impact of federal policy on pediatric health and education programs. In W. Dunn (Ed.), *Pediatric occupational therapy*. Thorofare, NJ: Slack.

of this text; however, the listing does serve as a starting point for further study and provides information on the history and sequence of federal legislation. Legislation specific to the education of children with disabilities has had a major impact on the provision of physical therapy services and is discussed in more detail in Chapters 10 and 11.

Changing Health-Care Delivery System

During the mid-20th century, many Americans had health insurance to cover hospital care, and, later, coverage for physicians and other out-of-hospital services. Outpatient physical therapy was one of the benefits of this expanded medical coverage. Before major medical coverage was available, outpatient therapy for children was paid for by the family, provided by charitable organizations, or provided under the federally supported Crippled Children's Services. Under the insurance fee-for-service system, the child's family selected their physicians and therapists and services were paid for in part (usually 80%) or totally by the insurance company. Aside from a large lifetime cap, there was

usually no limit on these services, and children with disabilities could receive comprehensive, long-term care. The family could select the physicians and physical therapists of their choice and go to specialists as necessary. Some insurance plans also included durable medical equipment such as wheelchairs.

In the 1950s, a number of small insurance companies began experimenting with what were called health maintenance organizations (HMOs). Groups of physicians and other health professionals provided comprehensive care that included the preventive care not covered under fee-for-service plans. The first such organizations were in Minnesota and California and were nonprofit. They remained relatively small until the 1980s, when there was a vast, nationwide expansion of what are now called managed care organizations. These organizations are now frequently for profit. Children with disabilities are included; however, the majority of families with children with special needs choose, when possible, to remain in the more costly fee-for-service plans that allow access to medical providers experienced in serving children with disabilities. In managed-care systems, approval to go to a specialist must first be obtained from the primary care provider, usually the pediatrician; then the child goes to a specialist who is part of the plan and who may or may not have experience in the care of children with disabilities.

The 1990s saw a dramatic, radical change in the health-care delivery system in the United States. Although we have one of the finest health-care systems in the world, we also have the most expensive. More and more employers found it cost effective to offer their employees only managed-care options, and many states converted to the less costly managed-care system for their citizens receiving Medicaid. These actions resulted in an increasing number of children with disabilities entering service delivery systems that might not allow them to continue with their previous physicians and other specialists skilled in meeting their complex needs.

In 1997, the State Children's Health Insurance Plan (SCHIP) was passed by the United States Congress to expand and initiate state health insurance coverage for uninsured, low-income children. Children whose parents earned too much to qualify for Medicare but could not afford private health insurance became eligible for state-run insurance programs. With 11.8% of all American children uninsured and 20.6% of children covered by Medicare or SCHIP (Maternal and Child Health Bureau, 2002, p. 66), therapists must face the reality that our services are costly, not always supported by outcome studies, and generally not critical to sustaining the life of the child, so reimbursement for services is not guaranteed. We must continue to seek evidence to support our interventions and advocate for the children and families we serve.

Family-Centered Care

One of the major changes in the delivery of physical therapy over the past decade has been the shift in focus from a child-centered to a family-centered approach. This shift has occurred throughout the practice of physical therapy and reflects not only changes in health-care service delivery but also an understanding of the importance of the entire family in the habilitative and rehabilitative processes. The input of families was always valued in pediatrics, but now families are considered partners in the habilitation and rehabilitation processes of a child with a disability. Therapists need to understand family systems, and be sensitive to the unique characteristics and needs of the culturally verse populations they serve. Throughout this text, we have incorporated issues related to family-centered care and understanding cultural diversity. All of Chapter 3 is devoted to these topics because of their importance in practice today.

Child Abuse and Neglect

Unfortunately, we would be remiss if we did not discuss the tragic issues of child abuse and neglect. An estimated 879,000 children were victims of abuse or neglect in 2000 (Maternal and Child Health Bureau, 2002, p. 28). Child abuse is a major cause of neurological trauma in children, and children who have a disability have a significantly increased likelihood of being abused or neglected. They may have difficulty communicating the abuse or neglect to others and may not be able to run away from an abuser. They may also have age-inappropriate dependency, be isolated, need affection and friendship, have a low self-image, and exhibit distressed behavior that could be attributed to their disorder and not to abuse or neglect (Hobbs, Hanks, & Wynn, 1999).

Physical therapists are in a unique position to observe child abuse or neglect first hand (Box 1.2). We frequently remove some of a child's clothing to observe muscle activity and movement, and this provides an opportunity to see the results of abuse such as scars and bruises. The small, round burn scars from being poked with cigarettes leave an all-too-common distinctive mark. When we handle a child, we may also note sensitive areas that have been traumatized. If unexplained burns, scars, or other signs of trauma are observed, we have an obligation to report suspected signs of child abuse to the authorities. The Federal Child Abuse and Prevention and Treatment Act (PL 93-247), and its amendments, requires every state to have a system for reporting suspected child abuse and neglect. The procedures vary from state to state, and therapists should be familiar with the laws in their state. Some states have one central agency and telephone number to contact; other states have the individual report the suspected case to their superior, who determines how the situation will be handled. Although our professional code of conduct says that the therapist/patient relationship is confidential and that information can be given only with written consent, child abuse mandates a breach of confidentiality that is supported by federal law.

Behavior Management

Somewhat unique to pediatric practice is the need to engage and play with the child to gain participation in the desired therapeutic activities and interventions. Infants, young children, and those with severe mental limitations are often unable to follow verbal commands. They must be

BOX 1.2 Common Manifestations of Child Abuse and Neglect

Signs of Abuse

- Impact injuries (bruises, abrasions, lacerations, and scars)
- Burns and scalding
- Fracture and joint injuries
- Head and brain injuries
- Internal injuries

Signs of Neglect

- Malnourishment
- Medical neglect (parental refusal to seek or maintain necessary medical intervention)
- Educational neglect (parental indifference to the child's school attendance or cognitive development)
- Emotional neglect (parental indifference to child's need for physical contact and psychological nurturance)
- Sexual abuse
- Emotional abuse

Source: From Gocha, V.A., Murphy, D.M., Dolakia, K.H., Hess, A.A., and Effgen, S.K. (1999). Child maltreatment: Our responsibility as health care professionals. *Pediatric Physical Therapy, 11*, 134. Copyright 1999 Lippincott Williams & Wilkins, Inc. Reprinted with permission of the author.

encouraged to perform activities using therapeutic play, interesting toys and activities, and significant creativity on the part of the therapist and parents. **Play** is the work of children, and it is the milieu in which intervention occurs for most children. Therapeutic play requires extraordinary work on the part of the therapist, and individuals who lack creativity and the ability to "play" will probably have a difficult time working with children.

Some children may choose not to participate in requested tasks, no matter how creative the therapist. These children might require a structured behavior management plan that not only assists with managing their behavior but also facilitates learning. Learning is believed to occur as a result of the consequences of behavior. **Behavioral programming** emphasizes manipulation of the environment through the use of positive reinforcement of desired behaviors and ignoring unwanted behaviors. **Positive rein-**

forcement might start as a primary reward such as food, then progress to secondary rewards such as toys, favorite activities, or tokens, and then, most important, progress to the nontangible natural rewards of social or natural reinforcers such as verbal praise or a smile. A hug from a parent after taking the first few independent steps encourages many more independent steps. Successfully accessing a computer is reinforcement enough to again perform the task.

Negative reinforcement, which is the removal of an aversive stimulus contingent on the performance of the desired behavior, is generally not an accepted technique in physical therapy. Unfortunately, negative reinforcement is occasionally used, such as when a child is allowed to end a therapy session if they perform a specific task. This is not the most appropriate way to reinforce behaviors. It would be far better to provide a positive reinforcement when the child performs a task than to tie performance with ending the session with the therapist.

Our goal is to increase the probability that the child will perform the desired behavior. To do this, it may first be necessary to use very frequent primary rewards in what is termed a *continuous schedule of reinforcement*. However, as soon as possible, the frequency of rewards should be decreased or "thinned" to an intermittent schedule of reinforcement and secondary rewards should be used until the behavior is naturally occurring without obvious reinforcement. There is an extensive body of literature on behavioral techniques and reinforcement schedules with which therapists should be familiar if they are going to work with children who are not likely to comply with requests or who have behavior disorders (summarized in Alberto & Troutman, 2002).

A behavior can be elicited and then improved and elaborated on by what are called **shaping** or **chaining techniques**. Shaping involves reinforcing behaviors that are increasingly closer to the desired behavior. Chaining links related behaviors to accomplish a more elaborate goal with sequenced elements. Chaining works best with discrete tasks that have a clear beginning and end, such as most activities of daily living, or selected serial tasks that are strung together, such as performing a sliding board transfer. Backward shaping involves teaching and reinforcing behaviors in a step-by-step progression in which the last step is learned first (e.g., performing the task of brushing teeth before learning to put the toothpaste on the brush).

Behavioral techniques should be considered in all areas of physical therapy intervention. Many of the children we serve require considerable time and effort to achieve even the smallest goal. They need to be encouraged and rewarded for their efforts, even if they do not achieve the desired goal. Positive reinforcement will encourage them to keep trying, just as an athlete values the encouragement received from a coach for a good play, even if the team loses the game.

Attaining and Maintaining Clinical Competence

There are numerous competencies a therapist must have to provide state-of-the-art physical therapy intervention to children, as elaborated throughout this text. As the body of knowledge regarding the art and science of pediatric physical therapy expands, it becomes more difficult for the generalist clinician to keep up with all areas of practice. Historically, pediatrics has been an area of specialization in medicine, although pediatrics is now considered general medical practice for children. Medical specialties, such as pediatric neurology and pediatric orthopedics, have become increasingly prominent in children's care. A similar evolution has occurred in physical therapy. Pediatric physical therapy was one of the first areas of physical therapy practice to be recognized by the APTA as a clinical specialty. Pediatric physical therapy is the general area of physical therapy to children, and there is increasing specialization among pediatric physical therapists, for instance, neurological pediatric physical therapy and cardiopulmonary pediatric physical therapy. Some therapists also have special skills and knowledge required to work in specific settings such as early intervention or sports programs.

To provide the most efficient and effective physical therapy to children, a therapist must work toward achieving clinical competence. Merely graduating from an entry-level physical therapy program does not fully prepare a therapist to provide quality care for most children. The recent graduate is prepared to serve some children independently, and others under supervision; however, therapists should develop a plan to achieve the competence necessary for independent practice with children.

There are published competencies and guidelines for therapists to review in their effort to achieve or maintain clinical competence in various areas of pediatric practice, such as neonatal intensive care nursery (Sweeney, Heriza, Reilly, Smith, & VanSant, 1999), early intervention (Chiarello, Effgen, Milbourne, & Campbell, 2003; Effgen, Bjornson, Chiarello, Sinzer, & Phillips, 1991), and school-based practice (APTA, 1990; Chiarello et al., 2003). The guidelines for pediatric clinical specialization also provide an excellent outline of important areas in which a therapist should achieve competence.

There are a number of ways to attain and maintain clinical competence. The most obvious is on-the-job training. Many clinical sites have excellent in-service training and mentoring programs for new staff. Unfortunately, with more children with disabilities appropriately served in community settings, therapists frequently find themselves working in total isolation or with a few professionals from other disciplines who are equally isolated. Therapists need to join or start journal clubs or special interest groups. Meeting and talking with colleagues is one way to gain and share information and recognize one's own limitations. One of the problems with working in isolation is that one can acquire a false sense of confidence because there is no one with expertise available to question the therapist's competence.

Therapists should attend educational programs. Continuing education programs are generally a few days long and centered on a specific topic. For more in-depth learning, therapists should consider postprofessional graduate education. Many universities are attempting to meet the needs of the working clinician by offering courses in the evening, on weekends, or through distance learning. Even if therapists have entry-level master's or entry-level doctoral degrees, they will still need to advance their professional competence in pediatrics. Formal education courses are an excellent way of achieving that goal.

Some states require physical therapists to acquire special certification beyond licensure to demonstrate that they have the skills necessary to work with specific pediatric populations, such as in school settings or early intervention programs. "Because of the structural, physiological, and behavioral vulnerabilities of neonates, pediatric physical therapists need postprofessional precepted training and experience before providing neonatal care" (Sweeney et al., 1999, p. 119).

Employers have begun to recognize that generalist licensure may not be sufficient to ensure competence to serve children with disabilities. Postprofessional degrees in specialty areas and clinical certification are ways of documenting advanced clinical competence. Recognized standards of competence in pediatric practice will become necessary as the supply of physical therapists finally meets the demand.

Summary

Pediatric physical therapy has a rich history since the beginnings of the profession. Pediatric physical therapy was one of the first areas of specialization recognized by the APTA in 1973, and the Section on Pediatrics now has more than 4,000 members. Serving children with disabilities and illnesses and their families is a challenging area of practice that requires diverse skills and knowledge as well as great flexibility and creativity. Therapists must not only be able to examine, evaluate, diagnose, make a prognosis, and provide complex intervention; they must also understand behavior management, developmental theory, family functioning, social trends, reimbursement issues, and the unique requirements of working in environments as diverse as a bone marrow transplant unit and the home of an impoverished inner-city infant born to drug-addicted parents.

The Bobaths have enlightened us to consider the whole child, the family, and the team of professionals when providing intervention. New developments in neuroscience, motor learning, and motor control are providing the scientific foundation for many of our new and old interventions. Recent models of intervention, such as the MOVE Curriculum, Conductive Education, and Task-Oriented Approach, are not technique based but rather are based on the principle that skill acquisition requires therapeutic practice of the skill in the environments where that skill is likely to be used. Although this text is divided on the basis of the major body systems, we must remember that rarely is only one system involved in children with disabilities. Therefore, a thorough understanding of all systems and their interactions is imperative.

DISCUSSION QUESTIONS

1. Why is the ICF model of disability becoming the preferred model?
2. Why might the ICF terminology of impairments in body functions lead to some confusion with the Nagi model terminology of impairments and functional limitations?
3. What are the four elements of good evidence-based practice?
4. Discuss the benefits of naturalistic observation.
5. Discuss the advantages of a transdisciplinary model in meeting the needs of a child with complex problems.
6. Why is collaboration so critical in meeting the needs of children?
7. What signs of child maltreatment should a physical therapist look for?
8. What is your plan for maintaining clinical competence in all areas where your license allows you to practice?

REFERENCES

Alberto, P.A., & Troutman, A.C. (2002). *Applied behavior analysis for teachers* (6th ed.). Englewood Cliffs, NJ: Merrill.

American Academy for Cerebral Palsy and Developmental Medicine (1996). *The history of the American Academy for Cerebral Palsy and Developmental Medicine.* Rosemont, IL: Author.

American Physical Therapy Association (APTA) (1990). *Practice in educational environments.* Alexandria, VA: Author.

American Physical Therapy Association (APTA) (1991). Standards for tests and measurements in physical therapy practice. *Physical Therapy, 71,* 589–622.

American Physical Therapy Association (APTA) (1997). Guide to physical therapist practice. *Physical Therapy, 77,* 1163–1650.

American Physical Therapy Association (APTA) (2001). Guide to physical therapist practice (2nd ed.). *Physical Therapy, 81,* 6–746.

American Psychological Association (APA) & World Health Organization (2003). *International classification of functioning, disability, and health procedural manual and guide for a standardized application of the ICF: A manual for health professionals.* Washington, DC: Author.

Ayres, A.J. (1979). *Sensory integration and the child.* Los Angeles: Western Psychological Services.

Bailey, D.B., & Wolery, M. (1992). *Teaching infants and preschoolers with disabilities* (2nd ed.). New York: Merrill.

Bidabe, L., & Lollar, J. (1990). *M.O.V.E., mobility opportunities via education manual.* Bakersfield, CA: Kern County Superintendent of Schools.

Blatt, B., & Kaplan, F. (1966). *Christmas in purgatory: A photographic essay on mental retardation.* Boston: Allyn & Bacon.

Bleck, E.E. (1975). Locomotor prognosis in cerebral palsy. *Developmental Medicine and Child Neurology, 17,* 18–25.

Bly, L. (1991). A historical and current view of the basis of NDT. *Pediatric Physical Therapy, 3,* 131–135.

Bly, L. (1999). *Baby treatment based on NDT principles.* San Antonio, TX: Therapy Skill Builders.

Bly, L., & Whiteside, A. (1997). *Facilitation techniques based on NDT principles.* San Antonio, TX: Therapy Skill Builders.

Bobath, B. (1971). *Abnormal postural reflex activity caused by brain lesions.* London: William Heinemann Medical Books Limited.

Bobath, B. (1980). The neurophysiological basis for the treatment of cerebral palsy. *Clinics in Developmental Medicine, No. 75.* Philadelphia: J.B. Lippincott.

Bobath, K., & Bobath, B. (1972). Cerebral palsy. In P.H. Pearson & C.E. Williams (Eds.), *Physical therapy services in the developmental disabilities* (pp. 31–185). Springfield, IL: Charles C Thomas.

Braddock, D. (1987). *Federal policy towards mental retardation and developmental disabilities*. Baltimore: Paul H. Brookes.

Campbell, P.H. (1991). Evaluation and assessment in early intervention for infants and toddlers. *Journal of Early Intervention, 15,* 36–45.

Capital Association for Conductive Education. (1997). *Conductive education fact sheet* [Brochure]. Arlington, VA: Author.

Chiarello, L., Effgen, S., Milbourne, S., & Campbell, P. (2003). Specialty certification program in early intervention and school-based therapy. *Pediatric Physical Therapy, 15,* 52–53.

Deming, W.E. (2000). *The new economics: For industry, government, education* (2nd ed.). Cambridge, MA: MIT Press.

Dormans, J.P., & Pellegrino, L. (Eds.). (1998). *Caring for children with cerebral palsy: A team approach.* Baltimore: Paul H. Brookes.

Dunn, W. (1991). Integrated related services. In L.H. Meyer, C.A. Peck, & L. Brown (Eds.), *Critical issues in the lives of persons with severe disabilities* (pp. 353–377). Baltimore: Paul H. Brookes.

Effgen, S.K. (1982). Integration of plantar grasp as an indicator of ambulation potential in developmentally disabled infants. *Physical Therapy, 4,* 433–435.

Effgen, S.K. (1991). Systematic delivery and recording of intervention assistance. *Pediatric Physical Therapy, 3,* 63–68.

Effgen, S.K. (2000a). Occurrence of gross motor behaviors in US preschools and conductive education preschools in Hong Kong [Abstract]. *Pediatric Physical Therapy, 12,* 211.

Effgen, S.K. (2000b). Factors affecting the termination of physical therapy services for children in school settings. *Pediatric Physical Therapy, 12,* 121–126.

Effgen, S.K. (2000c). The educational environment. In S.K. Campbell, D.W. Vander Linden, & R.J. Palisano (Eds.), *Physical therapy for children* (2nd ed.) (p. 920). Philadelphia: W.B. Saunders.

Effgen, S.K., Bjornson, K., Chiarello, L., Sinzer, L., & Phillips, W. (1991). Competencies for physical therapists in early intervention. *Pediatric Physical Therapy, 3,* 77–80.

Effgen, S.K., & Brown, D.A. (1992). Long term stability of hand-held dynamometric measurements in children who have myelomeningocele. *Physical Therapy, 72,* 458–465.

Evidence-based Medical Working Group (1992). Evidence-based medicine: A new approach to teaching the practice of medicine. *Journal of the American Medical Association, 268* (17), 2420–2425.

Federal Register, Part III, Department of Education, 32 CFR Part 303, Early Intervention Program for Infants and Toddlers with Handicaps; Final Regulations, June 22, 1989 (303.17, p. 26313).

Finnie, N.R. (1997). *Handling the young child with cerebral palsy at home* (3rd ed.). Boston: Butterworth-Heinemann.

Fleischman, K.E., Goldman, L., Johnson, P.A., Krasuski, R.A., Bohan, J.S., Hartley, L.H., & Lee, T. (2002). Critical pathways for patients with acute chest pain at low risk. *Journal of Thrombosis and Thrombolysis, 13*(2), 89–96.

Gocha, V.A., Murphy, D.M., Dolakia, K.H., Hess, A.A., & Effgen, S.K. (1999). Child maltreatment: Our responsibility as health care professionals. *Pediatric Physical Therapy, 11,* 133–139.

Gordon, J. (1987). Assumptions underlying physical therapy interventions: Theoretical and historical perspectives. In J.H. Carr & R.B. Shepherd (Eds.), *Movement science: Foundations for physical therapy rehabilitation* (pp. 1–30). Rockville, MD: Aspen Publishers.

Guralnick, M.J. (1997). *The effectiveness of early intervention.* Baltimore: Paul H. Brookes.

Hanft, B.E. (1991). Impact of federal policy on pediatric health and education programs. In W. Dunn (Ed.), *Pediatric occupational therapy* (pp. 273–284). Thorofare, NJ: Slack.

Harris, S.R. (1997). The effectiveness of early intervention for children with cerebral palsy and related motor disabilities. In M.J. Guralnick (Ed.), *The effectiveness of early intervention* (pp. 327–348). Baltimore: Paul H. Brookes.

Hobbs, C.J., Hanks, H.G., & Wynn, J.M. (1999). *Child abuse and neglect: A clinician's handbook.* London: Churchill Livingstone.

Horak, F.B. (1991). Assumptions underlying motor control for neurologic rehabilitation. In M.J. Lister (Ed.), *Contemporary management of motor control problems* (pp. 11–27). Alexandria, VA: Foundation for Physical Therapy.

Howle, J.M. (2002). *Neuro-developmental treatment approach: Theoretical foundations and principles of clinical practice.* Laguna Beach, CA: Neuro-Developmental Treatment Association.

Hunt, P., Soto, G., Maier, J., & Doering, K. (2003). Collaborative teaming to support students at risk and students with severe disabilities in general education classrooms. *Exceptional Children, 69*(3), 315–352.

Iowa Department of Education (2001). *Iowa guidelines for educationally related physical therapy services.* Des Moines: Author.

Kettenbach, G. (2001). *Writing SOAP notes* (3rd ed.). Philadelphia: F.A. Davis.

Knott, M., & Voss, D.E. (1968). *Proprioceptive neuromuscular facilitation: Patterns and techniques* (2nd ed.). New York: Harper & Row.

Kozma, I., & Balogh, E. (1995). A brief introduction to conductive education and its application at an early age. *Infants and Young Children, 8*(1), 68–74.

Law, M. (Ed.) (2002). *Evidence-based rehabilitation: A guide to practice.* Thorofare, NJ: Slack.

Linder, T.W. (1993). *Transdisciplinary play-based assessment: A functional approach to working with young children.* Baltimore: Paul H. Brookes.

Lindsey, D., O'Neal, J., Haas, K., & Tewey, S.M. (1980). Physical therapy services in North Carolina's schools. *Clinical Management in Physical Therapy, 4,* 40–43.

Lister, M.J. (Ed.) (1991). *Contemporary management of motor control problems*. Alexandria, VA: Foundation for Physical Therapy.

Mager, R.F. (1962). *Preparing instructional objectives*. Palo Alto, CA: Fearon Publishers.

Maternal and Child Health Bureau, US Department of Health & Human Services, Health Resources and Services Administration (2002). *Child health USA 2002*. Washington, DC: Author. Retrieved May 28, 2004 from http://www.hrsa.gov/chusa02.

McEwen, I. (Ed.). (2000). *Providing physical therapy services under Parts B & C of the Individuals with Disabilities Education Act (IDEA)*. Alexandria, VA: Section on Pediatrics, American Physical Therapy Association.

McLaughlin, J., & Bjornson, K.F. (1998). Quality of life and developmental disabilities. *Developmental Medicine and Child Neurology, 40*, 435.

Mead, S. (1968). Presidential address. The treatment of cerebral palsy. *Developmental Medicine and Child Neurology, 10*, 423–436.

Montgomery, P.C. (1987). Treatment planning: Establishing behavior objectives. In B.H. Connolly & P.C. Montgomery (Eds.), *Therapeutic exercise in developmental disabilities* (pp. 21–26). Chattanooga, TN: Chattanooga Corporation.

Montgomery, P.C. (1998). Predicting potential for ambulation in children with cerebral palsy. *Pediatric Physical Therapy, 10*(4), 148–155.

Montgomery, P.C., & Connolly, B.H. (Eds.). (2003). *Clinical applications for motor control* (pp. 1–23). Thorofare, NJ: Slack.

Murphy, W. (1995). *Healing the generations: A history of physical therapy and the American Physical Therapy Association*. Lyme, CT: Greenwich Publishing Group.

National Institutes of Health (1993). *Research plan for the National Center for Medical Rehabilitation Research*. NIH Publication No. 93–3509. Bethesda, MD: Author.

Nicholson, D. (2002). Practice guidelines, algorithms, and clinical pathways. In M. Law (Ed.), *Evidence-based rehabilitation: A guide to practice* (pp. 195–219). Thorofare, NJ: Slack.

Olson, L.J. (1999). Psychosocial frame of reference. In P. Kramer & J. Hinojosa (Eds.), *Frames of reference for pediatric occupational therapy* (2nd ed.) (pp. 323–375). Philadelphia: Lippincott Williams & Wilkins.

O'Shea, R.K. (2000). Conductive education in conjunction with inclusive education: Teaming physical and occupational therapists and conductors [Abstract]. *Pediatric Physical Therapy, 12*, 221.

Ott, D.A.D., & Effgen, S.K. (2000). Occurrence of gross motor behaviors in integrated and segregated preschool classrooms. *Pediatric Physical Therapy, 12*, 164–172.

Palisano, R.J., Campbell, S.K., & Harris, S.R. (2000). Decision making in pediatric physical therapy. In S.K. Campbell, D.W. Vander Linden, & R.J. Palisano (Eds.), *Physical therapy for children* (2nd ed.) (p. 204). Philadelphia: W.B. Saunders.

Prieto, G.M. (1992). Effects of physical therapist instruction on the frequency and performance of teacher assisted gross motor activities for students with motor disabilities. Unpublished master's thesis, MCP Hahnemann University, Philadelphia.

Rainforth, B. (1997). Analysis of physical therapy practice acts: Implication for role release in educational environments. *Pediatric Physical Therapy, 9*, 54–61.

Rainforth, B., & York-Barr, J. (1997). *Collaborative teams for students with severe disabilities: Integrating therapy and educational services* (2nd ed.) Baltimore: Paul H. Brookes.

Reddihough, D.S., King, J., Coleman, G., & Catanese T. (1998). Efficacy of programmes based on conductive education for young children with cerebral palsy. *Developmental Medicine and Child Neurology, 40*(11), 763–770.

Richardson, P.K. (2001). Use of standardized tests in pediatric practice. In J. Case-Smith (Ed.), *Occupational therapy for children* (4th ed.) (pp. 217–245). St. Louis: Mosby.

Richardson, P.K., & Schultz-Krohn, W. (2001). Planning and implementing services. In J. Case-Smith (Ed.), *Occupational therapy for children* (4th ed.) (pp. 246–264). St. Louis: Mosby.

Sackett, D., Rosenberg, W., Gray, J.A.M., Haynes, R.B., & Richardson, W.S. (1996). Evidence-based medicine: What it is and what it isn't. *British Medical Journal, 312*, 71–72.

Seamans, S. (1967). The Bobath concept on treatment of neurological disorders. In *Proceedings: An exploratory and analytical survey of therapeutic exercise* (pp. 732–788). Baltimore: Williams & Wilkins.

Soccio, C. (1991). Direct-individual versus integrated-group models of physical therapy service delivery. Unpublished master's thesis, MCP Hahnemann University, Philadelphia.

Spivack, F. (1995). Conductive education perspectives. *Infants and Young Children, 8*(1), 75–85.

Stockmeyer, S.A. (1967). An interpretation of the approach of Rood to the treatment of neuromuscular dysfunction. In *Proceedings: An exploratory and analytical survey of therapeutic exercise* (pp. 900–961). Baltimore: Williams & Wilkins.

Sweeney, J.K., Heriza, C.B., Reilly, M.A., Smith, C., & VanSant, A.F. (1999). Practice guidelines for the physical therapist in the neonatal intensive care unit. *Pediatric Physical Therapy, 11*(3), 119–132.

Thomson-O'Brien, M.A., & Moreland, J. (1998). Evidence-based practice information circle. *Physiotherapy Canada, 50*(3), 184–189.

Voss, D.E., Ionta, M.K., & Myers, B.J. (1985). *Proprioceptive neuromuscular facilitation: Patterns and techniques* (3rd ed.). New York: Harper & Row.

World Health Organization (1980). *International classification of impairments, disabilities and handicaps*. Geneva: Author.

World Health Organization (2001). *International classification of functioning, disability and health*. Geneva: Author.

Chapter *2*

Child Development and Appraisal

— Susan K. Effgen, PT, PhD

The development of a child is a fascinating and complex process of the interaction of inborn biology coupled with vast environmental influences and experiences. Philosophers and others have spent centuries debating the influence of nature versus nurture on the development of children. Theories of child development abound and numerous books have been written on the topic. The reader is urged to seek more in-depth information than is briefly summarized in this chapter. This chapter reviews theories of child development that have had the greatest impact on pediatric physical therapy. This is followed by an overview of the development of functional movement from birth through adolescence.

Physical therapists must understand child development in order to provide appropriate examination, evaluation, diagnosis, prognosis, and intervention. The examination and evaluation processes are complex, especially with children, because almost everything must usually be disguised as "play." Many of the tests and measurements used in examinations are specific to a body system and are presented in chapters on each system in this book. Tests and measures of neuromotor development, sensory integration, function, and quality of life are not system dependent and are reviewed in this chapter.

Theories of Child Development

There are numerous theories regarding child development. Theories, by definition, are hypotheses or conjectures to explain phenomena. Therefore, they change and evolve as new information becomes available. Theories of importance to physical therapists are reviewed briefly, since space limits more comprehensive and in-depth presentation. The theories presented are not mutually exclusive and they share different degrees of empirical support (Table 2.1).

Maturational View

The **maturational view** uses the framework of maturation of the central nervous system (CNS) as the foundation for development across all domains. Development was believed to occur in specific, invariant sequences. Shirley (1931), Gesell (1928, 1945, 1952), and McGraw (1932, 1935, 1945) carefully observed child behavior and recorded specific sequences and periods of motor skill development. They attempted to link the development of

Table 2.1 Child Development Theories

Theory	Basic Concepts	Proponents
Maturational	• Development follows a set, invariant sequence • Development is tightly tied to CNS development • Motor development is cephalocaudal and proximal to distal • Recent modifications acknowledge variations in the sequence and input from all systems	Gesell, McGraw, Bayley, Fiorentino, Bobath, Bly
Cognitive	• Thinking develops in stages of increasing complexity • Children organize mental schemes through the use of mental operations	Piaget, Montessori
Behavioral	• Behavior is shaped by the environment • The stimulus, response, and environmental consequence constitutes a contingency of behavior • Consequences of behavior influence future occurrences of the behavior	Skinner, Bandura
Psychodynamic/ psychoanalytic	• There are biologically determined drives and unconscious conflicts • The core of the conflicts is sexual • Initial drives are for survival; once basic needs are met, we seek self-actualization	Freud, Erickson, Maslow
Ecological, contextual	• The environment has a very strong influence on child development	Bronfenbrenner, Harris
Dynamic systems	• Movement emerges based on the internal milieu, the external environment, and task • Movement is not directed by one system, but many dynamic, interacting systems	Bernstein, Kelso, Thelen, Heriza, Shumway-Cook, Horak

motor behaviors with development of the CNS. Believing in a strict hierarchical system of control, they correlated the integration of reflexes and reactions with the time of myelinization of areas of the CNS. Pediatric physical therapy has been heavily influenced by the maturational viewpoint.

From the 1920s to 1950s, Gesell worked at the Yale Clinic of Child Development. As a physician, he understood neurological, anatomical, and physiological development. This understanding guided his observations and assumptions about the "role of maturation in the pattern of behavior" (Gesell & Thompson, 1934, p. 292). His description of behavior trends and many of his basic tenets have served as the foundation for pediatric physical therapy for the past 50 years. The tenets purport that development occurs in a cephalocaudal direction; development also occurs in a proximal-to-distal direction; development of

one motor skill leads to the development of another, more complex motor skill; motor milestones are invariant in their sequence; motor skills develop from gross to fine; and motor control progresses from reflexive to voluntary movement (Gesell, 1945; Scalise-Smith & Bailey, 1992, pp. 408–409).

In Gesell's later work, these tenets are no longer outlined, and he suggests that development occurs in successive epochs with variations that provide a spiral character to the progressions of development (1952, p. 66). The concept of spiral patterns has been further elaborated, and now it is recognized that the developmental sequence is *not* invariant and that his original tenets of development are *not* universal.

During this same period, McGraw (1935) engaged in an intensive, longitudinal study of the development of twins at Columbia University. She, like Gesell, used a new technology, cinematography, to record the development of movement, allowing greater analysis than in the past. She was not as concerned as Gesell with the timing of the achievement of specific skills, but with the sequence and patterns from which they developed. Her classic text, *The Neuromuscular Maturation of the Human Infant* (1945), is still a relevant source of information on the common sequential development of motor behaviors. The works of Gesell and McGraw were the foundation for many of the early neurophysiological or developmental physical therapy intervention approaches, such as those developed by Berta Bobath and Margaret Rood.

The maturational view supported a sequential pattern of development, and therefore a number of developmental scales were produced to assess infant development. Nancy Bayley (1936), who also performed longitudinal studies of infant mental and motor behaviors, published the *Bayley Scales of Infant Development*, now in its second edition (1993). This standardized test is still widely used in early intervention (Fewell & Glick, 1996). Gesell, in 1949, also published infant scales of motor, adaptive, language, and personal-social development. These comprehensive scales serve as the foundation for many of today's developmental tests.

Maturational concepts were expanded by an occupational therapist, Mary Fiorentino, who studied the stages of normal and abnormal development in relationship to reflex/responses and movement (Fiorentino, 1963, 1981). She believed that "our total postural behavior is the result of interaction of reflexes and the relative strength of each one of them" (Fiorentino, 1981, p. ix). Her reflex testing methods were standard procedures in pediatric physical and occupational therapy until the 1980s, when the functional and clinical significance of reflexes were seriously questioned and greater understanding of CNS development displaced the hierarchical view of the nervous system (see Chapter 6).

Recently, Lois Bly (1994) provided a comprehensive and balanced view of motor skill acquisition and the kinesiological aspects of motor development during the first year of life. She presented a sequential maturational perspective while acknowledging that a "global perspective in which maturation, environment, behavior, biomechanics, kinesiology, perception, learning, and goal direction are considered to be important" (1994, p. xii) in the developmental process. The research of Adolph and colleagues (Adolph, Vereijken, & Denny, 1998) now clearly indicates that the sequence of infant motor skill acquisition is indeed quite variable, with many infants skipping stages previously thought to be mandatory for achievement of independent walking.

Cognitive View

The **cognitive view** refers to the development of "age-appropriate mental functions, especially in perceiving, understanding, and knowing, that is, becoming capable of doing intellectual tasks" (Bowe, 1995, p. 552). As the maturational theories were developing in America, a number of Europeans were studying child development from a cognitive perspective. Piaget (1952), a Swiss psychologist, was interested in the genesis and theory of knowledge (genetic epistemology). He highlighted the importance of the child's active involvement in the environment, and not merely neurological maturation, as critical to the infant's development. Piaget's ideas have changed our understanding of human thinking and problem solving. He believed that thinking developed in stages of increasing complexity. In order to adapt, children must go through the processes of assimilation, accommodation, and equilibration. Patterns of thoughts, actions, and problem solving are referred to as schemas that assist a child in dealing with a challenge or situation. His observations of what he called the sensorimotor period of infant development were important in providing the rationale for some pediatric interventions. Piagetian principles and later variations that are compatible with learning theories are used throughout early childhood education today (Case, 1992).

In the early 1900s, Maria Montessori, an Italian physician, used cognitive and developmental theory to develop a revolutionary teaching strategy, first for children with mental retardation and later for all young children. In the Montessori approach (Montessori, 1964), a child is given freedom to interact independently with the environment and to choose activities from carefully developed materials. "Sensorial education" was encouraged, involving tasks that required both intelligence and movement. This encouragement of both mental and motor development was important for children with physical disabilities who have limited motoric options. Teachers act as facilitators of learning and not directors. This approach to early childhood education is still popular, although some believe it neglects the child's social development (Chattin-McNichols, 1992).

A new approach to early childhood learning is the Reggio Emilia Approach. This approach was developed over the past 40 years in the northern Italian city of Reggio Emilia, led by Loris Malaguzzi. The child is viewed as competent, capable, curious, creative, and full of potential. The child is encouraged to learn by investigating and exploring things of interest in a carefully prepared, stimulating environment. Development of problem-solving skills is critical as the child learns to predict and reflect. Parent participation is embraced, and the approach provides a supportive environment in which to learn. There is full inclusion of "children with special rights," and therapists work with the child within the school environment. Few, if any, sessions are one-to-one, and therapists instruct teachers on how to integrate therapy into daily classroom activities (Palsha, 2002). This approach is gaining in popularity in the United States as preschool educators and others learn more about this child-centered approach (Edwards, Gandini, & Forman, 1993).

Behavioral/Learning View

Almost simultaneous to the development of the previous theories, another group of individuals was studying human behavior from a very different perspective. In the early 1900s, Pavlov, a Russian physiologist, recognized the relationship between stimulus and responses in dogs and developed an understanding of what is called *classical conditioning*. B.F. Skinner (1953), an American psychologist, advanced the concept of *operant conditioning*. He studied the effects of the stimulus, response, and consequences in both animals and humans, and showed that environmental manipulation and reinforcement can condition some behaviors. This research provided a greater understanding of the importance of consequences of behaviors and the impact of consequences on recurrence of behavior.

The **behavioral view** assumes that behavior results from an interaction of genetic and environmental events and that most behaviors are learned responses. A behaviorist asserts that positively reinforced behaviors will occur with greater frequency than if the consequence of a behavior is punishment, because then there is decreased probability the behavior will reoccur. The primary concepts of the behavioral view, now commonly referred to as **applied behavior analysis**, include positive reinforcement, extinction (planned ignoring), negative reinforcement (the avoidance of an unpleasant event that increases the likelihood of the behavior), and punishment. Both positive and negative reinforcement are frequently used in therapy. We reward a child with praise, hugs, and perhaps stickers, toys, or food to reinforce positive behaviors. We also, unintentionally, use negative reinforcement when we allow a therapy session to end when a child is crying or uncooperative. By "giving in" to the child's behavior, we have reinforced this negative behavior and it is likely to occur again when the child wants to avoid an unpleasant situation.

Therapists also use Skinner's concept of shaping. In **shaping**, successive approximations of the desired behavior are reinforced until the individual can perform the desired behavior. This is a very useful methodology when working with young children learning new behaviors (Bailey & Wolery, 1992; Bowe, 1995, p. 3), and in constraint-induced movement therapy to advance the function of the impaired arm in adults and children having hemiplegia (Taub, Uswatte, & Pidikiti, 1999).

More recently, Bandura went beyond strict behaviorism to note that behaviors also cause changes in the environment. Reciprocal determinism reflects the premise that environment, behavior, and psychological processes interact to form personality. All learning need not be through reinforcement; we also learn by observation and modeling. This interest in processes also places Bandura with the cognitivists, and his theory is called the *social cognitive theory* (Bandura, 2002).

The behavioral view, applied behavior analysis, is used in education and rehabilitation. Target behaviors that need to be increased or decreased are carefully identified and described in measurable terms. Using the environmental manipulation of providing rewards or, in very selected, carefully controlled situations, punishment, has been successful with young children (Bailey & Wolery, 1992) and with individuals who have severe brain damage, serious behavior disorders, or other disabilities (Alberto & Troutman, 2002).

Psychoanalytical/Psychosocial View

Freud developed **psychoanalytic theories** regarding sexual development and the natural state of relationships between individuals of the opposite sex. He believed in biologically determined drives and unconscious conflicts, the core of which was sexual. Erickson expanded Freud's psychoanalytic theory with its emphasis on psychosexual stages into a theory based on psychosocial stages of emerging personality and development throughout the life span. Erickson believed changes are influenced by interrelated forces more than unconscious drives, including (1) the individual's biological and physical strengths and limitations, (2) the individual's life circumstances and history, and (3) the social, cultural, and historical forces during one's lifetime (Seifert & Hoffnung, 1997, p. 34). As with maturational and cognitive theories, psychoanalytic/psychosocial views share the concept of successive stages of development.

Maslow developed what is considered a humanistic hierarchical, not stage-dependent, theory of development. He believed that initial drives were for physiological survival and safety, followed by the need for love, affection, and esteem that culminated in self-actualization. He believed we are motivated not only by "deficiency drives" but also by the drive toward self-actualization. Self-actualization occurs through successful coping with problems in everyday life (Fidler & Fidler, 1978). Understanding a child's position in Maslow's scheme can help a therapist in understanding how to relate to a child. Highlighting an adolescent's dependence will not help develop self-esteem, and a child seeking safety, love, and affection might not appreciate opportunities for independence.

Developmental Task Concept

The developmental task concept mediates two opposing theories according to Havighurst (1972). The *theory of freedom*, in which the child will develop best if left free to develop, opposes the theory of constraint, in which the child learns to become responsible through the restraints imposed by society. The *developmental task concept* "assumes an active learner interacting within an active social environment" (Havighurst, 1972, p. vi). "A developmental task is a task which arises at or about a certain period in the life of an individual, successful achievement of which leads to his happiness and to success with later tasks, while failure leads to unhappiness in the individual, disapproval by society, and difficulty with later tasks" (Havighurst, 1972, p. 2). Developmental tasks have biological, psychological, and sociological bases. Havighurst's developmental tasks, based on a compilation of the work of others, are listed in Box 2.1.

Ecological, Contextual Views

The **ecological theory**, proposed by Bronfenbrenner (1995), includes a strong environmental view of child development. He proposes that the child is influenced by five interactive and overlapping ecological systems. As depicted in Figure 2–1, the *microsystem* is the setting in which the child lives. It is the physical and social situations with the family and peer group that directly affect the child. The *mesosystem* involves connections among the child's microsystems that influence the child because of the relationships, such as the relations of family experiences to school experiences and of family experiences to peer experiences. The *exosystem* involves the settings or situations that

---

BOX 2.1 Havighurst's Developmental Tasks

Tasks of Infancy and Childhood

1. Learning to walk.
2. Learning to take solid food.
3. Learning to talk.
4. Learning to control the elimination of body wastes.
5. Learning sex differences and sexual modesty.
6. Forming simple concepts and learning language to describe social and physical reality.
7. Getting ready to read.
8. Learning to distinguish right and wrong and beginning to develop a conscience.

Tasks of Middle Childhood

1. Learning physical skills necessary for ordinary games.
2. Building wholesome attitudes toward oneself as a growing organism.
3. Learning to get along with age-mates.
4. Learning an appropriate masculine or feminine social role.
5. Developing fundamental skills in reading, writing, and calculating.
6. Developing concepts necessary for everyday living.
7. Developing a conscience, morality, and a scale of values.
8. Achieving personal independence.
9. Developing attitudes toward social groups and institutions.

Tasks of Adolescence

1. Achieving new and more mature relations with age-mates of both sexes.
2. Achieving a masculine or feminine social role.
3. Accepting one's physique and using the body effectively.
4. Achieving emotional independence of parents and other adults.
5. Preparing for marriage and family life.
6. Preparing for an economic career.
7. Acquiring a set of values and an ethical system to guide behavior-developing ideology.
8. Desiring and achieving socially responsible behavior.

Source: From Havighurst, R.J. (1972). *Developmental tasks and education* (3rd ed.). New York: David McKay.

influence the child but in which the child does not necessarily have an active role. This might include the government's influence on the school system and, therefore, the child's education. The values, briefs, and policies of society and culture form the *macrosystem*. The *chronosystem* involves environmental events and transitions during life and sociohistorical conditions (Santrock, 1998, p. 50). Bronfenbrenner (1995) has recently added biological influences to his theory, although the ecological and environmental contexts still dominate. His theory has gained wide acceptance in both family therapy and special education, providing support for an ecological approach to family-centered intervention.

Harris (1998) elucidated the strong influence of the peer group over the parents and biology. This theory has recently caused some controversy, although it is not a new concept. Havighurst noted, "The most potent single influence during the adolescent years is the power of group approval.

The youth becomes a slave to the conventions of his age group" (1972, p. 45). The importance, and hopefully positive influence, of a peer group is one of the reasons for encouraging inclusive education of children with disabilities.

Dynamic Systems Theory

The **dynamic systems theory** is a theory of motor development across the life span and has replaced the maturational view as the theoretical framework for much of pediatric physical therapy. This is not one cohesive theory developed by an individual but rather reflects the work of many individuals (Buchanan & Horak, 2001; Heriza, 1991; Horak, 1991; Kelso & Tuller, 1984; Shumway-Cook & Woolacott, 2001; Thelen, Kelso, & Fogel, 1987; Thelen & Smith, 1994). The theory has its roots in the work of Nicolai

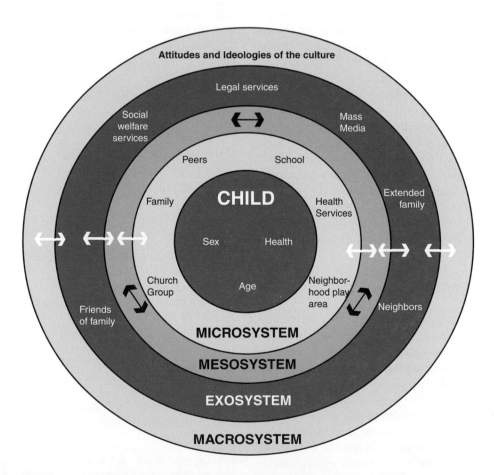

Figure 2–1 Bronfenbrenner's ecological system. (Adapted from Bronfenbrenner, U. (1979). *The ecology of human development.* Cambridge, MA: Harvard University Press.)

Bernstein, a Russian physiologist (1967). Various terms have been used, frequently interchangeably, to describe this theory, including systems, dynamic, dynamic action, task-oriented theory, systems approach (Shumway-Cook & Woolacott, 2001), and developmental biodynamics (Santrock, 1998, p. 153).

The dynamic systems theory assumes that the individual functions as a complex, dynamic system comprising many subsystems and that there is an innate organization that occurs between complex particles that is directed by no one system. Movement emerges based on the child's internal milieu, the external environment, and the motor task to be completed. The concepts about change in motor behaviors associated with development are derived from principles of nonlinear change that describe many biological and physical systems (Scholz, 1990). Universal milestones, such as crawling and walking, are learned through a process of adaptation, and movement patterns are modulated to fit a new task by exploring possible options. This and other current theories of motor development and motor learning are discussed more extensively in Chapters 6 and 7, because they now play a major role in determining our intervention strategies for children with neurological disabilities.

Influences on Child Development

Genetic Influences

At conception, the union of the mother's ovum and father's sperm starts an amazing and complex process of development that is beyond the scope of this text. The ovum and sperm each contain 23 chromosomes consisting of deoxyribonucleic acid (DNA). DNA is a combination of the nucleotide bases cytosine, thymine, adenine, and guanine that form a double-helix structure. These bases of DNA are organized into hundreds to thousands of units termed **genes**. Genes are encoded with the genetic code that determines our physical appearance and biochemical makeup. There are between 50,000 and 100,000 genes that code the proteins of our body. An error or a mutation in the production or translation of the genetic code may result in a genetic disorder.

There is a range of possible genetic disorders resulting from the addition or deletion of an entire chromosome or even the microdeletion of a gene within a chromosome. The clinical manifestations range from very severe limita-tions in function and activities, most commonly seen in the larger defects of an addition or a deletion of a chromosome, to relatively minor impairment in body structure seen in single-gene disorders. Chromosome disorders include **numerical** and **structural abnormalities**. In numerical abnormalities there is an additional chromosome (trisomy), where the individual has 47 chromosomes, or a deletion (monosomy), where there are 45 chromosomes. This is usually due to an error during early cell division, specifically a meiotic error during gametogenesis, and is not hereditary (Sanger, Dave, & Stuberg, 2001). The most common form of Down syndrome is a trisomy of the 21st chromosome. This trisomy, which causes mental retardation and other impairments, is discussed in Chapter 20. Other trisomies include Klinefelter syndrome (47XXY), a syndrome in which the male produces inadequate testosterone and has impairments in developing secondary male sexual characteristics, and trisomy 13 and 18, which are both rare with significant limitation in activities and participation, secondary to profound mental retardation and impaired body function and structure. Monosomy, or deletion of a chromosome, is usually not consistent with life, except for Turner syndrome (45X). This syndrome affects girls, who will have a short stature and webbed neck; 20% have obstruction of the left side of the heart. They usually have normal IQ scores but may have visual-perceptual impairments (Batshaw, 2002).

Structural abnormalities involve the deletion, translocation, inversion, or other rearrangement of chromosomes. In **deletions**, a portion of a chromosome is missing. In Cri-du-chat syndrome, a portion of the short arm of chromosome 5 is missing. The child will have microcephaly (small head size), an unusual facial appearance, and a high-pitched characteristic cry. **Translocations** involve a transfer of a portion of one chromosome to another. A form of Down syndrome that involves a partial trisomy of the 21st chromosome, it is caused by a translocation. Other rare rearrangements of chromosomes include inversions, when a chromosome breaks in two places and then reattaches in the reverse order, or a ring chromosome, when deletions occur at both tips of a chromosome and the ends stick together, forming a ring.

These numerical and structural abnormalities can have major consequences for a child's development. Approximately 0.7% of all babies are born with multiple malformations commonly due to genetic disorders (Jones, 1997, p. 1). In Table 2.2, there is a concise overview of genetic disorders commonly encountered by physical therapists. Several of these disorders are presented in more detail throughout the text.

Table 2.2 Common Genetic Disorders

Disorder	Etiology	Body Function and Structure Impairments	Potential Limitations in Activities and Participation Restrictions
Chromosomal Abnormalities			
Angelman syndrome	Partial deletion of chromosome 15q11q13 (maternal source)	Severe cognitive impairment, microcephaly, seizures, ataxic gait, and frequent laughter not associated with happiness.	Severe limitations in most activities of daily living (ADLs) and mobility, requires assistance throughout life.
Cri-du-chat syndrome	Partial deletion of short arm of fifth chromosome	Severe cognitive impairment, microcephaly, abnormal laryngeal development leads to characteristic high-pitched cry.	Severe limitations in most ADLs, requires assistance throughout life.
Klinefelter syndrome (47XXY)	Sex chromosome abnormality in males	Hypogonadism, long limbs, and slim stature; might have behavioral or psychiatric problems.	Poorly organized motor function, but ambulatory. Slight delay in language might mildly affect some activities, unless other limitations due to behavior.
Prader-Willi syndrome	Partial deletion of chromosome 15q11q13 (paternal source)	Mild cognitive impairment, hypotonia in infancy, short stature, and obesity.	Some activities might be limited depending on the degree of cognitive impairment and obesity.
Trisomy 13	Autosomal trisomy of 13th chromosome	Severe central nervous system abnormalities.	Severe limitations in most ADLs and mobility, requires assistance throughout life. Only 10% survive the first year of life.
Trisomy 18 (Edward's syndrome)	Autosomal trisomy of 18th chromosome	Severe cognitive impairment, most have significant cardiovascular, skeletal, urogenital, and gastrointestinal anomalies.	Severe limitations requiring extensive assistance. Frequently die during first year of life.
Trisomy 21 (Down syndrome)	Autosomal trisomy of 21st chromosome (95%), others due to translocation or mosaicism	Hypotonia, hyperflexibility, flat facial features, upslanted palpebral fissures, pelvic hypoplasia with shallow acetabular angle, single midpalmar crease (Simian crease), cognitive impairment, and frequent cardiac anomalies.	Delay in achieving most gross and fine motor skills and language. Will learn most ADLs, attend school with special education and related services; as young adult may work and live outside of home with supports.
Turner syndrome (45XO)	Sex chromosome abnormality in females	Weblike appearance of the lateral neck, small stature, transient congenital lymphedema, gonadal underdevelopment, hearing impairment, bone trabecular abnormalities, and perhaps visuoperceptual limitations.	Short stature might restrict some activities, otherwise few limitations.
Single-Gene Abnormalities			
Achondroplasia	Autosomal dominant	Disturbance of endochondral ossification at epiphyseal plate, resulting in short stature; bilateral shortness of humerus and femur; macrocephaly; may have spinal complications.	Gait deviations may cause reduced efficiency in activities. Short stature might require accommodations for some activities.

Disorder	Etiology	Body Function and Structure Impairments	Potential Limitations in Activities and Participation Restrictions
Cystic fibrosis (CF)	Autosomal recessive	Disorder of exocrine glands leading to pancreatic insufficiency, hyperplasia of mucus-producing cells in the lungs, excessive electrolyte secretion of sweat glands.	Endurance may be limited due to pulmonary involvement, but may participate in sports. Frequent need for removal of secretions from airways may limit time available for some activities. With advances in intervention, many live into adulthood.
Duchenne muscular dystrophy (MD)	X-linked (males)	Intrinsic muscle disease, creatine kinase elevated and dystrophin absent. Leads to progressive intrinsic muscle weakness commonly observed by 3 years of age, weakness from proximal to distal muscles.	Might have delay in early motor milestones. Then progressive loss of motor abilities during childhood leading to wheelchair use and further limitations in activities. Death in early adulthood.
Fragile X syndrome	X-linked, fragile site at Xq27	Hypotonia, moderate to borderline cognitive impairment, delayed motor milestones, and emotional lability.	Limitations depend on degree of cognitive impairment, but generally few restrictions in activities and participation related to motor skills.
Hemophilia	X-linked	Factor VIII (hemophilia A) or factor IX (hemophilia B) deficiency resulting in impaired blood clotting capability, can lead to reduced range of motion and muscle strength in joints into which bleeding occurs, especially the knee, ankle, and elbow.	Limitations of joint motion and pain can limit some activities, but are ambulatory and can perform ADLs. Contact sports are restricted. Intracranial hemorrhage can lead to death.
Hurler syndrome Mucopolysaccharidosis I Mucopolysaccharidosis II	Autosomal recessive X-linked recessive	Inborn error of metabolism resulting in abnormal storage of mucopolysaccharides in tissues; large skull with frontal bossing, heavy eyebrows, edematous eyelids, small upturned nose with flat nasal bridge, dwarfism, and usually cognitive impairment. Orthopedic deformities include flexion contractures, thoracolumbar kyphosis, genu valgum, hip dislocation, and claw hands.	Progressive loss of motor abilities during childhood leading to wheelchair use and further limitations in activities. Deterioration leads to death before adulthood.
Lesch-Nyhan syndrome	X-linked recessive	Excessive production of uric acid with serious damage to brain and liver. Choreoathetosis, spasticity, growth deficiency, autistic behaviors, and impaired cognitive functioning. Tendency to self-mutilate.	Serious limitations in all activities and participation including ambulation and ADLs.
Neurofibromatosis	Autosomal dominant, gene located in chromosome 17	Wide variance in expression, tumors may cause multiple system involvement, frequently in the central nervous system and skeletal system.	As tumors grow and affect more systems, there are increased limitations in activities and participation.

(Continued)

Table 2.2 **Common Genetic Disorders** (Continued)

Disorder	Etiology	Body Function and Structure Impairments	Potential Limitations in Activities and Participation Restrictions
Osteogenesis imperfecta (OI)	Autosomal dominant (types I and II) Autosomal recessive (types III and IV)	Problem with collagen development. Multiple fractures commonly of long bones, usually between 2 and 3 years and 10 and 15 years. Kyphosis and scoliosis. Hearing loss in young adults with type I and children with type III. Wide variability in expression.	Extent of fractures and secondary complications determine limitations in activities. Most all are ambulatory. Restrictions in sports, especially contact sports. Short stature might require accommodations for some activities.
Phenylketonuria (PKU)	Autosomal recessive	Absence of phenylalanine hydroxylase prevents conversion of phenylalanine to tyrosine, causing abnormal accumulation of phenylalanine. If untreated, leads to cognitive impairment, seizures, and autistic behaviors.	PKU can successfully be treated if detected at birth with no limitations. If untreated, serious limitations in most activities, although should be ambulatory.
Rett syndrome	X-linked dominant, gene *MECP2* (lethal in males)	Hypotonia and ataxia. Characteristic trunk rocking and stereotyped, repetitive hand wringing, tapping, or mouthing. Serious cognitive impairment.	Serious limitations in all activities and participation, although some girls can ambulate.
Spinal muscular atrophy (SMA)	Autosomal recessive	Anterior horn cell degeneration and flaccid paralysis: SMA 1 (Werdnig-Hoffmann disease) seen at birth. Proximal, symmetrical weakness, respiratory and feeding problems. SMA 2 (chronic Werdnig-Hoffmann disease), similar pattern as SMA 1 but slower progression, feeding not a problem. SMA 3 (Kugelberg-Welander disease) mild, progressive weakness of proximal muscles.	SMA 1: Severely limited motor development affecting all activities. Power mobility helps in participation. Rarely survive beyond 3 years. SMA 2: Not as severe as SMA 1, may learn to walk with assistance and do many ADLs. Computer keyboard use better than pencil use. SMA 3: Mild limitations in activities.
Tuberous sclerosis	Autosomal dominant, gene located on chromosome 9q34 or 16p13	Brain lesions consist of tubers, depigmented white birthmarks, and café-au-lait spots on skin. Usually develop seizures and may have cognitive impairment. Wide variability in expression.	Limitations in activities depend on control of seizures and degree of cognitive impairment.

Source: References include Behrman, Kliegman, & Arvin (1996); Jones (1997); Long & Toscano (2002).

The critical importance of genetic influences on our development is manifested in disorders that are inherited. In **autosomal dominant inheritance**, one parent provides the mutant gene and there is a 50% risk of the offspring inheriting the disorder. The abnormal gene overcomes the normal gene inherited by the other parent. There are thousands of autosomal dominant disorders; a common example is achondroplasia (short stature). In **autosomal recessive** **inheritance**, both parents carry the abnormal gene and the child must inherit the abnormal gene from both the mother and father to manifest the disorder. The parents will not have the disorder and usually there is no family history of the disorder, but there is a 25% chance that their child will inherit the autosomal recessive trait (McKusick, 1994). Cystic fibrosis, a disorder of the exocrine glands (see Chapters 8 and 19), is a common autosomal recessive disorder. The X-linked, or sex-linked, recessive disorders involve mutant genes located in the X (female) chromosome, generally affecting male offspring. Because males have only one X chromosome, the single dose of the abnormal recessive gene will cause the disease, such as hemophilia, Duchenne muscular dystrophy, and fragile X syndrome (see Table 2.2). In females with two X chromosomes, the single recessive gene should not cause the disease, although they may manifest the disease through a phenomenon termed *lyonization*, or unequal inactivation of the X chromosomes. **Multifactorial inheritance** is a result of the interaction of heredity and the environment. Therefore, environmental factors can influence the expression of genes. Multifactorial inheritance is thought to be responsible for some forms of diabetes, myelomeningocele (a neural tube defect), and cleft lip and palate.

A limited number of genetic disorders are due to alterations of small mitochondrial DNA fragments. Only the female's ova contain cytoplasm; therefore, all mitochondria are inherited from the mother. As a result, mitochondrial disorders are passed from unaffected mothers to all her children.

Mendelian genetics suggested that the appearance of a child would be the same whether a gene was inherited from the father or mother; however, genomic imprinting indicates that conditions will present differently depending on whether the trait is inherited from the mother or father. An example is a deletion of the long arm of chromosome 15. If it is inherited from the father, the child will have Prader-Willi syndrome (see Table 2.2). If it is inherited from the mother, the child will have Angelman syndrome, a much more serious disability affecting behavior and intelligence (Batshaw, 2002, p. 22). Another new aspect of genetic theory is termed *anticipation,* in which certain abnormalities will become more severe from generation to generation. The principles of Mendelian genetics have had to evolve to accommodate this new information.

Significant advances, which some call an explosion (Schaefer, 2001), are being made in understanding our genetic code though the Human Genome Project. Because therapists play a significant role in the examination, evaluation, diagnosis, and intervention of children with genetic diseases, they must work closely with genetic professionals (Sanger, Davc, & Stuberg, 2001). The rapid development of genetic information requires that therapists have access to accurate information. Information on the specific characteristics and traits coded on each gene are now available online (Online Mendelian Inheritance in Man, 2004).

The exponential increase in genetic knowledge can be overwhelming and is a major area of study and concern for the 21st century. A pressing issue now is how to handle the ethical, legal, and social issues of genetic information. The issues facing any health professional include, but are not limited to, genetic susceptibility, potential for genetic discrimination, access to information, and confidentiality. While the future holds great promise through genetic diagnosis and biopharmaceuticals, there is the potential for the use and abuse of information (Schaefer, 2001).

Environmental Factors

As important as the genetic factors are in development, the influences of the environment cannot be underestimated, from preconception through adulthood. The physiological well-being of mothers has an impact on fetal development, and the environment that both parents provide to their children has a significant impact on their development. Optimal development requires an appropriate level of external experience and the ability of the sensory mechanism to selectively attune to environmental stimulation (Reznick, 2000). While new empirical evidence regarding the impact of the environment on development continues to evolve, our understanding is still in its infancy.

Perinatal Environmental Factors

Even before conception, a mother's behavior has an influence on the future development of her child. Good nutrition, including a diet high in folic acid, and appropriate vaccinations before pregnancy help to improve the outcome of the pregnancy. Pregnant women must receive early and consistent prenatal care and avoid known threats to their fetus. Among pregnant women in the United States, approximately 5% to 14% abuse alcohol, 10% to 20% smoke cigarettes, 10% use marijuana, 1% use cocaine, and 0.5% use opiates (Center on Addiction and Substance Abuse, 1996, 2003), all of which can affect the outcome of the pregnancy.

Use of alcohol during pregnancy has been associated with a group of physical malformations and neurological complications termed **fetal alcohol syndrome (FAS)**. The criteria for diagnosis of FAS include prenatal and postnatal growth retardation, CNS abnormalities, and distinctive craniofacial abnormalities of microphthalmia (small eyes) and/or short palpebral fissure, thin upper lip, poorly developed groove in the midline of their lips (philtrum), and flat maxillae (Figure 2–2). Numerous abnormalities coupled with varying degrees of mental retardation provide a lifetime of challenges for children with FAS. Children with

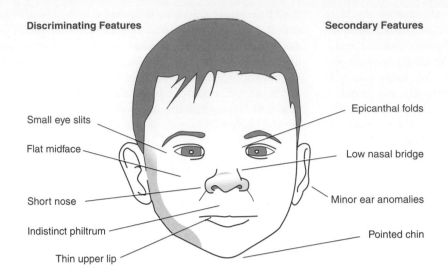

Discriminating Features

Small eye slits

Flat midface

Short nose

Indistinct philtrum

Thin upper lip

Secondary Features

Epicanthal folds

Low nasal bridge

Minor ear anomalies

Pointed chin

Figure 2–2 Characteristics of young child with fetal alcohol syndrome.

milder intellectual problems and few, if any, of the craniofacial malformations may have fetal alcohol effects (FAE) or alcohol-related neurodevelopmental disorder (ARND). These children frequently have intellectual functioning in the borderline-average range and subtle impairments in memory, language, fine motor, and perceptual motor skills (Wunsch, Conlon, & Scheidt, 2002); however, they appear to have the same degree of behavioral abnormalities as those having the more severe FAS (Steinhausen, Metzke, & Spohr, 2003).

The degree of manifestation of FAS, FAE, or ARND is influenced by the amount of alcohol consumed by the mother during pregnancy and the timing of consumption. High alcohol intake during the first trimester of pregnancy might lead to FAS; high intake later in the pregnancy might lead to FAE. Low or moderate intake during the entire pregnancy might lead to FAE. Hence, no amount of alcohol intake is considered safe during pregnancy (Jacobson & Jacobson, 1994).

Cocaine use during pregnancy has been associated with an increased risk of prematurity, low birth weight (LBW), placental abruptions, and neurobehavioral abnormalities. Cocaine is a highly addictive illicit drug and is frequently used concurrently with other drugs, so it is difficult to determine the effects of cocaine alone. Neonatal withdrawal can occur in newborn infants exposed to cocaine; symptoms might include irritability, restlessness, poor feeding, tremors, increased muscle tone, and lethargy. Withdrawal can last 2 to 3 days, followed by problems related to sleep, feeding, and attention. These infants tend to be irritable,

cry frequently, sleep poorly, and have disorganized motor behaviors, making their care often stressful (Wunsch et al., 2002).

Smoking during pregnancy increases the risk of preterm delivery and LBW. The effect of tobacco smoking on the fetus is directly related to the amount of smoking, coupled with the use of alcohol or other drugs. Infants prenatally exposed to tobacco average 200 g lighter than infants born to nonsmokers (Lee, 1998). Fortunately, cessation of smoking before and during pregnancy can prevent the reduction in birth weight (Li, Windsor, Perkins, Goldenberg, & Lowe, 1993). Smoking marijuana has not been shown to have the same adverse effects as tobacco smoking on the infant (Fried, Watkinson, & Gray, 1999; Lee, 1998); however, by age 10 years, prenatal marijuana exposure was significantly related to increased hyperactivity, impulsivity, and inattentiveness (Goldschmidt, Day, & Richardson, 2000) but not to impaired cognitive functioning (Fried, Watkinson, & Gray, 1998). Cigarette exposure was found to be associated with lower global intelligence scores at ages 9 to 12 years (Fried et al., 1998).

Other drugs can also cause abnormalities and problems in the fetus and infant. Heroin and phencyclidine (PCP), as well as certain prescription drugs, have been linked to perinatal abnormalities. Heroin-exposed neonates have severe withdrawal and frequently require pharmacological intervention to inhibit behavioral manifestations of drug exposure. These infants may have problems with sleep, be resistant to cuddling, or have decreased orientation to auditory and visual stimulation, and have growth retardation

(Wunsch, et al., 2002). The long-term effects of all drug exposure are being studied and are highly influenced by the environment in which the child is raised.

Maternal infections can also be passed to the fetus during pregnancy (transplacental infections) or during birth as the fetus passes through the vagina (ascending infections). These infections occur at a time when the fetus is least able to resist them. The most common maternal infections are known as the **STORCH** infections, also called TORCH or TORCHES. The letters stand for syphilis, toxoplasmosis, rubella, cytomegalovirus (CMV), and herpes (Table 2.3). Congenital syphilis can be transmitted during pregnancy or during delivery, whereas toxoplasmosis, rubella, and CMV are transplacental infections, and herpes is an ascending infection. Toxoplasmosis can be transmitted any time in the pregnancy through maternal ingestion of contaminated raw or improperly cooked meat or contact with the feces of infected cats. Stillbirth and death are common, and if the infant survives, there will be serious restrictions in all activ-

ities. There has been a significant reduction in rubella with the introduction of vaccination programs in the 1970s. Women can be tested for immunity to rubella before becoming pregnant. CMV is the most common cause of congenital viral infections, with an incidence of 0.2 to 2.2% of all live births in the United States (Hill & Haffner, 2002).

Another serious threat to the health and development of an infant is the presence of human immunodeficiency virus (HIV) infection or acquired immunodeficiency syndrome (AIDS). Transmission from the mother to the newborn can occur in utero, during the birth process, or through breast-feeding. The majority of infants born to infected mothers are not infected, and intensive use of antiretroviral therapy for the mother during pregnancy has continued to decrease the incidence (Fiscus et al., 2002) from 25% to 2% (National Institute of Child Health and Human Development, 2003). Those infants who do acquire the HIV infection generally follow two possible courses. Those

Table 2.3 STORCH (Intrauterine) Infections

Diagnosis	Etiology	Impairments of Body Functions and Structures	Potential Activity Limitations and Participation Restrictions
Syphilis	Parabacterial infection	Enlarged liver and spleen, jaundice, anemia, rash, oral lesions, inflammation of the eye, hearing loss	If the infant survives, limitations will depend on the extent of impairments in body function and structure.
Toxoplasmosis	Parasitic infection	Deafness, blindness, mental retardation, seizures, pneumonia, large liver, and spleen	Serious limitations in activities and participation.
Rubella	Virus	Meningitis, hearing loss, cataracts, cardiac problems, mental retardation; retinal defects	Serious limitations in activities and participation due to sensory impairments and limitations in cognitive functioning.
Cytomegalovirus	Virus	Hearing loss; in severe form, problems are similar to rubella	Serious limitations in activities and participation due to deafness and limitations in cognitive functioning.
Herpes simplex	Virus	*Disseminated form*: clotting disorder, liver dysfunction, pneumonia, and shock *Encephalitic form*: attacks CNS, causing mental retardation, seizures, and other problems *Localized form*: eye or skin lesions	Serious limitations in activities and participation with the disseminating and encephalitic forms. The localized form is usually successfully treated without limitations in activities.

Source: Hill & Haffner, 2002.

who develop symptoms of the infection in the first 12 months of life usually die by age 3 to 5 years (Abrams et al., 1995). They probably acquired the infection in utero before the immune system was fully developed. The other group of infants remains asymptomatic for the first 5 years of life. They probably acquired the infection at birth and they have a longer survival rate. In the mid-1990s, their median survival rate was more than 9 years (Barnhart et al., 1996), but the rate has continued to improve with advances in antiretroviral therapy. Infants infected with AIDS usually have slowed growth, delayed overall development, and frequent infections. Family-focused intervention is critical in their care.

Diseases, infections, medication, and radiation of the mother can also affect the outcome of the pregnancy. Drugs that successfully treat a disease in the mother can have devastating effects on the fetus. The most notorious example was the morning sickness pill, thalidomide, which caused major limb deficiencies in the fetus. Fortunately, thalidomide was not legal in the United States when its devastating effects were unknown. Recently, the very controlled use of thalidomide has been approved in the United States for the treatment of cancer. Pregnant women with medical problems must be under close medical supervision during pregnancy because the effect of all pharmacological agents on the fetus must be monitored carefully due to the potential of **teratogenic** (ability to cause physical defects in the developing fetus) effects on the fetus.

Recent research suggests that conditions present during the fetal period may program the individual's susceptibility to disease that occurs late in adult life. Women who were born weighing less than 2500 g were reported to have a 23% higher risk of cardiovascular disease than women born weighing more (Rich-Edwards et al., 1997). The small size at birth was reportedly not the problem. The factors in utero that created the suboptimal conditions that caused the infant to be born small for gestational age are thought to be the critical variables in these women who subsequently develop cardiovascular disease. Conversely, women who weighed more than 4000 g at birth had a greater likelihood of developing early breast cancer than those who weighed 2500 g at birth (Michels et al., 1996). Nathanielsz (1999), author of *Life in the Womb,* suggested that there is "compelling proof that the health we enjoy throughout our lives is determined to a large extent by the conditions in which we developed." This is a new and exciting frontier of scientific research and provides even more support for the need for healthy habits and excellent prenatal care of the mother.

Postnatal Environmental Factors

As noted by the developmental theorists, the environment plays a major role in the development of the child. Skinner (1953) emphasized the role of the environment in shaping behavior, and Piaget (1952) emphasized the role of the environment in the development of knowledge. They and others (Bailey & Wolery, 1992, p. 198) note that the critical element is not just the environment but also the child's interaction with the environment. Therein lies the major complication. Some children respond and learn very well in very stimulating environments, and others are overwhelmed and withdraw from the stimulation and do not interact. This variability in response to the environment is critical for therapists to understand and recognize. A clinical setting might be exciting for one child and totally overwhelming to another. The focus on home services for young children is based on the recognition that children generally respond best in their natural environment. However, not all natural or home environments are appropriately stimulating and supportive to children, and interventionists must recognize that, on occasion, other environments are more appropriate for the child's learning.

David and Weinstein (1987) recommend that the child's environment should fulfill five basic functions:

1. The environment should foster personal identity, and help children define their relationship to the world.

2. The environment should foster the development of competence by "allowing children opportunities to develop mastery and control over their physical surroundings" (p. 9).

3. The environment should be rich and stimulating.

4. The environment should foster a sense of security and trust.

5. The environment should provide opportunities for social contact and privacy.

For physical development, the child needs the opportunity to practice both universal skills, such as sitting, crawling, and walking, and advanced, culturally dependent skills, such as riding a bicycle or horse, playing tennis, or snow boarding. The amount of practice necessary to master a specific skill is dictated by innate ability and environmental variables.

For a child with disabilities, the physical environment can have a significant influence on performance. Not only should the environment be accessible, but it must also be responsive to the needs of the child. Historically, society and especially parents have been overprotective toward children with disabilities. This attitude can result in adults doing almost everything for the children and thereby imparting that the children have little control over their environment (Bailey & Wolery, 1992, p. 200; Ott & Effgen, 2000). Children easily perceive that they lack control over their lives and are unintentionally taught "learned helplessness" (DeVellis, 1977; Seligman, 1975). A physically responsive environment may help to increase perceptions of control (Bailey & Wolery, 1992, p. 200) that may carry over to other situations.

The child's physical environment is significantly influenced by the family's socioeconomic status (SES). Children raised in poverty are far less likely to have appropriate toys, reading material, and personal space than those raised by families having greater means, not to mention the basic necessities of food, clothing, and shelter. Children's success in school has a direct relationship to the educational attainment of their parents (Case, Griffin, & Kelly, 2001). In the United States, almost 20% of all children live in poverty, more than 25% of them in West Virginia, Louisiana, Mississippi, Arkansas, and New Mexico (Children's Defense Fund, 2003). This is almost twice as high as in other developed nations. Poverty is also unequally distributed across ethnic groups. Children raised in poverty are more likely than children raised in more affluent families (Morales & Sheafor, 2001) to:

- Have a disability
- Have no health insurance
- Have poor-quality child care
- Have inadequate housing
- Live in areas with high crime rates
- Change schools frequently
- Watch more television
- Not read
- Live in single-parent families

Their environments are frequently more chaotic and more stressful and lack the social and psychological supports needed to successfully develop. All of these factors are compounded if the child has a disability. Understanding the needs of the family and family-centered care is very important for physical therapists, and Chapter 3 is devoted to this important topic.

Nutrition

Nutrition plays an important part in normal growth and development. Culture, poverty, and lifestyle influence nutrition. During the first few years of life, children are completely dependent on their caregivers for their nutrition, as are some children with disabilities throughout their lives. For infants, breast milk is the best nourishment; it is more digestible than commercial infant formulas and provides some immunological protection (Cunningham, Jelliffe, & Jelliffe, 1991). Breast feeding during the first months of life is strongly recommended by the American Academy of Pediatrics, Committee on Nutrition (1998). Preterm infants and those with oral motor problems, who are unable to nurse adequately, can still be fed breast milk that has been expressed by the mother.

Undernutrition involves the underconsumption of nutrients and may lead to malnutrition. Malnutrition leads to severe failure to thrive and failure to meet expected growth standards. The inadequate intake of nutrition may lead to neurodevelopmental problems and lack of energy to explore and learn from the environment. The other extreme is the excessive intake of food relative to the metabolic needs of the child that leads to obesity. In developed countries of the world, increasing numbers of children are becoming obese (Steinberger & Daniels, 2003). This is caused by the increased consumption of fatty foods, increased time sitting watching television or playing video games, and decreased physical activity in general. Obesity also occurs in China, where the only child is indulged and fat-intensive Western foods are becoming popular.

Children with disabilities have a higher likelihood of becoming obese than the general population. Children with Down syndrome have lower metabolic rates that increase the likelihood of weight gain. Children with Prader-Willi syndrome have a compulsive eating problem. Those with muscular dystrophy or high-level myelomeningocele, disorders that can lead to restricted mobility and inactivity, also have problems with obesity. Obesity can lead to secondary medical problems associated with musculoskeletal pain, cardiopulmonary insufficiency, diabetes, and sleep apnea. Physical therapists should be supportive of proper nutrition and work closely with nutritionists, nurses, and physicians to make certain children have an appropriate balance of proper caloric input and exercise. Directing fitness programs for children with and without disabilities is becoming an expanded area of practice for physical therapists and is discussed in Chapters 8 and 12.

Culture and Ethnicity

Our most basic common link is that we all inhabit this planet. We all breathe the same air. We all cherish our children's future. (John F. Kennedy, address, The American University, 1963)

Child development is significantly influenced by the environmental factors of **culture** and **ethnicity**. "Culture is the behavior, patterns, beliefs and all other products of a particular group of people that are passed on from generation to generation" (Santrock, 1998, p. 579) and forms an "integrated system of learned patterns of behavior" (Low, 1984, p. 14). The characteristics of culture are complex and evolving. Adolescents and young adults might reject their cultural upbringing, only to embrace their culture when raising their own children. Cultural values influence child-rearing behaviors for children with and without disabilities.

Understanding cultural variations in child rearing will assist the therapist in providing culturally sensitive, competent intervention, as discussed in Chapter 3. One need only read Anne Fadiman's (1997) award-winning work, *The Spirit Catches You and You Fall Down*, to see what can go wrong when American physicians and health-care professionals fail to understand the collision of cultures. In this anthropology text, a young Hmong child, with a serious seizure disorder, eventually dies after years of misunderstanding and misinterpretation of the family and the family's culture by American health professionals.

Ethnicity is based not only on cultural heritage but also on nationality characteristics, race, religion, and language. There is wide diversity among individuals within those of a specific ethnic group. Failure to recognize this heterogeneity can result in inappropriate stereotyping. This stereotyping has, unfortunately, been common in research on ethnic minority children where the influences of SES have not been properly accounted for in drawing conclusions about ethnic issues. Researchers are only now beginning to document the strong influence of poverty on what were previously considered factors related to ethnicity (Low, 1984; Morales & Sheafor, 2001).

Sensitive Periods

Sensitive or critical periods in development have been discussed throughout the 20th century, and there is now renewed interest in this concept due to the revolution in neuroscience and greater understanding of neuroplasticity. Many use the terms "sensitive" or "critical" periods synonymously with "windows of opportunity." Some scientists use "critical periods" to define a time during which a system requires specific experiences if development is to proceed normally, whereas a "sensitive period" is a time when normal development is most sensitive to abnormal environmental conditions (Bruer, 2001). Regardless of the semantic confusion, the issue is that certain experiences at one point in development will have a profoundly different effect on future development than the very same experience at another point in time (Bruer, 2001). These periods are times during development when the individual is "especially sensitive to particular types of experiences" (Elman et al., 1997, p. 283), and before and after the experience there is reduced responsivity (Farran, 2001, p. 240). Common examples include the ease of learning a second language in the first decade of life compared with during adolescence or adult life and the classic work on effect of visual deprivation early in the life of kittens. Depriving kittens of visual input to one eye for the first 6 weeks of life led to blindness in that eye (Hubel & Wiesel, 1970).

Initially, scientists believed critical periods were short, well-defined periods of development. Now it is realized "that critical periods are rarely brief and seldom sharply defined; rather during a critical period the impact of experience peaks and then gradually declines" (Bruer, 2001, p. 8). Edward Taub, a distinguished rehabilitation researcher, has noted that the exciting aspect of his work is not merely that the immature brain has plasticity but that the mature brain also has plasticity (Bruer, 2001, p. 21). Taub and colleagues (Taub & Morris, 2001; Taub & Wolf, 1997) have successfully demonstrated the neuroplasticity of mature nervous systems in adults post stroke using constraint-induced movement therapy. Their work is now being replicated with children (Charles, Lavinder, & Gordon, 2001; Echols, DeLuca, Taub, & Ramey, 2000) where the results might be even more dramatic given the known neuroplasticity of the immature brain.

An excellent review of this evolving topic, of vital importance to pediatric physical therapy, can be found in *Critical Thinking About Critical Periods* (Bailey, Bruer, Symons, & Lichtman, 2001). In the conclusion of the book, Bailey and Symons write that "when a window of opportunity opens, we should take advantage of it, even if we don't have evidence that doing so now is necessarily better than later" (2001, p. 290). They note the need for further research but provide the following considerations for practice:

First, different windows open at different times . . . . Second, each child follows a unique developmental course . . . . Third, there is no point in trying to teach something if the window is not yet open . . . . Finally, it is clear that inequity exists in our society in the extent to which children have opportunities for access to various experiences after a certain window opens.

Development of Functional Movement

Any movement can be functional, depending on the context. A child with severely limited muscular activation produces functional movement with his eyes when he activates an environmental control unit that assists in operating his television. On the other hand, a child with autism who consistently runs in circles might not have true functional movement. Functional movement has been defined as a complex activity directed toward performing a behavioral task. Behaviors that are efficient in achieving the task are considered optimal (Shumway-Cook & Woolacott, 2001). Movement involves the complex interaction of the environment, individual, and task. The child generates a movement based on innate capabilities in response to the demands of the task within the limitations set by the environment. Movement is both proactive and reactive based on the needs of the task, the environment, and previous experience with that movement.

The study and discussion of the development of children are usually divided into specific age periods reflecting not only major periods of growth and development but also times of major transitions in the life of the child. Following this convention, the discussion of child development is divided into the following stages: prenatal, neonatal/infant, toddler, preschooler, school age, and adolescence. These are not mutually exclusive stages. An outline of the usual or customary development of functional movement, reflexes, and cognitive and language development in infants and children appears in Tables 2.4 to 2.8. The common age of attainment is provided; however, these are average ages and ranges of attainment, and it must be noted that there is a wide range of normal variability influenced by genetics, the environment, child-rearing practices, and cultural expectations.

Prenatal

Movement occurs during the earliest stages of embryonic development. Mothers first become aware of these movements of the fetus at about 16 to 18 weeks' gestation; however, ultrasound technology has documented extensive movement much earlier in fetal life. By 9 weeks' gestation, the embryo displays isolated arm and leg movement, and by 16 weeks, alternating leg movement is observed. Hand-to-mouth behaviors are also common. Movement continues to increase until 30 to 32 weeks' gestation, after which time the uterine environment restricts movement.

Neonate/Infant

The neonate does not look like the pictures in baby books; those adorable infants are generally 3 to 4 months old. The neonate's face is usually puffy and bluish; the ears and head may be pressed into odd shapes; the nose flattened; and the skin covered in a fine hair called lanugo. At birth the neonate fluctuates between bursts of energy and deep sleep.

The neonate is dependent on others for continued existence. Caregivers must provide nutrition and make certain that the neonate is kept clean and warm. Physical growth and development should be monitored carefully because extremely large and especially extremely small infants might indicate problems requiring medical attention. The U.S. growth standards have been changing, and the present standards for height and weight are documented in Figure 2–3. Reproducible and updated charts on the standards for infants and children's height, weight, head circumference, and body mass index are available on the Centers for Disease Control and Prevention–National Center for Health Statistics (2003) Websites. A child's measurements should be plotted on these growth charts and compared with the standards. Usually growth is consistent along a specific percentile. When there are radical fluctuations or consistent measures below the 10th percentile, malnutrition or other problems must be considered. It can be difficult to evaluate the growth of children with disabilities using the standard norms, so a number of specialized charts have been developed for children with disabilities such as Down syndrome (Cronk et al., 1988) and cerebral palsy (Krick, Murphy-Miller, Zeger, & Wright, 1996).

Gross Motor Development

The motor characteristics of neonates are limited and predictable, as outlined in Tables 2.4 to 2.7. Development of gross motor functional movement is shown in Table 2.4 and fine motor functional movement is shown in Table 2.5. Their reflexes (Figure 2–4; also see Table 2.6) are thought to be protective, allowing them to withdraw from noxious stimuli. In addition to responding reflexively to environmental stimuli, the neonate has independent responses to stimuli. Neonates will suck in a specific pattern once they learn that certain sucking patterns are reinforcing. They will kick in a particular way if a noise can be produced as when a bell is attached to their leg. They will respond in a similar vocal pattern to the rhythmic voice of their parents. Hand-to-mouth behavior, observed during fetal development, is used for self-calming in the postnatal period.

After the first few weeks of life, infants start to have longer periods of wakefulness and begin to amuse and

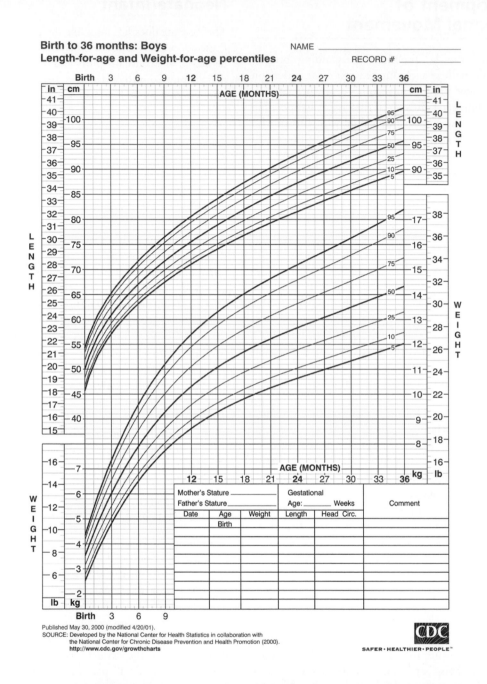

Figure 2–3 Growth charts for length/stature for age and weight for age for boys and girls from birth to age 20 years. (From Centers for Disease Control and Prevention [2003]. National Center for Health Statistics, National Health and Nutrition Examination Survey, CDC 2000 Growth Charts. Retrieved March 11, 2003, from *http://www.cdc.gov/nchs/about/major/nhanes/growthcharts/clinical_charts.htm*.)

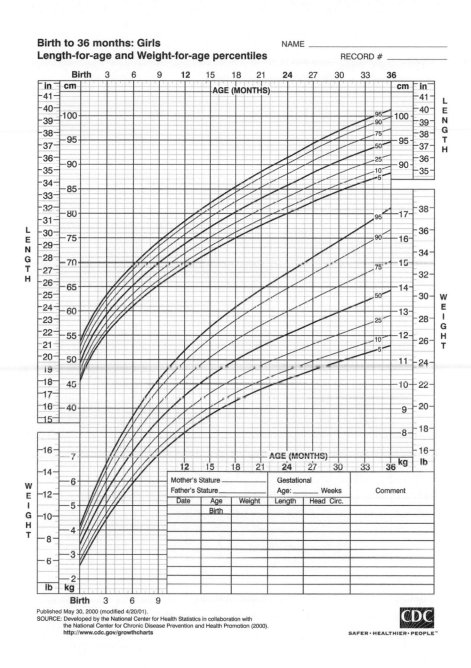

Birth to 36 months: Girls
Length-for-age and Weight-for-age percentiles

NAME _____

RECORD # _____

Published May 30, 2000 (modified 4/20/01).
SOURCE: Developed by the National Center for Health Statistics in collaboration with
the National Center for Chronic Disease Prevention and Health Promotion (2000).
http://www.cdc.gov/growthcharts

Figure 2–3 *(Continued)*

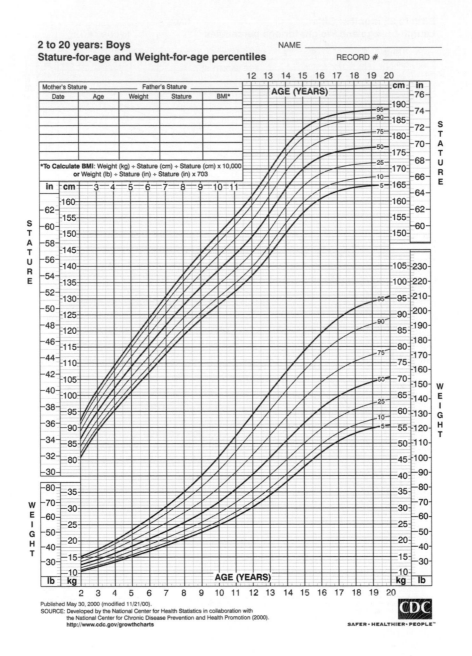

2 to 20 years: Boys
Stature-for-age and Weight-for-age percentiles

NAME _____

RECORD # _____

Published May 30, 2000 (modified 11/21/00).
SOURCE: Developed by the National Center for Health Statistics in collaboration with
the National Center for Chronic Disease Prevention and Health Promotion (2000).
http://www.cdc.gov/growthcharts

Figure 2–3 *(Continued)*

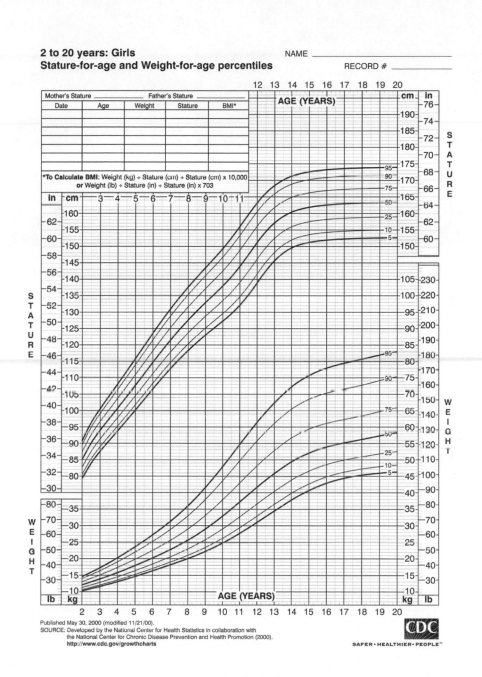

Figure 2–3 *(Continued)*

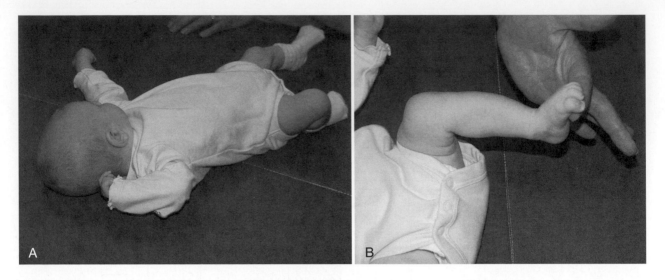

Figure 2–4   Reflexes commonly seen in infants. (*A*) Asymmetrical tonic neck reflex (ATNR). (*B*) Plantar grasp tested in supine position.

Table 2.4 Development of Gross Motor Functional Movement by Age and Position

Position/Age	Gross Motor Functional Movement
Rolling	
3–4 months	Rolls from supine to sidelying, rolls from prone to side accidentally
5–7 months	Rolls from prone to supine with right and left leg performing independent movements
6–14 months	Rolls segmentally prone to supine and back with roll initiated by the head, shoulder, or hips
Crawling/Creeping	
7 months	Crawls forward on belly; assumes quadruped position on hands and knees
7–10 months	Reciprocal creep on all fours (opposite/contralateral upper and lower extremities move simultaneously)
10–11 months	Creeps on hands and feet (plantigrade)
10–12 months	Creeps well, over, around, and on objects
Sitting	Very dependent on environmental affordances
0–3 months (held in sitting position)	Initially head bobs in sitting, back rounded, hips are apart, turned out, and bent; then head is steady; chin tucks; able to gaze at floor; sits with less support; hips are bent and shoulders are in front of hips
5–6 months (supports self in sitting position)	Sits alone momentarily with increased back extension, wide base, bent legs and periodic use of "high guard" position with arms; sits by propping forward on arms; protective responses with arms present when falling to the front

Position/Age	Gross Motor Functional Movement
5–10 months (sits alone)	Sits alone steadily, can flex head and keep cervical extension, initially wide base of support; able to play with toys in sitting position
6–11 months	Goes from sitting to quadruped or prone; gets to sitting position from prone
7–8 months	Equilibrium reactions are present; able to rotate upper body while lower body remains stationary; protective responses using arms are present when falling to the side; plays with toy in sitting
8–10 months	Sits well without support; legs are closer; full upright position, knees straight; increased variety of sitting positions, including "w" sit and side sit; difficult fine motor tasks may prompt return to wide base of support
9–18 months	Rises from supine position by rolling over to stomach then pushing up into four-point position, then to sitting
10–12 months	Protective extension backwards, first with bent elbows then straight elbows; able to move freely in and out of sitting position into other positions
11–12 months	Trunk control and equilibrium responses are fully developed in sitting, further increase in variety of positions
11–24+ months	Rises from supine by first rolling to side then pushing up into sitting position
Standing	
0–3 months	When held in standing position, takes some weight on legs
2–3 months	When held in standing position, legs may give way
3–4 months	Bears some weight on legs, but must be held proximally; head is up in midline, no chin tuck; pelvis and hips are behind shoulders; legs are apart and turned outward
5–10 months	Increased capability to bear weight; decreased support needed; may be held by arms or hands; legs spread apart and turned outward; bounces in standing position; stands while holding on to furniture
6–12 months	Pulls to standing position at furniture
8–9 months	Rotates the trunk over the leg; legs are more active when pulled to a standing position; pulls to standing by kneeling, then half-kneeling
9–13 months	Pulls to standing with legs only, no longer needs to use arms; stands alone momentarily
12 months	Equilibrium reactions are present in standing
31–32 months	Stands on one foot for 1–2 seconds
43–52 months	Stands on tiptoes
53–60 months	Stands on one foot for 10 seconds without swaying more than 20 degrees
Walking	
8 months	Cruises sideways at furniture using arms for support
8–18 months	Walks with two hands held
9–10 months	Cruises around furniture, turning slightly in intended direction

(Continued)

Table 2.4 Development of Gross Motor Functional Movement by Age and Position (Continued)

Position/Age	Gross Motor Functional Movement
9–17 months	Takes independent steps, falls easily; initial independent walking characterized by excessive hip flexion, external rotation, abduction with wide base of support, knee flexion through stance, no heel strike, hyperextension of swing leg, short stride length and swing phase and scapular adduction and high hand guard (Figure 2–5)
10–14 months	Walking: stoops and recovers in play
11 months	Walks with one hand held; reaches for furniture out of reach when cruising; cruises in either direction, no hesitation
18–20 months	Seldom falls; runs stiffly with eyes on ground
25–26 months	Walks backward 10 feet
27–28 months	Walks three steps on a taped line
29–30 months	Runs 30 feet in 6 seconds
41–42 months	Runs with arms moving back and forth, balls of feet used to push forward, high knee and heel lift and trunk leans forward
Stair Climbing	Very dependent on environmental affordances
8–14 months	Climbs up stairs on hands, knees, and feet
15–16 months	Walks up stairs while holding on
17–18 months	Walks down stairs while holding on
15–23 months	Creeps backwards down stairs
24–30 months	Walks up and down stairs without support, marking time
30–36 months	Walks up stairs, alternating feet
36–42 months	Walks down stairs, alternating feet
Jumping and Hopping	
2 years	Jumps down from step
2½+ years	Hops on one foot, few steps
3 years	Jumps off floor with both feet
3–5 years	Jumps over objects, hops on one foot
3–4 years	Gallops, leading with one foot and transferring weight smoothly and evenly
5 years	Hops in straight line
5–6 years	Skips on alternating feet, maintaining balance

Generally, age ranges start with the youngest reported average age and end with the oldest reported average age of typically developing children. All ages and sequences are approximations as there is wide individual variation.

Source: References include Bayley (1993); Bly (1994); Folio & Fewell (2000); Case-Smith (2001); and Knobloch & Pasamanick (1974).

Table 2.5 Development of Fine Motor Functional Movement by Age and Activity

Activity/Age	Fine Motor Functional Movement
Reaching	
0–2 months	Visual regard of objects
1–3 months	Swipes at objects
1–4^1/$_2$ months	Alternating glance from hand to object
2–6 months	Inspects own hands; reaches for, but may not contact, object
3^1/$_2$–4^1/$_2$ months	Visually directed reaching
3^1/$_2$–6 months	Hands are oriented to object, rapid reach for object without contact
4 months	Shoulders come down to natural level; hands are together in space; in sitting bilateral backhand approach with wrist turned so thumb is down
5 months	In prone bilateral approach, hands slide forward; two-handed corralling of object
5–6 months	Elbow is in front of shoulder joint; developing isolated voluntary control of forearm rotation
6 months	In prone, reaches with one hand while weight bearing on the other forearm; elbow is extended, wrist is straight, midway between supination and pronation
7 months	Prone: reaches with one hand while weight bearing on the other extended arm
8–9 months	Unilateral direct approach, reach and grasp single continuous movement
9 months	Controls supination with upper arm in any position, if trunk is stable
10 months	Wrist extended, appropriate finger extension
11–12 months	Voluntary supination, upper arm in any position
Grasp	
0–3 months	Hands are predominantly closed
2–7 months	Object is clutched between little and ring fingers and palm
3–3^1/$_2$ months	Hands clasped together often
4 months	Able to grasp rattle within 3 inches of hand
3–7 months	Able to hold a small object in each hand
4 months	Hands are partly open
4–6 months	Hands are predominantly open
4–8 months	Partial thumb opposition on a cube; attempts to secure tiny objects; picks up cube with ease
5–9 months	Rakes or scoops tiny objects using ulnar grasp
6–7 months	Objects held in palm by finger and opposed thumb (radial palmar grasp)

(Continued)

Table 2.5 **Development of Fine Motor Functional Movement by Age and Activity** *(Continued)*

Activity/Age	Fine Motor Functional Movement
6–10 months	Picks up tiny objects with several fingers and thumb
7–12 months	Precisely picks up tiny objects
8 months	Tiny objects are held between the side of index finger and thumb (lateral scissors)
8–9 months	Objects are held with opposed thumb and fingertips; space is visible between palm and object
9–10 months	Small objects are held between the thumb and index finger, first near middle of index (inferior pincer) finger; later between pads of thumb and index finger with thumb opposed (pincer)
10 months	Pokes with index finger
12 months	Small objects are held between the thumb and index finger, near tips, thumbs opposed (fine pincer)
12–18 months	Crayon is held in the fist with thumb up
2 years	Crayon is held with fingers, hands on top of tool, forearm turned so thumb is directed downward (digital pronate)
Release	
0–1 month	No release, grasp reflex is strong
1–4 months	Involuntary release
4 months	Mutual fingering in midline
4–8 months	Transfers object from hand to hand
5–6 months	Taking hand grasps before releasing hand lets go
6–7 months	Taking hand and releasing hand perform actions simultaneously
7–9 months	Volitional release
7–10 months	Presses down on surface to release
8 months	Releases above a surface with wrist flexion
9–10 months	Releases into a container with wrist straight
10–14 months	Clumsy release into small container; hand rests on edge of container
12–15 months	Precise, controlled release into small container with wrist extended
Feeding	Very dependent on environmental affordances
Birth–1 month	Rooting, sucking, and swallowing reflexes
3–4 months	Sucking–swallowing in sequence; mouth poises for nipple
4–6 months	Brings head to mouth; pats bottle or nibble; brings both hands to bottle

(Continued)

Activity/Age	Fine Motor Functional Movement
6–7½ months	Grasps and draws bottle to mouth; grasps spoon and pulls food off spoon with lips; sucks liquid from cup; keeps lips closed while chewing; explores things with mouth
9–10 months	Feeds self cracker; holds feeding bottle
10–12 months	Tries to feed self using spoon; holds and drinks from cup with spilling; lateral motion of tongue; pincer grasp of finger foods; choosy about food

Source: References: Bayley (1993); Erhardt (1982); Folio & Fewell (2000); Case-Smith (2001); Gesell & Amatruda (1947); Halverson (1931); Knobloch & Pasamanick (1974).

Generally, age ranges start with the youngest reported average age and end with the oldest reported average age of typically developing children. All ages and sequences are approximations as there is wide individual variation.

comfort themselves. Finger or hand sucking is common and the infant shows joy at the sight of a familiar face. Cycles of wakefulness and sleep are more established and the family settles into a routine that is very important for the infant.

During infancy, the primitive reflexes (Table 2.6) that dominated the first few weeks of life begin to lessen in prominence. The rooting reflex is replaced by an active visual search for the mother's breast or bottle. The asymmetrical tonic neck reflex (ATNR), which should never be dominant, might still be seen under stressful situations, such as when using maximal effort to lift something with one hand or in children with neurological dysfunction. The Moro reflex is no longer present; however, an infant might display a similar movement pattern to the Moro when startled by an irritating noise. Postural reactions that assist in the progression of movement begin to appear.

The infant joyously begins to discover and experience the environment and movement during the first few months of life (Figure 2–5, Table 2.7), first by a mere head turn, then by causing actions such as hitting an object with arms or legs. Tying a bell to an infant's hand or foot can produce endless enjoyment. Slowly the infant learns to turn his body to reach for an object and finally achieves the ability to roll over. This is a monumental event. The infant can now roll off the bed or changing table, much to the parents' concern! He can also start to roll to reach a desired object or person. This early experience in movement is soon followed by attempts to move on the stomach using random arm and leg movements.

At approximately 6 months of age, infants learn to sit independently when carefully placed using their arms as supports. Soon their heads and trunks become more erect and they can turn their heads. With practice, infants are able to slowly lift up one, then two hands, and then play with a toy in their lap while sitting. Their balance ability is controlled mainly by their hips, within their cone of stability. Eventually they will rotate in sitting to reach toys on either side and then behind themselves. They will also learn to protect themselves from falling by extending their arms using a protective (parachute) reaction. By 9 months, they can protect themselves in all directions, including backwards, the last protective reaction to emerge.

After infants develop skill in sitting, those in Western cultures frequently learn to move on their stomachs. They may learn a combat/amphibian crawl by flexing and extending all extremities or a homolateral crawling pattern where both the arm and leg on the same side of the body flex or extend in synchrony.* This is usually followed by the more advanced pattern of reciprocal arm and leg movements where the opposite arm and leg flex and extend together, also called contralateral crawling. Some infants never crawl on their bellies (Adolph, Vereijken, & Denny, 1998) but will learn to get up on hands and knees and rock, perhaps falling backward instead of forward. Soon they learn to creep on all fours. Creeping is far more efficient than rolling or crawling and probably less irritating for the infant. Initially they might move one limb at a time to maintain a stable posture, followed perhaps by a homolateral creep where both the arm and leg on the same side of the body flex or extend at the same time and then the reciprocal (also called diagonal or contralateral) creeping pattern where the opposite arm and leg flex and extend together.

---

* Historically, when reading international literature, the term *creeping* is used for movement on the belly and *crawling* is used for on all fours, which is the reverse of the usual U.S. professional terminology. In recent years, there is much greater inconsistency in U.S. professional terminology, and it is now best to add descriptive terms when discussing crawling and creeping, such as crawling on the belly or creeping on the hands and knees.

Figure 2–5(A–E)

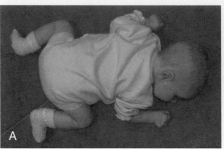
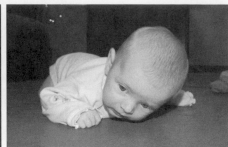

(*A*) A 2¹/₂-month-old is still generally flexed when prone (L), but can lift head (R).

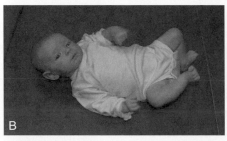
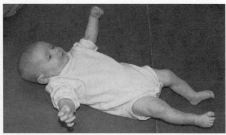

(*B*) A 2¹/₂-month-old can alternate between flexion (L) and extension (R) in supine position.

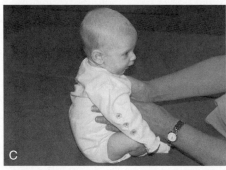
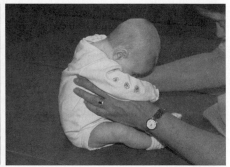

(*C*) In supported sitting at 2¹/₂ months, the back is still somewhat flexed, but the head is erect or flexed.

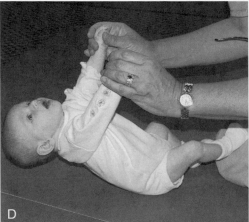
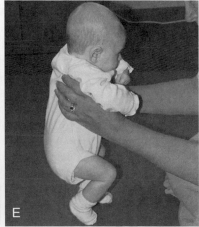

(*D*) Head lag is still present at 2¹/₂ months when infant is pulled to sitting.

(*E*) At 2¹/₂ months in standing position, the infant might choose to not bear weight. This is called *astasia*.

Figure 2–5(F–L) 69

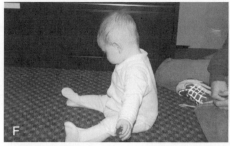
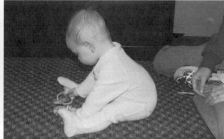

(*F*) At 6 months child can sit independently with erect trunk (L). Can also sit and reach for a toy within basis support (R).

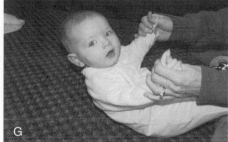
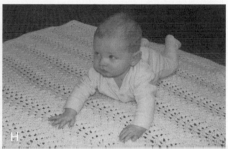

(*G*) At 6 months, when child is pulled to sitting, there is antigravity flexion of head, arms, and trunk.

(*H*) In prone position at 6 months, child is on open hands with extended arms, head erect, and trunk extended.

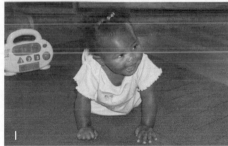
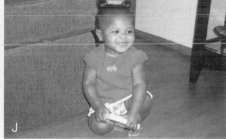

(*I*) Between 7 to 10 months of age, the infant starts to use creeping on all fours to explore the environment.

(*J*) By 11 months, a variety of erect sitting positions are possible, allowing easy and rapid transitions.

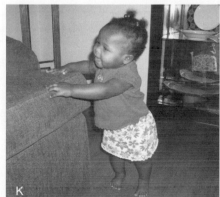
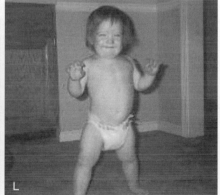

(*K*) Standing and beginning to cruise at a support surface are common for many, although not all, 11-month-old children.

(*L*) When the child is standing independently at 12 months, the arms and legs are abducted and externally rotated.

Table 2.6 Selected Primitive Reflexes

Reflex	Weeks of Gestation at Which Reflex Appears	Integrates After Birth*	Stimulus	Response
Asymmetrical tonic neck (ATNR)	20	4–5 months	Turning of head	Facial arm extends and abducts, occipital arm flexes and abducts
Rooting	28	3 months	Touch to perioral area of hungry infant	Turns head and lips toward stimulus
Suck-swallow	28–34	5 months	Touch to lips and inside mouth for suckling and liquid for swallowing	Rhythmic excursions of jaw; tongue rides up and down with jaw; then swallow
Palmar grasp	28	4–7 months	Pressure on palm of hand	Flexion of fingers
Plantar grasp	28	9 months	Supported standing on feet or pressure to sole of the foot just distal to metatarsal heads	Flexion of toes
Flexor withdrawal	28	1–2 months	Noxious stimulus to sole of foot	Flexion withdrawal of leg
Crossed extension	28	1–2 months, inconsistent	Noxious stimulus to sole of foot	Flexion of stimulated leg and then extension of opposite leg with adduction
Galant (trunk incurvation)	28	3 months, inconsistent	In prone, stroke paravertebral skin	Lateral curvature of trunk on stimulated side
Moro	28	3–5 months	Head drop backward (stimulus for the startle reflex is loud noise with same response)	Abduction and extension of arms, splaying of fingers, may be followed by arm flexion and adduction
Positive support	35	1–2 months, inconsistent	Balls of feet in contact with firm surface	Legs extend to support weight
Automatic walking/reflex stepping	37	3–4 months	Hold upright with feet on support	High stepping movements with regular rhythm
Symmetrical tonic neck (STNR)	4–6 months post full term delivery	8–12 months	Flexion or extension of head	With head flexion, arms flex and hips extend, with head extension arms extend and hips flex

*A weaker response to the stimulus might generally occur for a few more months.
Source: Classic references: Peiper (1963) and Touwen (1976).

Table 2.7 Customary Infant Development by Age

	Prone	Supine	Sitting	Upper Extremity	Locomotion	Social	Language
1 month	Slightly elevates and rotates head	Reciprocal and symmetrical kicking	Forward flexion of trunk; head in line with trunk	Opens and closes hands; reaching depends on body position and visual gaze on object	Turns head	Visual preferences for humans	Startle response to sound; moves in response to a voice
2–3 months	Elbows in line with shoulders for forearm support; lateral weight-shifting; arcs back in pivot prone (see Figure 2–5A)	Symmetrical posture precominates; kicking movements (see Figure 2–5B)	Midline head alignment; minimal head lag during pull-to-sitting; propped sitting with support (see Figure 2–5C)	Reaches and grasps with eye-hand coordination; finger play in mouth	May roll supine to prone	Listens to voices; may smile	Coos; cries to get attention; crying decreases with adult eye contact; vocalizes to express pressure
4–5 months	Weight-shifting to free arm and reach with one hand	Brings feet to mouth; attempts roll to side with leg or arm leading	No head lag when pulled to sit; static ring sitting emerging; attempts lateral weight-shift to support body with one arm and grasp toy with the other	Arms extend up in supine to reach in midline; palmar grasp on cube; holds toy with two hands	Pivot-prone rotation; may attempt rocking in quadruped and pushing backward; in standing bears weight	Laughs, excited by food	Turns head toward a voice; vocalizes; laughs and babbles
6–7 months	Elevates trunk with elbow extension; may rock on hands and knees; transitions to sitting; pushes backward (see Figure 2–5H)	Brings feet to chin or mouth; rolls to prone; attempts to raise self to sit	Static sitting while manipulating a toy; weight-shifting with lateral and anterior arm support (see Figure 2–5F)	Brings objects to midline; holds bottle with two hands; rakes for small objects; objects held in palm by fingers and opposed thumb (radial palmar grasp)	Moves forward with arms with or without abdomen elevated; rolls	Enjoys mirror; lively response to familiar people	Babbles; responds to name

Table 2.7 Customary Infant Development by Age (*Continued*)

	Prone	Supine	Sitting	Upper Extremity	Locomotion	Social	Language
8–9 months	Transitions in and out of sitting to quadruped or prone; pulls to stand with support	Raises self to sit	Manipulates toy in sitting position; anterior, lateral protective reactions present and backward emerging	Controlled release; transfers objects; radial digital grasp	Crawls; creeps; pulls to stand at support (see Figure 2–5I)	Shows initial separation concern; desires to be with people	Shouts or vocalizes to gain attention; vocalizes syllables
10–11 months	Pulls to stand through half-kneeling	Transitions to sitting and quadruped; rarely supine	Rotates or pivots while sitting to reach	Small objects held between thumb and middle of index finger (inferior pincer) later between pads of thumb and index finger (pincer)	Sidesteps or cruises with external support; walks with one hand held (see Figure 2–5K)	Plays peek-a-boo and patty-cake; waves bye-bye; has fear of strangers; performs for attention	Says repetitive consonant sounds like mama, dada; waves hi and bye; gives objects upon verbal request
12 months	Stands up through quadruped	Moves rapidly into sitting or quadruped to standing	Wide variety of sitting positions	Small objects held between tips of thumb and index finger (fine or superior pincer); rolls a ball; scoops with spoon; finger feeds	Independent walking with high hand guard and wide base of support; lowers self with control from standing; may move in and out of full squat position	Actively engages in play, understands and follows simple commands	Points to 3 body parts; imitates name of familiar objects; vocalizes with intent; uses a word to call a person

Source: References include Bly (1994); Case-Smith (2001); Folio & Fewell (2000); Long & Tosauno (2002); Rossetti (1990).

Recent research suggests that the sequence of skill acquisition of crawling and creeping is even more variable than previously believed. Adolph and colleagues (1998) studied longitudinally 28 healthy term infants. They found no strict, stagelike progression, although most infants did display most milestones. Some infants skipped expected stages such as crawling on their belly altogether, and there was a wide range of onset of belly crawling and creeping on hands and knees. Experience in belly crawling did not affect the age of onset of creeping on hands and knees. Smaller, slimmer, and more maturely proportioned infants did begin to creep on hands and knees earlier than bigger, fatter, top-heavy infants. They also found that infants used different crawling/creeping patterns from week to week and even test cycle to test cycle. Although infants who crawled on their bellies did not start to creep on hands and knees any earlier than those who never crawled, the former belly crawlers were more proficient on hands and knees compared with the non-belly crawlers. Superiority in velocity and cycle times lasted for 7 to 20 weeks after onset of creeping (Adolph, 2003). Thus, motoric experience did play a role in quality of the execution of the motor task but not in initial achievement of the task. Adolph (2003) also reports that infants who crawl or creep spend about 5 hours per day on the floor, and move 27 to 43 meters per hour, 60 to 188 meters per day, a total of about the length of two football fields! Compare that with the total dearth of movement activities, less than 10 minutes per morning, seen in children with disabilities in preschool classrooms (Effgen, 2001; Ott & Effgen, 2000).

In 1992, a correlation was made between sudden infant death syndrome (SIDS), and sleeping in prone. The American Academy of Pediatrics (1992) recommended that all healthy infants be positioned on their back for sleeping. As a result of this national effort to have all children sleep supine, there has been a decreased incidence of SIDS. An unexpected consequence of encouraging supine sleeping is that many infants have little, if any, time awake in prone. This has lead to secondary problems of head deformity and delayed development of the prone progression of rolling, crawling, and creeping (Davis, Moon, Sachs, & Ottolini, 1998; Dewey et al., 1998; Jantz, Blosser, & Fruechting, 1997; Mildred, Beard, Dallwitz, & Unwin, 1995). Prone positioning for play while awake is not a risk factor for SIDS, and parents need to be encouraged to play with their infants in prone during supervised "tummy time."

Once infants learn to creep, they will attempt to pull to standing at an object. The success of this effort will depend on the object selected, another instance of environmental

influence. Trying to pull to standing at a flat wall is usually unsuccessful, but the sides of a crib, low coffee table, or sofa are commonly the first places infants pull to standing. The problem is then how to get down! This is when infants call for help, either when they recognize they cannot get down, or after they have an uncontrolled fall from standing. These can be trying times for parents because infants insist on using their new skill of pulling to standing but require assistance to come safely down again.

While "stuck" in standing, infants will begin to shift weight and might even lift a leg. This weight shift is not only the start of upright balancing but also the start of upright mobility because infants will soon learn to cruise along a supporting surface. Cruising is an important developmental skill because of the unilateral weight bearing, balance, and synergistic hip abduction/adduction required for movement. Cruising, however, appears to be controlled by the arms, and infants do not take their legs and the floor into account to balance and respond adaptively (Adolph, 2003).

As infants freely creep and cruise, there are also initial attempts at standing independently, walking with support, and taking independent steps. There is great variability in achievement of these upright movements. Independent standing occurs around 10 to 11 months (Folio & Fewell, 2000; Piper & Darrah, 1994), although as many as 10% of infants may not stand alone at 13 months (Piper & Darrah, 1994). Independent walking occurs at about 12 months (Folio & Fewell, 2000; Sutherland, Olshen, Biden, & Wyatt, 1988), but African-American children walk at 10.9 months (Capute, Shapiro, Palmer, Ross, & Wachtel, 1985). Piper and Darrah (1994) found that 90% of children walk by 14 months. Some children do not walk until 16 months, which is still within the upper range of normal limits (Bayley, 1993). African-American children achieve these milestones slightly earlier than other children (Capute et al., 1985).

The infant's first steps are an exciting time for the infant and family, and this is an important milestone in most cultures. Sutherland, Statham, and their colleagues (Statham & Murray, 1971; Sutherland et al., 1988) note that **early walking** is characterized by a wide base of support, with wide step widths and small step lengths. The arms are held in "high hand guard" (abduction, external rotation, and flexion with scapular adduction), unless reaching forward for a parent. The hips are abducted, flexed, and slightly externally rotated; knee flexion occurs at foot contact and remains flexed through midstance and then knee extension occurs. At the ankle, there is no heel strike, and floor contact is usually with a flat foot followed by ankle dorsiflexion until midstance where it decreases. There is no plantar flexion for push-off. Sufficient extensor strength is considered critical for independent ambulation (Thelen, Ulrich, & Jensen, 1989). Shumway-Cook and Woolacott (2001, p. 343) believe there are three requirements for locomotion: (1) a rhythmic stepping pattern, (2) the ability to balance, and (3) the ability to modify and adapt gait to needs of the environment. Rhythmic stepping develops first and is even seen in the neonate. Then the stability required to balance develops as the child learns to walk during the end of the first year of life. In addition, the child must want to walk. There needs to be a reason or desire to use upright movement. Last, the adaptability required for generalization of ambulation across environments is refined during the second year of life.

As the child gains experience in walking and learns to control balance, the step length increases, the space width decreases, there is increased single limb support time, and the child can move slower and start and stop. Shortly after learning to walk unsupported, the infant will use walking as the primary means of locomotion and creeping will greatly decrease.

The ability of infants to adapt their movement to changes in the environment and their body dimensions has been studied by Adolph and Avolio (2000). They changed the infants' body dimensions by adding weights to their chests and had the infants walk down slopes. The infants generally overestimated their ability but were able to adjust their gait based on the degree of slope. The success rate decreased as the degree of slant increased; however, the more experienced walkers could handle the steeper slopes. In fact, experience in walking, not age, could predict their walking boundaries on the slopes. An interesting finding was that initially when wearing the weights, many babies weaved and staggered, but by the end of the first session they became "stiffer" and their gait appeared more normal. They adapted to the task by perhaps limiting their degrees of freedom and using more muscle cocontraction. Adolph and Avolio suggest that adaptation occurred on many levels, including behavioral, kinematic, and muscular, demonstrating the complex interacting processes of a dynamic system.

Fine Motor Development

Closely entwined with the development of gross motor skills is the development of upper extremity and fine motor skills as outlined in Table 2.5. The neonate, who initially bats at an object, soon learns directed hitting and is able to use a palmar grasp to hold appropriate-sized objects. By 6 months, the infant can transfer objects from hand to hand. The infant then progresses from a "raking and scooping" type of ulnar grasp to a more refined **radial palmar grasp** where objects are grasped from the radial side of the hand. Eventually the infant will only use fingers to grasp for small objects. By 10 months, a "three-jaw chuck" grasp is used involving the thumb and the index and middle fingers. By 12 months, the infant usually has a **superior pincer grasp** and can pick up small items such as pieces of cereal or raisins using the tips of the index finger and thumb. Parents must be very cautious about what is available in the environment for children to pick up and put in their mouths or other body openings. Noses and ears are all too common receptacles! Choking on small objects becomes a serious possibility.

During this period of infant development, there is great variability among infants. Some infants will display accelerated fine motor development while lagging behind in gross motor skills. Others display wonderful social skills while preferring to sit still in one place for extended periods. Great care must be taken when determining if there is a true deviation in development, delay in development, or merely typical variation. A number of standardized tests and measures are available to help examine all aspects of development and are discussed later in this chapter.

The critical importance of this early period of development has been highlighted by legislation in at least 120 countries, allowing for paid maternity leave from work so the mother can stay home with her infant. Many nations also allow paternal leave. The only developed nations of the world that do not provide paid maternity leave are Australia and the United States (Human Rights and Equal Opportunity Commission, 2003). In the United States, the Family Medical Leave Act of 1993 does allow for 12 weeks of unpaid leave for mothers or fathers.

Toddler

Toddlers, 1 to 3 years of age, are wonderful bundles of energy, trying even the most patient of parents. They want and need to explore everything! They learn by doing. Their ability to adapt to the demands of the environment continues to advance. In gait, the length of time in double limb support decreases, as does step width, pelvic tilt, abduction, and external rotation. Ankle dorsiflexion appears during swing phase, and by age 2 years, toddlers begin to have push-off in stance. Over the next several years, muscle amplitudes and durations increase and they will refine their gait until age 5 to 7 years, when their patterns become similar to adults.

Toddlers learn to run everywhere, climb up and over everything, and climb stairs and must be watched very carefully (Figure 2–6, Table 2.8; also see Table 2.4). Some, however, are content to sit and perform fine motor tasks or look through picture books for extended periods. Extremely active or sedentary behavior may just be a variation of typical development, may reflect the temperament common to their ethnic group, or may be an indication of possible abnormality. Children who prefer fine motor activities tend to excel in them and might need prompting to participate in gross motor activities. Additionally, recent research (Raine, Reynolds, Venables, & Mednick, 2002) suggests a relationship between high stimulation-seeking behaviors at age 3 years and higher IQs at 11 years of age. Perhaps toddlers who seek stimulation create an enriched environment that stimulates their cognitive development (Figure 2–6; see also Tables 2.4 and 2.8).

Preschooler

The preschool period is generally considered to be 3 to 5 years of age. Children are ready to experience the world beyond their home. In preschool, the curriculum's focus is usually social development along with a wide range of experiences in all domains. In some Asian cultures, 3-year-olds might begin to learn to read and write. The preschooler is a very social individual who is now making friends and exploring the world. Language skills, which are very closely tied to social ability, are developing exponentially. Children can understand past and future events, and they begin to emerge as conversational partners. Fine motor skills are advancing with more sophistication in fine motor play including pasting, coloring, and drawing. There is isolation of the thumb and fingers, rotation of the wrist, and progression from a static tripod to a dynamic tripod in the use of writing instruments.

Active movement throughout the environment characterizes the preschooler's play. Motor skills continue to be refined and are important in social interactions. However, many children are already spending too much time in sedentary activities, and they must not be allowed to become "couch potatoes" at this early age (Patrick, Spear,

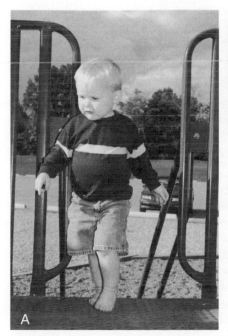
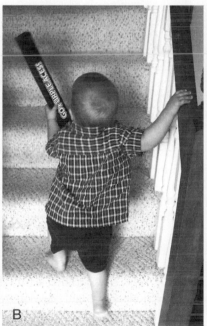
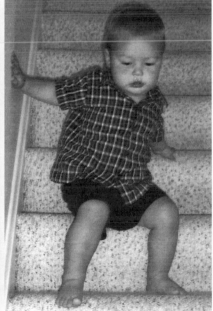

Figure 2–6   Toddler development. (*A*) Walking is mastered, with hands down at sides swinging, and a narrow base of support. (*B*) Going upstairs holding on and standing is easy, but going down is frequently more easily done in the sitting position.

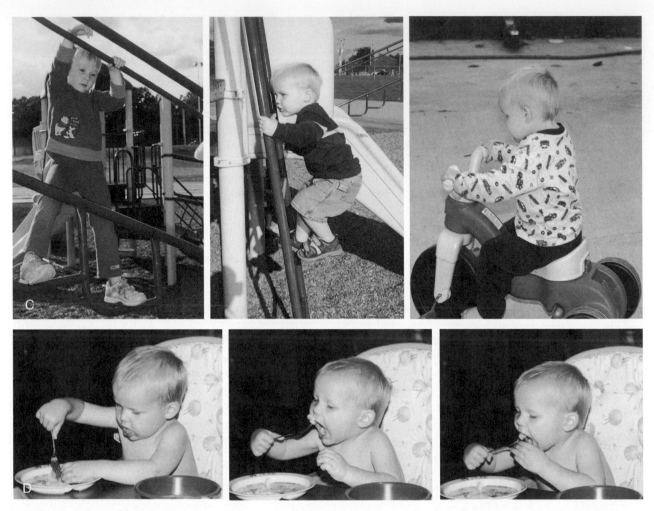

Figure 2–6 *(Continued)*   (*C*) Climbing and playing at the playground is fun and excellent for gross motor development. (*D*) Independent feeding is an important and enjoyable activity. Note the open mouth and protruding tongue as the child tries to get food on the fork. Then a bit of a miss before successfully getting the food in his mouth!

Holt, & Sofka, 2001). Exercise is important for fitness, and with obesity on the rise with children, therapists should be mindful of these very early signs of a sedentary lifestyle.

Play is the work of children (Figure 2–7), and three types of play have been identified in early childhood: (1) **dramatic** or **symbolic play** (the child pretends that dolls or figurines are real); (2) **constructive play** (involves building and constructing things); and (3) **physical** or **rough-tumble play** (active movement that includes jumping, running, and generally other children) (Case-Smith, 2001, p. 85). As children develop, their play becomes more elaborate and they concentrate for longer periods of time. Some children prefer play as a social activity, whereas others prefer solitary play. Understanding a child's preferences for play can assist the therapist in more easily establishing rapport with a child and gaining cooperation.

The preschool period is an excellent time for children with disabilities and typically developing children to learn about each other and interact in a playful environment. Children with disabilities learn to model typical behavior and develop friendships, typically developing children learn about children with special needs. Inclusive preschools have been shown to be beneficial for the development of social skills and other behaviors in children with disabilities (Buysse & Bailey, 1993; Guralnick, 1999, 2001) and for the development of sensitivity to the needs

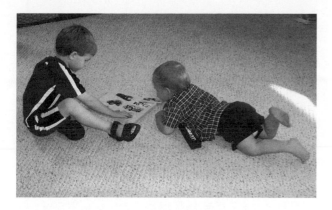

Figure 2–7 Play is the work of children. Note the different postures assumed for this activity.

of others by the typically developing children (Diamond & Carpenter, 2000).

School-Aged Child

Once the child enters school, all of the basic fine and gross motor skills are present and will be refined based on experiences and needs (Table 2.8). Children refine their writing and drawing throughout their school years, achieving varying degrees of competence. Children who participate in sports will learn the skills required of that sport. Children who take music lessons will learn the motor skills needed for their instrument. Practice is the critical factor in the level of skill development, although some children have a natural propensity for athletics or musical ability and will rapidly exceed the norm.

Some children will continue to have immature movement patterns, especially noticeable during physical education class or sports. Characteristics of **immature movement patterns** include *inconsistency* of performance; *perseveration*, the inability to stop when appropriate and having *extraneous movements; mirroring* or the inability to transpose right-left visual cues; *asymmetry* and difficulty in bilateral coordination; *loss of dynamic balance* and *falling* after finishing a motor task; *inability to maintain rhythm* or movement *pattern; inability to control force* whether unable to generate enough force or uses too much force; and *inappropriate motor planning* (Sherrill, 1993). Children with these problems may have a developmental coordination disorder, as discussed in Chapters 6 and 7, or other developmental disabilities.

In addition to the refinement of motor tasks,

Havighurst (1972) notes the following developmental tasks of middle childhood: (1) building wholesome attitudes toward oneself, (2) learning an appropriate masculine or feminine social role, (3) developing fundamental skills and concepts for everyday living, (4) developing conscience, morality, and a scale of values, and (5) developing attitudes toward social groups. How the child learns these tasks is a reflection of the physical, social, and cultural environment.

School-aged children having disabilities or special health-care needs should be attending their local school according to federal law and best practices. As discussed later, in Chapter 11, all children are to be educated in the least restrictive environment in their local school. Children are adaptable and accepting, and if the adults in the environment model behave appropriately, inclusive education has proved to be very successful for both children with disabilities and typically developing children (Giangreco, Dennis, Cloninger, Edelman, & Schattman, 1993; Hunt, Doering, Hirose-Hatae, Maier, & Goetz, 2001; Hunt, Soto, Maier, & Doering, 2003; Peck, Donaldson, & Pezzoli, 1990; Soto, Muller, Hunt, & Goetz, 2001).

Adolescent

Adolescence, usually ages 11 to 18 or up to 21 years, is a time of transition and desire for independence and separation from the family. The adolescent is seeking mature relationships with age-mates of both sexes, is learning an acceptable masculine or feminine role, is going through puberty, is achieving an adult physique, is seeking emotional independence from parents, and is preparing for adult life (Havighurst, 1972). This time of transition can be a trying time for both the adolescent and parents.

During adolescence there are numerous body changes, comparable only to those of the first year of life. The mean peak height velocity in females is at $11^1/_2$ years and menarche occurs around $12^1/_2$ years. Males begin their puberty growth spurt 2 years after the females, and their mean peak height velocity is at $13^1/_2$ years (Patrick et al., 2001).

Adolescents often find great enjoyment in sports participation or observation and community activities (Figure 2–8). Their motor skills continue to develop based on need and practice. Without proper training and fitness, there can be a tendency toward injury. Adolescents with injuries can be easy to motivate if they wish to return to their sport.

Table 2.8 Customary Child Development by Age Across Domains

Age	Gross Motor	Fine Motor	Cognitive	Language	Social-Emotional
13–18 months	Walks freely; creeps up stairs; stoops to pick up objects and regains standing	Imitative scribble; palmar-supinate grasp of pencil; precise release of pellet into small container	Understands and follows simple commands; includes others as recipients of play behaviors; points to three body parts	Uses expressive jargon; recessive language greater than expressive; shakes head "no"	Experiences peak of separation distress
18–24 months	Begins to run; creeps backwards down stairs or climbs stairs using railing (see Figure 2–6B)	Spontaneous scribble	Demonstrates invention of new means through mental combinations; finds hidden objects through invisible displacement; shows deferred imitation; activates toy or doll in pretend play	Understands multiword utterances; uses multiword utterance to express complex thoughts, e.g., "Mommy go," "Baby up"; 20–100+ word vocabulary; identifies pictures when named	Demonstrates less separation distress; begins to show empathic responses to another's distress
24–36 months	Jumps off low step; begins to ride a tricycle; kicks small ball; throws over hand (see Figure 2–6C)	Digital-pronate grasp of pencil; imitates vertical then horizontal stroke	Shows ability to substitute objects in pretend play; matches objects; responds to 2 or 3 commands; sings songs	Rapid increase in language; uses verb strategies to start a conversation; uses two-part sentences ("me go home"); demands response from others, 250+ word vocabulary	Begins to respond verbally to another's distress; includes others in pretend plan
3 years	Demonstrates true run, with both feet leaving ground; walks upstairs alternating feet; walks downstairs using marking time; jumps off step and over 2-inch object	Copies circle	Tells simple story; knows conventional counting words up to 5; tells action in pictures; puts together puzzle; follows a 3-step unrelated command	Is versatile in language use; speaks in more complete sentences; distinguishes graphics as writing versus picture graphics; begins to overgeneralize rules creating verb tenses and plurals; uses adult syntax and grammar	Uses physical aggression more than verbal aggression
3 1/2 years	Can hop a few steps on preferred foot; kicks ball; mounts, pedals and dismounts 3-wheel riding vehicle	Traces diamond with angles rounded	Can't easily distinguish reality from fantasy; can count 5 objects	Might use syllable hypothesis to create written words; rereads favorite storybooks using picture-governed strategies; often uses scribble-writing	Has difficulty generating alternatives in a conflict situation; will learn aggressive behavior rapidly if initially successful

Age	(gross motor)	(fine motor)	(cognitive)	(language)	(social/emotional)
4 years	Walks downstairs alternating feet; gallops; stands on tip toes; rotation of body follows throw of ball	Cuts straight line with scissors; copies cross; uses static tripod grasp of pencil	Makes row of objects equal to another row by matching; gives age; makes opposite analogies; matches and names 4 colors	Creates questions and negative sentences using correct word arrangement; imitation of parents' intonation pattern; voice well modulated and firm	Watches, on average, 2 to 4 hours of TV per day
4 1/2 years	Catches ball if prepared; jumps 2 to 3 inches; leans forward when jumping from a height	May begin to hold writing tool in finger grip; can button small buttons; copies square	Knows conventional counting up to 15; better able to distinguish reality from fantasy	Often reverses letter when writing; understands beside, between, and back; does not notice or grasp print conventions	
5 years	Can stop and change directions quickly when running; can hop 8 to 10 steps on 1 foot; throws ball and hits target at 10 ft; roller skates; rides bike	Uses dynamic tripod grasp of pencil; copies triangle	Appreciates past, present and future; creates classes of objects based on a single defining attribute; counts to 20	Understands passive sentences; may begin to use invented spellings	Is still poor at self-control; success depends on removal of temptation or diversion by others
6 years	Can skip	Can connect a zipper on a coat; may tie shoes; moves a writing tool with fingers while side of hand rests on table; copies diamond	Begins to demonstrate concrete operational thinking	Appreciates jokes and riddles based on phonological ambiguity	Feels one way only about a situation; has some difficulty detecting intentions accurately in situations where damage occurs
7 years		Makes small, controlled marks with pencils due to more refined finger dexterity	Begins to use some rehearsal strategies to aid memory; better able to play strategy games; may demonstrate conservation of mass and length	Appreciates jokes and riddles based on lexical ambiguity; might have begun to read	May express two emotions about one situation, but these will be same valence; understands gender constancy
8 years	Jumps rope skillfully; throws and bats a ball more skillfully	Plays games requiring considerable fine motor skill and good reaction time	Difficulty judging if a passage is relevant to a specific theme; may demonstrate conservation of area	Begins to sort out more complex syntactic difficulties such as "ask" and "tell"; might integrate cueing systems for smooth reading; becomes more conventional speller	May express 2 same-valence emotions about different targets simultaneously; understands people may interpret situation differently but thinks this is due to different information
9 years		Enjoys hobbies requiring high levels of fine-motor skill (sewing, model building)	May demonstrate conservation of weight	Interprets "ask" and "tell" correctly	Can think about own thinking or another person's thinking but not both at the same time.

Table 2.8 Customary Child Development by Age Across Domains (Continued)

Age	Gross Motor	Fine Motor	Cognitive	Language	Social-Emotional
10 years	Jumping distance continues to increase		Makes better judgments about relevance of a text; begins to delete unimportant information when summarizing	Becomes more sophisticated conventional speller	Can take own view and view of another as if a disinterested third party
11 years	Running speed stabilizes for girls		May demonstrate conservation of volume	Begins to appreciate jokes and riddles based on syntactic ambiguity	Still has trouble detecting deception; spends more time with friends
12 years	Plays ball more skillfully due to improved reaction time		Shows skill in summarizing and outlining		
13 years	Males continue to increase running speed and jumping distance		May demonstrate formal operational thinking	Speaks in longer sentences, uses principles of subordination; understands metaphors, multiple levels of meaning; increases vocabulary	Still has weak sense of individual identity, is easily influenced by peer group; spends more time with friends, usually of same sex; may begin sexual relationships, especially if male
14 years	Standing long jump distance continues to increase for males, but stabilizes for females		Continues to gain metacognitive abilities and improve study skills	Improves reading comprehension abilities; writes longer, more complex sentences	Seeks increasing emotional autonomy from parents
15 years	May reach fastest reaction time		Can think in terms of abstract principles; may demonstrate dogmatism-skepticism		Seeks intimate friendships and relationships
16 years	May reach peak performance level in sports		Can argue either side in a debate; shows growing interest in social and philosophical problems		Is actively involved in search for personal identity; is likely to be sexually active; may use alcohol and cigarettes

Source: References include: Erhardt (1982); Gallahue & Ozman (1995); Long & Toscano (2002); Rossetti (1990); Schickendanz, Schickendanz, Hansen, & Forsyth (1993).

However, they can be very difficult to motivate if the goal is improved physical fitness for obese teenagers or meeting the complex needs of teenagers with disabilities. Adolescents who participate in sports or who require fitness programs have unique physical therapy needs. In Chapter 12, the specific roles and responsibilities of therapists who work in this area are discussed.

For adolescents with disabilities this is an especially complicated period. As their bodies grow, they may face new limitations and restrictions due to increased body mass and shortening of muscles as bones grow. It is not uncommon for an adolescent with a disability, who was ambulatory at home and school, to decide that the effort and energy requirements of ambulation are too great, and a decision is made to use a wheelchair for the majority of the day (Dudgeon, Jaffe, & Shurtleff, 1991). They are also developing sexually. They and their parents must address issues of birth control and prevention of sexually transmitted diseases. This is particularly important for females, because they are especially vulnerable to sexual abuse. Participation in the community might become more restricted as the adolescent with a disability, who was once well accepted in the community, is no longer the "cute" little child, and inappropriate behaviors are no longer socially acceptable. This is also a time when integration into the general education curriculum might not continue

to be a realistic option. Teenagers frequently have a difficult time accepting each other and accepting a teenager with a disability may become more complex than when they were younger. The adolescent with a disability may now have to consider limitations in career options and ability to move away from the family. The stresses of school and determining future options can be a heavy burden on any adolescent.

Atypical Motor Behaviors

The majority of infants and children develop in the progressions noted in Tables 2.4 to 2.8. Their rates of development in various domains may differ and areas of early aptitude may continue throughout life. Some infants and children do not follow a customary developmental progression. This may be common in their culture or family and not a matter of concern. On the other hand, atypical or very delayed development may indicate a disability or detrimental environmental influences. The Bobaths (1980, 1984) and Bly (1994) have provided an outline of common atypical motor development (Figure 2–9 and Table 2.9) seen frequently in children later diagnosed with cerebral palsy and other developmental disabilities. Therapists should carefully determine the presence of atypical motor development. Its presence should be monitored and reported to the collaborative team working with the child. If it is observed during a developmental screening, then the child should receive a more comprehensive examination and, as appropriate, be referred to an early intervention program, and information be reported to the child's pediatrician.

Examination, Evaluation, and Intervention

The examination and evaluation of children, especially those with developmental delays and no obvious impairment of any specific system, include an appraisal of their developmental level and functional skills and, as appropriate, an examination and evaluation of each body system as outlined in the systems chapters of Section 2 of this text. Knowledge of the child's level of development and functioning can be critical in determining eligibility for services and the plan of care. In addition to the evaluations of developmental level, functional skills, and body systems, it is important to determine if there are problems with the

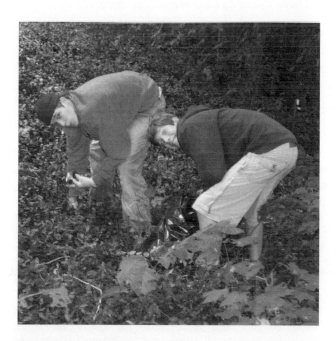

Figure 2–8   High school students participating in community service learning project.

Table 2.9 **Possible Indications of Atypical Motor Development**

Age	Possible Indications of Atypical Motor Development
Month 1	• Serious impairment of *body functions and structures*, such as intraventricular hemorrhage of grades III or IV, perinatal asphyxia, myelomeningocele, genetic abnormalities. • Impaired age-appropriate *activities*, such as feeding problems, lack of leg movement; being "stuck" in head, neck, and trunk hyperextension (opisthotonus); extremely floppy.
Month 4	• Serious impairment of *body functions and structures* will continue to affect motor development depending on the impairment. • Impaired age-appropriate *activities*, such as maintaining rigid postures; inability to alternate between flexion and extension; consistent asymmetrical postures; inability to achieve midline orientation of head and extremities; lack of reaching behaviors or only unilateral movement.
Month 6	• Serious impairment of *body functions and structures* will continue to affect motor development, such as strong hip extensor, adductor, internal rotation, and ankle plantar flexor activity, especially in combination when held in standing or the opposite combination of extreme external rotation, abduction, and dorsiflexion with eversion, especially in supine. • Impaired age-appropriate *activities*, such as lack of a wide variety of movements; inability to laterally flex in prone or side lying or bring feet to mouth in supine; inability to roll; rolling using extension; poor upper extremity weight bearing in prone; inability to maintain propped sitting; or problems reaching and grasping toy.
Month 9	• Serious impairment of *body functions and structures* will continue to affect motor development. • Impaired age-appropriate *activities* such as those mentioned above and inability to move forward in prone; get in or out of sitting or stand with support; use of a "bunny hopping" pattern in creeping; or lack of a controlled release of a cube.
Month 12	• Serious impairment of *body functions and structures* will continue to affect motor development. There should be balance of muscle activation and neither restricted nor excessive range of motion or strong asymmetrical postures. • Impaired age-appropriate *activities* such as those mentioned above including not walking with support with good weight shift; not climbing; lack of inferior pincer grasp; or stereotyped hand movements restricting function.
Month 15	• Serious impairment of *body functions and structures* will continue to affect motor development. • Impaired age-appropriate *activities* such as those mentioned above including not attempting to walk independently; or walking on toes with adducted legs; lack of a fine pincer grasp; or lack of controlled release of a pellet into a container.

Source: References include: Bly (1994) and Erhardt (1982).

child's sensory processing, if the child is experiencing any pain, and what the child's feelings are about quality of life. The areas that require examination and evaluation are addressed in the remainder of this chapter, along with an introduction to intervention.

Examination and Evaluation

There are a variety of terms used to describe what the American Physical Therapy Association (APTA) labels examination and evaluation in the *Guide to Physical Therapist Practice* (2001). As discussed in Chapter 1, many professionals, especially in pediatrics, continue to use the terms "examination," "evaluation," and "assessment" interchangeably. Others consider *evaluation* the process used to diagnose and identify atypical development or movement, whereas *assessment* is used to describe the process of collecting and organizing relevant information (Brenneman, 1999, p. 28), and some make no distinction at all (Campbell Vander Linden, & Palisano, 2000, p. 37). The Individuals with Disabilities Education Act (IDEA) (1997),

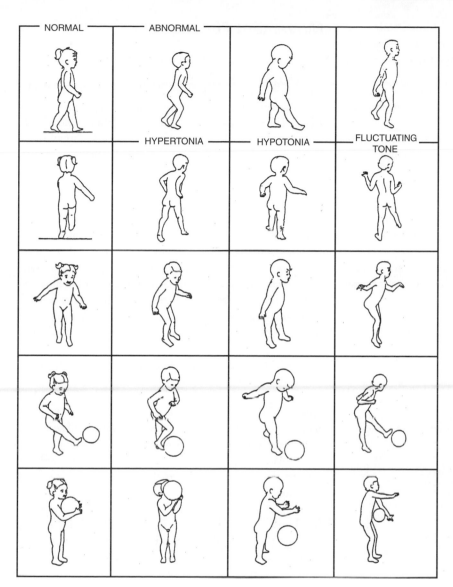

NORMAL — ABNORMAL —

HYPERTONIA — HYPOTONIA — FLUCTUATING TONE —

Figure 2–9 Common compensatory movement patterns seen in children with hypertonia, hypotonia, and fluctuating tone. (From Zelle, R.S., & Coyner, A.B. [1983]. *Developmentally disabled infants and children* [p. 372] Philadelphia: F.A. Davis. Copyright 1983 by F.A Davis Company. Reprinted with permission of the authors.)

the U.S. right-to-education law, uses the term *evaluation* to refer to the processes of examination and evaluation for eligibility for services, and *assessment* for program planning purposes. Throughout this text we have tried to use the APTA *Guide* (2001) terminology of *examination* for the physical process and *evaluation* for the dynamic, intellectual process of clinical decision making to determine the level of functioning of body functions and structures, activities, and participation. Under most situations both processes occur simultaneously, and throughout this text the terms "examination" and "evaluation" are usually used together, except when there is a real distinction between

the physical activity of the examination and the clinical judgment process of evaluation. In all settings, it is important to clarify the terminology used to avoid misunderstandings.

In pediatric practice, the outcome-driven, **top-down approach** (see Figure 1–4) to examination and evaluation, first elaborated by Pip Campbell (1991), has become the standard of practice (McEwen, 2000). The desired outcomes and goals of intervention are determined first, preferably with the parents and other team members, and then the examination is done to identify strengths that will assist in achieving the goals and the obstacles that must be overcome. The child and family are vital team members in this process. The traditional, deficit-driven model used a bottom-up approach in which the examination determined the needs and deficits, and then goals were developed based on the findings. This is rarely the approach of choice in pediatrics but is commonly used in other areas of physical therapy practice.

The purpose of the examination and evaluation is critical in determining the procedures and what tests and measures to use. The tests and measures used will be different for a screening examination, a diagnostic examination, or a prescriptive examination as discussed in Chapter 1. Frequently, there is overlap in the purposes of the examination, and some tests and measures might serve multiple purposes.

When working with preschoolers, Bailey and Wolery (1992, pp. 97–99) suggest that the evaluation process should achieve the following goals:

- Determine eligibility for services and the best place to receive those services
- "Identify developmentally appropriate and functional intervention goals" that are useful within the context of specific environments
- "Identify the unique styles, strengths, and coping strategies of each child"
- "Identify the parents' goals for their children and their needs for themselves," as in the top-down approach
- "Build and reinforce parents' sense of competence and worth"
- "Develop a shared and integrated perspective (across professionals and between professionals and family members) on the child and family needs and resources"
- "Create a shared commitment to the intervention goals" among the professionals and parents
- Evaluate the effectiveness and outcomes of the services and interventions

These goals of the evaluation process are not unique to preschoolers and can be applied across the pediatric age span. The focus on families noted by Bailey and Wolery (1992) has evolved since the enactment of Public Law 94–142, the Education for All Handicapped Children's Act, in 1976. This family-centered approach is now a clearly established orientation to serving children with disabilities and their families, as noted throughout Chapter 3.

Movement Functions

To examine and study movement dysfunction systematically, a framework and classification system are necessary to unify terminology and establish objective criteria. Under the *International Classification of Functioning, Disability and Health* (ICF), introduced in Chapter 1, the World Health Organization (WHO) (2001) has developed a broad-based definition of body functions that include the physiological and psychological functions of body systems. Body functions are divided into eight categories related to the systems of the body. The body function entitled *neuromusculoskeletal and movement-related functions* is the most critical to physical therapy intervention. This body function is divided into three sections: *functions of the joints and bones*, *muscle functions,* and *movement functions*. The functions of joints, bones, and muscles and their examination are discussed in Chapters 4 and 5; however, an understanding of *movement functions* (Table 2.10) is necessary to understand the development of functional movement.

The first movement functions are *motor reflex functions*. These are best displayed in the fetus and neonate. Many infant reflexes (see Table 2.6), such as the Moro reflex, ATNR, STNR, and palmar and plantar grasp reflexes, slowly fade until they are no longer observed in toddlers. Other motor reflexes, such as the stretch motor reflex, withdrawal reflex, and biceps and patellar reflexes, remain throughout life when the appropriate stimuli are presented.

The *involuntary movement reaction functions* are induced by body position, balance needs, and threatening stimuli. They include the postural reactions that develop during the first years of life. Facilitating the development and refinement of these reactions in a functional context is an important aspect of physical therapy intervention.

For a child to explore the environment, whether by rolling, crawling, or walking, a series of continual movements and postural adjustments are necessary. Adjustments allow a child to move freely and respond rapidly to the demands of the environment. As a child matures, a number of distinct movements and reactions develop, which orient the head and body in space, protect the child from falls, and assist in maintaining balance. The development of movement results from the complex interaction and evolution of the numerous subsystems and interactions with the environment. Postural reactions develop in infants in a relatively set sequence. Impaired development of these involuntary movement reactions may indicate neuromotor delay

Table 2.10 Specified Movement Functions

Motor reflex functions	"Functions of involuntary contraction of muscles automatically induced by specific stimuli"
Involuntary movement reaction functions	"Functions of involuntary contractions of large muscles or the whole body induced by body position, balance, and threatening stimuli"
Control of voluntary movement functions	"Functions associated with the control over and coordination of voluntary movement"
Involuntary movement functions	"Functions of unintentional, non- or semi-purposive involuntary contractions of a muscle or group of muscles"
Gait pattern functions	"Functions of movement patterns associated with walking, running or other whole body movement"
Sensations related to muscles and movement functions	"Sensations associated with the muscles or muscle groups of the body and their movement. Includes: sensations of muscle stiffness and tightness of muscles, muscle spasm or constriction and heaviness of muscles"

Source: Adapted from World Health Organization (WHO) (2001). *International classification of functioning, disability and health* (pp. 99–201). Geneva: Author.

or disability and aid in the diagnosis of CNS disorders. Testing for their presence is commonly part of a comprehensive examination.

Control of voluntary movement functions includes the control of simple and complex voluntary movement, and coordination of movements of the arms, legs, and eyes. Development of this control is an ongoing process throughout life; however, the peak developmental period is during the first several years of life, as previously discussed. Many of these voluntary movement functions are examined as part of the developmental and functional examination process.

Involuntary movement functions include nonpurposive movements such as tremors, tics, stereotypies, chorea, athetosis, dystonic movements, and dyskinesia. These involuntary movements can significantly interfere with functional movement. Under what conditions involuntary movement functions appear, or worsen, should be carefully considered. Some involuntary movements become worse during periods of stress or when performing difficult movement activities. They can be common symptoms of disabilities, such as the hand wringing seen in Rett syndrome, or the negative side effect of certain medications.

Acquiring the *gait pattern functions* and other *movement functions* is of primary importance to many parents and is the focus of much intervention. These abilities are impor-

tant for the next level of functioning—activities and participation. As discussed in Chapter 1, "Activity is the execution of a task or action by an individual," and "Activity limitations are difficulties an individual may have in executing activities." "Participation is involvement in a life situation," and "participation restrictions are problems an individual may have in executing activities" (WHO, 2001, p. 10). The nine major areas of Activities and Participation are listed in Appendix 2.A. These areas should be assessed based on the needs of the individual child, either by the system recommended by ICF (see Table 1.2) or by use of the available tests and measures. The Preferred Practice Patterns in the *Guide* (APTA, 2001) also provide recommendations to assist in examination of movement functions.

Tests and Measures

Physical therapists working in pediatrics have a long tradition of using tests and measures to assess the development and overall functioning of the children we serve. Therapists working at special centers serving children with disabilities have developed many "home-grown" tests. These tests may be useful but do not have the psychometric properties now required of our tests and measures as discussed in Chapter 1. Test construction is a very difficult, complex, time-consuming, and expensive task, and the rigor in the development of different tests and measures varies greatly. As a result, the reliability and validity of tests and measures also vary. Not all of the tests listed in Box 2.2 and Appendix 2.B would withstand rigorous review; however, because they are commonly used, therapists should be familiar with them. You must become knowledgeable regarding the strengths and weaknesses of the tests you administer. This is especially critical if the test is to be used for eligibility purposes, program evaluation, or research.

As noted in Chapter 1, before selecting a test or measure, the therapist must determine the purpose of the test. Will the test be used for screening, diagnosis, or prescriptive planning? Tests must be used for the purposes for which they were developed. The knowledge gained from appropriate tests and measures facilitates communication with parents and other professionals, assists in developing the plan of care, and is a preferred form of documentation.

In addition to determining the performance of each body system, it is frequently important to determine the level of neuromotor development and functional performance of the child in a systematic fashion. Using standardized tests and measures provides an excellent foundation for learning about child development for a therapist new to pediatrics. Numerous tests and measures have been developed to assist this process. Common tests and measures are listed by category of test in Box 2.2, and more detailed information is provided in Appendix 2.B. Several of these tests also cross categories but are listed in only one category. Some developmental or functional tests have very specific applications. The School Function Assessment (SFA) (Coster, Deeney, Haltiwanger, & Haley, 1998) provides an exemplary model of test development and application using a top-down, problem-solving approach based on the ICF model (Stewart, 2001). The child's current level of activity and participation in the school setting is determined, which provides an excellent guide for developing a plan of care specific to the needs of a child in a school setting. The Gross Motor Function Measure (GMFM) (Russell, Rosenbaum, Avery, & Lane, 2002) is an example of a test developed and validated for a specific population. This test is used to evaluate change in gross motor function, not quality of movement, in children with cerebral palsy. The GMFM has recently also been validated for children with Down syndrome (Russell et al., 1998).

In addition to determining the developmental and functional abilities of children, it is frequently important to determine their sensory processing/integration. The ability of our senses to work together is critical for the production of coordinated movement. Several tests that evaluate visual perception and visual motor skills are also included in Box 2.2 and Appendix 2.B.

Another aspect of child appraisal that should be part of any examination and evaluation is an assessment of pain. **Pain** has been called the fifth vital sign (American Pain Society, 1995), and its assessment is required under JCAHO Standard PE.1.1.10. Pain should be assessed in addition to the vital signs of pulse, blood pressure, core temperature, and respiration. Pain must be assessed for each child. Children with the same tissue damage will experience different levels of pain. The nature of the child's pain includes cognitive, behavioral; and emotional factors as outlined by McGrath (1995). Cognitive factors include the child's understanding of the source of the pain, ability to control what happened, and expectations regarding the pain. Behavioral factors include the child's overt actions such as crying, the response of parents and others, use of restraint, and the implications of the pain/injury in the child's life. The emotional factors include the ability to understand and cope with what has happened. All these factors have an impact on the child's perception of pain.

The assessment of a child's pain depends on the age and cognitive ability of the child. For infants and preverbal or nonverbal children, behavioral observation scales are used such as the Riley Infant Pain Scale (Schare, Joyce, Gerkensmeyer, & Keck, 1996). A number of pain intensity scales have been developed in which the child indicates perception of pain on a visual analog scale or selects a picture that best describes the pain level (Appendix 2.B). Self-report of pain is considered the "gold standard" of pain assessment (McGrath, 1995). Based on the level of pain indicated, appropriate pain management should be initiated by the child's medical team. Pain can significantly influence physical therapy intervention, and its management must be carefully monitored.

Another area of evaluation that should be considered is the child's perceived quality of life (QOL) and global measures of health-related outcomes for children. QOL closely parallels the ICF classification of participation. There are numerous myths about the QOL of individuals with disabilities, and an accurate understanding of a specific child's QOL and health-related outcomes is important. The number of QOL and health-related outcome measures for children is not as extensive as those for adults, but the number and quality are increasing (Lollar, Simeonsson, & Nanda, 2000) and several are listed in Appendix 2.B. In addition, a number of functional measures are consid-

BOX 2.2 Tests and Measures of Development, Function, Sensory Integration, Pain, and Quality of Life by Category*

Developmental Tests and Measures

- Ages & Stages Questionnaire (ASQ), 2nd ed.
- Alberta Infant Motor Scale (AIMS) and Motor Assessment of the Developing Infant
- Assessment, Evaluation, and Programming System (AEPS) for Infants and Children
- Battelle Developmental Inventory (BDI)
- Bayley Scales of Infant Development-II (BSID-II) and Bayley Infant Neurodevelopmental Screener (BINS)
- Brigance Inventory of Early Development, Revised Edition
- Bruininks Oseretsky Test of Motor Proficiency (BOTMP)
- The Carolina Curriculum for Infants and Toddlers with Special Needs (CCITSM), 2nd ed.
- Carolina Curriculum for Preschoolers with Special Needs (CPSN), 2nd ed.
- Denver Developmental Screening Test—II
- Developmental Hand Dysfunction, 2nd ed.
- Developmental Observation Checklist System (DOCS)
- Developmental Programming for Infants and Young Children—Revised (DPIYC)
- Firststep: Screening Test for Evaluating Preschoolers (FirstSTEP)
- The Infanib
- Inside the Hawaii Early Learning Profile (HELP)
- Merrill-Palmer Scale—Revised
- Motor Skills Acquisition in the First Year and Checklist
- Movement Assessment Battery for Children (MOVE-MENT ABC)
- Movement Assessment of Infants (MAI)
- Milani-Comparetti Motor Development Screening Test (MC), 3rd ed.
- Miller Assessment of Preschoolers (MAP)
- Neonatal Behavioral Assessment Scale (NBAS)
- Neonatal Individualized Developmental Care and Assessment Program (NIDCAP)
- Neurological Assessment of the Preterm and Full-term Born Infant (NAPFI)
- Neurological Exam of the Full Term Infant

- Peabody Development Motor Scales (PDMS-2), 2nd ed.
- Posture and Fine Motor Assessment of Infants
- Scales of Independent Behavior—Revised (SIB-R)
- Test of Gross Motor Development—2 (TGMD2)
- Test of Infant Motor Performance (TIMP)
- The T.I.M.E. Toddler and Infant Motor Evaluation
- Transdisciplinary Play-Based Assessment (TPBA)
- Vulpe Assessment Battery—Revised (VAB-R)

Functional Tests and Measures

- ABILITIES Index
- Canadian Occupational Performance Measure (COPM)
- Gross Motor Function Measure (GMFM)
- Pediatric Evaluation of Disability Inventory (PEDI)
- School Function Assessment (SFA)
- WEEFIM: Functional Independence Measure for Children

Sensory Integration Tests and Measures

- Clinical Observations of Motor and Postural Skills (COMPS), 2nd ed.
- Degangi-Berk Test of Sensory Integration (TSI)
- Developmental Test of Visual-Motor Integration (VMI-4), 4th ed.
- Developmental Test of Visual Perception (DTVP-2), 2nd ed.
- Sensory Integration and Praxis Tests (SIPT)
- Sensory Profile and Infant/Toddler Sensory Profile
- Test of Sensory Function in Infants (TSFI)
- Test of Visual—Motor Skills-Revised (TVMS-R)

Pain Scales

- Faces Pain Scale
- Oucher Scale
- Riley Infant Pain Scale
- Visual Analog Scale

Quality of Life/Health-Related Outcomes

- Child Health and Illness Profile—Adolescent Edition (CHIP-AE)
- Child Health Questionnaire (CHQ)
- POSNA Pediatric Musculoskeletal Functional Health Questionnaire
- Quality of Well-Being Scale (QWB)
- Youth Quality of Life Instrument—Research Version (YQOL-R)

---

*Information on each test can be found in Appendix 2.B.

ered indicators of health-related outcomes such as the SFA, Functional Independence Measure for Children (WeeFIM), and Pediatric Evaluation of Disability Inventory (Lollar et al., 2000).

Intervention and Plan of Care

As discussed in Chapter 1 and throughout the remainder of this text, intervention is based on the goals and desires of the child and family and on outcomes of the examination and evaluation. Intervention should not be predetermined based on assumptions about specific diagnoses. Every child presents with individual needs, and only after a thorough examination and evaluation can a plan of care and intervention be started. For some children with certain diagnoses, the plan of care might be very similar and based on a clinical pathway/guideline. However, based on individual variations and circumstances, intervention plans might be very different for children with the same diagnosis. Common impairments in body structure and function are more likely to require similar interventions than a broad diagnostic label. For that reason, this text is organized around the functioning of body systems and not diagnoses. Once the impairments in body structures and function in each of the systems are identified, along with restrictions in activities and participation, then an appropriate plan of care for intervention can be determined for an individual child. Children with disabilities generally present with complex problems involving many systems, all of which must be considered for intervention. Interventions for impairment of body systems are presented in each of the chapters of Section 2, along with interventions to improve limitations or restrictions in activities and participation.

Infants and toddlers who present with delay in development and no specific impairment in body structures and functions might have the most straightforward plan of care. They might need to learn the next level of skill in the developmental sequence. The therapist and parents would work on encouraging the performance and practice of that task. Whether it is better to break down the task into component parts or to teach the entire task at the same time is task dependent. This issue of whole or part practice is discussed in Chapter 7. Strict adherence to a developmental sequence is not appropriate, but as years of intervention by master clinicians has supported, it can be a useful frame of reference with face validity, especially for young children with no impairments of body structure and function. On the other hand, for usually older children who have had the time and opportunity to achieve developmental milestones and have not, achievement of functional skills in the natural environment is far more critical than achieving developmental milestones. Intervention for these older children should focus on achieving a specific motor skill that is important for the child's activity functioning. The older child, who has not achieved most motor milestones or has lost the ability to perform those milestones due to a disease process, probably has neuromotor dysfunction and the interventions discussed in Chapter 7 should be considered.

Summary

Maturational theory has provided us with important information regarding common, although not invariant, sequences of development in all domains. Our genetic base provides a foundation for our development, and the environment provides the stimulus and setting in which to learn and develop. Behavioral theory provides an understanding of our behavior and cognitive theory provides information on the process of development and learning. Dynamic systems theory is helping to reshape our intervention strategies for children with disabilities by emphasizing the interdependence and importance of all body systems.

The theories of development help us to shape our thinking regarding expectations in child development and to understand deviations in development, and thus influence our interventions. We need to recognize the importance of the preconception, prenatal, neonatal, infant's, and child's environment on all aspects of development. Environment is especially important for children with disabilities because they are frequently dependent on others for many environmental experiences. We must understand and appreciate the importance of the environment and use the opportunities afforded through enriched environments to maximize the child's learning and functioning.

The study of child development is a dynamic, ongoing process. To fully appreciate the complexity of development there are courses and excellent texts available. Physical therapists must not only be experts in motor development but also understand the overall development of a child and family dynamics to be able to perform a thorough examination and provide appropriate and effective intervention.

The examination of development, function, and sensory integration of children is exciting and challenging. The examination process with children is not easy and requires creativity and flexibility on the part of the therapist. A careful, comprehensive initial examination is mandatory. We must perform developmental and functional tests and measures of activities along with more traditional tests and measures of body structures and functions. Our goals, outcomes, and objectives should be based on the desires of the parents and child. The examination and evaluation lead to the diagnostic process, prognosis, plan of care, intervention, and outcomes. The specific examinations and interventions for each body system are presented separately in the major chapters of this text; however, children frequently have involvement of more than one system and require coordinated intervention to address impairments of body functions and structures of each system and restrictions in activities and participation. The separation of systems into chapters in this text is necessary for organizational purposes, but the child must be considered as a whole, with an understanding and appreciation that all systems interact at all times and that development is context dependent.

DISCUSSION QUESTIONS

1. What are the theories presently guiding physical therapy interventions? Why are they important to intervention?

2. Describe the most common features of the gait pattern of early walkers.

3. Why is knowledge of the customary sequence of early motor development important if there is so much variation in the sequence?

4. Discuss the criteria you would use to select a developmental test to administer to a child.

5. At a neighborhood get-together, several mothers ask you if their children are developing normally. What skills would you expect to see in infants at 4, 6, 9, or 12 months of age?

6. What are some of the limitations in body structures and functions and restrictions in activities that might indicate atypical motor development throughout the first year of life, besides minor delay in skill acquisition?

RECOMMENDED READINGS

Bailey, D.B., Bruer, J.T., Symons, F.J., & Lichtman, J.W. (Eds.). (2001). *Critical thinking about critical periods.* Baltimore: Paul H. Brookes.

Batshaw, M.L. (Ed.). (2002). *Children with disabilities* (5th ed.). Baltimore: Paul H. Brookes.

Bly, L. (1994). *Motor skills acquisition in the first year: An illustrated guide to normal movement.* San Antonio, TX: Therapy Skill Builders.

Cech, D.J., & Martin, S.T. (2002). *Functional movement development across the life span* (2nd ed.). Philadelphia: W.B. Saunders.

REFERENCES

Abrams, E.J., Matheson, P.B., Thomas, P.A., Thea, D.M., Krasinski, K., Lambert, G., et al. (1995). Neonatal predictors of infection and status and early death among 332 infants at risk of HIV-1 infection monitored prospectively from birth. *Pediatrics, 96,* 451–458.

Adolph, K. (2003). Advances in research on infant motor development. Paper presented at American Physical Therapy Association Combined Sections Meeting 2003, Tampa, FL (Cassette Recording No. CSM03-122). Englewood, CO: Sound Images. Handouts retrieved February 20, 2003, from *http://apta.org*

Adolph, K., & Avolio, A. (2000). Walking infants adapt locomotion to changing body dimensions. *Journal of Experimental Psychology: Human Perception and Performance, 26*(3), 1148–1166.

Adolph, K., Vereijken, B., & Denny, M.A. (1998). Learning to crawl. *Child Development, 69*(5), 1299–1312.

Alberto, P.A., & Troutman, A.C. (2002). *Applied behavior analysis for teachers* (6th ed.). Englewood Cliffs, NJ: Merrill.

American Academy of Pediatrics (AAP), Committee on Nutrition (1998). *Pediatric nutrition handbook.* Elk Grove Village, IL: Author.

American Academy of Pediatrics (AAP), Task Force on Infant Positioning and SIDS (1992). Positioning and SIDS. *Pediatrics, 89*(6 Pt 1), 1120–1126.

American Pain Society (1995). *Pain: The fifth vital sign.* Glenview, IL: Author

American Physical Therapy Association (APTA) (2001). Guide to physical therapist practice (2nd ed.). *Physical Therapy, 81*(1).

Bailey, D.B., Bruer, J.T., Symons, F.J., & Lichtman, J.W. (Eds.). (2001). *Critical thinking about critical periods.* Baltimore: Paul H. Brookes.

Bailey, D.B., & Symons, F.J. (2001). Critical periods. In D.B. Bailey, J.T. Bruer, F.J. Symons, & J.W. Lichtman (Eds). *Critical thinking about critical periods* (pp. 289–292). Baltimore: Paul H. Brookes.

Bailey, D.B., & Wolery, M. (1992). *Teaching infants and preschoolers with disabilities* (2nd ed.). New York: Merrill.

Bandura, A. (2002). Social cognitive theory in cultural context. *Applied Psychology: An International Review, 51(2),* 269–290.

Barnhart, H.X., Caldwell, M.B., Thomas, P., Mascola, L., Ortiz, I., Hsu, H., et al. (1996). Natural history of human immunodeficiency virus disease in perinatally infected children: An analysis from the pediatric spectrum of disease project. *Pediatrics, 97,* 710–716.

Batshaw, M.L. (2002). Chromosomes and heredity. In M.L. Batshaw (Ed.). *Children with disabilities* (5th ed.) (pp. 3–26). Baltimore: Paul H. Brookes.

Bayley, N. (1993). *Bayley Scales of Infant Development* (2nd ed.). San Antonio, TX: Psychological Corp.

Bayley, N. (1936). *The California Infant Scale of Motor Development.* Berkeley: University of California.

Behrman, R.E., Kliegman, R.M., & Arvin, A.M. (1996). *Nelson textbook of pediatrics* (15th ed.). Philadelphia: W.B. Saunders.

Bernstein, N. (1967). *The coordination and regulation of movement.* London: Pergamon Press.

Bly, L. (1994). *Motor skills acquisition in the first year: An illustrated guide to normal development.* San Antonio, TX: Therapy Skill Builders.

Bobath. K. (1980). The neurophysiological basis for the treatment of cerebral palsy. *Clinics in Developmental Medicine,* No. 75, Philadelphia: J.B. Lippincott.

Bobath, K., & Bobath, B. (1984). The neuro-developmental treatment. In D. Scrutton (Ed.). *Management of the motor disorders of children with cerebral palsy* (pp. 6–18). Philadelphia: J.B. Lippincott.

Bowe, F.G. (1995). *Birth to five: Early childhood special education.* New York: Delmar Publishers.

Brenneman, S.K. (1999). Assessment and testing of infant and child development. In J.S. Tecklin (Ed.). *Pediatric physical therapy* (3rd ed.) (pp. 28–70). Philadelphia: Lippincott Williams & Wilkins.

Bronfenbrenner, U. (1995). The bioecological model from a life course perspective. In P. Moen, G.H. Elder, & K. Lusher (Eds.). *Examining lives in context.* Washington, DC: American Psychological Association.

Bruer, J.T. (2001). A critical and sensitive period primer. In D.B. Bailey, J.T. Bruer, F.J. Symons, & J.W. Lichtman (Eds). *Critical thinking about critical periods* (pp. 1–26). Baltimore: Paul H. Brookes.

Buchanan, J.J., & Horak, F. B. (2001). Transition in a postural task: Do the recruitment and suppression of degrees of freedom stabilize posture? *Experimental Brain Research, 139,* 482–494.

Buysse, V., & Bailey, D.B. (1993). Behavioral and developmental outcomes in young children with disabilities in integrated and segregated settings: A review of comparative studies. *The Journal of Special Education, 26,* 434–461.

Campbell, P.H. (1991). Evaluation and assessment in early intervention for infants and toddlers. *Journal of Early Intervention, 15,* 36–45.

Campbell, S.K., Vander Linden, S.W., & Palisano, R.J. (Eds.). (2000). *Physical therapy for children* (2nd ed.). Philadelphia: W.B. Saunders.

Capute, A.J., Shapiro, B.K., Palmer, F.B., Ross, A., & Wachtel, R.C. (1985). Normal gross motor development: The influences of race, sex and socio-economic status. *Developmental Medicine and Child Neurology, 27,* 635–643.

Case, R. (1992). Potential contributions of neo-Piagetian theory to the art and science of instruction. In M. Carretero, M. Pope, R.J. Simons, & J.I. Pozo, *Learning and instruction: European research in an international context* (pp. 1–25). Elmsford, NY: Pergamon Press.

Case, R., Griffin, S., & Kelly, W.M. (2001). Socioeconomic differences in children's early cognitive development and their readiness for schooling (pp. 37–63). In S. Golbeck (Ed.). *Psychological perspectives on early childhood education: Reframing dilemmas in research and practice.* Mahwah, NJ: Lawrence Erlbaum Associates.

Case-Smith, J. (Ed.) (2001). *Occupational therapy for children* (4th ed.). St. Louis: Mosby.

Centers for Disease Control and Prevention (2003). National Center for Health Statistics, National Health and Nutrition Examination Survey, CDC 2000 Growth Charts. Retrieved March 11, 2003, from *http://www.cdc.gov/nchs/about/major/nhanes/growthcharts/clinical_charts.htm*

Center on Addiction and Substance Abuse (1996). *Substance abuse and the American woman.* New York: Columbia University.

Center on Addiction and Substance Abuse (2003). *The formative years: Pathways to substance abuse among young women ages 8–22* (pp 32–33). New York: Columbia University.

Charles, J., Lavinder, G., & Gordon, A. M. (2001). Effects of constraint-induced therapy on hand function in children with hemiplegic cerebral palsy. *Pediatric Physical Therapy, 13(2),* 68–76.

Chattin-McNichols, J. (1992). *The Montessori controversy.* Albany, NY: Delmar.

Children's Defense Fund (2003). *State of children in the states.* Retrieved March 20, 2003, from *http://www.childrensdefense.org*

Coster, W., Deeney, T., Haltiwanger, J., & Haley, S. (1998). *School Function Assessment.* San Antonio, TX: The Psychological Corporation.

Cronk, C., Crocker, A.C., Pueschel, S.M., Shea, A.M., Zackai, E., Pickens, G., et al. (1988). Growth charts for children with Down's syndrome: 1 Month to 18 years of age. *Pediatrics, 81,* 102–110.

Cunningham, A.S., Jelliffe, D.B., & Jelliffe, E.F.P. (1991). Breast feeding and health in the 1980s: A global epidemiologic review. *Journal of Pediatrics, 118,* 659–666.

David, T.B., & Weinstein, C.S. (1987). The built environment and children's development. In C.S. Weinstein & T.C. David (Eds.). *Spaces for children: The built environment and child development* (pp. 3–18). New York: Plenum Press.

Davis, B.E., Moon, R.Y., Sachs, H.C., & Ottolini, M.C. (1998). Effects of sleep position on infant motor development. *Pediatrics, 102(5),* 1135–1140.

DeVellis, R.F. (1977). Learned helplessness in institutions. *Mental Retardation, 15(5),* 10–13.

Dewey, C., Fleming, P., Golding, J., & the ALSPAC Study Team. (1998). Does the supine sleeping position have any adverse effects on the child? II. Development in the first 18 months. *Pediatrics, 101*(1), 1–5.

Diamond, K.E., & Carpenter, E.S. (2000). Participation in inclusive preschool programs and sensitivity to the needs of others. *Journal of Early Intervention, 23*(2), 81–91.

Dudgeon, B.J., Jaffe, K.M., & Shurtleff, D.B. (1991). Variations in midlumbar myelomeningocele: Implications for ambulation. *Pediatric Physical Therapy, 3*, 57–62.

Echols, K., DeLuca, S.C., Taub, E., & Ramey, S. (2000). Constraint-induced movement therapy in young children: A protocol and outcomes compared to traditional measures [Abstract]. *Pediatric Physical Therapy, 12*, 210.

Edwards, C., Gandini, L., & Forman, G. (Eds.) (1993). *The hundred languages of children: The Reggio Emilia approach to early childhood education.* Norwood, NJ: Ablex Publishing.

Effgen, S.K. (2001). Occurrence of gross motor behaviors in US preschools and conductive education preschools in Hong Kong. *Physical Therapy, 81*: A78.

Elman, J., Bates, E., Johnson, M., Karmiloff-Smith, A., Parisi, D., & Plunkett, K. (1997). *Rethinking innateness.* Cambridge, MA: The MIT Press.

Erhardt, R.P. (1982). *Developmental hand dysfunction: Theory, assessment, treatment.* Lauren, MD: RAMSCO.

Fadiman, A. (1997). *The spirit catches you and you fall down.* New York: The Noonday Press.

Farran, D.C. (2001). Critical periods and early intervention. In D.B. Bailey, J.T. Bruer, F.J. Symons, & J.W. Lichtman (Eds). *Critical thinking about critical periods* (pp. 233–266). Baltimore: Paul H. Brookes.

Fewell, R.R., & Glick, M.P. (1996). Program evaluation findings of an intensive early intervention program. *American Journal of Mental Retardation, 101*(3), 233–243.

Fidler, G.S., & Fidler, J.W. (1978). Doing and becoming: Purposeful action and self-actualization. *American Journal of Occupational Therapy, 32*, 305–310.

Fiorentino, M.R. (1963). *Reflex testing methods for evaluating C.N.S. development.* Springfield, IL: Charles C Thomas.

Fiorentino, M.R. (1981). *A basis for sensorimotor development—Normal and abnormal.* Springfield, IL: Charles C Thomas.

Fiscus, S.A., Adimora, A.A., Funk, M.L., Schoenbach, V.J., Tristram, D., Lim, W., McKinney, R., Rupar, D., Woods, C., & Wilfert, C. (2002). Trends in interventions to reduce perinatal human immunodeficiency virus type 1 transmission in North Carolina. *The Journal of Pediatric Infectious Disease, 21* (7), 664–668.

Folio, M.R., & Fewell, R.R. (2000). *Peabody Developmental Motor Scales* (PDMS-2). Austin, TX: Pro-ed.

Fried, P.A., Watkinson, B., & Gray, R. (1998). Differential effects on cognitive functioning in 9–12-year-olds prenatally exposed to cigarettes and marihuana. *Neurotoxicology and Teratology, 20*, 293–306.

Fried, P.A., Watkinson, B., & Gray, R. (1999). Growth from birth to early adolescence in offspring prenatally exposed to cigarettes and marijuana. *Neurotoxicology and Teratology, 21*, 513–525.

Gallahue, D.L., & Ozmun, J.C. (1995). *Understanding motor development: Infants, children, adolescents, adults.* Madison, WI: Brown & Benchmark.

Gesell, A. (1928). *Infancy and human growth.* New York: Macmillan.

Gesell, A. (1945). *The embryology of behavior* (p. 169). New York: Harper.

Gesell, A. (1949). *Gesell developmental scales.* New York: Psychological Corp.

Gesell, A. (1952). *Infant development.* Westport, CT: Greenwood Press.

Gesell, A., & Amatruda, C.S. (1947). *Developmental diagnosis: Normal and abnormal child development, clinical methods and pediatric applications.* New York: Harper & Row.

Gesell, A., & Thompson, H. (1934). *Infant behavior: Its genesis and growth.* New York: McGraw-Hill.

Giangreco, M.E., Dennis, R., Cloninger, C.J., Edelman, S., & Schattman, R. (1993). "I've counted Jon": Transformational experiences of teachers educating students with disabilities. *Exceptional Children, 59*, 359–372.

Goldschmidt, L., Day, N.L., & Richardson, G.A. (2000). Effects of prenatal marijuana exposure on child behavior problems at age 10. *Neurotoxicology and Tetralogy, 22*, 325–336.

Guralnick, M.J. (1999). The nature and meaning of social integration for young children with mild developmental delays in inclusive settings. *Journal of Early Intervention, 22*, 70–86.

Guralnick, M.J. (2001). *Early childhood inclusion: Focus on change.* Baltimore: Paul H. Brookes.

Halverson, H.M. (1931). An experimental study of prehension in infants by means of systematic cinema records. *Genetic Psychology Monographs, 10*, 107–286.

Harris, J.R. (1998). *The nurture assumption: Why children turn out the way they do.* New York: Free Press.

Havighurst, R.J. (1972). *Developmental tasks and education* (3rd ed.). New York: David McKay Company, Inc.

Heriza, C. (1991). Motor development: Traditional and contemporary theories. In M. Lister (Ed.). *Contemporary management of motor control problems. Proceedings of the II Step Conference* (pp. 99–126). Alexandria, VA: Foundation for Physical Therapy.

Hill, J.B., & Haffner, W.H.J. (2002). Growth before birth. In M.L. Batshaw (Ed.). *Children with disabilities* (5th ed.) (pp. 43–53). Baltimore: Paul H. Brookes.

Horak, F.B. (1991). Assumptions underlying motor control for neurologic rehabilitation. In M. Lister (Ed.). *Contemporary Management of motor control problems. Proceedings of the II Step Conference* (pp. 11–27). Alexandria, VA: Foundation for Physical Therapy.

Hubel, D.H., & Wiesel, T.N. (1970). The period of susceptibility to the physiological effects of unilateral eye closure in kittens. *Journal of Physiology, 206*, 419–436.

Human Rights and Equal Opportunity Commission (2003). Goward applauds introduction of 12 weeks paid parental leave in New Zealand. Retrieved April 10, 2003, from *http://www.hreoc.gov.au/media releases/2002/4102.html*

Hunt, P., Doering, K., Hirose-Hatae, A., Maie J., & Goetz, L. (2001). Across-program collaboration to support students with and without disabilities in a general education classroom. *Journal for the Association for Persons with Severe Handicaps, 26,* 240–256.

Hunt, P., Soto, G., Maier, J., & Doering, K. (2003). Collaborative teaming to support students at risk and students with severe disabilities in general education classrooms. *Exceptional Children, 69*(3), 315–332.

Individuals with Disabilities Education Act Amendments of 1997, PL 105–17, 20 U.S.C. §§1400 et seq.

Jacobson, J.L., & Jacobson, S.W. (1994). Prenatal alcohol exposure and neurobehavioral development: Where is the threshold? *Alcohol Health and Research World, 18,* 30–36.

Jantz, J.W., Blosser, C.D., & Fruechting, L.A. (1997). A motor milestone change noted with a change in sleep position. *Archives of Pediatrics and Adolescent Medicine, 151,* 565–568.

Jones, K.L. (1997). *Smith's recognizable patterns of human malformation* (5th ed.). Philadelphia: W.B. Saunders.

Kelso, J.A.S., & Tuller, B. (1984). A dynamical basis for action systems. In M. Gassaniga (Ed.). *Handbook of cognitive neuroscience.* New York: Plenum Press.

Knobloch, H., & Pasamanick, B. (Eds.) (1974). *Gesell and Amatruda's manual of developmental diagnosis* (3rd ed.). New York: Harper & Row Publishing.

Krick, J., Murphy-Miller, P., Zeger, S., & Wright, E. (1996). Patterns of growth in children with cerebral palsy. *Journal of the American Dietetic Association, 96,* 680–685.

Lee, M. (1998). Substance abuse in pregnancy. *Obstetrics and Gynecology Clinics, 25,* 65–83.

Li, C.Q., Windsor, R.A. Perkins, I., Goldenberg, R.L., & Lowe, J.B. (1993). The impact on infant birth weight and gestational age of cotinine-validated smoking reduction during pregnancy. *Journal of the American Medical Association, 269,* 1519–1524.

Long, T.M., & Toscano, K. (2002). *Handbook of pediatric physical therapy* (2nd ed.). Philadelphia: Lippincott Williams & Wilkins.

Lollar, D.J., Simeonsson, R.J., & Nanda, U. (2000). Measures of outcomes for children and youth. *Archives of Physical Medicine and Rehabilitation, 81*(12), 46–52.

Low, S.M. (1984). The cultural basis of health, illness and disease. *Social Work in Health Care, 9*(3), 13–23.

McEwen, I.R. (2000). Children with cognitive impairments. In S.K. Campbell, D.W. Vander Linden, & R.J. Palisano (Eds.). *Physical therapy for children* (2nd ed., pp. 502–532). Philadelphia: W.B. Saunders.

McGrath, P.A. (1995). Pain in the pediatric patient: Practical aspects of assessment. *Pediatric Annals, 24*(3), 126–138.

McGraw, M.B. (1932). From reflex to muscular control in the assumption of erect posture and ambulation in the human infant. *Child Development, 3,* 291–297.

McGraw, M.B. (1935). *Growth: A study of Johnny and Jimmy.* New York: Appleton-Century.

McGraw, M.B. (1945). *The neuromuscular maturation of the human infant.* New York: Columbia University Press.

McKusick, V.A. (1994). *Mendelian inheritance in man: Catalogs of autosomal dominant, autosomal recessive, and X-linked phenotypes* (11th ed.). Baltimore: Johns Hopkins University Press.

Michels, K.B., Trichopoulos, D., Robins, J.M., Rosner, B.A., Manson, J.E., Hunter, D.J., et al. (1996). Birthweight as a risk factor for breast cancer. *Lancet, 348*(9041), 1542–1546.

Milani-Comparetti, A., & Gidoni, E.A. (1967). Routine developmental examination in normal and retarded children. *Developmental Medicine and Child Neurology, 9,* 631–638.

Mildred, J., Beard, K., Dallwitz, A., & Unwin, J. (1995). Play position is influenced by knowledge of SIDS sleep position recommendations. *Journal of Paediatric Child Health, 31,* 499–502.

Montessori, M. (1964). The *Montessori method.* New York: Schocken Books.

Morales, A.T., & Sheafor, B.W. (2001). *Social work* (9th ed.). Needham Heights, MA: Pearson Education.

Nathanielsz, P. (1999). *Life in the womb: The origins of health and disease.* Ithaca, NY: Promethean Press.

National Institute of Child Health and Human Development (2003). The NICH's 40th anniversary. Retrieved September 9, 2003, from *http://www.nichd.nih.gov/40th/*

Online Mendelian Inheritance in Man (2004). Retrieved May 31, 2004, from *http://www.ncbi.nlm.nih.gov/entrez/query.fcgi?bd=Omim/*

Ott, D.A.D., & Effgen, S.K. (2000). Occurrence of gross motor behaviors in integrated and segregated preschool classrooms. *Pediatric Physical Therapy, 12,* 164–172.

Palsha, S. (2002). An outstanding education for ALL children: Learning from Reggio Emilia's approach to inclusion. In V.R. Fu, A.J. Stemmel, & L.T. Hill (Eds.). *Teaching and learning: Collaborative exploration of the Reggio Emilia approach* (pp. 109–130). Upper Saddle River, NJ: Merrill Prentice Hall.

Patrick, K., Spear, B., Holt, K., & Sofka, D. (Eds.) (2001). *Bright futures in practice: Physical activity.* Arlington, VA: National Center for Education in Maternal and Child Health.

Peck, C.A., Donaldson, J., & Pezzoli, M. (1990). Some benefits nonhandicapped adolescents perceive for themselves from their social relationships with peers who have severe handicaps. *Journal of the Association for Persons with Severe Handicaps, 15,* 241–249.

Peiper, A. (1963). *Cerebral function in infancy and childhood.* New York: Consultants' Bureau.

Piaget, J. (1952). *The origins of intelligence in children.* New York: International University Press.

Piper, M.C., & Darrah, J. (1994). *Motor assessment of the developing infant.* Philadelphia: W.B. Saunders.

QOLID (2003). Quality of life instruments database. Retrieved April 4, 2003, from *http://www.qolid.org*

Raine, A., Reynolds, C., Venables, P.H., & Mednick, S. (2002). Stimulation seeking and intelligence: A prospective longitudinal study. *Journal of Personality and Social Psychology, 82*(4), 663–674.

Reznick, J.S. (2000). Biology versus experience: Balancing the equation. *Developmental Science, 3,* 133–134.

Rich-Edwards, J.W., Stampfer, M.J., Manson, J.E., Rosner, B., Hankinson, S.E., Colditz, G.A., Willett, W.C., & Hennekens, C.H. (1997). Birthweight and risk of cardiovascular disease in a cohort of women followed up since 1976. *British Medical Journal, 315*(7105), 396–400.

Rossetti, L. (1990). *The Rossetti Infant-Toddler Language Scale.* East Moline, IL: Lingui Systems, Inc.

Russell, D., Palisano, R., Walter, S., Rosenbaum, P., Gemus, M., Gowland, C., Galuppi, B., & Lane, M. (1998). Evaluating motor function in children with Down syndrome: Validity of the GMFM. *Developmental Medicine and Child Neurology, 40,* 693–701.

Russell, D., Rosenbaum, P., Avery, L., & Lane, M. (2002). Gross Motor Function Measure (GMFM-66 & GMFM-88) User's Manual. *Clinics in Developmental Medicine, No. 159,* London, England: MacKeith Press.

Sanger, W.G., Dave, B., & Stuberg, W. (2001). Overview of genetics and role of the pediatric physical therapist in diagnostic process. *Pediatric Physical Therapy, 13,* 164–168.

Santrock, J.W. (1998). *Child development* (8th ed., pp. 35–71). Boston: McGraw-Hill.

Scalise-Smith, D., & Bailey, D. (1992). Facilitating motor skills. In D.B. Bailey & M. Wolery (Eds.). *Teaching infants and preschoolers with disabilities* (2nd ed.). New York: Merrill.

Schaefer, G.B. (2001). Clinical genetics in pediatric physical therapy practice? The future. *Pediatric Physical Therapy, 13,* 182–184.

Schare, J., Joyce, B., Gerkensmeyer, J., & Keck, J. (1996). Comparison of three preverbal scales for postoperative pain assessment in a diverse pediatric sample. *Journal of Pain and Symptom Management, 12*(6), 348–359.

Schickendanz, J., Schickendanz, D., Hansen, K., & Forsyth, P.D. (1993). *Understanding children.* Mountain View, CA: Mayfield Publishing.

Scholz, J.P. (1990). Dynamic pattern theory—Some implications for therapeutics. *Physical Therapy, 70*(12), 827–843.

Seifert, K.L., & Hoffnung, R.J. (1997). *Child and adolescent development* (4th ed., pp. 29–55). New York: Houghton Mifflin Co.

Seligman, M.E.P. (1975). *Helplessness: On depression, development, and death.* San Francisco: W.H. Freeman.

Sherrill, C. (1993). *Adapted physical activity, recreation and sport: Cross disciplinary and life span* (Chapters 5, 10, 11, and 12). Dubuque, IA: W.C. Brown.

Shirley, M.M. (1931). *The first two years: A study of twenty-five babies,* Vol. I. Minneapolis: University of Minnesota Press.

Shumway-Cook, A., & Woolacott, M. (2001). *Motor control theory and practical applications* (2nd ed.). Philadelphia: Lippincott Williams & Wilkins.

Skinner, B.F. (1953). Science and human behavior. New York: Macmillan.

Soto, G., Muller, E., Hunt, P., & Goetz, L. (2001). Critical issues in the inclusion of students who use AAC: An educational team perspective. *Augmentative and Alternative Communication, 17*(3), 62–72.

Statham, L., & Murray M. (1971). Early walking patterns of normal children. *Clinical Orthopaedics and Related Research, 79,* 8–24.

Steinberger, J., & Daniels, S.R. (2003). Obesity, insulin resistance, diabetes, and cardiovascular risk in children: An American Heart Association scientific statement from the Atherosclerosis, Hypertension, and Obesity in the Young Committee (Council on Cardiovascular Disease in the Young), and the Diabetes Committee (Council on Nutrition, Physical Activity, and Metabolism). *Circulation, 107*(10), 1448–1453.

Steinhausen, H., Metzke, C.W., & Spohr, H. (2003). Behavioral phenotype in foetal alcohol syndrome and foetal alcohol effects. *Developmental Medicine and Child Neurology, 45,* 179–182.

Stewart, K.B. (2001). Purposes, processes and methods of evaluation. In J. Case-Smith (Ed.). *Occupational therapy for children* (4th ed.) (pp. 190–213). St. Louis: Mosby.

Sutherland, D., Olshen, R., Biden, E., & Wyatt, M. (1988). The development of mature gait. *Clinics in Developmental Medicine,* No. 104/105. Philadelphia: J.B. Lippincott.

Taub, E., & Morris, D.M. (2001). Constraint-induced movement therapy to enhance recovery after stroke. *Current Atherosclerosis Reports, 3,* 279–286.

Taub, E., & Wolf, S.L. (1997). Constraint-induced (CI) movement techniques to facilitate upper extremity use in stroke patients. *Topics in Stroke Rehabilitation, 3,* 38–61.

Taub, E., Uswatte, G., & Pidikiti, R. (1999). Constraint-induced movement therapy: A new family of techniques with broad application to physical rehabilitation—A clinical review. *Journal of Rehabilitation Research and Development, 36*(3), 237–251.

Thelen, E., Kelso, J.A., & Fogel, A. (1987). Self-organizing systems and infant motor development. *Developmental Review, 7,* 39–65.

Thelen, E., & Smith, L.B. (1994). *A dynamic systems approach to the development of cognition and action.* Cambridge, MA: The MIT Press.

Thelen, E., Ulrich, B.D., & Jensen, J.L. (1989). The developmental origins of locomotion. In M.H. Woollacott & A. Shumway-Cook (Eds.). *Development of posture and gait across the life span* (pp. 25–47). Columbia, SC: University of South Carolina Press.

Touwen, B. (1976). Neurological development in infancy. *Clinics in Developmental Medicine,* No. 58, Philadelphia: J.B. Lippincott.

World Health Organization (WHO) (2001). *International classification of functioning, disability and health.* Geneva: Author.

World Health Organization (WHO) (2003). ICF Checklist, version 2.1a, Clinician form. For *International classification of functioning, disability and health.* Geneva: Author. Retrieved on September 29, 2003, from *http://www.who.int/classification/icf*

Wunsch, M.J., Conlon, C.J., & Scheidt, P.C. (2002). Substance abuse. In M.L. Batshaw (Ed.). *Children with disabilities* (5th ed.) (pp. 107–122). Baltimore: Paul H. Brookes.

Appendix *2.A*

Activities and Participation (from *International Classification of Functioning, Disability and Health)*

Learning and Applying Knowledge (ICF Checklist: Shortlist of Activities and Participation Domains, WHO, 2003)
  Watching
  Listening
  Learning to read
  Learning to write
  Learning to calculate
  Solving problems

General Tasks and Demands (ICF Checklist: Shortlist of Activities and Participation Domains, WHO, 2003)
  Undertaking a single task
  Undertaking multiple tasks

Communication (ICF Checklist: Shortlist of Activities and Participation Domains, WHO, 2003)
  Communicating with–receiving–spoken messages
  Communicating with–receiving–nonverbal messages
  Speaking
  Producing nonverbal messages
  Conversation

Mobility (Complete list of Activities and Participations for Mobility from ICF, WHO, 2001, pp. 138–148)
  CHANGING AND MAINTAINING BODY POSITION
   Changing basic body positions
    Lying down
    Squatting
    Kneeling
    Sitting
    Standing
    Bending
    Shifting the body's center of gravity
    Changing basic body position, other specified
    Changing basic body position, unspecified
   Maintaining a body position
    Maintaining a lying position
    Maintaining a squatting position
    Maintaining a kneeling position
    Maintaining a sitting position
    Maintaining a standing position
    Maintaining a body position, other specified
    Maintaining a body position, unspecified
   Transferring oneself
    Transferring oneself while sitting
    Transferring oneself while lying
    Transferring oneself, other specified
    Transferring oneself, unspecified
   Changing and maintaining body position, other specified and unspecified

(Continued)

CARRYING, MOVING, AND HANDLING OBJECTS
   Lifting and carrying objects
      Lifting
      Carrying in the hands
      Carrying in the arms
      Carrying on shoulders, hip, and back
      Carrying on the head
      Putting down objects
      Lifting and carrying, other specified
      Lifting and carrying, unspecified
   Moving objects with lower extremities
      Pushing with lower extremities
      Kicking
      Moving objects with lower extremities, other specified
      Moving objects with lower extremities, unspecified
   Fine hand use
      Picking up
      Grasping
      Manipulating
      Releasing
      Fine hand use, other specified
      Fine hand use, unspecified
   Hand and arm use
      Pulling
      Pushing
      Reaching
      Turning or twisting the hands or arms
      Throwing
      Catching
      Hand and arm use, other specified
      Hand and arm use, unspecified
   Carrying, moving, and handling objects, other specified and unspecified
WALKING AND MOVING
Walking
   Walking short distances
   Walking long distances
   Walking on different surfaces
   Walking around obstacles
   Walking, other specified
   Walking, unspecified
Moving around
   Crawling
   Climbing
   Running
   Jumping
   Swimming
   Moving around, other specified
   Moving around, unspecified
Moving around in different locations
   Moving around within the home
   Moving around within buildings other than home
   Moving around outside the home and other buildings
   Moving around in different locations, other specified
   Moving around in different locations, unspecified
Moving around using equipment
Walking and moving, other specified and unspecified

MOVING AROUND USING TRANSPORTATION
Using transportation
Using human-powered vehicles
Using private motorized transportation
Using public transportation
Using transportation, other specified
Using transportation, unspecified
Driving
Driving human-powered transportation
Driving motorized vehicles
Driving animal-powered vehicles
Driving, other specified
Driving, unspecified
Riding animals for transportation
Moving around using transportation, other specified and unspecified
Mobility, other specified
Mobility, unspecified

Source: From World Health Organization (WHO) (2001). *International classification of functioning, disability and health*. Geneva: Author. and World Health Organization (WHO) (2003). ICF Checklist, version 2.1a, Clinician form. For *International classification of functioning, disability and health*. Geneva: Author. Retrieved on September 29, 2003, from *http://www.who.int/classification/icf*.

Appendix *2.B*

Tests and Measures of Development, Function, Sensory Integration, Pain, and Quality of Life

Test/Measure and Author/ Reference or Publisher	Age Range	Areas Tested	Primary Use
ABILITIES Index Simeonsson, R.J., Bailey, D., Smith, T., & Buyssee, V. (1995). Young children with disabilities: Functional assessment by teachers. *Journal of Developmental Physical Disabilities, 7,* 267–284.	36–69 months	Index of 9 domains: audition, behavior, intelligence, limbs, intentional communication, tonicity, integrity of health, eyes, and structure.	Documents the nature and extent of the functional characteristics of childhood disability. Has potential to identify discrete profiles of functional characteristics.
Ages & Stages Questionnaire (ASQ), 2nd ed. Diane Bricker, Jane Squires, and Linda Mounts *Paul H. Brookes Publishing Co.* *PO Box 10624* *Baltimore, MD 21285-0624*	4–60 months	Norm-referenced, standardized parent report of communication, gross motor, fine motor, problem-solving and personal-social development.	Screening tool to determine if areas require further testing. Encourages family participation, commonly used in Early Head Start programs.
Alberta Infant Motor Scale (AIMS) and Motor Assessment of the Developing Infant Martha Piper and Johanna Darrah *WB Saunders Co.* *The Curtis Center* *Independence Mall West* *Philadelphia, PA 19106*	Birth–18 months	Standardized observation of spontaneous gross motor skills in four positions: prone, supine, sitting, and standing.	Identifies infants and toddlers with gross motor delay and evaluates gross motor skill maturation.
Assessment, Evaluation, and Programming System (AEPS) for Infants and Children Diane Bricker *Paul H. Brookes Publishing Co.* *PO Box 10624* *Baltimore, MD 21285-0624*	1–36 months and 3–6 years	Criterion-referenced assessment done through observation of naturally occurring activities. Areas observed include fine motor, gross motor, cognitive, adaptive, social-communication, and social.	Identifies skill attainment and assist in program planning and monitoring of outcomes. No standard scores or age equivalents provided; it is linked to a curriculum.
Battelle Developmental Inventory (BDI) Jean Newborg, John Stock, Linda Wnek, John Guidubaldi, and John Svinicki *Riverside Publishing Co.* *8420 Bryn Mawr Avenue* *Chicago, IL 60631*	Birth–8 years	Norm-referenced, standardized assessment of personal-social, adaptive, motor, communication, and cognition skills completed by interview or observation. A screening tool is also available.	Commonly used tool to determine developmental delay or dysfunction in infants and young children for eligibility for early intervention services. Unfortunately, there are few items in each domain at each age level.

Test/Measure and Author/ Reference or Publisher	Age Range	Areas Tested	Primary Use
Bayley Scales of Infant Development-II (BSID-II) and Bayley Infant Neurodevelopmental Screener (BINS) Nancy Bayley *Psychological Corporation 19500 Bulverde Rd. San Antonio, TX 78259-3701*	1–42 months (BSID-II) 3–24 months (BINS)	Norm-referenced, standardized assessment of cognitive and motor development and criterion-referenced behavioral scale. Motor scale includes fine and gross motor function.	Commonly used assessment in early intervention and research to determine developmental delay. Requires training in assessment. BINS is a quick screening tool.
Brigance Inventory of Early Development, revised ed. Albert Brigance *Curriculum Associates 5 Esquire Road North Billerica, MA 01862-2589*	Birth–7 years	Criterion-referenced test of: psychomotor, self-help, speech and language, general knowledge and comprehension, early academic skills, and social-emotional development.	Commonly used assessment in early intervention and preschool programs to determine developmental delay in several domains and for program planning.
Bruininks Oseretsky Test of Motor Proficiency (BOTMP) Robert Bruininks *American Guidance Service Publisher's Bldg. PO Box 99 Circle Pines, MN 55014-1796*	4.5–14.5 years, mainly for children who are ambulatory	Norm-referenced, standardized test of gross and fine motor skills. Subscales for running speed and agility, balance, bilateral coordination, strength, upper limb coordination, response speed, visual-motor control, and upper limb speed and dexterity.	Common assessment tool for higher level motor skills and to evaluate motor training programs.
Canadian Occupational Performance Measure (COPM) Mary Law, Sue Baptiste, Anne Carswell, Mary Ann McCall, Helene Polatajko, and Nancy Pollock *CTTC Building, Suite 3400 1125 Colonel By Drive Ottawa, Ontario K1S 5RI*	All ages	Child identifies areas of concern regarding perception of self-care, productivity, and leisure occupations.	Functional, client-centered approach, especially useful with child or adolescent who is able to participate in program planning.
The Carolina Curriculum for Infants and Toddlers with Special Needs (CCITSN), 2nd ed. Nancy Johnson-Martin, Kenneth Jens, Susan Attermeier, and Bonnie Hacker *Paul H. Brookes Publishing Co. PO Box 10624 Baltimore, MD 21285-0624*	Birth–24 months, developmental range 2–5 years, developmental range	Criterion-referenced test of cognition, communication, social adaptation, and fine and gross motor skills.	Assesses infants, toddlers, and preschoolers with disabilities to determine developmental level and assist in curriculum planning. Not used for eligibility because there is no standardized score.
Child Health and Illness Profile—Adolescent Edition (CHIP-AE) Starfield, B., Berger, M., Ensminger, M., Riley, A., Ryan, S., Green, B., et al. (1993). Adolescent health status measurement: Development of the Child Health and Illness Profile. *Pediatrics, 91,* 430–435.	11–17 years	Self-administered questionnaire of health assessment. Domains covered: comfort, satisfaction with health, risk, disorder, achievement of social expectations, and resilience.	Detects differences in health status among children with chronic illness.

(Continued)

Test/Measure and Author/ Reference or Publisher	Age Range	Areas Tested	Primary Use
Child Health Questionnaire (CHQ) Jeanne Landgraf, Linda Abetz, and John Ware *Quality Metric Inc.* *640 George Washington Highway, Suite 201* *Lincoln, RI 02865*	2 months–5 years 5–15 years, Parents	Questionnaire covers concepts of physical functioning; bodily pain; limitations in schoolwork and activities due to behavioral difficulties; mental health; general behavior; and self-esteem.	Measures general health and emotional impact of the child's health on the parent and family activities.
Clinical Observations of Motor and Postural Skills, (COMPS), 2nd ed. Brenda Wilson, Nancy Pollack, Bonnie Kaplan, and Mary Law *Therapro* *225 Arlington Street* *Framingham, MA 01702-8723*	5–9 years	Tests subtle motor coordination during slow movements, arm rotation, finger-nose touching, prone extension posture, asymmetrical tonic neck reflex, and supine flexion posture.	Screens for subtle motor coordination problems.
DeGangi-Berk Test of Sensory Integration (TSI) Georgia DeGangi and Ronald Berk *Western Psychological Services* *12031 Wilshire Blvd.* *Los Angeles, CA 90025*	3–5 years	Criterion-referenced test of postural control, bilateral motor integration, and reflex integration.	Screens for sensory integration dysfunction in preschoolers.
Denver Developmental Screening Test—II William Frankenburg, Josiah Dodds, Phillip Archer, Beverly Bresnick, Patrick Maschka, Norman Edelman, and Howard Shapiro *Denver Developmental Materials, Inc.* *PO Box 6919* *Denver, CO 80206-0919*	1 week–6$\frac{1}{2}$ years	Norm-referenced, standardized test of development in: personal-social, fine motor-adaptive, language, gross motor, and behavior.	Commonly used screening test to determine developmental delay, although the specificity is weak and the sample population may be biased.
Developmental Hand Dysfunction, 2nd ed. Rhonda Erhardt *Therapy Skill Builders* *19500 Bulverde Rd.* *San Antonio, TX 78259-3701*	Birth–5 months	Criterion-referenced assessment of prehension including positional-reflexive, cognitively directed movement, and prewriting skills.	Used to determine delay or dysfunction in prehension skills, but without standardized scores. Useful tool in intervention planning.
Developmental Observation Checklist System (DOCS) Wayne P. Hresko, Shirley Miguel, Rita Sherbenou, and Steve Burton *PRO-ED, Inc.* *8700 Shoal Creek Blvd.* *Austin, TX 78757-6897*	Birth–6 years	Norm-referenced checklist covering language, motor, social, and cognitive development. Also includes adjustment behavior and parent stress and support.	Provides general developmental assessment.

Test/Measure and Author/ Reference or Publisher	Age Range	Areas Tested	Primary Use
Developmental Programming for Infants and Young Children—Revised (DPIYC) Sue Schafer, Martha Moersch, and Diane D'Eugenio *University of Michigan Press* *389 Green Street* *Ann Arbor, MI 48104*	0–36 months: Early Intervention Developmental Profile (EIDP) 36–60 months: Preschool Developmental Profile (PDP)	Criterion-referenced test of cognition, gross motor, fine motor, language, social-emotional, and self-care.	Used to describe the developmental status of a child with a disability across domains. Used for program planning, not to determine eligibility.
Developmental Test of Visual-Motor Integration (VMI-4), 4th ed. Keith Beery *PRO-ED, Inc.* *8700 Shoal Creek Blvd.* *Austin, TX 78757-6897*	3–8 years (short form) 3–18 years (long form)	Norm-referenced test of visual perception, motor coordination, and integration.	Easy test to determine problems in visual-motor integration important in writing and reading.
Developmental Test of Visual Perception (DTVP-2), 2nd ed. Donald Hammil, Nils Person, and Judith Voress *PRO-ED, Inc.* *8700 Shoal Creek Blvd.* *Austin, TX 78757-6897*	4–10 years	Norm-referenced test of form consistency, figure ground, position in space, and spatial relation.	Assists in distinguishing between problems in visual perception versus visual-motor problems.
Faces Pain Scale Bieri, D., Reeve, R., Addicoat, L., and Ziegler, J. (1990). The Faces Pain Scale for the self-assessment of the severity of pain experienced by children. *Pain, 41,* 139–150.	>6–8 years	Pain intensity rating scale using pictures of faces.	Measures self-reporting of pain intensity, although probably a better measure of child's emotional distress.
Firststep: Screening Test for Evaluating Preschoolers (FirstSTEP) Lucy Jane Miller *The Psychological Corporation* *19500 Bulverde Road* *San Antonio, TX 78259-3701*	2.9–6.2 years	Norm-referenced screening test of cognition, communication, motor, social-emotional, and adaptive behavior.	Determines delay in all developmental areas.
Gross Motor Function Measure (GMFM) Russell, D., Rosenbaum, P., Avery, L., & Lane, M. (2002). *Clinics in Developmental Medicine, No. 159,* London, England: MacKeith Press	5 months–16 years for children with cerebral palsy (probably best at 1–5 years)	Gross motor function along the dimensions of lying and rolling, sitting, crawling, standing, and walking, running, and jumping.	Common assessment to determine quantity of movement in children with cerebral palsy.
The Infanib Patricia H. Ellison *Therapy Skill Builders* *19500 Bulverde Rd.* *San Antonio, TX 78259-3701*	4–18 months, at-risk infants, including those born prematurely	Tests spasticity, vestibular function, head and trunk control, French angles, and legs.	To determine normal and abnormal neuromotor function.

(Continued)

Test/Measure and Author/ Reference or Publisher	Age Range	Areas Tested	Primary Use
Inside the Hawaii Early Learning Profile (HELP) Stephanie Parks *VORT Corporation PO Box 6032 Palo Alto, CA 94306*	Birth–36 months	Criterion-referenced assessment of regulatory/sensory organization, cognition, language, gross motor, fine motor, social-emotional, and self-help.	Complements the very popular HELP curriculum and assessment materials by providing guidelines for administration and scoring. Used to determine delay and program planning, but without a standardized score.
Merrill-Palmer Scale— Revised (2003) *Stoelting Co. 620 Wheat Lane Wood Dale, IL 60191*	2–78 months	Norm-referenced, standardized measure of cognitive (reasoning, memory, visual, etc.), language and motor (fine and gross), self-help/adaptive, and social-emotional development. Patterns of development are assessed. Includes supplemental parent and examiner ratings.	The new addition of the motor measures makes this a comprehensive assessment that can be used from birth to kindergarten to determine delay or dysfunction and evaluate intervention effectiveness.
Milani-Comparetti Motor Development Screening Test, 3rd ed. A. Milani-Comparetti and E.A. Gidoni (Wayne Stuberg, revised edition) *Media Resource Center Meyer Children's Rehabilitation Institute University of Nebraska Medical Center 444 South 44th Street Omaha, NE 68131-3795*	Birth–2 years	Standardized screening of spontaneous motor behaviors including locomotion, sitting, and standing, and evoked responses, including equilibrium reactions, protective reactions, righting reactions, and primitive reflexes.	Helpful in describing an infant's motor development, but no total score obtained. Relies on the integration of primitive reflexes for the development of postural control.
Motor Skills Acquisition in the First Year and Checklist Lois Bly *Therapy Skill Builders 19500 Bulverde Rd. San Antonio, TX 78259-3701*	Birth–12 months	Detailed explanation with photographs and checklist of gross motor development and indications of possible disturbances in motor development.	To monitor motor development and assist in intervention planning for infants with motor delays or dysfunction.
Movement Assessment Battery for Children (MOVEMENT ABC) Sheila Henderson and David Sugden *The Psychological Corporation 19500 Bulverde Road San Antonio, TX 78259-3701*	4–12 years	Norm-referenced standardized performance test of manual dexterity, ball skills, and static and dynamic balance. Also included is a checklist of daily routine activities, consideration of the context of performance, and behavioral attributes.	Identifies impairments in motor function of children with milder movement disorders. Includes qualitative and quantitative information.
Movement Assessment of Infants (MAI) Lynnette Chandler, Mary Andrews, and Marcia Sanson *Infant Movement Research PO Box 4631 Rolling Bay, WA 98061*	Birth–12 months	Criterion-referenced assessment of muscle tone, reflexes, automatic reactions, and volitional movement.	A risk score is calculated for identification of infants at risk for motor dysfunction. High-risk profiles are provided for only 4- and 8-month-old infants.

Test/Measure and Author/ Reference or Publisher	Age Range	Areas Tested	Primary Use
Miller Assessment of Preschoolers (MAP) Lucy Jane Miller *The Foundation for Knowledge in Development 1855 West Union Avenue Suite B-8 Englewood, CO 80110*	2 years 9 months–5 years 8 months	Norm-referenced test of sensory and motor foundations and coordination, verbal and nonverbal cognitive skills, and complex tasks.	Determination of preschoolers, without major problems, who are at risk for preacademic problems.
Neonatal Behavioral Assessment Scale (NBAS) T. Berry Brazelton and J. Kevin Nugent *Clinics in Developmental Medicine, No. 137 Cambridge University Press 40 W. 20th Street New York, NY 10011*	Full-term neonates 37–48 weeks post conceptional age	Criterion-referenced test of habituation, motor-oral responses, truncal and vestibular function, and social-interactive behaviors.	Provides information on the infant's interactive patterns that can be used to assist parents and caregivers. Training program recommended to become reliable in test administration.
Neonatal Individualized Developmental Care and Assessment Program (NIDCAP) Heidelise Als *National NIDCAP Training Center Enders Pediatric Research Laboratories The Children's Hospital 320 Longwood Avenue Boston, MA 02115*	Neonates–4 weeks postterm	Criterion-referenced assessment of physiological and behavioral responses in the areas of autonomic, motor, and attention.	Used to determine the infant's physiological and behavioral responses to the environment to assist parents and caregivers. Training program recommended to become reliable in test administration.
Neurological Assessment of the Preterm and Full-term Born Infant (NAPFI) Lilly Dubowitz and Victor Dubowitz *Clinics in Developmental Medicine, No. 79 Cambridge University Press 40 W. 20th Street New York, NY 10011*	Full-term infants up to 3rd day of life and stable preterm infants	Criterion-referenced test of neurological maturation. Tests habituation, movement and tone, reflexes, and neurobehavioral responses.	Classic assessment to determine maturation and deviations in neurological development of infants. Commonly used though limited psychometric data available.
Neurological Exam of the Full Term Infant Heinz Prechtl *Clinics in Developmental Medicine, No. 63 Cambridge University Press 40 W. 20th Street New York, NY 10011*	Full-term and preterm infants 38–42 weeks gestation	Norm-referenced, standardized examination of posture, eyes, power and passive movement, spontaneous and voluntary movements, and state.	Classic test to determine neurological dysfunction in young infants.
Oucher Scale Beyer, J.E. (1984). The Oucher: A user manual and technical report. Evanston, IL: The Hospital Play Equipment Co.	5–12 years	Pain intensity rating scale using actual pictures.	Measures self-reporting of pain intensity.

(Continued)

Test/Measure and Author/ Reference or Publisher	Age Range	Areas Tested	Primary Use
Peabody Development Motor Scales (PDMS-2), 2nd ed. M. Rhonda Folio and Rebecca R. Fewell *PRO-ED, Inc.* *8700 Shoal Creek Blvd.* *Austin, TX 78757–6897*	1–72 months	Norm-referenced, standardized assessment of gross motor and fine motor skills divided into 6 subtests: reflexes, stationary, locomotion, object manipulation, grasping, and visual-motor integration.	Motor quotients are determined to estimate overall motor abilities. Commonly used in early intervention programs to determine eligibility for services. Has accompanying Motor Activities Program to assist in teaching skills.
Pediatric Evaluation of Disability Inventory (PEDI) Stephen M. Haley, Wendy J. Coster, Larry H. Ludlow, Jane T. Haltiwarger, and Peter J. Andrellas *The Psychological Corporation* *19500 Bulverde Road* *San Antonio, TX 78259-3701*	6 months–7 years and those whose functional abilities are lower than those of a 7-year-old	Norm-referenced, standardized assessment based on parent interview to determine self-care (eating, grooming, dressing, bathing, and toileting); mobility including transfers; social function (communication, social interaction, household and community tasks); and need for modifications and assistance.	Identifies the functional and activity capabilities of infants and children with disabilities. Used to monitor change in activities and functional skills and evaluate program outcomes.
POSNA Pediatric Musculoskeletal Functional Health Questionnaire Daltroy, L.H., Liang, M.H., Fossel, A.H., & Goldberg, M.J. (1998). Pediatric Outcomes Instrument Development Group. Pediatric Orthopaedic Society of North America. *Journal of Pediatric Orthopedics, 18*, 561–571.	2–18 years with musculoskeletal disorders	Scales completed by child and parent to measure upper extremity function, transfers and mobility, physical function and sports, comfort (pain free), happiness and satisfaction, and expectations for treatment.	Used to assess functional health outcomes, generally postorthopedic surgery. Can also examine child-parent agreement.
Posture and Fine Motor Assessment of Infants Jane Case-Smith and Rosemarie Bigsby *Therapy Skill Builders* *19500 Bulverde Rd.* *San Antonio, TX 78259–3701*	2–12 months	Fine motor scales addressing infant's reaching and grasping patterns, finger and thumb movements, release, and manipulation.	Assists in intervention planning and documenting progress over brief periods of time.
Quality of Well-Being Scale (QWB) Kaplan, R.M., Bush, J.W., & Berry, C.C. (1976). Health status: Types of validity and the index of well-being. *Health Services Research, 11*, 478–507.	14+ years	Four scales focus on the physical impact of an illness related to symptoms, functions, and social and mobility levels.	Summarizes health across symptoms, problems, and functional states.
Riley Infant Pain Scale Schare, J., Joyce, B., Gerkensmeyer, J., & Keck, J. (1996). Comparison of three preverbal scales for postoperative pain assessment in a diverse pediatric sample. *Journal of Pain and Symptom Management, 12*(6), 348–359.	Infants and preverbal or nonverbal children	Behavioral observation as an indication of pain.	Indication of pain in infants and preverbal or nonverbal children.

Test/Measure and Author/ Reference or Publisher	Age Range	Areas Tested	Primary Use
Scales of Independent Behavior—Revised (SIB-R) Robert Bruininks, Richard Woodcock, Richard Weatherman, and Bradley Hill *Riverside Publishing Co.* *8420 Bryn Mawr Avenue* *Chicago, IL 60603*	3 months– adulthood	Norm-referenced, standardized test using interviews to determine motor skills, social interaction and communication skills, personal living skills, and problem behaviors.	Measure functional independence and adaptive functioning across settings. Is used with the Adaptive Living Skills Assessment Intervention System.
School Function Assessment (SFA) Wendy Coster, Theresa Deeney, Jane Haltiwanger, and Stephen Haley *The Psychological Corporation* *19500 Bulverde Road* *San Antonio, TX 78259-3701*	Children with disabilities in grades K–6	Criterion-referenced, standardized, judgment-based interview to determine the child's participation in all aspects of the school environment; task supports needed to function in school; activity performance of school-related activities; physical tasks such as changing position, manipulation, using materials, eating, and written work; and cognitive and behavioral tasks.	Comprehensive assessment of activity and functional capabilities of children with disabilities in school setting. While not tied to a curriculum, information obtained assists in determining eligibility for service and in development of educationally relevant objectives
Sensory Integration and Praxis Tests (SIPT) A. Jean Ayres *Western Psychological Services* *12031 Wilshire Blvd.* *Los Angeles, CA 90025*	4 years–8 years 11 months	Measure sensory integration of form and space perception, somatic and vestibular processing, praxis, and bilateral integration and sequencing.	Determine presence and type of sensory integrative disorder. Require advanced training to properly administer and interpret.
Sensory Profile and Infant/ Toddler Sensory Profile Winnie Dunn *The Psychological Corporation* *19500 Bulverde Road* *San Antonio, TX 78259-3701*	3–10 years and birth–36 months (Infant/ Toddler)	Questionnaire used to determine basic sensory processing in daily life; sensory processing modulation and behavioral and emotional responses.	Links strengths and barriers in sensory processing with daily life
Test of Gross Motor Development—2 (TGMD2) Dale Ulrich *Pro-ed* *8700 Shoal Creek Blvd.* *Austin, TX 78757-6897*	3–10 years	Norm-referenced test of 12 gross motor skills involving locomotion and object control.	Used to identify children who are significantly behind their peers in gross motor skill development.
Test of Infant Motor Performance (TIMP) Suzann Campbell *Infant Motor Performance Scales, LLC* *1301 W. Madison St. #526* *Chicago, IL 60607-1953*	Prematurely born infants 34 weeks post conceptual age–4 months post term	Functional movements of head and trunk control in prone, supine and upright positions. 28 items scored dichotomously and 31 scaled items.	Discriminates infants with risk of poor motor outcome; sensitive to effects of intervention.
Test of Sensory Function in Infants (TSFI) Georgia DeGangi and Stanley Greenspan *Western Psychological Services* *12031 Wilshire Blvd.* *Los Angeles, CA 90025*	4–18 months	Criterion-referenced test of reactivity to tactile pressure, adaptive motor function, visual-tactile integration, ocular motor control, and reactivity to vestibular stimulation.	Identifies sensory processing and reactivity dysfunction in infants.

Test/Measure and Author/ Reference or Publisher	Age Range	Areas Tested	Primary Use
Test of Visual-Motor Skills-Revised (TVMS-R) Morrison Gardner *Psychological and Educational Publications, Inc. PO Box 520 Hydesville, CA 95547-0520*	3–14 years	Norm-referenced tests of eye-hand coordination, motor accuracy, motor control, motor coordination, and the child's interpretation.	Simple test of visual-motor skills.
The T.I.M.E. Toddler and Infant Motor Evaluation Lucy Jane Miller & Gale Roid *The Psychological Corporation 19500 Bulverde Road San Antonio, TX 78259-3701*	4 months–3½ years with suspected motor delay or dysfunction	Comprehensive qualitative assessment of mobility, motor organization, stability-functional performance, and social-emotional abilities. Items indicating motor organization are observed during parent-child interaction.	Track development over time to determine extent of motor delay or dysfunction and to link function with quality of movement.
Transdisciplinary Play-Based Assessment (TPBA), Revised Edition Toni W. Linder *Paul H. Brookes Publishing Co. PO Box 10624 Baltimore, MD 21285-0624*	6 months–6 years	Criterion-referenced assessment based in observations of the child at play. Areas observed include cognitive, social-emotional, communication and language, and sensorimotor development.	Used to identify intervention needs and evaluate progress of children with disabilities. Scores do not compare the child to others. An intervention volume is also available.
Visual Analog Scale Shields, B., Cohen, D., Harbeck-Weber, C., Powers, J., & Smith, G. (2003). Pediatric pain measurement using a visual analogue scale. *Clinical Pediatrics,* April.	5 years and above, over 11 years	Pain intensity rating scale using numerical scale on a vertical or horizontal continuum.	Measures self-report of pain intensity.
Vulpe Assessment Battery—Revised (VAB-R) Shirley German Vulpe *Slosson Educational Publications, Inc. PO Box 280 East Aurora, NY 14052*	Birth–6 years for children with disabilities	One of the first criterion-referenced tests with enough items/task analysis to be useful in assessing children with significant delay or dysfunction. Includes assessment of basic senses and function, development behavior, environment and performance analysis system.	Identifies areas of skill performance, strengths, and needs for children with moderate to severe disability. Includes environment's influence on task performance. Psychometric data are incomplete.
WEEFIM: Functional Independence Measure for Children Carl Granger, Susan Braun, Kim Griswood, Nancy Heyer, Margaret McCabe, Michael Msau, & Byron Hamilton *Uniform Data System for Medical Rehabilitation State Univ. of New York Research Foundation 82 Farbert Hall SUNY South Campus Buffalo, NY 14214*	6 months–8 years, but can be used up to 12 years with children with disabilities	Comprehensive, criterion-referenced assessment based on observation of motor function of 18 items in 6 subscales including self-care, sphincter control, tranfers, locomotion, and cognitive function including communication and social cognition. This is the child version of the Functional Independence Measure (FIM).	Determines degree of a child's disability, ability to accomplish tasks, and caregiver assistance required. Must use their data collection and outcome reporting system.

Test/Measure and Author/ Reference or Publisher	Age Range	Areas Tested	Primary Use
Youth Quality of Life Instrument-Research Version (YQOL-R) The Association for Professionals in Services for Adolescents *Elsevier Science Ltd.* *360 Park Ave, South* *New York, NY 10010–1710*	12–18 years with and without disabilities	Self-report measure in four domains: sense of self, social relationships, environment, and general quality of life.	To assess quality of life with an emphasis on aspects of positive health.

Resources: Test manuals; test catalogs; Lollar, Simeonsson, & Nanda (2000); Long & Toscano (2002); QOLID (2003).

Chapter 3

Family-Centered Intervention

— Lisa Ann Chiarello, PT, PhD, PCS

Overview of Family-Centered Intervention

The physical therapy profession has historically acknowledged that family involvement is essential to the success of physical therapy. This is especially true for the pediatric population. However, in the present health-care arena, the family's role in health care is changing. Consumers' rights and responsibilities and functional outcomes are becoming crucial elements in issues regarding health-care service delivery. Family-centered intervention is a process that respects the rights and roles of family members while providing intervention to achieve child and family outcomes that promote well-being and quality of life. The purpose of this chapter is to provide an introduction to issues related to **family-centered care** to support physical therapists in their interactions and interventions with the children and families they serve.

Family-centered intervention is not restricted to the pediatric specialty area; it is a life-span approach. The World Health Organization's model on functioning, disability, and health supports a family-centered approach (2001). Cherry (1991) identified that in pediatric physical therapy, "there is a greater need for a holistic approach that encompasses the total child, the family, and the natural settings where children live, learn, and play" (p. 70). This need especially continues during the transition into adulthood (Rubin & Quinn-Curran, 1983). Family-centered care provides an opportunity for a preventive and supportive approach to wellness across the life span. Practicing

physical therapists have identified the need for family information to be included in entry-level coursework (Cochrane & Farley, 1990). Entry-level physical therapy curricula are becoming committed to teaching a family-centered care approach (Sparling & Sekerak, 1992).

The foundation for family-centered practice is based on the synthesis of many theoretical frameworks. The fundamental premise of family-centered care is that a person does not exist in isolation but functions within a family as well as within larger and more complex social systems. Social systems, including the family unit, influence the function of that person and that person subsequently influences the function of the systems in which he or she belongs. This proposition is central to systems theory. The **family systems theory** views individual and family functioning as an interactional dynamic process (Becvar & Becvar, 1988). Interventions for the family can indirectly influence the child's development.

In pediatric physical therapy, the needs of children can best be met by involving their families. The **transactional model of development** emphasizes the reciprocal relationship between the child and caregiving environment. A supportive environment may minimize the effects of biological risks (Sameroff & Chandler, 1975). The child's characteristics and the environment work together to determine functional outcomes. The importance of an appropriate match between the child and the environment is emphasized. The **ecological model of human development** discusses the role that larger social systems have on the function of the family unit (Bronfenbrenner, 1977).

Support from social networks and the political and economical culture can influence how a family interacts and cares for their child. Recent research in early intervention has emphasized that family patterns (parent-child relationship, family arranged experiences, and health and safety) have the greatest impact on child outcomes (Guralnick, 1998). Family-centered care in pediatrics is based on the philosophy that the family plays the central role in the life of a child.

To develop an understanding of family-centered care, it is essential to understand what is meant by a family. Therapists must broaden their conceptualization of the traditional family configuration, for the contemporary family in America is diverse (Sparling, 1991). Family is defined more by emotional or functional elements than by structural or legal elements. A family is a group of people who love and care for each other. The family is the base for caring and nurturing, and is the place where values are taught and learned.

Edleman defined *family-centered care* "as a collaborative relationship between families and professionals in the continual pursuit of being responsive to the priorities and choices of families" (cited in Leviton, Mueller, & Kauffman, 1992, p. 1). There are four primary goals of family-centered care. The first goal is to support the family unit (Brewer, McPherson, Magrab, & Hutchins, 1989). This includes protecting the integrity of the family and respecting and supporting the subunits of the family, and the developmental goals of each of its members. These subunits include the adult-adult relationship, caregiver-child relationship, sibling-sibling relationship, and extended family relationship. The second goal of family-centered care is to enhance **family competence** (Dunst, Johanson, Trivette, & Hamby, 1991). This process includes strengthening family function by proactively helping families identify and mobilize resources and support. Establishing a sense of community, including both informal and formal community sources of support, is an essential part of this process. Living at home and participating within the community are supported. Providing information and consultation to the family and child are also crucial. The professional's role is to be the family's assistant. The third goal of family-centered care is the goal with which therapists are most akin—enhancing the growth, development, and functional independence of the child through a **partnership** with the family and child. This partnership entails a commitment of shared responsibility toward the accomplishment of an outcome. Care directed toward goals that are important and relevant to the family and child is the fourth goal. The therapist's role is to match these goals of family-centered care with actual program practices. Therapists bring part of themselves to any partnership, and the **therapist-family/child relationship** is the avenue through which family-centered practice is provided.

History of Family-Centered Services

Historically, services for children with disabilities were limited and families were solely responsible for their children's care, education, and treatment. In the early part of the 20th century, families were encouraged to institutionalize children with disabilities. From the middle of the 20th century, through humanitarian efforts, charitable organizations began providing services to children (Newman, 1983), but most families had a passive role. In the 1960s, Head Start programs and similar intervention projects were instituted to address the needs of select groups. During this time, families organized major advocacy groups and fought for rights and services for their children.

Traditionally, the medical model was a child-centered approach and parents did not assume an active role. The professional was viewed as the expert and was responsible for developing and implementing the intervention plan. Intervention techniques were aimed at enhancing the development of the child, and outcomes were based on achievement of developmental skills (Bricker & Veltman, 1990).

Caregiver-focused intervention programs became popular in the 1970s, and interventions were aimed at training caregivers to promote their child's development. This decade was marked with increased caregiver involvement, as well as advocacy. In many cases, caregivers were leading advocates for the rights and services for children with disabilities. The passage of landmark federal legislation in the United States, the **Education of All Handicapped Children Act of 1975**, included a mandate for caregiver involvement in their children's education. According to the legislation, caregivers were to be involved in the decision-making process, to help plan and coordinate their child's education, to be advocates for their child's rights, and to assume a teaching role at home. Caregiver training and home programs became an integral component of intervention programs (Bazak, 1989). Caregivers wanted to have opportunities for decision making, be kept informed of their child's test results and progress, and actively participate in their child's intervention (Redman-Bentley, 1982). Some caregivers began to publish articles and books and participate in support groups in which they shared their personal experiences and provided guidance for other families. While this legislation acknowledged the competence and importance of caregivers, negative consequences were also realized. The federal mandate set forth the practices that public agencies must do to involve caregivers; however, caregiver response and level of involvement are individual. The degree of involvement can be overwhelming to caregivers, and there is a controversy of how much responsibility should be put on the caregivers (Turnbull & Turnbull, 1982). Caregivers assuming the primary roles of teacher and therapist may negatively influence the **caregiver-child relationship**. Another concern has been that the practice of caregiver involvement was a formality on paper only and that the actual degree of caregiver/professional partnership was limited.

As models of service delivery evolved into a family-centered approach, a model developed in early intervention that was identified as relationship focused. The goal of the relationship-focused model was to guide caregivers in understanding and responding to their child's behaviors, interests, and needs. The relationship-focused model in early intervention strove to enhance positive caregiver-child interactions and emphasized that these interactions provide the foundation for a satisfying relationship, as well as the development of the child and caregiver (Affleck, McGrade, McQueeney, & Allen, 1982; Bromwich, 1981). Family-centered intervention emerged with a shift of emphasis from only the child or caregiver to the larger context of the family and social environment.

In early intervention, the Education of the Handicapped Act Amendments of 1986 and its reauthorizations clearly mandate services to meet the needs of the family related to enhancing their child's development. Assessment of the family's concerns, priorities, and resources; family training and counseling; intervention in the child's natural environment; and social work were some of the services identified in the law that particularly relate to this concept of family-centered care. Physical therapists need to be familiar with federal and state laws and their rules and regulations to provide service that reflects legal, ethical, and best-practice standards (see Chapters 1, 10, and 11).

A family-centered philosophy can still be integrated with more traditional client-centered approaches (Deardorff, 1992). Recent trends in child-centered intervention emphasize approaches that are more aligned with a family-centered philosophy. These approaches include child-initiated activities, use of daily routines, and natural contexts (Bricker & Veltman, 1990). Caregivers acknowledge that they want some portion of the intervention to be child centered. Child-centered intervention does not have to be viewed as though it is at the opposite end of the spectrum from a family-centered approach. Health-care professionals can provide direct intervention to the child and still assist the family in using their resources. Caregiver education is a vital component of family-centered care when it is practiced in a respectful manner and there is a reciprocal exchange of information. Child-centered, caregiver-centered, and family-centered models each have their own values and limitations. In practice, therapists use a variety of models throughout a child's intervention because it is very difficult to provide service to only the child without involving the caregivers or to only the caregivers without involving the child. Family-centered intervention is the most comprehensive model of service delivery. When family-centered care is individualized, it may include aspects of both child- and caregiver-centered service delivery models to meet the needs of the family and promote the child's development and function (Figure 3–1).

In summary, family participation is an integral component of most pediatric intervention programs. Families have long been recognized as an important environmental variable in the response of patients to physical therapy. Family information is collected at initial assessment and is used to guide intervention planning, family education, home programs, and discharge planning. Physical therapists are concerned about the structure of the home environment, the family's understanding of the disability, and the family's daily routines. In a meta-analysis of the effectiveness of early intervention, Shonkoff and Hauser-Cram (1987) concluded that the programs that focused intervention on the caregiver and child together appeared to be the most effective. The question for therapists becomes, how is it most appropriate to foster caregiver involvement and family-centered care? The most effective approach involves flexibility and individualization based on the family's concerns, priorities, and resources and on the strengths and needs of the child.

Factors in a Family Unit That Influence Family-Centered Intervention

The concept of family is broad, and family structure, family function, and a **family's life cycle** are very individual. Awareness of this variability is important when developing a family-centered intervention plan. Family structure and function may be identified by the family as a strength or a need in terms of influencing the intervention process. If

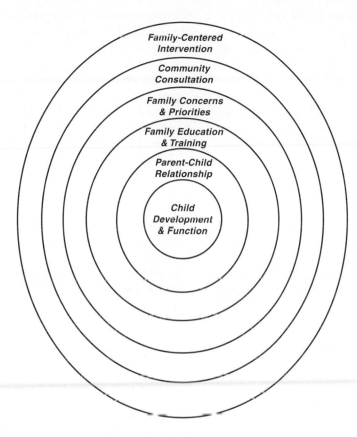

Figure 3–1 Family-centered intervention.

these factors are identified as strengths, family structure and function could be capitalized on to promote opportunities to enhance the child's development and function. If these factors are identified as concerns, professionals and the family can work collaboratively to access avenues of resources and support.

The structure of the family can include family members, caregivers, and extended family and friends. Some families include a large number of people resources, and in others the number may be very small. Demographic statistics revealed the decrease in family size across all ethnic groups in the United States, an increase in the number of children living with only their mothers, and an increase in the number of children with working mothers (U.S. House of Representatives, 1989). In addition to the human resources in a family, the structure of the home, the material resources, and the neighboring environment are also changing. Inner-city environments, housing conditions, and poverty are dimensions of family life that influence family function. Material resources may or may not be adequate to

provide the necessities for daily function and development. Socioeconomic status and the organization of the home, including the provision of appropriate play materials, have been shown to positively correlate with child development (Poresky & Henderson, 1982; Ramey, Mills, Campbell, & O'Brien, 1975). Professionals need to be aware of the influence that family members, home environment, and material resources may have on the intervention process to recommend appropriate intervention strategies that promote family-identified outcomes.

In addition to the actual constitution of a family and home, how a family functions needs to be considered when developing a family-centered intervention plan. In discussing the transition from child-centered to family-centered care, Stuberg and Harbourne (1994) stated that therapists need to understand how **family dynamics** influence functional outcomes. Therapists first need an understanding about the roles and responsibilities of family members as defined by each individual family. In addition, an awareness of individual family members' attitudes toward themselves and others in the family will help the therapist guide the intervention process. For example, a parent with low self-esteem regarding his or her parenting skills may benefit from a therapist acknowledging his or her appropriate carrying and holding of the child.

Therapists need to be aware of the mother's, father's, and siblings' other caregivers' roles in child care. Numerous studies have documented the positive influence that maternal involvement has on child development (Ainsworth & Bell, 1974; Clarke-Stewart, 1973; Mahoney, Finger, & Powell, 1985; Yarrow, Rubenstein, Pedersen, & Jankowski, 1972). However, it is important to remember that both mothers and fathers influence their child's development (Lamb, 1983). Paternal involvement is increasing in child care tasks. The role that the father plays in the family is diverse and changing. In addition, professionals need to acknowledge the importance of the sibling bond. Seligman and Darling (1989) emphasized that siblings have a need for accurate and appropriate information, a balance between caregiving responsibility and age-appropriate tasks, and individual parental attention. Professionals need to consider that the appropriate amount of involvement of a sibling will vary from family to family and that the intervention plan may need to include steps to foster sibling adjustment. With family consent, it may be appropriate to include the mother, father, siblings, or other "family members" in the intervention plan.

Family function and personal development of all family members are interdependent with the family's life cycle (Minuchin, 1985). The life-span process is no longer viewed just as the traditional stages that persons pass through as they marry, establish a career, have children, send their children off into the world, and retire. The pattern of the family life cycle is variable and depends on many life events and life circumstances. Factors such as culture, economics, political contexts, health, lower birth rate, longer life expectancy, changing role of women, and increasing divorce and remarriage rates shape an individual family's life cycle pattern (Carter & McGoldrick, 1989). The family life cycle involves several generations and the process influences each individual member. Where a family is in the life-span process, as well as the developmental tasks of the individual family members, will influence how they make meaning of their life circumstances and how they respond to the disability and intervention. Knowing and respecting the developmental tasks of the family as a whole, as well as the individual members, and how these two interrelate will make the intervention process more meaningful to the family.

A family's **culture** provides a foundation for their expectations and actions. Low (1984, p. 14) defined *culture* as "the integrated system of learned patterns of behavior." A person's cultural identify is influenced by many variables, including ethnicity, race, age, gender, family, vocation, religion, and disability. An earnest assessment of a family's culture will provide valuable information that may be a resource for intervention. Culture affects intervention through three processes: (a) communication of information between the family and the provider, (b) life style of the family and the provider, and (c) societal environment in terms of regulations for health care (Hill, Fortenberry, & Stein, 1989). The family's ethnic heritage, lifestyle, child-rearing practices, values, and beliefs make the process and content of intervention very individual.

The family ecology of ethnic minority groups and the traditional American lifestyle have been generalized, compared, and contrasted (McGoldrick, 1989; Sparling, 1991). While it is helpful to be aware that differences may be present in terms of relationships, extended family, role flexibility, and rules of family life, families deserve our respect to allow them to teach us about their individual family perspective. Gerhard (1995) recommended that therapists demonstrate respect for individual family culture by careful observation and by following the lead of the family. An awareness of the family's communication and problem-solving style will help a therapist to optimize sharing of information and learning. A therapist may choose to use an interpreter to help bridge language barriers but may want to become skillful in appropriate nonverbal communication methods to develop a relationship with the family.

It is particularly important for therapists to explore and acknowledge the family's values regarding childhood, independence, work ethics, health care, decision making, and disability and to be aware of how these values may have an impact on intervention outcomes. Child-rearing practices and parental expectations are of particular importance to physical therapists because these factors have been related to motor development (Cintas, 1995). The family practices of ethnic groups, including African-Americans, Hispanic-Americans, Asian/Pacific Islanders, and Native Americans/Alaskan natives have more heavily emphasized the role of the extended family as a resource and support compared to traditional European-American practices. In addition, child-rearing philosophy has promoted interdependency and cooperation as opposed to independence and competitiveness (Harrison, Wilson, Pine, Chan, & Buriel, 1990). The family's values may guide a therapist's recommendations for resources, such as extended family members, as well as for intervention strategies, such as independent play activities versus interactive play activities.

Hanson (1992) recommended that interventionists need to consider (1) how a family views their child's disability, (2) how receptive a family is to intervention, and (3) the family's preferences for location, method, type, agent, and style of service delivery. In reference to the current model of family-centered care, therapists need to be sensitive to the family's beliefs about family participation. As emphasized by Lynch (1992), family-professional partnership is not common in many cultures and families may not be ready to fully participate in a collaborative process. Therapists need to respect the position of the family while at the same time provide informal opportunities for the family to share their opinions and priorities. Case Example 3–1 provides a clinical scenario regarding the influence that culture has on the intervention process.

CASE EXAMPLE 3–1 . . . . .

Family Culture and Physical Therapy Intervention

A physical therapist went to conduct an initial home visit for a 1-year-old girl with Down syndrome and her family, who were of Asian descent. The visit was scheduled at midday and the older sibling, a preschooler, and the mother were present. When the therapist entered the home, she noticed that shoes were lined up in the foyer by the door. The therapist quietly slipped off her shoes when she entered the foyer. After introductions were made, the mother offered the therapist some lunch. The therapist politely declined the offer; however, the mother persisted. The mother, although very quiet, was able to explain to the therapist that it was important to her to be able to share some food with the therapist as a way of showing her appreciation. The therapist decided that it was more important to build a trusting relationship with the family than to abide by policy, which required that therapists did not accept gifts of any nature from clients. The therapist sat down at the table that was prepared and shared a brief meal with the mother.

During the initial meeting, the therapist encouraged family input as well as participation from the mother. However, the mother always placed herself several feet behind the therapist and commented that the therapist should do what she felt was right. The therapist did not push the matter any further and spent the rest of the session playing with the child. The therapist made sure to make an occasional connection with the mother by commenting on the child's abilities. During subsequent visits, the therapist was able to make comments on mother-child interactions, as the therapist observed the mother carry and comfort the child. The therapist was able to convey to the mother that she respected the mother's abilities and would be happy if the mother felt comfortable participating in part of the sessions. The mother's participation started out very slowly, but collaboration was developing. After several weeks, the mother asked if it would be okay if the father came home for lunch so that he could be part of the therapy session. The therapist and family achieved a trusting partnership that was founded on mutual respect.

Therapists must make a commitment to achieve **cultural competence**. Thorpe and Baker (1995) defined *cultural competence* as "the ability to think and behave in ways that enable a member of one culture to work effectively with members of another culture" (p. 143). An awareness of one's own beliefs will help therapists be open and respectful of cultural variations. Therapists then need to make a concerted effort to gain knowledge of the culture of the families that they serve. Lynch (1992) recommended avenues through which to gain this information: reading, talking, and working with individuals from other cultures, sharing the daily routines of another culture, and learning other languages. This knowledge then needs to be put into action as the therapist learns the skills to most effectively interact with each family as well as using cultural resources as part of the intervention process.

Family stress and **coping skills** influence a family's ability to function and develop. While it is necessary to acknowledge a family's daily stress, it is important to be aware that family stress is not necessarily related to raising a child with a disability (Chiarello, 1993; Hanson & Hanline, 1990). The presence of a child with a disability does not necessarily mean the family will have problems (Petersen & Wikoff, 1987). The family's role in society has changed, and contemporary family life has many challenges that can be a source of stress (Petersen & Wikoff, 1987; Sparling, 1991). The range of these challenges includes dual-career families, teenage pregnancy, single-parent families, violence and substance abuse in the family, absence of extended family, geographic mobility, and financial constraints. Time constraints may limit family members' rests, fitness activities, social interactions, and leisure activities. All these factors may influence the family's overall satisfaction and happiness.

Even though physical therapists are not the primary professionals dealing with the issues of daily stress and coping, physical therapists do come in contact with these issues because they interact with the family on a routine and frequent basis. Physical therapists can be helpful by providing the family opportunities to articulate concerns, supporting the family's coping strategies, respecting the family's privacy, and being flexible. However, the field of psychology and family therapy is beyond the scope of the practice of physical therapy. Specialized study is needed in these fields to truly have the in-depth knowledge to intervene at that level of professional practice, and physical therapists should refer families when appropriate.

The process of **family adaptation** when a child has a special health-care need is beyond the scope of this chapter. The therapist should be cognizant that the process is complex and influenced by many variables, including the nature of the disability, the time of onset, the family's personal belief system, and the family's support network and resources (Roberts, 1984; Yau & Li-Tsang, 1999). It is important to remember that family members will vary in how they perceive and react to a stress. In addition, the number and quality of stressors as well as the extent of the **family's resources and support systems** will influence the family's response to any particular stress. As indicated by Sparling, Kolobe, and Ezzelle (1994), "support for family members appears to be an important mediating variable in adaptation, yet generic support is not easily described. The unique constellation of stressors experienced by contemporary families requires a combination of support ranging from financial and intellectual support to social support" (p. 830). Social support has been defined as "mutually rewarding personal interactions from which an individual derives feelings of being needed, valued, and esteemed" (p. 832). Dunst, Trivette, and Cross (1986) found that social support had a positive influence on parent and family well-being, parent-infant play opportunities, and child development for families with young children in early intervention. The interrelationship between stress and support influences how a family adapts and how they are able to participate in an intervention program.

Three common stresses often associated with raising a child with a disability have been acknowledged. These are lack of information, dealing with the health-care system, and extended caregiving (Dura & Kiecolt-Glaser, 1991). Limited knowledge of their child's condition and standards of care creates an uncertainty that can be stressful. Parents may not be aware of federal, state, and local resources. Dealing with the complexity of the health-care system, school environment, and special services requires energy, time, and skills. The complexities of daily care management can add to the primary stresses of contemporary life. Prolonged caregiving can dramatically alter the family's way of functioning and may have negative physiological and psychological effects (Dura & Kiecolt-Glaser, 1991). The family must balance the amount of time needed to care for a child with special needs with the amount of time for other family members and work responsibilities. Issues such as loss of privacy and freedom to individuate must be handled. In addition, the parents must cope with their own fears regarding the child's health and future. The degree to which the caregiving "burden" influences family function and development appears to be more related to a family's subjective perception, as opposed to direct objective issues of caregiving. An understanding of this relationship is helpful for a therapist to avoid a judgment or a direct comparison between families. For example, some families may decide on residential care for their children. Therapists need to be supportive and respectful of each family's personal decision and not view the decision as a failure of the family or the service-delivery system.

Transitional periods in the family life cycle have also been identified as stressful times. How a family adapts to a transition can be influenced by their personal family history; the nature, duration, and timing of the transition itself; and the family's perception of the transition (Elder, 1991). Special birthdays, events, and celebrations may evoke mixed feelings—happiness for the occasion but sadness for the loss of normalcy. Therapists can acknowledge the normal aspects of the developmental transition and create the opportunity for the family to celebrate the event (Roberts, 1984). Therapists can assist with preparations for attending a dance or the first day at a new school. Adapting to a new school, classroom, teacher, classmates, therapists, and administrators can be overwhelming. Parents have to deal with the uncertainty regarding the appropriateness of the educational placement, the philosophy of care, intervention services, and equipment needs. In the educational system, transition plans are now required to be proactive in helping families meet these challenges.

Guidelines for Family-Centered Intervention

To provide family-centered care, therapists must respect family rights and abilities (Rosenbaum, King, Law, King, & Evans, 1998; Viscardis, 1998). Professionals need to respect the caregiver's primary role as the child's caregiver, a source of nurturing and love, not as teacher or therapist. In family-centered care, the family is recognized as the key member of the intervention team. The family is the consumer of services and retains the ultimate decision-making authority. Historically, there had been an erroneous assumption that experts were better able to decide what was in the best interest of the child and family. In family-centered care, it is the professionals' responsibility to provide information that the caregivers can use to make informed decisions and to give informed consent. This concept has been referred to as **empowering** (Dunst, Trivette, Davis, & Cornwell, 1988). Information on federal and state legislation and local policies related to service provision for children with disabilities is to be provided to families. Professionals provide families with appropriate and individualized options and thorough explanations. Caregiver-professional partnership forms the foundation of service delivery. This partnership includes learning from each other, sharing responsibility, and accepting each other's perspective.

Communication is a crucial key to establishing the caregiver-professional partnership. Caregivers have acknowledged that they respect the professionals' knowledge and clinical expertise regarding recommendations for their children. However, it is important for professionals to value the caregiver's expertise in knowing if the recommendation is appropriate for their individual circumstances (Leviton et al., 1992). Caregivers know their child in the most intimate way and have valuable information to share. When professionals acknowledge family competence, they help create an environment in which the family can be successful. This concept has been referred to as **enabling** (Dunst et al., 1988). Through empowering and enabling, therapists acknowledge the family's competence, strengths, and ability to mobilize resources to meet their needs (Dunst et al., 1988). The relationship between the professional and family will change and develop over time. Andrews and Andrews (1995) viewed this evolution "as the family teaching the clinician how to help them even as the clinician is teaching the family how to help their child. The process is a mutual one, each teaching the other, and each learning to be more effective in carrying out his or her responsibility relative to the child with a disability" (p. 66).

Providing support for families is a critical component of family-centered care. Therapists can strive to achieve a balance between acknowledging a family's unique realities and acknowledging their right to be a "normal" family. Therapists show respect by accepting families as they balance their many responsibilities at home and work. The role of the professional in this process is to be flexible because the degree and type of professional involvement will vary depending on the family's needs at any particular time (Leviton et al., 1992; Strickland, 1983). Support may include being an active listener, accompanying caregivers to meetings, providing information, providing guidelines on accessing community services and collaboration strategies, conducting a variety of training programs, providing direct service for their child, and making referrals to appropriate community resources. Pediatric physical therapists must advocate for the needs of children with disabilities and their families (Cherry, 1991) and support the involvement of all family members in the intervention process (Rosenbaum et al., 1998).

In a family-centered model, it is important not to lose sight of the therapist's role in providing support for the child (Bazak, 1989). The child is respected as an individual and is involved in intervention planning and decision making. The child's roles as a member of a family, as a sibling, as a friend, and as a student need to be acknowledged and promoted (Bazak, 1989).

The guidelines presented are based on the philosophical model of family-centered service delivery. Research has begun to look at the process and outcomes of family-centered care. In early intervention, the philosophies and behaviors of service providers who strive to be family centered have been examined. The components of family-centered services that were identified were (1) family orientation, positiveness, thinking the best of families; (2) sensitivity, putting themselves in the parents' shoes; (3) responsiveness, doing whatever needs to be done; (4) friendliness, treating parents as friends; and (5) child and community skills (McWilliam, Tocci, & Harbin, 1998). Family-centered care for families of children with chronic illness resulted in greater parent satisfaction with care and child adjustment than standard care (Stein & Jessop, 1984). Family-centered intervention is complex. It is the foundation for all service-delivery systems and an approach through which physical therapists can embed their unique skills. Research is needed to identify family-centered intervention processes that promote improved outcomes for children and their families.

Family-Centered Physical Therapy

Sokoly and Dokecki (1992) reminded us that "despite the expressed willingness of professionals to regard families as partners in the care of children with developmental disabilities, partnership thinking has not always prevailed at the level of practice" (p. 23). This is the challenge for the professional today, that is, to apply current philosophy regarding respect for and partnership with families to actual, meaningful practice.

Pediatric Physical Therapy Competencies

The Section on Pediatrics of the American Physical Therapy Association (APTA) (1990) has adopted practice guidelines for physical therapists practicing in the neonatal intensive care unit (Sweeney, Heriza, Reilly, Smith, & VanSant, 1999), in early intervention, and in the school system. All of the documents include competencies related to family-centered care. The Competencies for Physical Therapists in Early Intervention has an entire section on this topic (Effgen, Bjornson, Chiarello, Sinzer, & Phillips, 1991). Even though the competencies were focused on early intervention, they can be generalized to other areas of pediatric practice. In the position statement that introduced the competencies, the task force of the Section on Pediatrics of APTA acknowledged that family-centered services provide for maximum intervention. The competencies can serve as a guide for therapists as they strive to develop the knowledge and skills necessary to provide quality service. The main competency stated that "The physical therapist can demonstrate knowledge of the importance of family systems theory and is able to provide family-focused services" (p. 79). The subcompetencies are listed in Box 3.1.

Physical Therapy Examination and Evaluation

There are many points to consider when applying the principles of a family-centered framework to the performance of a physical therapy examination. The first point is that the purpose and process of the child and **family assessment** need to be discussed and agreed on before the examination and evaluation begin. In today's health-care arena, therapists may not be able to meet all the requests of caregivers, but caregivers should have the opportunity to provide their recommendations regarding the format, content, time, and place of the examination and evaluation. Therapists also need to ask families how they want to be involved in the actual examination. Do family members want to be the facilitator, assist with activities, observe, or exchange ideas (Leviton et al., 1992)? Families provide accurate and valid

---

BOX 3.1 **Family-Centered Intervention Competencies for Physical Therapists in Early Intervention**

1. Demonstrate knowledge of family systems theory and its application to early intervention.

2. Discuss the impact of a child with special needs on a family unit.

3. Discuss, design, and implement basic strategies to support the family unit, including the marital dyad, parental competence, parent-child relationships, and sibling subsystems, and demonstrate skill in empowering the family.

4. Support the parents' primary roles as mother and father to the child.

5. Advocate for the right of parents to be decision makers in the early intervention process, including providing them with the information and options needed for informed decisions.

6. Identify and discuss cultural, socioeconomic, ethical, historical, and personal values and factors affecting a child's and family's development and early intervention program.

7. Demonstrate communication skills needed to establish a collaborative relationship with the child and the family.

8. Acknowledge the value of the family as the most significant member of the team and collaborate with family members to identify their priorities, strengths, needs, and goals.

9. Develop an individualized family-focused intervention program to enhance the growth and development of the child through a partnership with the family.

10. Assist the family in identifying and developing internal and external resources, a social support network, and advocacy skills.

11. Respect the family and demonstrate personal characteristics that enhance successful interaction with team members, the child, and the family.

Source: Effgen, S.K., Bjornson, K., Chiarello, L., Sinzer, L., & Phillips, W. (1991). Competencies for physical therapists in early intervention. *Pediatric Physical Therapy, 3*(2), 79–80.

information regarding their children and this information is valuable to the team (Long, 1992; Wilson, Kaplan, Crawford, Campbell, & Dewey, 2000).

If the child's development is being examined in more than one area, the team may consider an **arena model** for the examination and evaluation (Connor, Williams, & Siepp, 1978). This model is consistent with many family-centered principles. One team member may lead the examination, thus not overwhelming the child, whereas other team members observe. The child is typically observed in a variety of contexts, such as interactive play and feeding, allowing the child's abilities to be viewed in natural situations. The family does not have to repeat background information to a variety of professionals and the arena model fosters team interactions. However, a family may be uncomfortable if many professionals are in the room. Such factors as the child's age and degree of impairment may also influence the decision regarding an appropriate format for the examination and evaluation. Providers need to be flexible in their approach.

A second point to consider when applying the principles of family-centered care to physical therapy examination concerns respect for the child's rights and sensitivity to the child's age and temperament. Therapists need to think about the child's interests and how these interests can be used to promote motor function. Ideally, some portion of the examination should be in the child's **natural setting** during activities of daily living, play, interactions between the child and the family members, and interactions between the child and his or her peers (Comfort & Farran, 1994). Practically, simulating natural situations may be more feasible, but therapists need to obtain information regarding the child's home, school, and community environment. Observing family-child interactions during play or snack time will provide valuable information regarding the child's sensorimotor function and the family's strengths and needs. Therapists are concerned about how a child uses his or her skill to function, which is to play and interact with his or her environment, not just the ability to perform the skill. Multiple observations and sources of information will provide a more representative picture of the child and family (Comfort & Farran, 1994). Physical therapy examination reflects the expertise of the physical therapist in physical and adaptive development and is child centered. However, recognition during the examination of the way that the child uses those physical and adaptive skills within his or her environment reflects the family-centered approach to physical therapy.

A third point to consider is the need for a family assessment. Family assessment is a voluntary, interactive process between the professionals and family members to determine the concerns, priorities, and resources of the family related to enhancing the development of the child. The focus of the assessment is determined by the concerns of the family, the relevance of the information to the family's ability to enhance the child's development, and the scope of practice of the professional. A physical therapist will be involved in some aspects of family assessment and will recommend consultation with other professionals or human service agencies when it is appropriate (Chiarello, Effgen, & Levinson, 1992; Effgen & Chiarello, 2000).

Family assessment is generally performed by way of a personal interview and/or self-report survey instruments. Typically, the family assessment and child examination are not two different entities but are often interwoven. As a therapist is observing the child at play, she or he will ask the family about a typical day, the home environment, the child's interests and preferences, the child's strengths, and what they would like the child to accomplish. The therapist usually guides the interview, but it is important for the therapist to be an active listener and let the family do the talking. Communication style needs to be tailored to capture both mothers and fathers (Turbiville, Turnbull, & Turnbull, 1995). Box 3.2 provides information on important interviewing skills.

Caregivers and professionals have identified information as one of the primary needs of families (Summers et al., 1990). Therefore, in a family assessment it is crucial to ascertain what knowledge the family has regarding their child's condition and what additional information they want. It is important to discuss the family's awareness and use of, and satisfaction with, medical, therapeutic, and educational services. In addition, professionals need to inquire about which family members are involved in care-

---

BOX 3.2 Recommended Interviewing Skills

- Be aware of eye contact.
- Respect personal space.
- Use inviting facial expressions and gestures.
- Give your full attention to the speaker.
- Ask for clarification or examples.
- Acknowledge caregiver concerns and suggestions.
- Provide requested information.
- Adapt interviewing skills to respect the family's culture.

giving and about what strategies the family is using to help their child (Kolobe, Sparling, & Daniels, 2000). Andrews and Andrews (1995) recommended asking families to describe what they have done that appears most helpful for the child. This question acknowledges the family's abilities and provides the therapist with vital information for intervention planning. The family assessment includes having the caregivers identify their formal, informal, and material supports as well as their competing needs (Seligman & Darling, 1989). Knowledge of the family's basic needs in regard to nutrition, health care, clothing, and shelter, as well as the availability of professional and informal support networks, provides a realistic and essential starting point for any intervention plan. Box 3.3 provides examples of specific interview questions that reflect a family-centered approach.

Many family-oriented assessments that measure areas of family support, strengths, resources, and stress are available. Some of these assessments are self-report paper and pencil questionnaires. As therapists review these instru-

ments to determine the appropriateness for their setting, they will also gain an awareness of the variety of issues that may be important to an intervention program. If a standardized assessment is used, clinicians need to become knowledgeable in administration and interpretation of the information. The team collaboratively interprets the information from family assessments in context with other child and family information. Assessments include the Family Routines Inventory (Gallagher, Beckman, & Cross, 1983), Family Needs Survey (Bailey & Simeonsson, 1988), Family Celebrations, Traditions, Routines, and Strengths Questionnaire (McCubbin, Thompson, Pirner, & McCubbin, 1988), Family Resource Scale (Dunst & Leet, 1987), and Parenting Stress Index (Abidin, 1990).

Intervention Planning

In a family-centered approach, intervention planning is a collaborative effort among the child, family, and professionals to design an intervention process that is suited to the child's and family's needs and style. Before the plan is delineated, therapists need to provide the family with information obtained from the examination. The family's concerns, priorities, strengths, and resources, as well as the child's strengths and needs, are reviewed with the family. Professionals acknowledge the child's strengths so caregivers can celebrate the typical aspects of their child's abilities. Relaying the information from the examination is crucial because it will help families make informed recommendations and decisions. Verbal feedback should be given to the family immediately after the examination, and more detailed information can be given to the family during the intervention planning process. During this process professionals also need to ask the family how they perceived the examination, what information they gained from the examination, and if they have any additional information not addressed in the examination. Caregivers' observations of their child's abilities have validity and need to be respected (Leviton et al., 1992).

Professionals need to set a positive tone for **collaboration**. All team members, including the family, should be addressed with the same degree of formality or informality (Leviton et al., 1992). Eliciting the perspectives of all those involved may expand the intervention options and provide opportunities for family participation (Andrews & Andrews, 1995, Leviton et al., 1992). Caregivers will vary in their ability to participate, and professionals need to

---

BOX 3.3 Sample Family-Centered Interview Questions

- "Tell me about your child."
- "Tell me about your family and friends who are an important part of your child's life."
- "What is a typical day like for your family and your child?"
- "How would you describe your child's personality?"
- "How does your child like to interact with other people?"
- "How does your child like to play?"
- "What are your child's interests and preferences?"
- "What are your family's interests?"
- "Share with me something your child does that you like."
- "What is the one thing that has helped your child the most?"
- "What would you like your child to learn to do in the immediate future?"
- "What would you like help with in the immediate future?"
- "What supports and resources can you rely on?"

encourage all families to provide their input. An effective approach is to directly ask the caregivers how they want to be involved, what they see as their role, and how they want the professionals to be involved (Leviton et al., 1992). Families are invited to provide their requests and recommendations. Collaboration should not be viewed as negotiation, but that does not mean that negotiations will not be part of the process. Professionals need to be active listeners. If therapists are uncertain about information the family provides, clarification or examples are requested instead of making assumptions. When talking to families, the therapist must avoid using jargon. The therapist may present options for the intervention plan, but when making a recommendation, it is important to phrase it as an "I statement" (Meilahn, 1993). For example, "I believe that Susan would benefit from a preschool program" is more acceptable than "You need to put Susan into preschool." Professionals need to present themselves in a dignified manner, but at the same time they need to establish a relaxed and friendly environment. Courteous conversation and light humor can be used effectively to accomplish this goal.

Discussions for intervention planning should be **solution focused** as opposed to problem focused (Andrews & Andrews, 1995, Deardorff, 1992). Globally, the plan includes services necessary to enhance the development of the child and the capacity of the family to meet the needs of the child. Leviton and colleagues (1992) recommended the use of exploratory questions to inquire what resource would be the most helpful for families to reduce stress. In a family-centered framework, the plan may include use of family and community resources, consultative services between professionals and the family (Hanft, 1989), and direct professional service for the child or family.

Community resources that may benefit both the child and family should be identified. "Children with special health care needs should have the opportunity to live at home and to share in the everyday family and community experiences that those without such needs take for granted" (Brewer et al., 1989, p. 1056). These may include recreation activities such as YMCA programs, swimming, horseback riding, dance, fitness programs, music, and sports organizations, in addition to special resources such as therapeutic services, special education, nutrition, family-to-family networking, vocational rehabilitation, transportation, housing, and financial assistance.

The intervention plan is specific enough to provide the family with the following information: summary of the child's present level of functioning, type and method of service delivery, payment arrangement, location of inter-vention, frequency, intensity, duration, strategies, and expected outcomes. Efforts must be made to ensure that the method and location of service delivery are family oriented. Intervention in natural community environments, as well as the least restricted environment, are preferred and supported by federal legislation (Education for All Handicapped Children Act, 1975; Individuals with Disabilities Education Act (IDEA) Amendments of 1997). Outcomes should be meaningful to the child and family. They should not be goals that address impairments but rather functional goals and objectives. There is an important difference between "the child will be able to hold his arms antigravity" and "the child will be able to reach his arms towards his parents when indicating that he wants to be picked up from the crib." If during the course of the upcoming year the child will be transitioning from one agency to another, a specific plan on the transitioning process must be included. This plan includes procedures to (1) review service options with the family, (2) communicate information between agencies, (3) orient the child and family to the new agency, and (4) determine what abilities are needed before the transition. The goal of the plan is to avoid disruption of services, ensure appropriate placement, ease the process for the family, and enhance adaptation. This transition plan is especially crucial when a child is transitioning from a pediatric to an adult care agency.

A written intervention plan serves as a communication vehicle among team members, a guide for intervention, and a standard for program evaluation. The family needs to be involved in an informative monitoring plan to evaluate program effectiveness (Strickland, 1983). Caregivers need assurance that the intervention plan will be implemented and that the family will be informed and involved with revisions when circumstances change. Written communication, telephone calls, and meetings can be used to exchange information on an ongoing basis.

Presently in early intervention, the intervention planning process is outlined and mandated as an **Individualized Family Service Plan (IFSP)** (IDEA, 1997). The mandate includes guidelines for the child examination and family assessment, an annual meeting with the family, persons involved with the evaluation, persons who will be providing service, and an assigned service coordinator. As part of the collaboration process, the family has the opportunity to decide who they wish to invite to the meeting. This option is especially important for families of cultures where other family or community members are valued in the decision-making process. Even though the intervention planning process is most clearly defined for the early intervention years, family collaboration during this process is crucial for all ages and establishes a family-professional partnership of mutual trust and respect.

While the legislation related to early intervention clearly requires family participation, and current practice endorses family empowerment, the process of family-centered intervention is not meant to imply that the family is to take sole responsibility for the education and therapeutic needs of their child. Caregivers have the option of deciding on their level of involvement and professionals must not be judgmental.

Physical Therapy Intervention

Family-centered physical therapy intervention begins with **prevention**. In addition to early identification, early and appropriate referrals, and comprehensive child examinations and family assessments, therapists need to make a commitment to developing community-based prevention programs. Prevention programs vary in structure, content, and process. Many community hospitals provide families of newborns with a gift bag that includes information on child care, immunization schedules, and developmental milestones, as well as sample baby products such as a toy tester that alerts parents of the choking hazards of small toys. Typically, physical therapists consult to neonatal intensive care units and high-risk follow-up clinics to provide preventive information and guidance to caregivers on motor and functional development and early warning signs of developmental problems. Their role as a consultant also includes conducting screenings to identify infants who need to be monitored or referred to early intervention. Physical therapists may also be involved in community- or school-based prevention programs to promote fitness or identify musculoskeletal problems such as scoliosis. Health-care objectives now emphasize the importance of prevention efforts. Physical therapists need to make the commitment to put these programs into practice.

Family-centered intervention does not preclude **direct service delivery** from a professional (Hanft, 1989). Direct physical therapy service is indicated to address neuromuscular, musculoskeletal, and cardiopulmonary impairments that limit function and to enhance neurobehavioral organization to promote balance and movement. Direct service is especially indicated when specialized intervention procedures are needed and when the child is learning a new skill. Family-centered intervention does mean that direct service

is provided in a manner that fosters and respects child and family competence. Family members and the child are active participants during therapy sessions.

The initial focus of intervention should be in an area where success is most likely. Achievement of outcomes acknowledges the family's and child's competence and may give them the confidence to work on more challenging tasks (Andrews & Andrews, 1995). The initial focus should also be on an area that is important to the child and family, and not necessarily the therapist's first priority. Therapeutic goals and activities address functional skills needed for the child to be an active participant in social relationships. For example, functional cruising for a 6-year-old may provide the child with the responsibility for a household chore, such as setting the table or the ability to collect lunch money at school.

The content and process of physical therapy sessions need to be family centered. Interventions are provided within the natural environment of the child. The natural environment goes beyond the actual location of the intervention and requires that the intervention be provided within the context of the family and child's daily activities and routines while promoting learning opportunities for the child (Dunst, Bruder, Trivette, Hamby, Raab, & McLean, 2001; Dunst & Bruder, 2002). The settings where children live and play afford opportunities to address family and caregiver interests and priorities related to providing care for the child (Dunst et al., 2001; McWilliam & Scott, 2001). Therapists provide the family with the skills and resources needed for specialized daily care for their children. When therapists work with young children, therapists can involve the family by setting up opportunities for reciprocal and enjoyable caregiver-child interactions. For preschool and school-aged children, opportunities for developmentally appropriate sibling and **peer interactions** and application of their motor behaviors in meaningful contexts become important. Providing guidance for playground and extracurricular activities will enable children to more fully participate in their natural environments. Law et al. (1998) performed a single group pilot study on the effects of family-centered functional therapy for young children with cerebral palsy and reported that children improved in functional performance. Upon analysis of the interventions, the authors recommended further development of specific intervention strategies that focus on the task and environment.

Therapists promote **motor function, playfulness**, and **self-esteem** by using play as a context for therapy (Chiarello, 1993; Fewell & Glick, 1993; Schaaf & Mulrooney, 1989). Play includes sensory, neuromuscular, and mental processes. Play with motion is an integral part of physical therapy. Play makes therapy more meaningful; it elicits a child's attention, motivation, cooperation, and initiation. A motor skill for a play activity is an understandable goal for the child. Play provides an avenue for motor learning and also affords a relaxed and enjoyable atmosphere. More importantly, through play, physical therapists support children's playfulness, their enjoyment, and their engagement with activities (Bundy, 1997). Physical therapists provide the caregiver with the physical resources, such as positioning equipment and adaptive switches, to make play time happen at home. Therapists encourage active participation of the child and sensitivity to the child's interests, cues, and needs. When choices are available, they should be offered to the child. Even simple choices provide the child with the opportunity to direct an interaction and to be a leader. Physical therapists are concerned with not only teaching a child a motor skill but also helping the child gain the confidence to use that skill in his or her daily interactions. A range of activities should be used to provide a balance among interactive play, exploration, and independent play.

Another aspect of family-centered physical therapy is communication. Communications during therapy need to be respectful. It is unacceptable to talk in front of children without acknowledging them. This rule is frequently abused when discussing issues with the family, other healthcare/educational professionals, or student interns. During the course of a session, communications with the family often include general social conversation as well as opportunities to share information. Mothers have identified communication skills as a necessary factor for promoting positive outcomes for families and children (Washington & Schwartz, 1996). Therapists need to ask families how they would like information presented to them. Some families like to keep a journal notebook and others prefer written information such as books or articles. Explanations and demonstrations are two important ways to help make information meaningful to the family. When therapists see children in a school setting, it is very important to send short notes home to the families because in this setting, families can feel isolated from the day-to-day interactions between their children and the therapists.

When and where intervention sessions take place represent another issue related to family-centered care. The availability of appointments, such as the option of some evening and weekend hours, respects the family's lifestyle and may provide the opportunity for a variety of family members and caregivers to participate in the intervention. As health-

care providers, therapists need to put consumer-focused services into practice. Federal legislation supports the provision of early intervention services in the natural environment. With infants and toddlers, the context of learning is their home or child care facility. These environments foster spontaneous use of skills by providing natural cues and reinforcement (Grabowski, 1991). Even though home-based services may not be feasible in all instances, home visits should be an integral component to an intervention plan. Caregivers have acknowledged that home visits are one of the most helpful aspects of early intervention (Upshur, 1991). During home visits, therapists can gain valuable information about the child's natural environment that can guide intervention plans and recommendations for environmental adaptations and adaptive equipment. In addition to home visits, therapists may need to consult in a variety of settings in the child's community, such as child care or school. In the clinic, therapists can set up simulations to address functional skills needed in the home, school, and community. As an example, caregivers may be asked to measure the height of furniture at home so that transfer training in the clinic can simulate the chair to bed transfer that is needed in the home.

Home recommendations are essential if an intervention plan is to incorporate practice and to promote generalization of skill into the natural environment. In a family-centered philosophy, therapists do not prescribe home programs (Bazak, 1989); rather, home programs are established in collaboration with the family. Therapists need to be sensitive to the unique situations within each family. An elder caregiver may not be able to participate in a program geared to play time on the floor, or a single parent may have limited time and energy. Home activities should be functional and incorporated into activities of daily living and the family's daily routine (Rainforth & Salisbury, 1988). Therapists collaborate with the family to identify naturally occurring intervention opportunities (Kaiser & Hancock, 2003). The family and child choose program activities that are realistic and meaningful to them. Playtime may be an avenue to capture a father's preference for participation (Turbiville et al., 1995). It is the therapist's responsibility to ensure that the family is comfortable with the techniques and activities. Therapists need to ask the family how they would best learn a therapeutic technique. The many avenues of learning include modeling, participatory demonstrations, photographs, videos, diagrams, and written instruction. It is important to remember to find out if the activity worked. Bazak (1989) urges therapists to stop using the term *noncompliance*. If the activity has not been used at home, then the therapist and family need to revisit appropriate and realistic home activities.

Case Examples 3–2 and 3–3 provide clinical scenarios highlighting some of the family-centered principles discussed.

CASE EXAMPLE 3–2 . . . . .

Family-Centered Intervention for a Young Child

A therapist was providing service for a 5-year-old boy with a diagnosis of global developmental delay. His gross motor age equivalent was 12 months, and the child had limited standing balance and was not ambulating independently. He had limited expressive communication. His parents worked and he had two older siblings. The *first step* in developing an intervention plan was to determine the family's goals and objectives. The family identified four skills for the child to learn that were important to them: (1) the ability to stand up from the potty chair, (2) the ability to climb into the bathtub, (3) the ability to walk safely in the house and outside in the yard, and (4) the ability to shake hands. The *second step* was to discuss the method of intervention. The family requested home-based services in the early evening or Saturday morning. They expressed their desire to participate during part of the session, but they also believed that their son should work alone with the therapist for part of the time. This balance enabled the family members to participate in some positive play and functional activities but also to have some independent time while their son was working one-on-one with the therapist during a challenging activity. The therapist was able to try new interventions and determine their success before teaching the family. The *third step* was to discuss the family's typical routine to identify opportunities for integrating intervention techniques. The family acknowledged their busy schedule but identified Saturday morning as a relaxed time when the children sometimes climbed into the parents' bed for some cuddling and play. This time was hallmarked as a fun way to work on climbing. The home setting enabled the therapist to work on functional mobility on the stairs, in the bathroom, and outside in the yard.

CASE EXAMPLE 3–3 . . . . .

Family-Centered Intervention for an Adolescent

A 15-year-old boy with a diagnosis of juvenile rheumatoid arthritis was referred to outpatient pediatric rehabilitation. During the intake telephone call, a description of the facility and pediatric rehabilitation program was provided to the mother. The therapist requested that this information be shared with her son. Both the mother and son made an informed decision that the son would be comfortable being served in a pediatric facility. The therapist made an effort to redesign a portion of the therapy gym to respect the interests of older children.

During the initial evaluation, the adolescent was asked what he wanted to gain from therapy, what he enjoyed most about therapy in the past, and what he enjoyed least about therapy in the past. The adolescent was able to clearly identify three goals: (1) he wanted to maintain his range of motion to avoid surgery, (2) he wanted to be able to walk short distances in his home, but he was comfortable using his wheelchair for long distances, and (3) he wanted to have enough energy to participate in after-school activities such as throwing some basketball shots. The adolescent was very open in his communication style and shared that he had been angry during previous episodes of therapy when the therapist did not believe his subjective reports of pain. The therapist and adolescent agreed on a contract in which the therapist would stop any activity if the adolescent used a designated time-out signal. This agreement was upheld throughout the therapy process and was an essential element in building a trustful relationship. Based on the adolescent's goals, an intervention program consisting of range of motion, positioning, ambulation activities, strengthening, and endurance training was developed.

The therapist discussed with the family how other family members wanted to be involved. The adolescent wanted to be treated without his parents present, but it was agreed that at the end of the session the adolescent and therapist would provide the parents with an update on any changes in status or recommended activities for home. The mother and adolescent did discuss involving the younger sister during an occasional session. The mother believed that it was important for her daughter to be involved in a positive experience with her brother. At the end of therapy sessions, his sister was often invited to participate in a sport activity with her brother. A brief, daily, home range-of-motion program was recommended. The rest of the movement activities were integrated into the adolescent's responsibilities and routines, such as clearing the dinner table and eventually walking to the mailbox to get the mail each day. This approach respected the adolescent's academic demands and social needs.

The adolescent was followed for periodic therapy over the course of the next few years. During his senior year in high school, he was involved in the decision-making process of obtaining powered mobility in preparation for the locomotion demands of a college campus. The therapist, parents, and adolescent talked openly of transitioning his care to the college health center as well as to an adult rheumatologist. The family scheduled several consultation visits before selecting an adult specialist. After the discharge from the pediatric facility, the therapist made a follow-up call to both the young adult and the parents to make sure that there were no gaps in the service-delivery process. The young adult was on his way to being an advocate for himself to receive appropriate, respectful care.

Coordination and Collaboration of Service

Agencies' policies and procedures for referral process and service delivery should reflect a family-centered philosophy (Leviton et al., 1992; Shelton & Stepanek, 1995) and ensure that families receive appropriate services and documentation in a timely manner. **Coordination** of services is crucial to family-centered care and is economically more cost effective (Brewer et al., 1989). Services for families and children with special needs are often complex, dispersed through a variety of agencies, organizations, and facilities, and have varying eligibility and financial requirements. Administrative bureaucracy can undermine an atmosphere of support and respect. "Appropriate, flexible, and reasonable ways must be found to link them together to provide maximum benefit to these children and their families" (Brewer et al., 1989, p. 1056). Meaningful **documentation** of services communicates vital information to the family, service providers, and agencies to promote coordination. Families can participate in the documentation process to ensure that it accurately reflects their child's and family's status, accomplishments, and needs.

In educational systems, service coordinators and case managers organize services for children and their families; however, throughout all areas of pediatrics, physical therapists can be instrumental in promoting coordinated care and ease of entry into their community's intervention systems. Physical therapists can consult with local agencies to help establish an efficient and effective system for service delivery with appropriate health care, education, and recreational providers. Physical therapists can help form the link between the social worker or case manager in the health-care center with the service coordinator in the educational center. Coordination of services is an important function of family-centered care. Time constraints often leave this job undone, and families and professionals may be frustrated by gaps in the care plan.

Respite care, which is temporary care for a person with a disability or chronic illness, that provides rest for the primary caregiver is one service often needed and requested by families, and should be part of family-centered service coordination. Family-centered care supports children living in their home; however, this process must be assisted and must not just be a philosophical agreement. Physical therapists can become involved in a respite program on many levels including being aware of community programs and making referrals, assisting with the development or administration of a respite program, being on the advisory board of a respite program, educating staff involved with the program, and providing direct service in a respite program (Short-DeGraff & Kologinsky, 1988; Warren & Cohen, 1986).

Physical therapists can be instrumental in increasing professional and community awareness of the needs of families. Political involvement is needed to support legislation that assists families with financing and availability of services. Physical therapists can provide consultation to community-based rehabilitation programs, and they can become involved in developing resource directories and conducting parent workshops. Topics frequently requested by parents include availability of financial resources, legislative mandates affecting service delivery, and how to collaborate within the school system. While successful support groups are led by the participants, physical therapists can be instrumental in helping families develop parent, sibling, and peer support groups.

Continuous quality improvement needs to be an essential part of the coordination process. Use of customer satisfaction surveys may be an effective method of collecting information on the family's perspective on intervention services they receive. It is important to share the results of the surveys with the families and to develop and implement action plans to modify the program to meet the identified needs from the survey. This process is effective in identifying and improving issues that are important to families, such as a door for the waiting room, greater ease in accessibility, and decreased waiting time for appointments (Odle, 1988).

Summary

Family-centered intervention takes time and consideration. It is challenging. In the clinical arena, with the never-ending demands of high caseloads, productivity standards, and funding, it is at times difficult to meet all the responsibilities; however, not using a family-centered approach is a disservice to the children and families. Therapists need to consider how their belief system matches accepted state-of-the-art practice principles of family-centered care, as well as how to integrate these practices in a clinical arena with many payor constraints. Therapists must focus on quality standards. Family-centered care gives the family and child the chance to develop to their fullest.

The theory of family-centered intervention can guide practice and research endeavors to document the effectiveness of this approach. Harris (1990) promoted efficacy research in pediatric physical therapy on family-focused outcomes. Many of these outcomes have not been studied specifically, but clinicians and researchers have expressed their subjective insights that physical therapy appears to positively affect a family's well-being (Ferry, 1986; Wright & Nicholson, 1973). In discussing future considerations for pediatric physical therapy practice, Stuberg and Harbourne (1994) stated, "It is becoming clearer that pediatric physical therapy can no longer focus primarily on the developmental and neuromotor aspects of patient care. We must now address all levels of the disablement continuum and health-related quality of life issues. Family-centered services with a focus on the consumer and not the provider will be the trend of the future; new theoretical concepts, assessment methods; and perhaps new physical therapy intervention techniques need to address this area of practice" (p. 124). Family-centered care requires the integration of the science of family systems with other behavioral, biological, and clinical sciences (Sparling & Sekerak, 1992). "Only through collaborative efforts between parents, professionals, and service providers can the goal of family-centered, community-based, coordinated care for these families and their children become a reality" (Odle, 1988, p. 85). It is well worth the effort.

DISCUSSION QUESTIONS

1. How do your values and behaviors reflect a family-centered perspective?

2. What are some stumbling blocks that could prevent a therapist-family partnership from developing? What are some communication skills we can use to prevent this from happening? What can we do to prevent or minimize additional stressors that a family may be facing? What administrative supports or policies are needed to assist you in implementing family-centered care in your practice?

3. What is our role when presented with other team members who do not embrace this philosophy?

RECOMMENDED READINGS

Dunst, C.J., Trivette, C.M., Davis, M., & Cornwell, J. (1988). Enabling and empowering families of children with health impairments. *Children's Health Care, 17*(2), 71–81.

Rosenbaum, P., King, S., Law, M., King, G., & Evans, J. (1998). Family-centered service: A conceptual framework and research review. *Physical and Occupational Therapy in Pediatrics, 18*(1), 1–20.

Shelton, T.L., & Stepanek, J.S. (1995). Excerpts from family centered care for children needing specialized health and developmental services. *Pediatric Nursing, 21*(4), 362–364.

Viscardis, L. (1998). The family-centered approach to providing services: A parent perspective. *Physical and Occupational Therapy in Pediatrics, 18*(1), 41–53.

REFERENCES

Abidin, R. (1990). *Parenting Stress Index* (3rd ed.). Charlottesville, VA: Pediatric Psychology Press.

Affleck, G., McGrade, B. J., McQueeney, M., & Allen, D. (1982). Promise of relationship-focused early intervention in developmental disabilities. *Journal of Special Education, 16*, 413–430.

Ainsworth, M.D., & Bell, S.M. (1974). Mother-infant interaction and the development of competence. In K. Connolly & J. Brunner (Eds.). *The growth of competence* (pp. 97–118). New York: Academic Press.

American Physical Therapy Association (1990). *Physical therapy practice in educational environments.* Alexandria, VA.: American Physical Therapy Association.

Andrews, J.R., & Andrews, M.A. (1995). Solution-focused assumptions that support family-centered early intervention. *Infants and Young Children, 8(1)*, 60–67.

Bailey, D.B., & Simeonsson, R.J. (1988). Assessing needs of families with handicapped infants. *Journal of Special Education, 22,* 117–127.

Bazak, S. (1989). Changes in attitudes and beliefs regarding parent participation and home programs: An update. *American Journal of Occupational Therapy, 43*(11), 723–728.

Becvar, D.S., & Becvar, R.J. (1988). *Family therapy: A systemic integration.* Boston: Allyn and Bacon.

Brewer, E.J., McPherson, M., Magrab, P.T., & Hutchins, V.L. (1989). Family centered, community-based, coordinated care for children with special health care needs. *Pediatrics, 83*(6), 1055–1060.

Bricker, D., & Veltman, M. (1990). Early intervention programs: Child-focused approaches. In S.J. Meisels & J.P. Shonkoff (Eds.). *Handbook of early childhood intervention* (pp. 373–399). New York: Cambridge University Press.

Bromwich, R. (1981). *Working with parents and infants: An interactional approach.* Baltimore: University Park Press.

Bronfenbrenner, U. (1977). Toward an experimental ecology of human development. *American Psychologist, 32,* 513–531.

Bundy, A. (1997). Play and playfulness: What to look for. In L. Parham & L. Fazio (Eds.). *Play and occupational therapy for children.* (pp.52–66). Philadelphia: Mosby.

Carter, B., & McGoldrick, M. (1989). Overview: The changing family life cycle: A framework for family therapy. In B. Carter & M. McGoldrick (Eds.). *The changing family life cycle: A framework for family therapy* (2nd ed., pp. 3–28). Boston: Allyn & Bacon.

Cherry, D. (1991). Pediatric physical therapy: Philosophy, science, and techniques. *Pediatric Physical Therapy, 3,* 70–76.

Chiarello, L. (1993). Influence of physical therapy on the motor and interactive behaviors of mothers and their children with motor delay during play (Doctoral dissertation, MCP Hahnemann University). *Dissertation Abstracts International, 54/07-B,* 3572.

Chiarello, L. (1993, May). Innovative approaches in working with families and their children. In Family-Centered Early Intervention Conference. Symposium conducted at Hahnemann University, Philadelphia, PA.

Chiarello, L., Effgen, S., & Levinson, M. (1992). Parent-professional partnership in evaluation and development of individual family service plans. *Pediatric Physical Therapy, 4,* 64–69.

Cintas, H.L. (1995). Cross-cultural similarities and differences in development: Impact of parental expectations on motor behavior. *Pediatric Physical Therapy, 7*(3), 103–111.

Clarke-Stewart, K.A. (1973). Interactions between mothers and their young children: Characteristics and consequences. *Monographs of the Society for Research in Child Development, 38*(6–7, Serial # 153).

Cochrane, C.C., & Farley, B.G. (1990). Preparation of physical therapists to work with handicapped infants and their families: Current status and training needs. *Physical Therapy, 70,* 372–380.

Comfort, M., & Farran, D.C. (1994). Parent-child interaction assessment in family-centered intervention. *Infants and Young Children, 6*(4), 33–45.

Connor, F.P., Williamson, G.G., & Siepp, J.M. (1978). *Program guide for infants and toddlers with neuromotor and other developmental disabilities.* New York: Teachers College Press.

Deardorff, C.A. (1992). Use of the double ABCX model of family adaptation in the early intervention process. *Infants and Young Children, 4*(3), 75–83.

Dunst, C.J., & Bruder, M.B. (2002). Valued outcomes of service coordination, early intervention, and natural environments. *Exceptional Children, 68*(3), 361–375.

Dunst, C.J., Bruder, M.B., Trivette, C.M., Hamby, D., Raab, M., & McLean, M. (2001). Characteristics and consequences of everyday natural learning opportunities. *Topics in Early Childhood Special Education, 21*(2), 68–92.

Dunst, C.J., Bruder, M.B., Trivette, C.M., Raab, M., & McLean, M. (2001). Natural learning opportunities for infants, toddlers, and preschoolers. *Young Exceptional Children, 4*(2), 18–25.

Dunst, C.J., Johanson, C., Trivette, C.M., & Hamby, D. (1991). Family-oriented intervention policies and practices: Family-centered or not? *Exceptional Children, 58*(2), 115–126.

Dunst, C.J., & Leet, H.E. (1987). Measuring the adequacy of resources in households with young children. *Child: Care, Health and Development, 13,* 111–125.

Dunst, C.J., Trivette, C.M., & Cross, A. H. (1986). Mediating influences of social support: Personal, family, and child outcomes. *American Journal of Mental Deficiency, 90,* 403–417.

Dunst, C.J., Trivette, C.M., Davis, M., & Cornwell, J. (1988). Enabling and empowering families of children with health impairments. *Children's Health Care, 17*(2), 71–81.

Dura, J.R., & Kiecolt-Glaser, J.K. (1991). Family transitions, stress, and health. In P.A. Cowan & M. Hetherington (Eds.). *Family transitions* (pp. 59–76). Hillsdale, NJ: Lawrence Erlbaum Associates.

Education for All Handicapped Children Act (PL 94–142). (1975), 20 U.S.C. 14.

Education of Handicapped Act Amendments of 1986 (PL 99–457). 20 U.S.C. 1400–1485.

Effgen, S.K., Bjornson, K., Chiarello, L., Sinzer, L., & Phillips, W. (1991). Competencies for physical therapists in early intervention. *Pediatric Physical Therapy, 3*(2), 77–80.

Effgen, S.K., & Chiarello. L.A. (2000). Physical therapist education for service in early intervention. *Infants and Young Children, 12*(4), 63–76.

Elder, G.H. (1991). Family transitions, cycles, and social change. In P.A. Cowan & M. Hetherington (Eds.). *Family transitions* (pp. 31–57). Hillsdale, NJ: Lawrence Erlbaum Associates.

Ferry, P.C. (1986). Infant stimulation programs: A neurological shell game? *Archives of Neurology, 43,* 281–282.

Fewell, R., & Glick, M.P. (1993). Observing play: An appropriate process for learning and assessment. *Infants and Young Children, 5,* 35–43.

Gallagher, J., Beckman, P., & Cross, A. (1983). Families of handicapped children: Sources of stress and its amelioration. *Exceptional Children, 50,* 10–19.

Gerhard, M. (1995). Perspective: Home-based early intervention in a multicultural community. *Pediatric Physical Therapy, 7*(3), 133–134.

Grabowski, K. (1991). *Best practices for therapy in preschool settings.* Morgantown, NC: North Carolina Division for Early Childhood of the Council for Exceptional Children.

Guralnick, M.J. (1998). Effectiveness of early intervention for vulnerable children: A developmental perspective. *American Journal of Mental Retardation, 102*(4), 319–345.

Hanft, B.E. (1989). Early intervention: Issues in specialization. *American Journal of Occupational Therapy, 43*(7), 431–434.

Hanson, M.J. (1992). Ethnic, cultural, and language diversity in intervention settings. In E. Lynch & M. Hanson (Eds.). *Developing cross-cultural competence* (pp. 3–18). Baltimore: Paul H. Brookes.

Hanson, M.J., & Hanline, M.F. (1990). Parenting a child with a disability: A longitudinal study of parental stress and adaptation. *Journal of Early Intervention, 14,* 234–248.

Harris, S. (1990). Efficacy of physical therapy in promoting family functioning and functional independence for children with cerebral palsy. *Pediatric Physical Therapy, 2*(3), 160–164.

Harrison, A.O., Wilson, M.N., Pine, C.J., Chan, S.Q., & Buriel, R. (1990). Family ecologies of ethnic minority children. *Child Development, 61,* 347–362.

Hill, R.F., Fortenberry, J.D., & Stein, H.F. (1989). Culture in clinical medicine. *Southern Medical Journal, 83*(9), 1071–1080.

Individuals with Disabilities Education Act (IDEA) Amendments of 1991, Public Law 102–119, 105 STAT, 587.

Individuals with Disabilities Education Act (IDEA) Amendments of 1997, Public Law 105–17.

Kaiser, A.P., & Hancock, T.B. (2003). Teaching parents new skills to support their young children's development. *Infants and Young Children, 16*(1), 9–21.

Kolobe, T.H.A., Sparling, J., & Daniels, L.E. (2000). Family-centered intervention. In S.K. Campbell, D.W. Vander Linden, & R.J. Palisano (Eds.). *Physical therapy for children* (2nd ed.). Philadelphia: W.B. Saunders Company.

Lamb, M. (1983). Fathers of exceptional children. In M. Seligman (Ed.). *The family with a handicapped child: Understanding and treatment* (pp. 125–146). New York: Grune & Stratton.

Law, M., Darrah, J., Pollock, N., King, G., Rosenbaum, P., Russell, Palisano, R., Harris, S., Armstrong, R., & Watt, J. (1998). Family-centered functional therapy for children with cerebral palsy: An emerging practice model. *Physical and Occupational Therapy in Pediatrics, 18*(1), 82–102.

Leviton, A, Mueller, M, & Kauffman, C. (1992). The family-centered consultation model: Practical applications for professionals. *Infants and Young Children, 4*(3), 1–8.

Long, T.M. (1992). The use of parent report measures to assess infant development. *Pediatric Physical Therapy, 4*(2), 74–77.

Low, S.M. (1984). The cultural basis of health, illness and disease. *Social Work Health Care, 9*(3), 13–23.

Lynch, E.W. (1992). From culture shock to culture learning. In E. Lynch & M. Hanson (Eds.). *Developing cross-cultural competence* (pp. 19–34). Baltimore: Paul H. Brookes.

Mahoney, G., Finger, I., & Powell, A. (1985). Relationship of maternal behavioral style to the development of organically impaired mentally retarded infants. *American Journal of Mental Deficiency, 90,* 296–302.

McCubbin, H., Thompson, A., Pirner, P., & McCubbin, M. (1988). *Family types and strengths: A life cycle and ecological perspective.* Edina, MN: Bellwether Press.

McGoldrick, M. (1989). Ethnicity and the family life cycle. In B. Carter & M. McGoldrick (Eds.). *The changing family life cycle: A framework for family therapy* (2nd. ed., pp. 69–90). Boston: Allyn & Bacon.

McWilliam, R.A., & Scott, S. (2001). A support approach to early intervention: A three-part framework. *Infants and Young Children, 13*(4), 55–66.

McWilliam, R.A., Tocci, L., & Harbin, G.L. (1998). Family-centered services: Service providers' discourse and behavior. *Topics in Early Childhood Special Education, 18*(4), 206–221.

Meilahn, K. (1993). Promoting partnerships between health care providers and parents of children with special health care needs. *Nutrition Focus, 8*(3), 1–6.

Minuchin, P. (1985). Families and individual development: Provocations from the field of family therapy. *Child Development, 56,* 289–302.

Newman, J. (1983). Handicapped persons and their families: Philosophical, historical, and legislative perspectives. In M. Seligman (Ed.). *The family with a handicapped child: Understanding and treatment* (pp. 3–25). New York: Grune & Stratton.

Odle, K. (1988). In my opinion…Partnership for family-cen-tered care: Reality or fantasy? *Children's Health Care, 17*(2), 85–86.

Petersen, P., & Wikoff, R.L. (1987). Home environment and adjustment in families with handicapped children: A canonical correlation study. *Occupational Therapy Journal of Research, 7*(2), 67–82.

Poresky, R.H., & Henderson, M.L. (1982). Infants' mental and motor development: Effects of home environment, maternal attitudes, marital adjustment, and socioeconomic status. *Perceptual and Motor Skills, 54,* 695–702.

Rainforth, B., & Salisbury, C.L. (1988). Functional home programs: A model for therapists. *Topics in Early Childhood Education, 7*(4), 33–45.

Ramey, C.T., Mills, P., Campbell, F.A., & O'Brien, C. (1975). Infants' home environments: A comparison of high-risk families and families from the general population. *American Journal of Mental Deficiency, 80,* 40–42.

Redman-Bentley, D. (1982). Parent expectation for professionals providing services to their handicapped children. *Physical and Occupational Therapy in Pediatrics, 2,* 13–27.

Roberts, J. (1984). Families with infants and young children with special needs. In J.C. Hansen & E.I. Coppersmith (Eds.). *Families with Handicapped Members* (pp. 1–17). Rockville, MD: Aspen.

Rosenbaum, P., King, S., Law, M., King, G., & Evans, J. (1998). Family-centered service: A conceptual framework and research review. *Physical and Occupational Therapy in Pediatrics, 18*(1), 1–20.

Rubin, S., & Quinn-Curran, N. (1983). Lost, then found: Parents' journey through the community service maze. In M. Seligman (Ed.). *The family with a handicapped child: Understanding and treatment* (pp. 63–94). New York: Grune & Stratton.

Sameroff, A.J., & Chandler, M.J. (1975). Reproductive risk and the continuum of care taking casualty. In F.D. Horowitz, M. Hetherington, S. Scarr-Salapatek, & G. Siegel (Eds.). *Review of child development research* (vol. 4). Chicago: University of Chicago Press.

Schaaf, R.C., & Mulrooney, L.L. (1989). Occupational therapy in early intervention: A family-centered approach. *American Journal of Occupational therapy, 43*(11), 745–754.

Seligman, M., & Darling, R. B. (1989). *Ordinary families, special children*. New York: Guilford Press.

Shelton, T.L., & Stepanek, J.S. (1995). Excerpts from family centered care for children needing specialized health and developmental services. *Pediatric Nursing, 21*(4), 362–364.

Shonkoff, J.P., & Hauser-Cram, P. (1987). Early intervention for disabled infants and their families: A quantitative analysis. *Pediatrics, 80*, 650–658.

Short-DeGraff, M.A., & Kologinsky, E. (1988). Respite care: Roles for therapist in support of families with handicapped children. *Physical and Occupational Therapy in Pediatrics, 7*(4), 3–18.

Sokoly, M.M., & Dokecki, P.R. (1992). Ethical perspectives on family-centered early intervention. *Infants and Young Children, 4*(4), 23–32.

Sparling, J.W. (1991). The cultural definition of the family. *Physical and Occupational Therapy in Pediatrics, 11*(4), 17–29.

Sparling, J.W., Kolobe, T., & Ezzelle, L. (1994). Family-centered intervention. In S.K. Campbell (Ed.). *Physical therapy for children* (pp. 823–846). Philadelphia: W.B. Saunders Company.

Sparling, J.W., & Sekerak, D.K. (1992). Embedding the family perspective in a physical therapy curriculum. *Pediatric Physical Therapy, 4*, 116–121.

Stein, R.E.K., & Jessop, D.J. (1984). Does pediatric home care make a difference for children with chronic illness? Findings from the pediatric ambulatory care treatment study. *Pediatrics, 73*, 845–853.

Strickland, B. (1983). Legal issues that affect parents. In M. Seligman (Ed.). *The family with a handicapped child: Understanding and treatment* (pp. 27–59). New York: Grune & Stratton.

Stuberg, W., & Harbourne, R. (1994). Theoretical practice in pediatric physical therapy: Past, present, and future considerations. *Pediatric Physical Therapy, 6*, 119–125.

Summers, J.A., DellOliver, C., Turnbull, A.P., Benson, H.A., Santelli, E., Campbell, M., & Siegel-Causey, E. (1990). Examining the individualized family service plan process: What are family and practitioner preferences? *Topics in Early Childhood Special Education, 10*, 78–99.

Sweeney, J.K., Heriza, C.B., Reilly, M.A., Smith, C., & VanSant, A.F. (1999). Practice guidelines for the physical therapist in the neonatal intensive care unit. *Pediatric Physical Therapy, 11*(2), 119–132.

Thorpe, D.E., & Baker, C.P. (1995). Perspective: Addressing "cultural competence" in health care education. *Pediatric Physical Therapy, 7*(3), 143–145.

Turbiville, V.P., Turnbull, A.P., & Turnbull, H.R. (1995). Fathers and family-centered early intervention. *Infants and Young Children, 7*(4), 12–19.

Turnbull, A.P., & Turnbull, H.R. (1982). Parent involvement in the education of handicapped children: A critique. *Mental Retardation, 20*, 115–120.

United States House of Representatives Select Committee on Children, Youth, and Families (1989). *U.S. Children and Their Families: Current Conditions and Recent Trends, 1989*. Washington, DC: U.S. Government Printing Office.

Upshur, C.C. (1991). Mothers' and fathers' ratings of the benefits of early intervention services. *Journal of Early Intervention, 15*, 345–357.

Viscardis, L. (1998). The family-centered approach to providing services: A parent perspective. *Physical and Occupational Therapy in Pediatrics, 18*(1), 41–53.

Warren, R.D., & Cohen, S. (1986). Respite care services: A role for physical therapist. *Clinical Management, 6*, 20–23.

Washington, K., & Schwartz, I.S. (1996). Maternal perceptions of the effects of physical and occupational therapy services on caregiving competency. *Physical and Occupational Therapy in Pediatrics, 16*(3), 33–54.

Wilson, B.N., Kaplan, B.J., Crawford, S.G., Campbell, A., & Dewey, D. (2000). Reliability and validity of a parent questionnaire on childhood motor skills. *American Journal of Occupational Therapy, 54*(5), 484–493.

World Health Organization (2001). *International classification of functioning, disability, and health*. Geneva, Switzerland.

Wright, T., & Nicholson, J. (1973). Physiotherapy for the spastic child: An evaluation. *Developmental Medicine and Child Neurology, 15*, 146–163.

Yarrow, L.J., Rubenstein, J.L., Pedersen, F.A., & Jankowski, J.J. (1972). Dimensions of early stimulation and their differential effects on infant development. *Merril-Palmer Quarterly, 18*, 205–218.

Yau, M.K., & Li-Tsang, C.W.P. (1999). Adjustment and adaptation in parents of children with developmental disability in two-parent families: A review of the characteristics and attributes. *British Journal of Developmental Disabilities, 45*(88), 38–51.

Systems

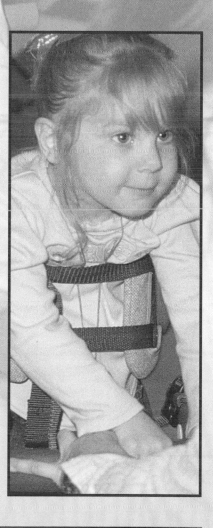

Chapter *4*

Musculoskeletal System: Structure, Function, and Evaluation

— Margo N. Orlin, PT, PhD, PCS, and
Linda Pax Lowes, PT, PhD, PCS

This chapter is designed to present information on the musculoskeletal system in childhood and adolescence and to relate this information to pediatric disorders commonly seen by the physical therapist. The chapter is divided into three main sections. The first section contains information on developmental biomechanics, including principles of growth and musculoskeletal development during childhood and adolescence. The second section reviews the histology and anatomy of the main musculoskeletal tissue systems—connective tissue, bone, and muscle—relating each to specific pediatric disorders. The third section discusses the comprehensive pediatric musculoskeletal examination process, including specific procedures and their evaluation.

Developmental Biomechanics

Developmental biomechanics is defined as "the effects of forces on the musculoskeletal system during the entire life span" (LeVeau & Bernhardt, 1984, p. 1874). Understanding how the musculoskeletal system changes and reacts to internal and external forces provides a framework to evaluate musculoskeletal examination data and develop a plan of care. This section highlights the major principles of musculoskeletal growth and discusses the changes that occur from birth and throughout childhood.

Principles of Growth and Development

During development and, to a lesser extent, throughout life, biological tissue is created, shaped, and remodeled through external or internal forces. Tissues respond not only to the different types of forces to which they are exposed in the intrauterine and extrauterine environments but also to the direction and amount of force. Force is only one factor that influences body size; shape, genetics, nutrition, drugs, and hormones also influence body structure. The basic structure and function of three key tissues in the musculoskeletal system—connective tissue, bone, and muscle—are discussed as they affect child development and function. An appreciation of the typical sequence of development and the impact of pathological influences will assist the physical therapist in identifying deviations from typical development and may allow prevention or remediation of impairments and limit disability. In this section, principles of growth and development will also be applied to the key musculoskeletal tissue systems.

Musculoskeletal Tissue Systems

Connective Tissue

There are two general types of connective tissue—dense ordinary connective tissue and cartilage. **Dense ordinary**

connective tissue can have a regular or irregular arrangement. Tendons and ligaments have regular arrangements of dense ordinary connective tissue, which is best suited to withstand tension in only the direction of the fibers. This makes them strong to resist the pull of muscles. The connective tissue that surrounds the bones, muscles, heart, and other areas is irregularly aligned and withstands tension in a number of directions.

Tendons are composed of tightly packed bundles of parallel collagen fibers. If the tendon rubs over a bone or other friction-producing surface, *synovia* (synovial fluid) acts as a lubricant. The synovial sheath is made up of an inner sheath that is attached to the tendon and an outer sheath that attaches to the object that is rubbing against the tendon. Synovial fluid fills the space between the two sheaths and allows the surfaces to glide past one another.

Ligaments are composed primarily of tightly packed parallel bundles of collagen, but they also have elastic fibers interwoven within the main fibers. This construction provides the stability for strong support around articulating joints while allowing flexibility to permit appropriate joint motion.

Both tendons and ligaments can heal if torn or surgically cut. Tendon regeneration is mediated by the fibroblasts in the inner tendon sheath or surrounding loose connective tissue. The new fibroblasts become oriented along the tendon axis, and then collagen is produced. A common complication of tendon regeneration is the development of fibrous adhesions between the tendon and surrounding tissues. These adhesions can prevent the return of normal movement. Early, gentle range of motion (ROM) can disrupt production of adhesions in undesired directions and speed recovery (Mortensen, Skov, & Jensen, 1999).

Cartilage, the second type of connective tissue, is found at the site of articulating joints and provides a smooth surface for movement. Cartilage provides the initial prenatal structure for bone development. Cartilage is a gel-like substance with fine collagen fibrils distributed in the gel to add tensile strength.

Bones

Bone is similar to cartilage except that bone has more collagen, is heavily mineralized, and is covered by a fibrous connective tissue called **periosteum**. These differences make bone much harder and less supple than cartilage. Bone cells, or osteocytes, are found in lacunae (little caves) throughout the rigid bone. The heavy mineralization of bone precludes long-range diffusion of nutrients; therefore, osteocytes must be in close proximity to blood capillaries. Canaliculi are narrow, fluid-filled channels that interconnect the osteocyte lacunae with nutrients from the capillaries.

Most bones develop from a cartilaginous model formed of mesenchyme early in the embryonic period. Mesenchyme is part of the mesoderm layer of the embryo found between the outer ectoderm and inner endoderm layers. Bone, cartilage, and muscle are all derived from the mesoderm. Bone growth occurs through apposition, or the deposition of additional bone on preexisting surfaces. There are two methods of bone appositional growth. The clavicle, mandible, and facial and cranial flat bones develop directly in vascularized mesenchyme through a process called intramembranous ossification. Intramembranous ossification begins near the end of the second month of gestation.

The remaining bones of the body develop through endochondral ossification, or the deposition of bone on a cartilaginous model. A limb bud, or mesodermal outgrowth, develops on the embryo where the extremities are going to form. The mesenchymal cells condense and determine the shape of the future bone and then begin the process of bone development by differentiating into chondroblasts that produce a framework of hyaline cartilage. Mesenchymal cells can differentiate into either chondroblasts or osteoblasts. Determination of the type of cells produced is dependent on vascularization. The differentiation of mesenchymal cells into osteoblasts, or bone precursor cells, is dependent on the availability of oxygen. Therefore, bone is produced only in areas that are vascularized, whereas cartilage can be produced in avascular areas. Around the end of the second month of gestation, periosteal capillaries begin to invade the cartilage near the middle of the model, bringing with it osteogenic cells. This area begins the process of bone matrix deposition over the cartilage and is the primary center of ossification. As the bony matrix is deposited, the central portion of the model undergoes resorption and the medullary cavity is developed. The middle section, or diaphysis, of the bone is therefore formed first while the ends of the bone, or epiphysis, are still cartilaginous. Calcification of fetal bone increases as the fetus increases in weight. Neonates born prematurely therefore have significantly less calcified bones (Walker, 1991). Long bones will eventually develop secondary centers of ossification in the epiphyseal region. The majority of secondary centers of ossification develop postnatally. The secondary centers in the lower end of the femur and the upper end of the tibia are the only centers present at birth. Following the development of the secondary centers of ossification, the epiphysis begins the process of conversion to bone, except that cartilage remains on the articulating surfaces of the bone and a transverse disc of hyaline cartilage remains on the border of the diaphysis. These regions of cartilage, called the *epiphyseal plates*, allow the bone to grow until adult stature is attained.

Postnatal longitudinal bone growth occurs on the diaphyseal sides of both epiphyseal plates. During this process, capillaries are sprouting and invade the spaces vacated by the chondrocytes. The capillaries can be injured as they grow and a small amount of blood can leak into the lacunae. If a child has a bacterial infection in another part of the body, it may be transmitted to the bone and result in juvenile osteomyelitis, which commonly begins at the diaphysis.

The width of the epiphysis is wider than the width of the diaphysis. The tapered area that connects the wide epiphysis to the narrow diaphysis is referred to as the *metaphysis*. The metaphysis retains a tapered shape through the process of resorption. As the shaft is lengthened, bone is resorbed in the area that was previously adjacent to the epiphysis to match the diameter of the diaphysis (Figure 4–1). Resorption is also involved in the process of growth in the diameter of the bone. Successive layers of osteoblasts are deposited to the outer surface of the diaphysis. This is accompanied by absorption on the inner surface, which allows widening of the medullary cavity to prevent the bone from becoming too thick and heavy. Mechanical forces influence the rate of bone deposition or resorption. Early in the prenatal period the role of mechanical forces on the fetus is minimal because the uterus and embryonic fluid suspend the fetus in a "weightless" environment. As the fetus grows, the confines of the uterus can have an impact on development, especially if there is a size discrepancy between a small uterus and large baby or if the fetus is positioned atypically. Abnormal facies and talipes equinovarus (congenital clubfoot) are examples of atypical bone structure caused by uterine crowding (Walker, 1991). Breech positioning also puts atypical stresses on the fetus and has been related to musculoskeletal changes such as torticollis and hip dysplasia (Davids, Wenger, & Mubarak, 1993). Decreased joint movement also affects the developing fetus and may delay the formation of secondary ossification centers (Trueta, 1968). This could result in fragile, misshapen bones.

After initial development, bone shape can be changed through a process called **modeling,** which includes bone formation and resorption. These two factors serve to increase the amount of bone and determine its shape. Remodeling is a process that replaces immature and old bone with no net gain but possibly a decrease in bone. These processes of bone formation and adaptation are influenced by several factors, including nutrition and

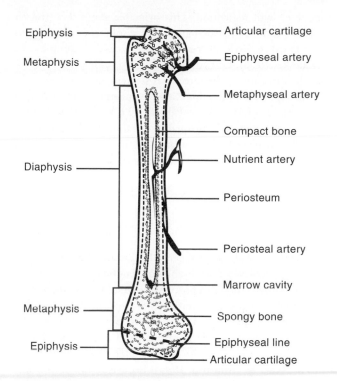

Figure 4–1   Schematic drawing of parts of a bone. (From Pratt, N [1991] *Clinical musculoskeletal anatomy* [p. 6]. Philadelphia: J.B. Lippincott. Copyright 1991 by the J.B. Lippincott Company. Reprinted with permission.)

heredity. Another factor is expressed by **Wolff's law,** first proposed in the 1870s, which suggested that bones develop a particular internal trabecular structure in response to the mechanical forces that are placed on them (Mullender & Huiskes, 1995). The type of loading and stress (or force per bone area) in different situations affect bones differently.

Loading a bone longitudinally, parallel to the direction of growth, results in either compression or tension. Either type of loading, applied intermittently with appropriate force, such as with weight bearing or muscle pull, stimulates bone growth. Intermittent compression forces appear to stimulate more growth than tension (LeVeau & Bernhardt, 1984; Nigg & Grimston, 1994). Animal studies have also shown that weight bearing has a beneficial effect on fracture healing (O'Sullivan, Bronk, Chao, & Kelly, 1994) and improves the density and trabecular network of osteopenic bone when coupled with active exercise (Bourrin, Palle, Genty, & Alexandre, 1995).

Constant or excessive static loading, however, causes bone material to decrease, and thus can be detrimental to bone integrity and strength (Lanyon & Rubin, 1984). This is demonstrated by the **Hueter-Volkmann principle** of bone growth regulation. This principle states that growth plates produce increased growth in response to tension and decreased growth in response to excessive compression (Zaleske, 1996). Growth plates line up to be perpendicular to the direction of the forces across them, and in the case of a malaligned fracture, this is a mechanism for remodeling to take place (Grasco & de Pablos, 1997). Therefore, if the forces are directed unequally or abnormally across an epiphyseal plate because of malalignment, growth may be uneven and increase the malalignment. In the lower extremities, this could result in genu valgum ("knock-knees") or genu varum ("bowlegs"). In the spine, this mechanism has been shown to contribute to the uneven grown of the vertebrae in scoliosis, a lateral curvature of the spine (Stokes, 1997).

Asymmetrical growth can also occur during fracture healing. However, bone is able to straighten some degree of malalignment though a process known as **flexure drift**. This remodeling mechanism outlined by Frost in 1964 describes a process whereby strain on a curved bone wall applied by repeated loading tends to move the bone surface in the direction of the concavity to straighten the bone (Cusick, 1990; Nigg & Grimston, 1994). Bone is resorbed from the convex side and laid down on the concave side. This process is seen in the femur and tibia during development as the child loses the initial genu valgum posture (Figure 4–2).

In addition to stimulating growth, dynamic mechanical loading promotes bone density and normal developmental remodeling. Children who do not participate in normal physical activities can experience osteopenia, or decreased bone density, which leads to weaker bones (Apkon, 2002; Bourrin, et al., 1995; King, Levin, Schmidt, Oestreich, & Heubi, 2003). Frequently, children with neuromuscular disorders, such as cerebral palsy (CP), do not participate in as much physical activity as do peers without disorders (Van Den Berg-Emons, Van Baak, Speth, & Saris, 1998). A lack of weight bearing is also one of the risk factors for faulty hip joint alignment in CP (Bleck, 1987). Chronic inflammatory diseases such as rheumatoid arthritis can lead to osteoporosis (Cimaz, 2002). Intervention strategies for maintaining and improving bone mineralization are discussed in Chapter 5.

Alignment

The principles of reshaping the musculoskeletal system will now be applied to the developing fetus and child. A neonate has a skeletal structure and alignment that is uniquely different from that of an adult. Intrauterine positioning for 40 weeks and the posture of "**physiological flexion**" profoundly affect the alignment of the newborn. Physiological flexion refers to the normal hip, knee, and elbow flexion contractures or "physiological limitation of motion" seen in newborns (Walker, 1991, p. 887). The term *contracture*, as used here, is not pathological but refers to the normal flexed posture that develops toward the end of gestation as the fetus grows and becomes cramped in the uterus. Compare the infant in Figure 4–3, who was born

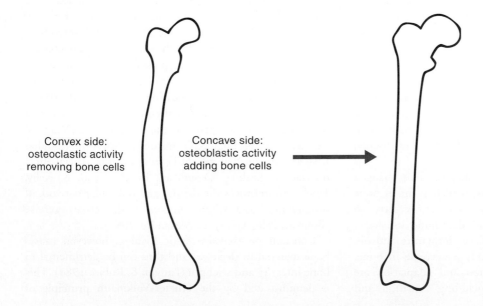

Convex side:
osteoclastic activity
removing bone cells

Concave side:
osteoblastic activity
adding bone cells

Figure 4–2 Schematic drawing of the process of flexure drift using an example of a femur in varus alignment.

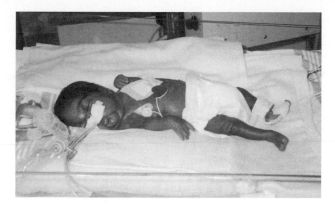

Figure 4–3   Infant born prematurely. Note extended posture.

prematurely, with the infant in Figure 4–4, who was born at full term. The preterm infant has not had the full 40-week gestation to develop the flexed posture of the full-term infant. Note how the upper and lower extremities of the infant in Figure 4–3 are more extended, with fewer "normal" joint restrictions than the full-term infant.

The physical therapist must always be aware of the wide variability of reported norms for ROM within typical populations. Average values of joint ROM vary within different samples of children, and with measurement methodology. Understanding musculoskeletal development is more important than knowing specific joint ROM values. Age-based ROM values are available (Staheli, 1992) for the therapist to evaluate examination findings relative to normative samples when making a differential diagnosis or planning intervention.

Spine

The infant's spine is initially in a kyphotic position, but as the infant begins to hold its head up and prop on its forearms in prone position, cervical and lumbar lordosis begin to develop. The lumbar lordosis is further accentuated as the infant begins to attain the quadruped position with gravity pulling down on the normally weak abdominal area (LeVeau & Bernhardt, 1984).

Pelvis

At birth, the neonate's hip is unstable. Both the acetabulum and the femur contribute to this instability. The acetabulum is largely cartilaginous and shallow (Walker, 1991), whereas the femoral head is flat, has a high femoral neck-shaft angle, and is anteverted. Despite this instability, the

femoral head is normally seated within the acetabulum at birth because of bony structure as well as the surface tension of the synovial fluid (Weinstein, 1996). The modeling process is described in more detail in Chapter 5.

Hip and Femur

Neonates present with a hip flexion contracture of about 30° as a result of intrauterine positioning (Cusick, 1990; Drews, Vraciu, & Pellino, 1984). The range of contracture reported at birth varies between 50° and 120° because of measuring differences and tester variability (Hensinger & Jones, 1982). In a study of 86 typical healthy infants, the hip flexion contracture diminished from a mean of 10° (SD = 2.6°) at 9 months to 9° (SD = 4.8°) at 12 months, 4° (SD = 3.2°) at 18 months, and 3° (SD = 3.0°) at 24 months (Phelps, Smith, & Hallum, 1985). It is interesting to note that the standard deviations increase as the children age, suggesting that variability may increase with age. Sutherland and colleagues (1987) report that during gait, 1-year-old children lack approximately 8° of hip extension, 1½- year-olds lack approximately 4°, and by age 2, the hip reaches 0° flexion. The change in hip ROM occurs as the young child attempts to attain and maintain positions against gravity. As the iliopsoas muscle stretches out, the anterior hip joint capsule also elongates, allowing anterior glide of the head of the femur and permitting increasing extension (Bleck, 1987; Cusick, 1990). Action of the major hip extensor, the gluteus maximus, during antigravity activities is also essential for decreasing the normal hip flexion contracture of the infant.

In the frontal plane, neonates have large amounts of hip abduction, again because of the influence of intrauterine positioning. The amount of hip abduction differs depending on whether the hip was held in a more extended posi-

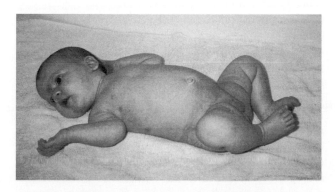

Figure 4–4   Infant born at full term.

tion (within the limits of available extension) or in a flexed position. In a flexed position, more hip abduction is available. Published hip abduction mean values range between 69° and 76° (Drews et al., 1984; Haas, Epps, & Adams, 1973). Hip abduction range decreases to a mean of 60° at age 2 years (Phelps et al., 1985) and continues to decrease over time to the typical adult value of 45°. This extreme abduction range decreases in conjunction with the development of upright postures, such as quadruped (all fours), kneeling, standing, and walking, and the need for the lower extremity to be in a position that will support weight bearing (Hensinger & Jones, 1982) with a stable pelvis.

In the transverse plane, more lateral rotation than medial rotation is present in the first few months of life. The reported mean for lateral hip rotation in the newborn is between 89° (Haas et al., 1973) and 114° (Drews et al., 1984). Medial rotation means are reported between 62° (Haas et al., 1973) and 80° (Drews et al., 1984). The large amount of lateral hip rotation is quite apparent in supported standing when the young child stands with toes pointed outward. During the first 2 years of life, lateral rotation decreases to a mean value of 47° and medial rotation increases to a mean value of 52° (Drews et al., 1984). Decreased lateral rotation is related to increased hip extension. As the hip joint stretches out into extension, this lateral rotation pull diminishes (Phelps et al., 1985). The mechanism for the decrease in lateral rotation is similar to that of hip abduction. As the infant assumes standing, decreasing lateral rotation allows the greater trochanter to lie in a more lateral position, so that the hip abductors work more efficiently to stabilize the pelvis in standing (Pitkow, 1975).

At birth, the femur is in a position of **coxa valga**, which is defined as an increased angle of inclination or neck-shaft angle. The **angle of inclination** is the angle formed by the long axis of the femur and an axis drawn through the head and neck of the femur (Figure 4–5). The typical neonatal value ranges from 135° to 145° (McCrea, 1985), and decreases to the adult value of 125° to 135° during late adolescence (Staheli, 1992). This angle decreases as a result of the compression and tension forces placed on the proximal end of the femur through normal weight bearing and muscle pull (LeVeau & Bernhardt, 1984).

To understand the position of the femur, the terms *version* and *torsion* require discussion. **Torsion** refers to the normal amount of rotation present in a long bone (Figure 4–6). Femoral torsion is the angle formed by an axis drawn through the head and neck of the femur and an axis through the femoral condyles. The easiest way to visualize this angle is to actually look down the long axis of a femur.

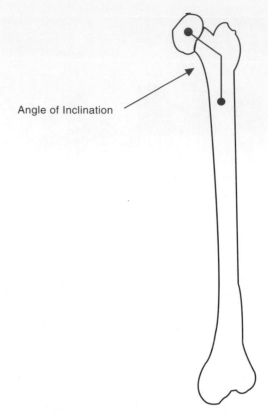

Figure 4–5   Femoral angle of inclination.

Line up the posterior surfaces of the femoral condyles with a horizontal surface such as a table. Then look down the bone toward the head of the femur and you will notice that the head and neck of the femur are angled upward or from the table approximately 15°. This is the angle of torsion.

Antetorsion occurs when the head and neck of the femur are rotated forward in the sagittal plane relative to the axis through the femoral condyles. If the head and neck of the femur are backwardly rotated, the femur is said to be in **retrotorsion**. The femur has maximum antetorsion, approximately 30° to 40°, at birth (McCrea, 1985; Phelps et al., 1985; Rang, 1993c; Staheli, 1992). This angle decreases from birth through adolescence. The derotation progresses rapidly between birth and the first year, more slowly between 1 and 8 years, and then rapidly again through adolescence to reach an adult mean of 16° by approximately age 14 to 16 years (Staheli, 1992). The femur is said to "untwist" through the process of growth, muscle action, reduction of the coxa valga angle, and reduction of the hip flexion contracture (Bleck, 1987).

Femoral antetorsion can cause a lower extremity posture of **in-toeing**. In-toeing is not seen in an infant when the

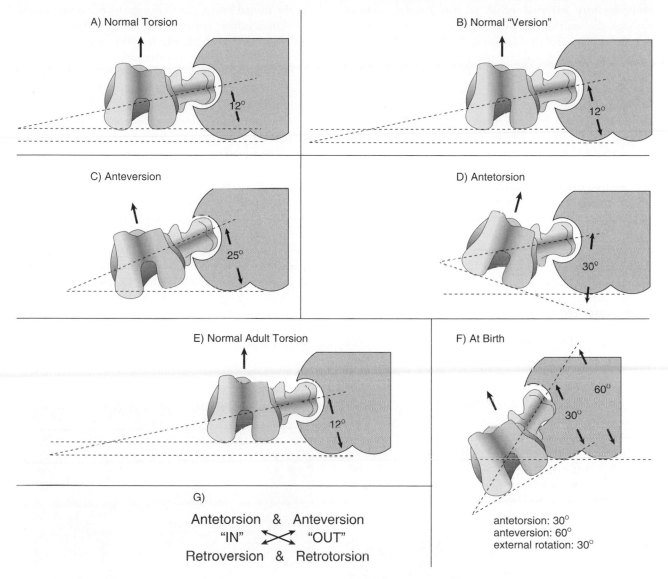

A) Normal Torsion

B) Normal "Version"

C) Anteversion

D) Antetorsion

E) Normal Adult Torsion

F) At Birth

antetorsion: 30°
anteversion: 60°
external rotation: 30°

G)
Antetorsion & Anteversion
"IN" ⤫ "OUT"
Retroversion & Retrotorsion

Figure 4–6 Schematic drawing of femoral version.

infant is placed in supported stance because the excessive lateral hip rotation and femoral anteversion overcompensate for the inward rotation of the shaft of the femur and result in an appearance of out-toeing. If the normal antetorsion does not reduce with development, the child may have an in-toeing gait pattern when the normal reduction in the lateral rotation occurs with age. The majority of children with in-toeing caused by a normal amount of "persistent fetal antetorsion," in the absence of other disease processes, will improve as the hips spontaneously realign (Rang, 1993c; Staheli, 1992). In less than 1% of these children, antetorsion fails to resolve and the children warrant

treatment (Staheli, 1992). In children with CP, however, persistent fetal antetorsion is a causative factor in the development of hip instability. This is discussed later in this chapter.

Unlike persistent fetal antetorsion, in which the child starts out with a normal amount of antetorsion but it does not reduce over time, some infants have excessive fetal femoral antetorsion. In a large follow-up study, these children retained a higher amount of femoral torsion through skeletal maturity. However, the in-toeing that accompanies excessive femoral antetorsion disappeared over time in 50% of the children. This is attributed to the development of compensatory external tibial torsion (lateral rotation through the shaft of the tibia) rather than to a decrease in femoral torsion (Fabry, MacEwen, & Shands, 1973). This compensatory tibial rotation tends to lead the foot to an out-toed posture even though the femur continues to have excessive antetorsion.

Femoral **version** refers to the position of the head of the femur in the acetabulum relative to the posterior pelvis (frontal plane). Anteversion positions the head of the femur anteriorly in the acetabulum and results in a position of thigh external rotation. Conversely, retroversion positions the head of the femur posteriorly in the acetabulum and results in thigh internal rotation. At birth, a neonate has 60° of anteversion. By adulthood, femoral version has reduced to 12°. At birth, anteversion (60°) is greater than antetorsion (30°) with a net result of an external rotated femur. This is why a newborn has an externally rotated lower extremity posture at rest.

Knee and Tibia

In the sagittal plane, the newborn demonstrates a knee flexion contracture of approximately 20° to 30° (Drews et al, 1984; Hensinger & Jones, 1982), as demonstrated in Figure 4–7. Again this is caused by physiological flexion as a result of intrauterine positioning. This will gradually stretch out with elongation of the hamstrings through activities, such as the infant bringing hands to feet and feet to mouth in supine position, positions such as the three-point position (weight bearing on both extended arms, one foot, and one knee), and bear walking (weight bearing on both extended arms and both feet).

In the frontal plane, the tibia appears outwardly bowed in a position called "**apparent physiological bowing.**" The entire tibia is rotated slightly forward, which places the larger lateral head of the gastrocnemius muscle in a more forward position. This gives the appearance of a bowed tibia even though the bone itself is only mildly bowed. This "apparent bowing," caused by the forwardly rotated position of the tibia, results from the contracture of the medial knee structures due to intrauterine positioning (Wilkins, 1986). The tibiofemoral angle of the infant is in a varus position, also called genu varum. The tibiofemoral angle is formed by the longitudinal axes of the femur and the tibia (Engel & Staheli, 1974) (Figure 4–8). The apex of the angle is the knee with the femur and tibia forming the distal segments. The angle may be in **genu varum** (bowing [the distal segments are more medial than the apex]), **genu valgum** (knock-knee [the distal segments are more lateral than the apex]), or neutral. Figure 4–7 shows a child in a position of slight genu valgum. As can be seen, the distal portion of the tibia is more lateral than the apex of the angle.

A natural progression of this angle has been documented. At birth, genu varum may be as high as 15° but decreases

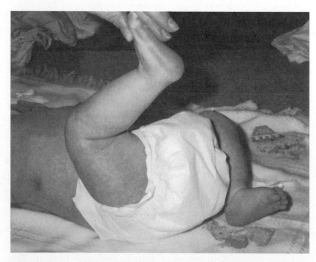

Figure 4–7   Maximum knee extension in a newborn infant.

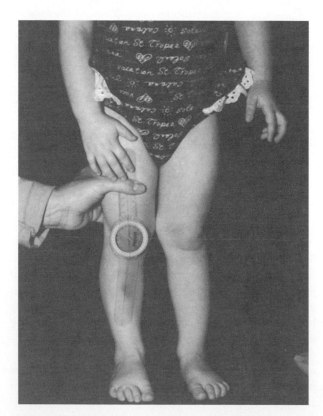

Figure 4–8   Tibiofemoral angle measurement.

approximately 5° during the first year of life (Salenius & Vankka, 1975). Bowing of the knee joint during the first 1 to 2 years of life is likely because of a number of factors, including medial knee joint capsule tightness caused by intrauterine positioning, coxa valga angle of the femur, and lateral hip rotation contracture (Beeson, 1999; Cusick, 1990; Hensinger & Jones, 1982). As weight bearing on the lower extremities increases between 12 and 24 months of age, during standing, both the **coxa valga** angle of the femur (distal end of the femur is more lateral/bowleg) and the femoral anteversion resolves. Additionally, between 3 and 4 years of age, the genu varum shifts into about 10 to 15° of genu valgum (Beeson, 1999; Hensinger & Jones, 1982). After this peak of valgus, the knee angle decreases until it stabilizes at approximately 6 to 7 years of age, at about 5° valgus (Bleck, 1982; Salenius & Vankka, 1975). In prepubescent children, there is no gender difference in angulation; however, during puberty, males typically tend to have more coxa valga (bowlegged) posture than females (Beeson, 1999).

There are various opinions about when or if genu varum or valgum in young children warrants treatment. Both Bleck (1982) and McDade (1977) state that if the varus position of the knees is not decreasing by age 18 months to 2 years, either bilaterally or unilaterally, further investigation is warranted, particularly if the value is at or beyond 25° (Bleck, 1982). Likewise, if the genu valgum position does not reduce to the typical value of 5 to 7° but remains excessive bilaterally or presents unilaterally, further evaluation may be necessary.

The neonatal tibia is in a position of slight external torsion (approximately 5°). The distal end is externally rotated with respect to the proximal end. The external torsion increases to 18° by age 14 years (Engel & Staheli, 1974) and 23 to 25° of external rotation by skeletal maturity (LeVeau & Bernhardt, 1984). Therefore, since the tibia begins in a position of slight external torsion that continues to increase, internal tibial torsion is not a common finding during typical development. If internal tibial torsion is found during childhood, adolescence, or adulthood, it may have resulted from a lack of progression of typical tibial external rotation during early childhood or may be a compensation for rotational malalignment in the femur, hip, or foot.

Ankle and Foot

In general, the newborn foot is very flexible. The newborn talocrural (talus articulation with ankle mortice) joint rests in dorsiflexion and may have a plantar flexion limitation (Cusick, 1990). This dorsiflexed position is, again, the

result of intrauterine posture, particularly during the last 2 to 3 months of gestation (LeVeau & Bernhardt, 1984). As gravity begins to have an effect on ankle motion, and as the child begins to move the ankle joint, the amount of plantar flexion increases quickly during the first year of life (Cusick, 1990).

The calcaneus and talus in the newborn foot are inclined medially as a result of intrauterine positioning and shortening of the medial structures (Cusick, 1990). The foot follows this medial slant so that the forefoot is also slightly inverted in the non–weight-bearing position (Bernhardt, 1988; McCrea, 1985). Therefore, both the rear foot and the forefoot are in varus positions in non–weight bearing. Despite this inverted posture, the infant's foot will appear everted when in supported stance. This appearance is caused by the medial forces placed on the foot in standing caused by the posture of hip abduction and lateral rotation, tibiofemoral varus, and the normal fat pad in the midfoot area.

The foot should have a straight lateral border regardless of its weight-bearing status. A foot that has a lateral border that is curved like a "C" has a metatarsus adductus, with an atypical adduction of the metatarsals. This is called a "packaging" problem attributed to intrauterine positioning and is differentiated from a "manufacturing" problem with a structural malformation or genetic cause (Williams, 1982).

Newborns have **flat feet** because of a thick fat pad covering the longitudinal arch of the midfoot and laxity of the joints of the midfoot (Staheli, Chew, & Corbett, 1987). The arch develops through early childhood and is generally observable in stance by approximately 4 years of age (Engel & Staheli, 1974). Flat feet in children up to 4 to 5 years of age are normal and do not require intervention; however, there is a great deal of controversy about whether to intervene in older children. The child with flatfoot along with a neuromuscular or musculoskeletal disorder such as Down syndrome or cerebral palsy may require intervention, and this flatfoot should be differentiated from the typical flatfoot of a young child or that of an older child with no other disability. Figure 4–9 is a picture of a child aged 4 years who is just beginning to show a longitudinal arch but still has a slight flatfoot typical of this age. Generally, intervention is not warranted unless the feet are painful or are affecting the child's balance.

Muscle

There are three general types of muscle tissue: skeletal, cardiac, and smooth. Skeletal muscle, also known as striated or voluntary muscle, is the focus of this section. Skeletal muscle fibers are developed from embryonic myoblast cells.

The majority of human muscle fibers are present before birth, with the remainder being formed during the first year of life. After the first 4 years of life, the muscles need to continue to grow to match increasing skeletal size; however, this is done entirely through hypertrophy of the existing muscle fibers, rather than addition of more fibers. Each muscle fiber is made up of smaller myofibrils. Additional myofibrils can be added to individual muscle fibers, and this process accounts for the majority of the circumferential growth of a muscle. New myofibrils are added to the periphery, expand, and then split to create more myofibrils. In addition to the genetic predetermination, the demands put on the muscle through exercise will ultimately determine the muscle size. Longitudinal growth of muscle fibers is accomplished by adding additional sarcomeres to the muscle fiber at the ends of the muscle. A sarcomere is the contractile unit of a muscle and is composed of actin (thin) and myosin (thick) filaments.

There are two basic types of muscle fibers, which are classified by the speed of contraction and method for generating energy to perform the contraction. Type 1, slow-twitch oxidative, fibers have a slow contraction time and have a low level of anaerobic energy production. Type 1 fibers primarily use oxidative activity, which is best suited for low-level sustained activity. In contrast, type 2 muscle fibers have faster contraction speeds. The type 2 fibers are subdivided into two groups. Type 2A fibers are considered intermediate fibers because they use both aerobic and anaerobic energy production and have a greater resistance to fatigue than the type 2B fibers. Type 2B fibers are the most rapidly contracting fiber type and use primarily anaerobic energy production.

The percentage of each fiber type in any given muscle is dependent on the function of the muscle. The soleus muscle, for example, is primarily a postural muscle, which requires it to perform slow, prolonged contraction rather than bursts of high-intensity activity. The soleus muscle therefore has a higher concentration of type 1 fibers (Haggmark & Eriksson, 1979). The distribution of fiber types differs between individuals. Elite athletes have a higher proportion of the fiber type best suited for their sport. For example, sprinters have a higher proportion of type 2 fibers, whereas distance runners have more type 1 fibers (Pitman & Peterson, 1989). Genetic predisposition of fiber type distribution may be partially responsible for the natural selection of elite athletes (Pitman & Peterson, 1989).

Although there can be a mixture of fiber types in each muscle, a single nerve branch innervates only one fiber type. The impulse a muscle receives from a nerve appears to

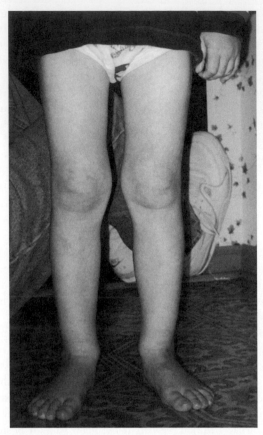

Figure 4–9   Slightly flat feet typical of a 4-year-old child.

influence the type of muscle fiber. Sending external electrical impulses through a nerve (Munsat, McNeal, & Waters, 1976) or surgically transecting the nerve from one muscle to another (Dubowitz, 1967) has been shown to change fiber type orientation. This would suggest that fiber type distribution might be changed therapeutically to optimize motor performance.

Musculoskeletal Examination

There are many examination procedures for the child with musculoskeletal concerns. This portion of the chapter will discuss procedures used across many different impairments and the most important procedures for particular disorders. It is not possible to detail all available procedures and the reader is encouraged to review the suggested readings at the end of the chapter.

There are several principles that should be followed regardless of the procedure. The examination should follow a consistent, logical sequence that is dictated by a careful, detailed history, observation of the child, discussion of present and historical symptoms, and the child's and caregiver's goals. Children may not always be forthcoming with information, so the therapist must pay attention to the child's expressions and behavior during the examination to detect pain or discomfort with any procedures and ask questions if the child is able to answer.

The examination should be comprehensive, but focused, so all salient procedures can be performed. This requires knowledge of the natural history of pediatric conditions so the therapist can focus the examination on critical areas. The age and developmental expectations of the child should form a framework for the examination, to ensure there is appropriate evaluation of examination data. For example, when examining a neonate, the therapist must take into account the normal ROM limitations seen in newborns, to avoid erroneous conclusions. In addition, the therapist needs to develop unusual and entertaining ways to keep the child engaged during the examination process. This involves establishing a rapport with the child before beginning the examination. Preferably the examination can be done in the child's home or other familiar environment or, if a natural environment is not possible, a clinic area with age-appropriate decorations and toys to help put the child at ease. Getting onto the floor and playing with a young child, or talking to an older child about school or hobbies before the examination also helps develop rapport.

Once the examination has begun, the therapist must develop a systematic way of accurately recording and evaluating the data. Time is often limited by the child's endurance or clinic scheduling, so information must be gathered efficiently. The therapist must accurately document the examination results while trying to keep the child engaged. Having equipment readily available and a flexible strategy outlined will help the therapist proceed quickly from one activity to the next while keeping the child's attention and cooperation.

The therapist working with children must recognize that the examination and intervention will both need to be performed in ways that make the child feel as comfortable as possible. When a child is uncooperative, it is difficult to determine whether the child cannot or simply will not perform the activity. The use of games, toys, stickers, songs, and other age-appropriate activities will significantly improve cooperation and provide a more representative picture of the child's abilities. The caregiver can give you an idea of a young child's personality and favorite toys or activities so that you can best tailor the examination to the child. Finally, it is important when giving directions to talk directly to the child at a level appropriate for his or her age and understanding. In the following discussion of specific examination procedures, some ideas for implementation with children will be presented to assist in making the examination process a success.

Child and Family Goals

Family-centered care will allow the therapist to complete a succinct evaluation by first determining the child's and family's goals for the therapy. Leading questions will enable the entire family to articulate their concerns, rather than just repeating something they were told by another professional. For example, a child is rarely worried about decreased ROM but could be bothered by difficulty putting on a shirt. Making the evaluation and intervention meaningful to the child should improve cooperation and adherence. The therapist must also be culturally sensitive and family focused. Except in cases of abuse or neglect, the family is entitled to make decisions for the child that best meet the needs of the family, regardless of whether these decisions are in line with the therapist's values. The family is in the best position to take into account all factors surrounding the current situation and to make the best overall decision. The therapist's job is to provide information about the medical condition, treatment potential, and complications. The therapist may try to guide the family toward a decision by providing information but must respect the family's decision unless the child is being put in danger.

History

A detailed history includes information gathered from many sources. In a pediatric examination, the therapist must listen carefully to the parents or other caregivers and, if the child is able to answer questions, ask questions at the developmentally appropriate level. The therapist should allow enough time for the interview so that it can be done in a sympathetic, caring, and sensitive manner. Many families go through a grieving period when a child is diagnosed with a disorder and may display a range of emotions, such as sadness or anger. Sensitive interview techniques will allow the therapist to gain information without unnecessarily distressing the family.

Birth history and developmental history are particularly important if the child has a multisystem disorder such as CP, Down syndrome, or myelomeningocele. However, even in a child with a specific segment disorder, such as limping, in- or out-toeing, torticollis, or knee pain, the birth and developmental histories may assist in differential diagnosis of the problem. Determining developmental and functional status, as addressed in Chapter 2, is an important part of a comprehensive examination. The therapist must be sure to document pertinent historical information such as illnesses, medications, operations, school history, and previous therapies.

Observation

Before beginning any musculoskeletal examination, the child should be observed while playing. This will help the therapist determine how the child's musculoskeletal status may be affecting functional activities and will allow the child time to acclimate to the examination setting. The therapist should interact with the child while playing to establish a nonthreatening rapport. An astute, knowledgeable observer is able to quickly assess the child's movements and determine the most important tests and measures to perform.

Specific Musculoskeletal Tests and Measures

Leg Lengths

Leg length is an important measurement when the child presents with a limp, a pelvic obliquity, back pain, or an asymmetrical gait pattern. Leg length asymmetries are frequently seen in children with neuromuscular involvement.

Physical therapists traditionally have used either a tape measure or the block method for assessing leg length discrepancy. The most accurate method for documenting limb length is to use a tape measure (Figure 4–10). Beattie, Isaacson, Riddle, and Rothstein (1990) compared tape measurements with measurements obtained through radiographs and found the tape measurement technique yielded valid results. The child lies supine with hips and knees extended and the measurement is taken between the most prominent point on the anterior superior iliac spine and the medial malleolus. It is important that the child lie quietly for tests of leg length, so before beginning, give the child a quiet toy to manipulate or a video to watch during the test. It may be helpful to talk to the child, tell a story, or sing a

song to make sure that the supine position is maintained throughout the measurements. To improve accuracy, use a washable marker to identify bone landmarks, and use the average of two measurements (Beattie et al., 1990).

The block method is not advocated because of its poor reliability. In the block method, the child stands with his or her back to the therapist. The therapist palpates the iliac crests and determines visually if they are level. In a study by Mann, Glasheen-Wray, and Nyberg (1984), therapists were unable to consistently identify which side was higher. After the tape measure method is used to identify a leg length discrepancy, blocks might provide supplemental information about the combined effects of other factors contributing to a functional leg length discrepancy, such as posture or lower extremity joint contractures.

The **Galleazi sign,** or Allis test, is a quick screening method to assist in the determination of leg length equality. The Galleazi sign is performed with the child supine with

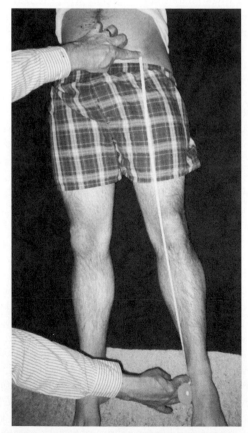

Figure 4–10   Measurement of leg length with a tape measure.

the hips and knees flexed and the feet flat on the table (Figure 4–11). The anterior-superior iliac spines are held level so a pelvic obliquity does not appear to cause a difference in the knee heights. Look to see if one knee is higher than the other; if so, this may be evidence that the legs need to be measured to quantify the difference. The therapist can also use a gravity-assisted angle finder placed across the knees to determine whether the knees are level. The Galleazi sign is also used as one indication of hip joint integrity. If a child has a dislocated hip, the femur will slide posteriorly when the child is in the testing position and therefore the femur will appear shorter than the other side. Tape measurements can be used to differentiate between a leg length discrepancy and a dislocated hip.

Range of Motion

Joint ROM is an important component of any musculoskeletal examination. The therapist is attempting to find joints that have motion limitations, contractures, or excessive motion. A ROM examination can be difficult to achieve in children who are very young, apprehensive, and active or who generally have difficulty with the demands of the examination process. There are some ways in which the therapist can help the child tolerate the testing situation. One, as mentioned earlier, is to distract the child with songs, to provide small toys, and to enlist the help of caregivers to provide distraction. Another is to structure the ROM examination to cover all tests in one position before moving the child to another position. For example, perform all supine ROM tests and additional tests such as leg length measurements before moving to prone. In addition, if the examination is performed in a consistent order, it is less likely that tests will be missed or forgotten even when working with distractible youngsters. This is particularly important for the novice clinician.

Children with hypertonicity frequently have ROM deficits. Hypertonicity presents unique measurement difficulties. Illness, temperament, medication, and speed of movement can all affect the ROM of a child with hypertonicity (Gajdosik & Bohannon, 1987; Harris, Harthun-Smith, & Krukowski, 1985; Stuberg, Fuchs, & Miedaner, 1988). Both interrater and test-retest reliability in children with CP is difficult to achieve. Harris and colleagues (1985) examined goniometric reliability on a child with spastic quadriplegia. Measurements were within 10° of each other 57 to 100% of the time. Often clinical decisions are made based on a change of ROM of 10° or less. This study suggests that decisions based on ROM should be considered carefully, as the data may not be accurate. This study also suggests that therapists must evaluate their goniometric reliability.

Frequently, the therapist is measuring an angle to indicate the severity of the limitation and how it compares with a normative sample. Because there are age-related changes, measurements must be compared with an appropriate-age sample. Understanding that there is a wide range of normal values is critical. ROM tests relevant to children with common musculoskeletal disabilities will be discussed by segment, beginning proximally with the hip.

Spine

The spine should always be screened for scoliosis, a lateral spinal curvature, and excessive kyphosis, a forward curvature of the spine. The spine should be examined in standing and using the **Adams forward bend test** (Figure 4–12).

To perform the forward bend test, the child bends forward with his or her arms hanging in front and the knees straight. The therapist stands behind and then in front of

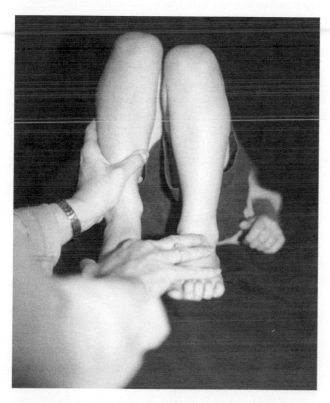

Figure 4–11   The Galleazi sign, or Allis test. The lower knee of this child may indicate a leg length discrepancy and should be measured using the tape measure method.

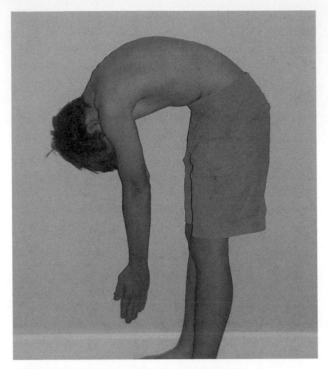

Figure 4–12 The Adams forward bend test.

the child and assesses back symmetry. Asymmetry may be indicated by a prominence on one side of the back or the spine appearing curved when viewed from the top to the bottom. The forward bend is a screening procedure, not a definitive diagnostic test, so children with asymmetries should be referred to a pediatric orthopedic surgeon (Lonstein, 1996). Additional findings on observation may be uneven iliac crest heights or shoulder heights. The child should also be viewed from the side to determine if excessive kyphosis is seen. Some forward curvature is normally present, as is seen in the young man in Figure 4–12. However, excessive kyphosis is seen when the curve is more severe and angular.

Idiopathic scoliosis refers to scoliosis of an unknown cause, and it may occur at any age in children without specific disabilities. Idiopathic scoliosis accounts for a majority of scoliosis cases; however, scoliosis may be indicative of an underlying cause such as a spinal tumor or congenital malformation (Lonstein, 1996). Scoliosis also frequently develops in children with neuromuscular disorders, such as CP, Down syndrome, or myelomeningocele, so it is important that children with these disorders always be screened for scoliosis. Many school districts in the United States regularly screen school children for scoliosis,

and a physical therapist employed by a school district may be involved in administering scoliosis screening.

Hip

In the sagittal plane, lack of hip extension is often a problem in children with CP caused by the tightness of the iliopsoas muscle group. Hip flexion contractures may also occur in children with juvenile rheumatoid arthritis and myelomeningocele. The presence of hip flexion contractures may be tested with the **Thomas test** or the **prone hip extension test** (Staheli, 1977). The Thomas test is done with the child in supine with the leg being tested hanging off of the table at the height of the knee. The opposite hip is flexed toward the abdomen and held there to flatten out the lumbar spine and the resulting angle that the other thigh makes with the surface is the amount of hip flexion contracture (Figure 4–13).

The Thomas test is commonly used, but may be difficult to do reliably in children with CP (Bleck, 1987). The **prone hip extension test** (Staheli, 1977) can also be used to assess hip flexion contracture. In this test, the child is in the prone position on a table with the opposite leg hanging over the edge of the table. In this position, the lumbar spine is flattened. The examiner holds the pelvis down at the level of the posterior superior iliac spines and pulls the leg being examined into hip extension until the pelvis begins to move anteriorly. At that point, the angle between the femur and the surface is measured and reflects the degree of hip flexion contracture (Bleck, 1987; Gross, 1995). There are several limitations to this test. It can be difficult to perform

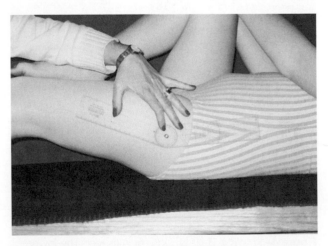

Figure 4–13 The Thomas test for hip flexion contracture.

this test with large children because the therapist needs to hold the leg while simultaneously holding the goniometer and measuring the angle. However, this test has been shown to have better reliability compared to the Thomas test in children with spastic diplegic CP (Bartlett, Wolf, Shurtless, & Staheli, 1985) (Figure 4–14).

Hip abduction and adduction ROM are both frontal plane motions. Hip adduction contractures (limitations in hip adduction), seen in certain types of CP, can result from spasticity in the hip adductor muscles, often adductor longus and gracilis. These limitations can interfere with sitting balance, hygiene, and activities of daily living (Bleck, 1987). Hip abduction limitation is an important factor in the development of spastic hip disease and subluxed or dislocated hips in the child with CP (Miller, Dias, Dabney, Lipton, & Trianna, 1997; Reimers, 1980). The mechanics of hip problems in children with CP are discussed in more detail in Chapter 5. Adequate hip abduction allows the head of the femur to move into the acetabulum, and is frequently limited in children with slipped capital femoral epiphysis and Legg-Calvé-Perthes disease.

Hip adduction limitations are frequently seen in juvenile rheumatoid arthritis (Scull, 2001). One method of assessing the amount of hip adduction is the **Ober test,** which indirectly measures contracture of the iliotibial band. The iliotibial band is the large flat band of thick fascia on the lateral border of the thigh that extends from the gluteal fascia from the iliac crest and the inferior border of the tensor fasciae latae muscle caudally to the fascia surrounding the popliteal area. This fascia may become tight and restricted with excessive hip external rotation or hip abduc-

tion, as seen in the gait of children with juvenile rheumatoid arthritis.

To perform the Ober test, the child is in sidelying position with the bottom hip flexed toward the chest. The top hip being measured is slightly flexed and abducted. The knee is either in extension or flexed to 90°. The hip is then pulled into extension and allowed to fall into adduction. If contracture is present, the hip is unable to adduct. As with many orthopedic tests, achieving adequate reliability depends on using a consistent protocol. In adults, if the knee is flexed to 90°, it limits adduction more than if the knee is extended (Gajdosik, Sandler, & Marr, 2003; Melchione & Sullivan, 1993). Allowing the hip to move into flexion also distorts results. Therapists need to develop a consistent protocol for testing and document this with their results.

Measurement of the Ober test using a goniometer is shown in Figure 4–15. Instead of a goniometer, this may also be done with a gravity-referenced angle finder, as is shown in Figure 4–16. This gravity reference is very helpful in referencing either the horizontal or vertical axis or abduction.

Hip internal and external rotations are transverse plane motions that may be measured with the child in sitting, supine, or prone. The prone position, with the hip extended and the knees flexed to 90° with the tibia vertical, is the preferred position. In prone, the pelvis can be held down, avoiding inaccurate rotation measures caused by

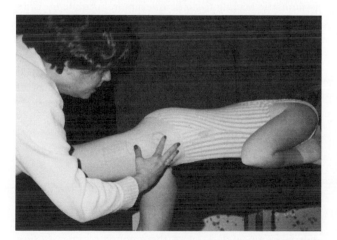

Figure 4–14 The Staheli test for hip flexion contracture.

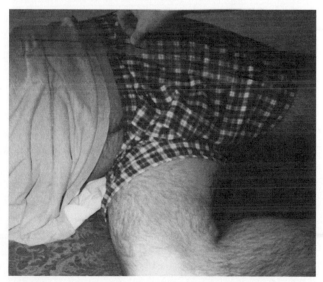

Figure 4–15 The Ober test measurement using a goniometer.

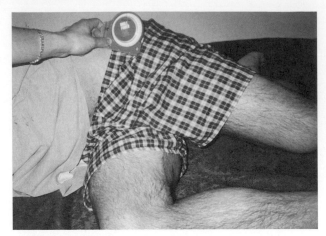

Figure 4–16   The Ober test measurement using a gravity-assisted angle finder.

upward and downward rolling of the pelvis during leg movement. The examiner holds one hand across the pelvis while the leg is rotated and the ranges are measured. A gravity-assisted angle finder may be used (Figure 4–17).

Ryder's test, also called **Craig's test**, is an estimation of the amount of femoral torsion. The objective of this test is to rotate the hip until the head and the neck of the femur are on the frontal plane and then to measure the resulting hip rotation. To perform this test, the child may be prone, supine, or sitting. Figure 4–18 shows this test being performed in the sitting position. The hip may be flexed or extended, but the knee is flexed to 90°. The examiner holds the leg proximal to the ankle and rotates the hip medially and laterally while palpating the greater trochanter. When the trochanter reaches its most prominent lateral position, it is assumed that the head and the neck of

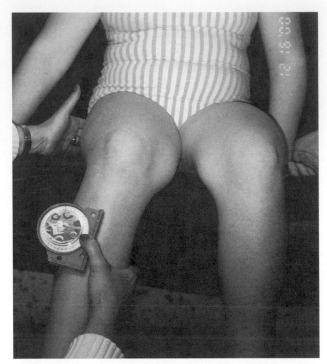

Figure 4–18   Ryder's test done sitting at the edge of a table.

the femur are on the frontal plane. The amount of hip rotation is measured at this point. Comparisons between this technique and computed tomography scans have shown that there is actually 20° more medial femoral torsion than the value obtained from this test (Cusick & Stuberg, 1992; Stuberg, Koehler, Witicha, Temme, & Kaplan, 1989), so 20° of internal rotation is added to the goniometric reading to determine a more accurate measure of femoral torsion. Therefore, if the obtained reading was 10° of internal rotation, the estimated measurement would be 30° femoral antetorsion. Similarly, if the examiner measures 25° of external hip rotation when the lateral trochanter is at its most prominent point, then when 20 is added, it would result in a negative number. This would be interpreted as –5° of femoral antetorsion or 5° of retrotorsion.

Knee

In the sagittal plane at the knee joint, it is important to measure knee extension because hamstring flexibility may be a problem. To measure the length of the hamstring muscle group and estimate the amount of knee flexion contracture, the straight leg test, popliteal angle test, or hamstring length test may be performed. The **popliteal**

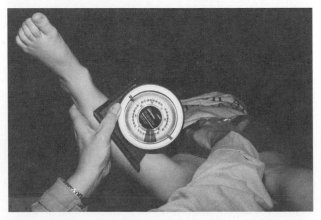

Figure 4–17   Measurement of hip internal rotation using gravity-assisted angle finder.

angle test is typically done with neonates and is a measure of physiological flexion. The test is performed in supine with the hip and knee of the leg being measured flexed to 90° (Figure 4–19). The other hip is stabilized against the surface while the testing leg is extended up into the air. The goniometer is placed with the axis at the knee joint and the arms along the long axes of the leg and thigh. The angle that is measured is that between the leg and the thigh.

The procedure for the **hamstring length test** is the same as the popliteal angle test with the exception that the angle recorded is the amount of ROM that is *missing* or lacking from full knee extension. The angle measured by the goniometer is subtracted from 180° to yield the hamstring length test. This test measures the length of the hamstring muscles because they are stretched over both the hip and knee joints in this test.

When there is a limitation in knee flexion ROM, the hamstring test evaluates the contribution of the hamstring length to the problem. To evaluate the contribution of

other structures in the knee to the limitation, the **straight-leg test** can be used. In neutral hip extension, the hamstrings are in a slackened state and the knee flexion contracture is attributed to other causes (Figure 4–20). The child is placed in a relaxed supine position with the hips in neutral rotation. The knee should rest against the table except in the young infant, who will have a normal, temporary flexion contracture as discussed previously.

In the frontal plane at the knee joint, varus and valgus should be measured. This test should begin with an observation of the knees in the supine position to delete the effects of rotation, weakness, and knee flexion (Rang, 1993a). There are two methods for measuring varus and valgus. In the standing position, if valgus is present, the distance between the medial malleoli is measured with a tape measure with the patella directly forward and the knees touching; if varus is present, the distance between the femoral condyles is measured with the malleoli touching (Figure 4–21).

Another method in standing or supine position is to line up the patellae facing forward with the axis of the goniometer over the knee joint. One arm of the goniometer is placed over the long axis of the thigh pointing toward the anterior superior iliac spine (ASIS) and the other arm along the long axis of the tibia pointing toward the middle of the ankle (Cahuzac, Vardon, & Sales de Gauzy, 1995; Heath & Staheli, 1993) (Figure 4–22).

In the transverse plane, tibial torsion should be measured. Tibial torsion is the normal rotation between the proximal and distal ends of the tibia and, again, values greater than two standard deviations from the mean for an age group are considered atypical. This is measured in two ways. The **thigh-foot angle test** is an estimate of tibial torsion because it actually measures the angular difference

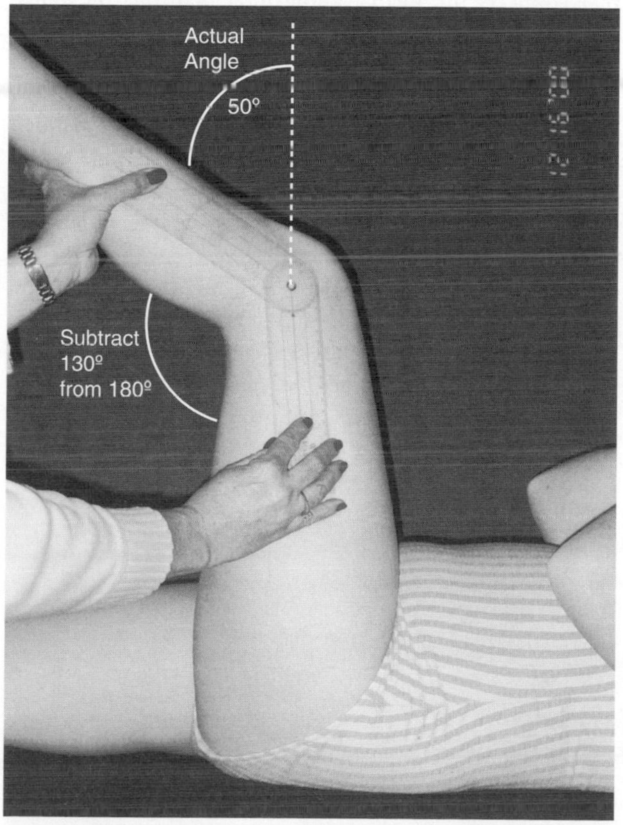

Figure 4–19 Measurement of hamstring length test. The measured angle is subtracted from the full vertical of 180° to yield the actual angle. In this case, the angle would be 50°.

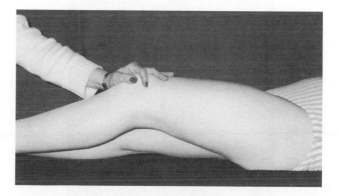

Figure 4–20 Example of knee flexion contracture seen with hip extension to slacken hamstrings.

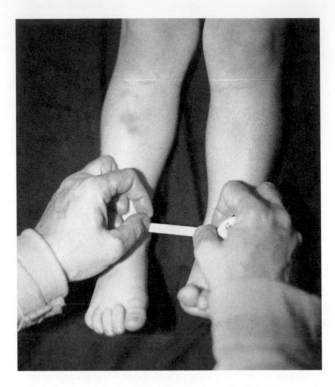

Figure 4–21   The distance between malleoli is measured with the knees touching in the standing position, yielding a measure of knee valgus.

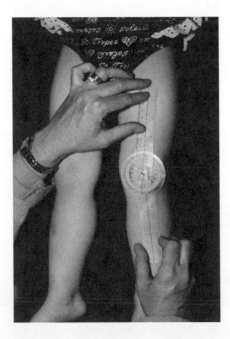

Figure 4–22   Measurement of knee valgus using a goniometer in supine position.

between the thigh and foot axes (Bleck, 1987; Staheli, 1992). The child is in the prone position with the thighs parallel, in neutral rotation, the hips extended, and the knee flexed to 90° and the ankle is allowed to fall into a neutral position of 90° (Staheli, 1992). The axis of the goniometer is placed over the center of the calcaneus, the stationary arm is placed along a visual bisection of the thigh, and the moveable arm is placed on the long axis of the foot along the second metatarsal (Figure 4–23). The resulting angle is measured. The convention is to assign a negative value to a measurement that points in toward the midline (internal tibial version or torsion) and a positive value to a measurement that points away from the midline (external tibial version or torsion).

The thigh-foot angle test, although it is a quick and relatively accurate screen, may present validity problems if there is a forefoot disorder (such as a metatarsus adductus) (Tolo, 1996). In this case, the **transmalleolar angle test** should be performed. The transmalleolar angle test uses the same position but different landmarks. A line is drawn that connects the medial and lateral malleoli (the transmalleolar axis). A second line perpendicular to the first that bisects the calcaneus is drawn and a line through the long axis of the femur is visualized. Figure 4–24 shows the landmarks drawn onto a schematic of the foot and thigh and the resulting angle that is measured. This angle would be measured with a goniometer. The angle measured is between the long axis of the femur and the bisection of the calcaneus. This eliminates the forefoot from the measurement so that forefoot problems will not cause an invalid measurement. The negative and positive conventions are the same as for the thigh-foot angle test; that is, a measurement that points toward the midline is a negative value and a measurement that points away from the midline is a positive value.

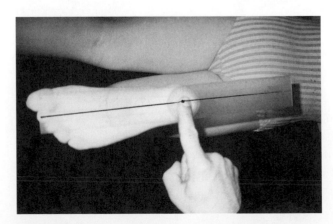

Figure 4–23   Measurement of the thigh-foot angle.

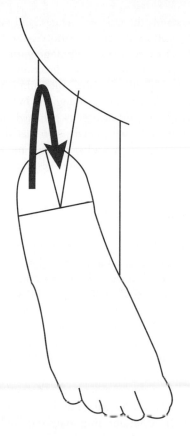

Figure 4–24   Landmarks for the measurement of the transmalleolar angle indicated by the black arrow.

Foot and Ankle

Measurements of a child's foot and ankle can be difficult to make. Ankle dorsiflexion is measured as in adults; however, extra care should be taken to hold the foot in slight inversion and not allow the midfoot to move independently of the rear foot. If there is a limitation in the length of the gastrocnemius-soleus complex, the foot may bend at the midfoot (talocalcaneonavicular and calcaneocuboid joints) and incorrectly appear as dorsiflexion. Holding the ankle in slight inversion locks the midtarsal joint so that midfoot bending will not occur (Bleck, 1987; Sullivan, 1996). If there is a limitation of motion with the knee extended, then the test should also be performed with the knee flexed. This will assist in differentiating whether the limitation is in the soleus, the gastrocnemius, or the talocrural joint. If the ROM is more limited with the knee in extension, the gastrocnemius muscle is responsible for the limitation (Bleck, 1987; Gage, 1991).

There are many ways to examine the foot. In general, the foot posture should be observed in both weight bearing and non–weight bearing. The lateral border of the foot should be straight, not curved. A curvature may indicate a metatarsus adductus that occurs when the metatarsals are adducted toward the midline. The amount of metatarsus adductus can be classified by drawing a straight line that bisects the heel and continues through the long axis of the foot (Bleck, 1987). In a normally aligned foot, this line should pass between the second and third toes. In metatarsus adductus, the toes are medial to the line. If the distal projection of the line passes between the third and fourth toes, it is considered moderate, and if the line passes through the fourth and fifth toes, it is considered severe metatarsus adductus. In mild cases, there is often a spontaneous resolution; however, in moderate or severe cases, intervention with stretching, corrective shoes, or casting may be required (Staheli, 1992; Wenger, 1993a). These are used to reverse the excessive compressive forces on the tarsal and metatarsal bones because, according to the Heuter-Volkmann principle discussed earlier, these abnormal compressive forces will alter growth (Wenger, 1993a).

The position during weight bearing should be observed for arch development and position of the rear foot. As discussed in developmental biomechanics, children younger than 3 to 4 years will not have a longitudinal arch, so flat feet are typical in this age group. Flat feet in older children may be flexible or rigid. Flexible flat feet have little or no arch when standing caused by calcaneal valgus. Extension of the great toe or standing on tiptoes will cause the arch to reappear (Sullivan, 1996) and the heel will realign into slight varus (Wenger, 1993b). If an arch cannot be elicited and there is limited subtalar ROM, it is a rigid flatfoot. A rigid flatfoot signals a problem such as a vertical talus or a tarsal coalition, and should be examined in more detail by an orthopedic surgeon.

A *congenital vertical talus,* a rare condition in children (Scoles, 1988), is more prevalent in children with CP or myelomeningocele and is defined as a superior dislocation of the talonavicular joint (Rang, 1993b). The head of the talus lies below the navicular bone producing what is termed a "rocker-bottom foot deformity." In a **rocker-bottom foot deformity,** there is no arch and the foot curves downward where the arch would typically be present. This deformity should be evaluated by an orthopedic surgeon and is generally treated by surgery. A **tarsal coalition** (also called a bar) is a congenital fusion of tarsal bones and may involve several different tarsal bones. The two most common tarsal coalitions are calcaneonavicular and talocalcaneal (Rang, 1993b). Tarsal coalitions, although rare (Stormont & Peterson, 1983), can cause foot pain and are the most common causes of rigid flat feet in children. (Rang, 1993b)

The decision to treat a flexible flatfoot is somewhat controversial; however, there is little scientific evidence that intervention for asymptomatic flat feet is warranted (Wenger, Mauldin, Speck, Morgan, & Lieber, 1989). If persistent pain is present or gross motor skills are affected, further examination is necessary to rule out a deformity such as a tarsal coalition or a vertical talus, as discussed in the preceding paragraph. Providing a stabilizing insert to children with flat feet who have gross motor delays may improve the child's balance and promote improved skills. It is important to measure the ROM of the gastrocnemius-soleus complex in children with flat feet, because limitation is shown to be a causative factor in the development of flat feet with calcaneal valgus (Harris & Beath, 1948). If limitations are noted, the parents and child should be instructed in passive and self-stretching techniques.

Strength

Strength is an extremely important component of function and the ability of the child to perform the gross motor activities that are age appropriate. In children with typical development, many skills have a component of strength that is needed for competency in that task. For example, the ability of a young child to ride a tricycle is partly attributed to having the strength to push the pedals. The abilities to jump, hop, and climb stairs all need muscular strength for achievement in addition to all of the other components needed, such as adequate ROM, balance, and sensory processing. Improvement in strength has been shown to improve ambulation ability in children with CP (Damiano, Kelly, & Vaughn, 1995; Kramer & MacPhail, 1994). In addition, children with CP were able to show improvements in gross motor abilities (Kramer & MacPhail, 1994) after strength training, indicating the importance of strength to daily activities.

The examination of strength capabilities gives the therapist more information for a physical therapy diagnosis. There are many ways to test strength. In very young babies, movement against gravity, such as kicking in the air, the pull-to-sit maneuver, and the ability to lift the head in the prone positions, are all indications of strength. In the toddler and preschool child, strength-assessing maneuvers include getting up from the floor in a mature fashion, jumping, standing on one foot, the ability to ascend and descend stairs, and standing on tiptoes. It is useful to look at these functional measures of strength because they give the examiner an idea of how the child uses his or her strength. Games such as "Simon Says" help ensure that the child understands the task, cooperates, and gives the most representative effort. A demonstration is also helpful.

Manual muscle testing can be done with children who are old enough to understand the directions and remain in test positions. This may be when the child is as young as 3 to 4 years old. When testing young children, the grades of 0 (no activity), 1 (contraction is palpated but no movement), 2 (full ROM with gravity eliminated), and 3 (full ROM), are used as with adults. There is more subjectivity in grades 4 (full ROM with some resistance) and 5 (full ROM with full resistance), because force must be adjusted based on the child's age. If more objective measurement is needed, handheld dynamometry is preferred (Connolly, 1995).

Children aged 3 to 4 years may be tested reliably with a standard handheld dynamometer as long as they understand the directions and are given verbal praise to help them put forth their best effort (Gajdosik, Nelson, & Gleason, 1994). It has also been shown to be reliable in children with CP (Pax Lowes, Westcott, Palisano, Effgen, & Orlin, 2004), spina bifida (Effgen & Brown, 1992), juvenile rheumatoid arthritis (Wessel et al., 1999), spinal muscular atrophy (Merlini, Mazzone, Solari, & Morandi, 2002), muscular dystrophy (Stuberg & Metcalf, 1988), and adolescents with intellectual disabilities (Horvat, Croce, & Roswal, 1994). Again, it is important the child understands the directions. Handheld dynamometry eliminates the need to estimate resistance based on the child's age and is therefore more objective than manual muscle testing. Average values for handheld dynamometry for a small sample of children aged 4 to 16 years without motor impairment are presented in Table 4.1. The study had only a small sample at each age (n = 9 to 13) so the values should be used only as a general guideline. The size of the standard deviation should also be noted. A large standard deviation suggests that there is variability in the normal sample. In general, a child would have to fall two standard deviations below the mean to be considered "abnormal." In a small sample size, the standard deviations may be unusually large. So again, the numbers and standard deviations are only general guidelines until a more normative database is generated. In general, force abilities in this study were similar between girls and boys until about age 14 years, with the exception that 10-year-old girls showed a growth spurt and were stronger (Beenakker, van der Hoeven, Fock, & Maurits, 2001). The authors found a strong correlation between force and the child's weight (Beenakker et al., 2001). This should be considered when testing children with disabilities because they can be significantly lighter than typically developing peers.

Table 4.1 Force Output in Newtons (kg. m. s²) For Boys and Girls Aged 4 to 16 Years

Muscle Group		Age (yr)												
		4	5	6	7	8	9	10	11	12	13	14	15	16
Neck flexors	Boys			48 (9)*	64 (11)	56 (8)	66 (9)	74 (20)	67 (13)	70 (16)	98 (40)	129 (42)	143 (36)	141 (33)
	Girls			55 (8)	60 (7)	56 (10)	55 (2)	55 (25)	67 (15)	76 (15)	92 (17)	96 (15)	108 (27)	87 (14)
Shoulder abductors	Boys	62 (20)	55 (10)	97 (27)	92 (29)	98 (9)	110 (31)	136 (26)	110 (39)	118 (29)	159 (46)	205 (44)	219 (36)	253 (54)
	Girls	68 (26)	47 (9)	75 (17)	91 (18)	94 (25)	91 (27)	81 (17)	129 (25)	123 (27)	154 (26)	178 (18)	173 (29)	173 (38)
Elbow extensors	Boys			73 (8)	85 (16)	90 (18)	89 (22)	120 (18)	103 (31)	104 (31)	128 (42)	158 (42)	175 (46)	182 (64)
	Girls			73 (8)	85 (14)	82 (10)	91 (24)	84 (20)	108 (25)	117 (24)	118 (26)	129 (23)	141 (37)	107 (36)
Elbow flexors	Boys	78 (24)	70 (12)	103 (21)	121 (32)	124 (23)	134 (24)	173 (19)	153 (30)	160 (25)	195 (26)	253 (50)	287 (55)	276 (68)
	Girls	69 (21)	66 (12)	105 (9)	103 (20)	115 (16)	125 (28)	134 (21)	172 (25)	168 (28)	201 (23)	193 (32)	198 (48)	215 (30)
Wrist extensors	Boys			77 (11)	89 (26)	87 (15)	97 (5)	121 (21)	100 (19)	108 (21)	153 (42)	195 (41)	218 (49)	237 (58)
	Girls			66 (6)	74 (13)	75 (11)	80 (1)	80 (17)	112 (16)	127 (23)	152 (14)	155 (6)	166 (26)	147 (28)
Hip flexors	Boys			182 (39)	182 (57)	225 (40)	232 (53)	261 (74)	245 (65)	198 (38)	289 (60)	337 (66)	301 (69)	395 (102)
	Girls			162 (31)	184 (50)	175 (36)	195 (48)	177 (25)	264 (55)	232 (61)	308 (51)	281 (72)	288 (70)	301 (42)
Hip abductors	Boys			128 (40)	124 (32)	131 (30)	153 (33)	174 (47)	151 (63)	158 (41)	225 (58)	306 (83)	356 (87)	312 (106)
	Girls			109 (26)	122 (24)	117 (18)	124 (35)	104 (25)	140 (22)	171 (44)	227 (52)	244 (30)	257 (68)	244 (59)
Knee extensors	Boys			156 (33)	157 (38)	185 (41)	194 (30)	267 (47)	239 (65)	225 (43)	296 (70)	370 (61)	362 (76)	396 (90)
	Girls			148 (24)	177 (47)	166 (30)	173 (57)	198 (57)	265 (36)	250 (71)	346 (49)	280 (69)	325 (79)	373 (81)
Knee flexors	Boys	111 (15)		158 (38)	180 (45)	185 (20)	195 (40)	268 (48)	218 (64)	201 (34)	273 (59)	307 (64)	327 (76)	382 (80)
	Girls	92 (25)		154 (33)	171 (35)	160 (23)	180 (54)	175 (29)	246 (52)	221 (54)	301 (38)	271 (76)	282 (61)	336 (57)
Ankle dorsiflexors	Boys	71 (22)	105 (20)	104 (11)	130 (26)	137 (24)	141 (31)	154 (18)	149 (26)	170 (28)	218 (55)	257 (60)	267 (50)	291 (60)
	Girls	75 (20)	99 (15)	95 (17)	114 (18)	121 (17)	137 (32)	130 (21)	178 (25)	177 (34)	214 (29)	207 (31)	220 (40)	232 (30)

*Values given as mean (SD) in Newtons (kg • m • s²) (n = 7 to 13 per age group).

Source: From Beenakker, E.A., van der Hoeven, J.H., Fock, J.M., & Maurits, N.M. (2001). Reference values of maximum isometric muscle force obtained in 270 children aged 4–16 years by hand-held dynamometry. *Neuromuscular Disorders, 11*(5), 441–446. Copyright 2001 by Elsevier. Reprinted with permission.

Summary

The musculoskeletal system is an integral part of the overall health and well-being of children both with and without neurological complications. A systematic assessment of the musculoskeletal system, guided by patient complaints, will allow the therapist to formulate orthopedic-based intervention strategies that will complement neurological techniques.

Working with children requires organization so that the therapist can maximize the child's attention span, assess as many items as possible, and remain flexible to change the routine if the child is hesitant to cooperate. By establishing a rapport with the child and performing assessments in the natural environment or at least a child-friendly environment, the therapist can use play to evaluate the child's typical performance.

DISCUSSION QUESTIONS

1. How would you organize an initial assessment of a 2-year-old child?

2. Describe how decreased lower extremity weight bearing would affect hip joint development.

3. How would you assess a 4-year-old with flat feet? What factors would influence your recommendations to the family?

4. Discuss the role of stretching and passive ROM in children with cerebral palsy.

REFERENCES

Apkon, S.D. (2002). Osteoporosis in children who have disabilities. *Physical Medicine and Rehabilitation Clinics of North America, 13*(4), 839–855.

Bartlett, M.D., Wolf, L.S., Shurtless, D.B., & Staheli, L.T. (1985). Hip flexion contractures: A comparison of measurement methods. *Archives of Physical Medicine and Rehabilitation, 66,* 620–625.

Beattie, P., Isaacson, K., Riddle, D.L., & Rothstein, J. (1990). Validity of derived measurements of leg-length differences obtained by use of a tape measure. *Physical Therapy, 70*(3), 150–157.

Beenakker, E.A., van der Hoeven, J. H., Fock, J.M., & Maurits, N.M. (2001). Reference values of maximum isometric muscle force obtained in 270 children aged 4–16 years by hand-held dynamometry. *Neuromuscular Disorders, 11*(5), 441–446.

Beeson, P. (1999). Frontal plane configuration of the knee in children. *The Foot, 9,* 18–26.

Bernhardt, D. (1988). Prenatal and postnatal growth and development of the foot and ankle. *Physical Therapy, 68*(12), 1831–1839.

Bleck, E.E. (1982). The shoeing of children: Sham or science. *Developmental Medicine and Child Neurology, 13,* 188–195.

Bleck, E. (1987). *Orthopaedic management in cerebral palsy.* Oxford: MacKeith Press.

Bourrin, S., Palle, S., Genty, C., & Alexandre, C. (1995). Physical exercise during remobilization restores a normal bone trabecular network after tail suspension-induced osteopenia in young rats. *Journal of Bone and Mineral Research, 10*(5), 820–828.

Cahuzac, J.P., Vardon, D., & Sales de Gauzy, J. (1995). Development of the clinical tibiofemoral angle in normal adolescents: A study of 427 normal subjects from 10 to 16 years of age. *Journal of Bone and Joint Surgery (British), 77*(5), 729–732.

Cimaz, R. (2002). Osteoporosis in childhood rheumatic diseases: Prevention and therapy. *Best Practice & Research in Clinical Rheumatology, 16*(3), 397–409.

Connolly, B. (1995). Testing in infants and children. In H.J. Hislop & J. Montgomery (Eds.). *Daniels and Worthingham's muscle testing* (6th ed., pp. 235–260). Philadelphia: W.B. Saunders.

Cusick, B. (1990). *Progressive casting and splinting for lower extremity deformities in children with neuromotor dysfunction.* Tucson, AZ: Therapy Skill Builders.

Cusick, B.D., & Stuberg, W.A. (1992). Assessment of lower-extremity alignment in the transverse plane: Implications for management of children with neuromotor dysfunction. *Physical Therapy, 72,* 3–15.

Damiano, D.L., Kelly, L.E., & Vaughn, C.L. (1995). Effects of quadriceps femoris muscle strengthening on crouch gait in children with spastic diplegia. *Physical Therapy, 75,* 658–667.

Davids, J.R., Wenger, D.R., & Mubarak, S.J. (1993). Congenital muscular torticollis: Sequela of intrauterine or perinatal compartment syndrome. *Journal of Pediatric Orthopedics, 13,* 1–7.

Drews, J.E., Vraciu, J.K., & Pellino, G. (1984). Range of motion of the joints of the lower extremities of newborns. *Physical and Occupational Therapy in Pediatrics, 4*(2), 49–62.

Dubowitz, V. (1967). Pathology of experimentally re-innervated skeletal muscle. *Journal of Neurology, Neurosurgery and Psychiatry, 30*(2), 99–110.

Effgen, S.K., & Brown, D.A. (1992). Long term stability of hand-held dynamometric measurements in children who have myelomeningocele. *Physical Therapy, 72,* 458–465.

Engel, G.M., & Staheli, L.T. (1974). The natural history of torsion and other factors influencing gait in childhood. *Clinical Orthopedics and Related Research, 99,* 12–17.

Fabry, G., MacEwen, G.D., & Shands, A.R., Jr. (1973). Torsion of the femur. A follow-up study in normal and abnormal conditions. *Journal of Bone and Joint Surgery, 55-A*(8), 1726–1738.

Frost, H.M. (1964). *The laws of bone structure.* Springfield, IL: Charles C Thomas Publishers.

Gage, J.R. (1991). *Gait analysis in cerebral palsy.* New York: Cambridge University Press.

Gajdosik, R.L., & Bohannon, R.W. (1987). Clinical measurement of range of motion: Review of goniometry emphasizing reliability and validity. *Physical Therapy, 67,* 1867–1872.

Gajdosik, C.G., Nelson, S.A., & Gleason, D.K. (1994). Reliability of isometric measurements of girls ages 3-5 years: A preliminary study. *Pediatric Physical Therapy, 6,* 206.

Gajdosik, R.L., Sandler, M.M., & Marr, H.L. (2003). Influence of knee positions and gender on the Ober test for length of the iliotibial band. *Clinical Biomechanics, 18*(1), 77–79.

Grasco, J., & de Pablos, J. (1997). Bone remodeling in malunited fractures in children. *Journal of Pediatric Orthopedics, Part B, 6,* 126–132.

Gross, M.T. (1995). Lower quarter screening for skeletal malalignments: Suggestions for orthotics and shoewear. *Journal of Orthopedics and Sports Physical Therapy, 21,* 389–405.

Haas, S.S., Epps, C.H., & Adams, J. P. (1973). Normal ranges of hip motion in the newborn. *Clinical Orthopedics, 91,* 114–118.

Haggmark, T., & Eriksson, E. (1979). Hypotrophy of the soleus muscle in man after Achilles tendon rupture. Discussion of findings obtained by computed tomography and morphologic studies. *American Journal of Sports Medicine, 7*(2), 121–126.

Harris, R.I., & Beath, T. (1948). Hypermobile flat-foot with short tendon Achilles. *Journal of Bone and Joint Surgery, 30-A,* 116–150.

Harris, S.R., Harthun-Smith, L., & Krukowski, L. (1985). Goniometric reliability for a child with spastic quadriplegia. *Journal of Pediatric Orthopedics, 5,* 348–351.

Heath, C.H., & Staheli, L.T. (1993). Normal limits of knee angle in white children—genu varum and genu valgum. *Journal of Pediatric Orthopedics, 13*(2), 259–266.

Hensinger, R.N., & Jones, E.T. (1982). Developmental orthopedics. I: The lower limb. *Developmental Medicine and Child Neurology, 24,* 95–116.

Horvat, M., Croce, R., & Roswal, G. (1994). Intratester reliability of the Nicholas Manual Muscle Tester on individuals with intellectual disabilities by a tester having minimal experience. *Archives of Physical Medicine and Rehabilitation, 76,* 808–811.

King, W., Levin, R., Schmidt, R., Oestreich, A., & Heubi, J.E. (2003). Prevalence of reduced bone mass in children and adults with spastic quadriplegia. *Developmental Medicine and Child Neurology, 45*(1), 12–16.

Kramer, J.F., & MacPhail, A. (1994). Relationships among measures of walking efficiency, gross motor ability, and isokinetic strength in adolescents with cerebral palsy. *Pediatric Physical Therapy, 6,* 3–8.

Lanyon, L.E., & Rubin, C.T. (1984). Static vs dynamic loads as an influence on bone remodelling. *Journal of Biomechanics, 17,* 897–905.

LeVeau, B.F. Bernhardt, & D.B. (1984). Developmental biomechanics. *Physical Therapy, 64*(12), 1874–1881.

Lonstein, J.E. (1996). Scoliosis. In R.T. Morrissey & S.L. Weinstein (Eds.). *Lovell and Winter's pediatric orthopedics* (pp. 625–685). Philadelphia: Lippincott-Raven Publishers.

Mann, M., Glasheen-Wray, M., & Nyberg, R. (1984). Therapist agreement for palpation and observation of iliac crest heights. *Physical Therapy, 64*(3), 334–338.

McCrea, J.D. (1985). *Pediatric orthopedics of the lower extremity. An instructional handbook.* Mount Kisco, NY: Futura Publishing Co.

McDade, W. (1977). Bow legs & knock knees. *Pediatric Clinics of North America, 24*(4), 825–839.

Melchione, W.E., & Sullivan, M.S. (1993). Reliability of measurements obtained by use of an instrument designed to indirectly measure iliotibial band length. *Journal of Orthopaedic and Sports Physical Therapy, 18*(3), 511–515.

Merlini, L., Mazzone, E.S., Solari, A., & Morandi, L. (2002). Reliability of hand-held dynamometry in spinal muscular atrophy. *Muscle and Nerve, 26,* 64–67.

Miller, F., Dias, R.C., Dabney, K.W., Lipton, G., & Trianna, M. (1997). Soft-tissue release for spastic hip subluxation in cerebral palsy. *Journal of Pediatric Orthopaedics, 17*(5), 571–584.

Mortensen, H.M., Skov, O., & Jensen, P.E. (1999). Early motion of the ankle after operative treatment of a rupture of the Achilles tendon. A prospective, randomized clinical and radiographic study. *Journal of Bone and Joint Surgery (American), 81*(7), 983–990.

Mullender, M.G., & Huiskes, R. (1995). Proposal for the regulatory mechanism of Wolff's law. *Journal of Orthopedic Research, 13*(4), 503–512.

Munsat, T.L., McNeal, D., & Waters, R. (1976). Effects of nerve stimulation on human muscle. *Archives of Neurology, 33*(9), 608–617.

Nigg, B.M., & Grimston, S.K. (1994). Bone. In B.M. Nigg & W. Herzog (Eds.). *Biomechanics of the musculoskeletal system.* Chichester, England: Wiley & Sons.

O'Sullivan, M.E., Bronk, J.T., Chao, E.Y.S., & Kelly, P.J. (1994). Experimental study of the effect of weight bearing on fracture healing in the canine tibia. *Clinical Orthopedics and Related Research, 302,* 273–283.

Pax Lowes, L., Westcott, S.L., Palisano, R.J., Effgen, S.K., & Orlin, M.N. (2004). Muscle force and range of motion as predictors of standing balance in children with cerebral palsy. *Physical and Occupational Therapy in Pediatrics, 24* (1/2), 57–77.

Phelps, E., Smith, L.J., & Hallum, A. (1985). Normal ranges of hip motion of infants between nine and 24 months of age. *Developmental Medicine and Child Neurology, 27,* 785–792.

Pitkow, R.B. (1975). External rotation contracture of the extended hip. *Clinical Orthopedics and Related Research, 110,* 139–145.

Pitman M.I., & Peterson, L. (1989). Biomechanics of skeletal muscle. In M. Nordkin & V.H. Frankel (Eds.) *Basic biomechanics of the musculoskeletal system* (pp. 89–107). Philadelphia: Lippincott.

Rang, M. (1993a). Bow-legs and knock knees. In D.R. Wenger & M. Rang (Eds.). *The art and practice of children's orthopedics* (pp. 201–219). New York: Raven Press.

Rang, M. (1993b). Other feet. In D.R. Wenger & M. Rang (Eds.). *The art and practice of children's orthopedics* (pp. 168–200). New York: Raven Press.

Rang, M. (1993c). Toeing in and toeing out: Gait disorders. In D.R. Wenger & M. Rang (Eds.). *The art and practice of children's orthopedics* (pp. 50–76). New York: Raven Press.

Reimers, J. (1980). The stability of the hip joint in children. A radiological study of the results of muscle surgery in cerebral palsy. *Acta Orthopaedica Scandinavica Supplementum, 184,* 1–100.

Salenius, P., & Vankka, E. (1975). Development of the tibiofemoral angle in children. *Journal of Bone and Joint Surgery, 57-A,* 259–261.

Scoles, P.V. (1988*). Pediatric orthopedics in clinical practice* (2nd ed.). Chicago: Year Book Medical Publishers, Inc.

Scull, S. (2001). Juvenile rheumatoid arthritis. In S.K. Campbell, R.J. Palisano, & D.W. Vander Linden (Eds.). *Physical therapy for children* (2nd ed., pp. 227–246). Philadelphia: W.B. Saunders.

Staheli, L.T. (1992). *Fundamentals of pediatric orthopedics.* New York: Raven Press.

Staheli, L.T. (1977). The prone hip extension test. *Clinical Orthopedics and Related Research, 12,* 12–15.

Staheli, L.T., Chew, D.E., & Corbett, M. (1987). The longitudinal arch. *Journal of Bone and Joint Surgery, 69-A*(3), 426–428.

Stokes, I.A. (1997). Analysis of symmetry of vertebral body loading consequent to lateral spinal curvature. *Spine, 22*(21), 2495–2503.

Stormont, D.M., & Peterson, H.A. (1983). The relative incidence of tarsal coalition. *Clinical Orthopedics and Related Research, 181,* 28–35.

Stuberg ,W.A., & Metcalf, W.K. (1988). Reliability of quantitative muscle testing in healthy children and in children with Duchenne muscular dystrophy using a hand-held dynamometer. *Physical Therapy, 68,* 977–982.

Stuberg, W.A., Fuchs, R.H., & Miedaner, J.A. (1988). Reliability of goniometric measurements of children with cerebral palsy. *Developmental Medicine and Child Neurology, 30,* 657–666.

Stuberg, W.A., Koehler, A., Witicha, M., Temme, J., & Kaplan, P. (1989). Comparison of femoral torsion assessment using goniometry and computerized tomography. *Pediatric Physical Therapy, 1,* 115–118.

Sullivan, J.A. (1996). The child's foot. In R.T. Morrissey & S.L. Weinstein (Eds.). *Lovell and Winter's pediatric orthopedics* (pp. 1077–1135). Philadelphia: Lippincott-Raven.

Sutherland, D.H., Olshen, R.A., Biden, E.N., & Wyatt, M.P. (1987). *The development of mature walking.* Oxford: MacKeith Press.

Tolo, V. (1996). The lower extremity. In R.T. Morrissey & S.L. Weinstein (Eds.). *Lovell and Winter's pediatric orthopedics* (pp. 1047–1075). Philadelphia: Lippincott-Raven.

Trueta, J. (1968). *Studies of the development and decay of the human frame* (p. 37). Philadelphia: W.B. Saunders.

Van Den Berg-Emons, R.J., Van Baak, M.A., Speth, L., & Saris, W.H. (1998). Physical training of school children with spastic cerebral palsy: Effects on daily activity, fat mass and fitness. *International Journal of Rehabilitation Research, 21,* 179–194.

Walker, J. (1991). Musculoskeletal development: A review. *Physical Therapy, 71*(12), 878–889.

Weinstein, S.L. (1996). Developmental hip dysplasia and dislocation. In R.T. Morrissey & S.L. Weinstein (Eds.). *Lovell and Winter's pediatric orthopedics.* Philadelphia: Lippincott-Raven.

Wenger, D.R. (1993a). Calcaneovarus and metatarsus varus. In D.R. Wenger & M. Rang (Eds.). *The art and practice of children's orthopedics* (pp. 103–136). New York: Raven Press.

Wenger, D.R. (1993b). Flatfoot and children's shoes. In D.R. Wenger & M. Rang (Eds.). *The art and practice of children's orthopedics* (pp. 77–102). New York: Raven Press.

Wenger, D.R., Mauldin, D., Speck, G., Morgan, D., & Lieber, R.L. (1989). Corrective shoes and inserts as treatment for flexible flatfoot in infants and children. *Journal of Bone and Joint Surgery (American), 71*(6), 800–810.

Wessel, J., Kaup, C., Fan, J., Ehalt, R., Ellsworth, J., Speer, C., Tenove, P., & Dombrosky, A. (1999). Isometric strength measurements in children with arthritis: Reliability and relation to function. *Arthritis Care Resource, 12*(4), 238–246.

Wilkins, K. (1986). Bowlegs. *The Pediatric Clinics of North America, 33*(6), 1429–1438.

Williams, P.F. (1982). *Orthopedic management in childhood.* London: Blackwell Scientific Publications.

Zaleske, D.J. (1996). Metabolic and endocrine abnormalities. In R.T. Morrissey & S.L. Weinstein (Eds.). *Lovell and Winter's pediatric orthopedics* (pp. 137–201). Philadelphia: Lippincott-Raven.

Chapter *5*

Musculoskeletal System: Considerations and Interventions for Specific Pediatric Pathologies

— Linda Pax Lowes, PT, PhD, PCS

— Margo N. Orlin, PT, PhD, PCS

In this chapter, we apply principles of musculoskeletal development to common pediatric conditions and discuss intervention strategies. For educational purposes, this book is divided into systems. The human body, however, operates through an interaction of all the systems. Individuals with neurological impairment are affected by the musculoskeletal system and, in contrast, individuals with musculoskeletal impairment can make improvements through refinements in the nervous system. For example, someone who repeatedly injures a joint may alleviate the problem by educating the nervous system to move in a new pattern. In addition, functional abilities of an individual with neurological impairment can be enhanced through improvements in range of motion (ROM) or force production. In this chapter, we will address only the musculoskeletal aspects of disease. For information on the neurological components, please refer to Chapters 6 and 7. The end of the chapter provides more in-depth information and intervention suggestions for three common pediatric conditions with significant musculoskeletal concerns: cerebral palsy (CP), Down syndrome, and scoliosis.

Musculoskeletal Pathologies of Connective Tissue

Both **Ehlers-Danlös syndrome (EDS)** and osteogenesis imperfecta are characterized by connective tissue abnormalities. Children with osteogenesis imperfecta have ligamentous laxity; however, bone abnormalities are the main problem, so it will be discussed in the section on bone in this chapter. Table 5.1 provides information on the etiology, pathology, impairment, and limitations associated with EDS. There are several subclassifications of EDS that vary in the combination of symptoms and severity. The degree of impairments and limitations associated with EDS is also highly variable, so each child must be assessed individually.

Physical therapy intervention duration and frequency for a child with EDS vary according to the severity of the disease and the needs of the child and family. The child and family require information about the disease and assistance in developing a preventive health plan to optimize the child's functional skills and independence while avoiding injury. This could include assistance in selecting appropriate activities for promoting the child's health and fitness, and peer interaction. Recommended activities should be based on the child's interests and the nature of the impairments and should minimize the risk of injury. They might include swimming, cycling, dancing, tennis, or golf. Rough-house play and contact sports should be avoided.

The child should be instructed in joint preservation techniques. Assistive devices could be recommended to maximize the child's independence while preserving joint integrity. When selecting assistive devices, it is important to remember that compliance is often low in children unless they are included in the decision-making process and value the device. For children to value a device, it must enhance the performance of an important task or the child must understand the importance of preventive medicine. The concept of preventive medicine may be difficult for children, many of whom go through a natural period of feeling invincible or are unable to project themselves several decades into the future. Devices that are prescribed for preventive health purposes but diminish performance or speed are frequently discarded. For example, a child is unlikely to continue to use a walker or cane to improve movement patterns and reduce stress on joints if he or she can walk faster unaided (see Table 5.1).

Table 5.1 Pediatric Diseases Affecting Connective Tissue

Diagnosis	Etiology	Pathology	Impairments of Body Functions and Structures	Potential Activity Limitations and Participation Restrictions	Potential Interventions
Ehlers-Danlös syndrome (Grahame, 2000; Sacheti et al., 1997)	Genetic mutation	Autosomal dominant inheritance is most common	• Hyperextensibility of the skin • Soft, velvetlike skin • Bone and soft tissue fragility with easy bruising • Frequent joint dislocation or subluxation • Calcification of soft tissues • Slow wound healing • Joint hypermobility • Osteopenia (reduced bone mass) • Nearsightedness • High occurrence of chronic pain, most often in shoulders, hands, and knees	• ADL skills such as dressing • Need to avoid physical activities that put bones and joints at risk	• Child and family education to minimize injury • Strengthening and fitness programs to reduce injuries • Pain management as needed • Assistive devices and functional training as needed
Juvenile rheumatoid arthritis (JRA)—Systemic onset	Cause unknown	• Joint inflammation involving few or many joints • Joint synovium proliferates, causing a massive overgrowth (pannus), which can erode the adjacent cartilage and bone • Joint adhesions and osteophytes (bony spurs) possible	• ROM limitations • Joint space narrowing and/or destruction • Significant pain	• May limit mobility and self-care activities • May impair handwriting	• Child and family education • ROM • Strengthening and fitness programs • Pain management • Environmental and lifestyle modification • Splinting • Assistive device and mobility aid selection

Diagnosis	Etiology	Pathology	Impairments of Body Functions and Structures	Potential Activity Limitations and Participation Restrictions	Potential Interventions
JRA—Pauciarticular onset	Cause unknown	• Joint inflammation involving four or fewer joints • Pannus can erode the adjacent cartilage and bone • Joint adhesions and osteophytes possible	• ROM limitations: most commonly the knee, ankle, and fingers • Joint space narrowing and/or destruction • 20% have chronic iritis, which may lead to blindness	• May limit mobility and self-care activities • May impair hand-writing	Same as above
JRA—Polyarticular onset	Cause unknown	• Joint inflammation involving five or more joints • Pannus can erode the adjacent cartilage and bone • Joint adhesions and osteophytes possible	• ROM limitations, generally of bilateral knees, wrists, and ankles • Joint space narrowing and/or destruction	• May limit mobility and self-care activities • May impair hand-writing if finger involvement	Same as above

Juvenile rheumatoid arthritis (JRA) affects cartilage and is the most common chronic childhood rheumatoid disease. The cause of JRA is unknown. Hypothetical causes include a viral infectious agent, an immunological abnormality, or a combination of the two. Three subgroups of JRA are typically identified, based on the distribution of the symptoms or onset characteristics. **Systemic-onset JRA** is the least common but generally most painful form. It is characterized by a febrile onset with a temperature of greater than 103° F accompanied by a characteristic rash. Other systemic manifestations can include heart infections, swollen glands, an enlarged spleen, abdominal pain, anemia, and growth retardation (Rhodes, 1991). It occurs in boys and girls equally, generally between the ages of 5 and 15 years. The prognosis for children with systemic onset JRA varies. If the arthritis continues after the systemic symptoms subside, there is a greater possibility of developing persistent arthritis that can lead to marked disability. Severe degeneration of the hip joint is the major cause of chronic functional limitations and pain.

The next two types of JRA do not involve fever and are based on the distribution of the disease. **Pauciarticular-onset JRA** is the most common form and is defined as affecting 4 or fewer joints after the first 6 months of the disease. It is 4 times more common in girls and is most often diagnosed around 2 years of age (Sherry & Mosca, 1996). The prognosis for pauciarticular JRA varies, but one study found only 47% of the children in remission 10 years after onset (Oen et al., 2002). Permanent joint space narrowing is frequently seen after remission but most of the young adults who had JRA do not have severe chronic disability.

Polyarticular JRA is defined as involvement in five or more joints. As with pauciarticular JRA, it occurs predominantly in girls, but onset peaks at age 1 to 3 years and again in early adolescence. After the first year of the disease, there is often a symmetrical distribution pattern. The prognosis for children with polyarticular JRA ranges from 6 to 23% of the children in remission 10 years after onset (Oen et al., 2002). If the disease is contracted in the adolescent years, however, the prognosis is poor, with up to 50% developing severe destructive arthritis (Schaller, 1997).

In all three types of JRA there can be periarticular changes as a result of the inflammatory process. Capsular hypertrophy, ligamentous laxity, irregular bone growth, and osteoporosis are all possible sequelae of inflammation. Periods of inflammation and swelling can stretch the surrounding ligaments and lead to joint instability when the swelling subsides. The adjacent muscles and tendons may also become inflamed and lead to further restrictions in ROM caused by pain. Secondarily, a lack of movement can cause articular cartilage damage. Movement bathes the articular cartilage in synovial fluid, which contributes to nourishment and health. Decreased movement compounds the destructive forces. All of the periarticular changes can destroy the normal skeletal alignment of the body and lead to further destructive force being applied.

Inflammation can also change the growth rate of bones. **Inflammatory hyperemia** can stimulate adjacent growth plates and cause overgrowth, or cause early physeal closure and subsequent limb shortening (Sherry & Mosca, 1996). The effect can be unilateral or bilateral and may be symmetrical or asymmetrical within the growth plate. Therefore, leg length discrepancy (LLD) is a common complication of monoarticular and pauciarticular JRA. Most commonly, LLD is caused by disease of the knee. Three growth abnormality patterns have been identified (Simon, Whiffen, & Shapiro, 1981). If the disease onset is earlier than 9 years of age, overgrowth of the involved knee and premature growth arrest of the acetabulum and femoral head are most often noted. Generally, the overgrowth in the knee does not exceed 3 cm. Conversely, if the disease onset is after 9 years of age, premature closure of the growth plate with subsequent shortening of the involved extremity is most common. Early physeal closure can result in more severe deformity with a discrepancy of up to 6 cm.

Foot deformities are extremely prevalent in children with JRA (Spraul & Koenning, 1994). A sample of 144 consecutive JRA clinic patients was evaluated and more than 80% had some degree of foot dysfunction. The most common problems were pronated rear foot (73%) and midfoot (72%). Toe valgus and ankle ROM limitations (35%) were also prevalent (Spraul & Koenning, 1994). Pressure distribution under the foot when walking can also be indicative of pathology. Foot pressure analysis equipment has shown that children with JRA do not load the great toe during terminal stance as much as do children without JRA. This is likely because of joint stiffening at the metatarsophalangeal joint, and it can affect push-off (Dhanendran, Hutton, Klennerman, Witemeyer, & Ansell, 1980). Significant radiographic changes can also be seen in the cervical spine, including subluxations or ankylosing (fusing). This can lead to limited neck ROM, particularly in extension.

Examination of the child with JRA needs to include an evaluation of functional skills (Miller, Kress, & Berry, 1999), strength (Giannini & Protas, 1993; Wessel et al., 1999), bony deformities, ROM, fatigue, and pain, as all of these symptoms are common. Not only can symptoms vary between children, but also individual complaints can vary within 1 day, week, or year. For example, children often report increased pain and stiffness in the morning and with cold temperatures, whereas functional skills may decline at the end of the day because of fatigue. A thorough examiner will inquire into the child's typical day, week, and even year to assess the patterns of impairment.

Intervention objectives for children with JRA include pain relief; prevention/remediation of ROM, strength, and deformity; and maintenance or improvement of functional abilities. This is best accomplished through a team with the child and the family as center. Team members may include a pediatric rheumatologist, orthopedic surgeon, physical therapist, occupational therapist, case manager, nurse specialist, educator, psychologist, and nutritionist. The chronic and variable nature of the disease will cause the members of the team to change as the child's disease changes.

The goal of medical management is remission of the disease. Controlling the inflammation can help prevent permanent joint problems. The swelling associated with inflammation can stretch the joint ligaments. When the swelling subsides, the stretched ligaments can cause joint instability. Many drugs are used to promote disease remission, and control symptoms such as pain and inflammation. These drugs include nonsteroidal anti-inflammatory drugs (NSAIDs); slow-acting antirheumatic drugs (SAARDs); and cytotoxic agents, of which methotrexate is the most common. Etanercept (Enbrel), which is an anti–tumor necrosis factor (TNF)-α biological drug, has been successfully used in children with polyarticular JRA. Intra-articular injected steroid drugs are also used, particularly with pauciarticular JRA (Lovell, Passo, Giannini, & Brunner, 2001).

Therapy intervention should include child and family education, pain management, deformity prevention, promotion of functional abilities, and physical fitness. The child, if old enough, should be given information about the disease and allowed to participate in determining the plan of care. In addition to pharmacological pain management, a program of joint protection and therapeutic exercise can help to prevent or reduce pain. Self-guided ROM activities spaced throughout the day can prevent stiffening from prolonged lack of movement. Movement and stretching can be painful at first, but most children report that regular gentle movement helps alleviate pain.

Pain often causes the child to decrease physical activity, which frequently leads to deconditioning and weakness. Community-based exercise programs have been shown to improve endurance and decrease joint symptoms (Klepper, 1999; Klepper & Giannini, 1994). Eighty percent of the children with polyarticular JRA who participated in an 8-week/24-session program of low-impact aerobics, strengthening, and flexibility exercises reported a significant improvement in joint pain, and all had improved endurance.

Because physical fitness is so important to maximizing health, efforts should be made to enhance lifelong participation. Selection of activities should be based on the child's interests while minimizing risk to the joints and maximizing therapeutic benefit. An activity that provides ROM, strengthening, and cardiovascular endurance would be optimal. The level of stress the activity puts on the joints must be evaluated before initiating a program. The child should also be advised of the need to include preactivity and postactivity stretching. Aquatic therapeutic exercise has been shown to improve ROM (Bacon, Nicholson, Binder, & White, 1991) and can be performed in a group setting. Tepid pool water can help motion and minimize fatigue. Additional activities such as swimming, Tai Chi, low-impact aerobics, and cycling may be good choices.

Education about **joint protection** may also help reduce pain. Joint protection minimizes the stress on the joints by avoiding end-range positions and high-torque movements. The use of aides to help with activities of daily living (ADLs) is one way to limit joint stress. Large-handled items can improve grip strength while reducing joint stress. School-age children should avoid carrying heavy stacks of books throughout the school day. The student might require two sets of books. The appropriate book could be left in each classroom and another set could remain at home for completing homework. Items that need to go with the child from room to room could be kept in a backpack for ambulatory children or in a bag attached to a walker or wheelchair.

Splinting is also an important consideration in children with JRA. A splint can provide stability, maintain the extremity in an optimal position for function, and reduce degenerative deformity. An ankle-foot orthosis provides stability for ambulation while maintaining ankle integrity. A wrist extension splint might increase the grip force through use of the tenodesis effect. Night splints are used to increase or maintain ROM.

Conditions Affecting Bone

The initial limb bud undergoes a remarkable process of growth and modeling in response to in utero movement and stresses. This process is clearly illustrated in the hip joint. Early in gestation, the fetal femoral head is almost completely surrounded by a deep acetabulum. With fetal growth, the diameter of the acetabulum surpasses the increase in acetabular depth, resulting in a shallower acetabulum. In addition, the femoral head is initially spherical but becomes more flattened by constriction in the uterus as the fetus grows. It is hypothesized that the unstable hip joint facilitates the passage of the fetus through the birth canal; however, it also may lead to a dislocated or subluxated hip (Walker, 1991). Postnatally, the depth of the acetabulum increases over time and the femoral head returns to a more spherical shape to form a congruent stable joint.

Developmental dysplasia of the hip (DDH) is a condition of pathological hip instability. A subluxable hip is seen in 1 in 100 neonates; more severe instability is seen in 1 to 1.5 of 1000 neonates who have a dislocation (Goldberg, 2001) (Table 5.2). Hip abduction limitation or asymmetry is the most consistent sign of hip dysplasia in neonates. Typically, a neonate has between 75° and 90° abduction in each hip. If a significant limitation or even a small asymmetry (5° to 10°) exists, developmental hip dysplasia should be considered. Other clinical signs can include skinfold asymmetry, pistoning, or an apparent LLD as the child is examined using the Galleazi sign (see Figure 4–11).

The **Ortolani** and **Barlow signs** are the two primary clinical tests used to assess hip stability in neonates less than 1 month of age. The Ortolani sign (Figure 5–1) is the palpable sensation of the femoral head gliding over the neolimbus (cartilaginous ridge) as it moves back into the acetabulum. The infant's hips and knees are flexed 90°. The thigh is gently abducted, which brings the femoral head from its dislocated posterior position forward into the acetabulum, reducing the femoral head back into the acetabulum. In a positive finding, there is generally a palpable and audible "clunk" as the hip reduces.

The Barlow maneuver (Figure 5–2) is a more aggressive maneuver in which the hip is flexed and adducted while the examiner palpates the femoral head as it exits the acetabulum (Wenger, 1993). The hip is flexed and the thigh adducted while pushing posteriorly in the line of the shaft of the femur, causing the femoral head to dislocate posteriorly from the acetabulum. Dislocation is palpable as the femoral head slips out of the acetabulum.

Both the Ortolani and Barlow signs must be performed on one leg at a time, when the infant is completely relaxed, because muscle contractions can hide the instability. During both tests, the examiner's thumb is on the anterior surface of the thigh while the fingers are palpating the posterior joint space. Both the Ortolani and Barlow signs require training with an experienced mentor to ensure reliability. A physical therapist working with neonates in a neonatal intensive care unit, nursery, or outpatient program should be able to perform the tests accurately and reliably.

Table 5.2 Congenital Joint Anomalies

Diagnosis	Etiology	Pathology	Impairments of Body Functions and Structures	Potential Activity Limitations	Potential Interventions
Talipes equinovarus	Unknown Speculated multifactorial: • Genetic component • Arrested embryonic development • Neuromuscular abnormalities • Mechanical uterine constriction	Displacement of the navicular, calcaneus, and cuboid bones around the talus	Hindfoot equinus with varus of the forefoot and heel and adducted forefoot	• Interferes with standing, ambulation, and other upright activities • Difficulty fitting shoes • Cosmesis	• PT intervention: taping, stretching, parent education on home stretching, developmental stimulation • Health-care team intervention: if other measures are unsuccessful or too severe, child may need casting or surgery
Developmental dysplasia of the hip (DDH)	• Multifactorial • Genetic predisposition; firstborn; 80% female • Ethnic: higher incidence in Native Americans, lower incidence in Chinese and Africans • Mechanical: breech position, oligohydramnios (insufficient amniotic fluid) • Neuromuscular • Myelomeningocele	• Subluxation, dislocation, or dysplasia of the hip • Hypertrophied ridge of cartilage in the superior, posterior, and inferior aspects of the acetabulum, called a neolimbus	• Unstable hip joint • Limited hip abduction • Poor weight-bearing surface • Apparent leg length discrepancy if femur not residing in the acetabulum • Poor hip socket development	• Can interfere with motor milestone acquisition • Impedes ambulation and other upright activities • Leg length inequality may be cosmetically displeasing and require increased energy expenditure for ambulation • Painful degenerative changes over time	• Parent education • Developmental stimulation program • Positioning and gentle ROM

The unstable hip joint should be considered when positioning or performing ROM with all neonates, not just those showing clinical signs of joint instability. Positions of extreme or forceful extension should be avoided because they may lead to dislocation. In addition, a relationship between sleeping position preferences and hip dysplasia has been reported. In a sample of 41 infants with a preferred sidelying position, hip dysplasia was seen in the upper hip of 19 of the children (Heikkilä, Ryoppy, & Laihimo, 1985). It was hypothesized that the position of adduction and medial rotation of the upper hip reduced the remolding stimulus of the acetabulum.

The most common intervention for DDH in a neonate or an infant is the **Pavlik harness,** shown in Figure 5–3. The harness maintains the hip in a position of flexion and abduction that can promote acetabular development while avoiding the subluxing positions of extension and adduction. The harness is preferable over casting because it allows spontaneous movement; however, hip spica casts are sometimes used if adequate containment cannot be achieved using the harness. The Pavlik harness has a success rate of approximately 95% for subluxed hips and 85% for dislocations if used correctly (Cashman, Round, Taylor, & Clarke, 2002). Although complications associated with the use of the Pavlik harness are infrequent, periodic monitoring of the hips is required to avoid avascular necrosis, femoral

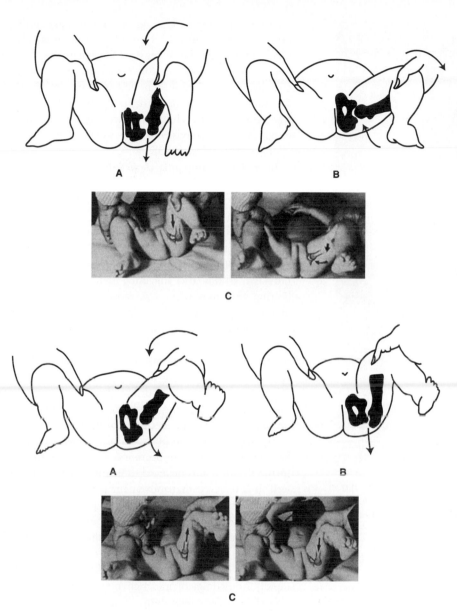

Figure 5-1 Ortolani sign for suspected developmental dysplasia of the hip. *(A)* Start with the hip in flexion and adduction. *(B)* Gently distract and abduct the hip to feel a reduction. *(A* and *B* from Wenger, D.R, & Rang, M.C. (1993). *The art and practice of children's orthopedics* [p. 265]. New York: Raven Press, with permission. *C* reprinted from *Advances in Neonatal Care, 3*(2), Witt, C., Detecting developmental dysplasia of the hip, pp. 65–75, copyright 2003, with permission from The National Association of Neonatal Nurses.)

Figure 5-2 Barlow maneuver for suspected developmental dysplasia of the hip. *(A)* Start with the hip in flexion and abduction. *(B)* Gently adduct and compress the hip to feel a subluxation. *(A* and *B* from Wenger, D.R., & Rang, M.C. (1993). *The art and practice of children's orthopedics* [p. 264]. New York: Raven Press, with permission. *C* reprinted from *Advances in Neonatal Care, 3*(2), Witt, C., Detecting developmental dysplasia of the hip, pp. 65–75, copyright 2003, with permission from The National Association of Neonatal Nurses.)

nerve palsy, or inferior dislocations. If the dysplastic hip is not detected in the neonatal or infancy period, the prognosis is less favorable. Infants older than 9 months may need to have a closed hip reduction and then be placed in a hip spica cast. Often the cast can be fabricated to allow weight bearing and ambulation. If the closed reduction is unsuccessful, an open reduction and containment may be warranted (Guille, Pizzutillo, & MacEwen, 2000). Surgical reduction may be preceded by 2 to 3 weeks of traction to avoid avascular necrosis (bone death caused by inadequate blood supply). Generally, home traction can be used to avoid a lengthy hospital stay (see Table 5.2).

The development of an upright posture and subsequent stress on the bones contributes to the normal postnatal developmental changes in bony alignment. If the normal developmental sequence of upright activities is absent, delayed, or performed in atypical ways, the stresses to the bone will be different and can lead to abnormal bone development. For example, the delayed developmental sequence and abnormal movement patterns seen in children with neurological impairment, such as occurs with CP or spina bifida, contribute to differences in their bone development and alignment. Movement and posture also influence bone changes in children with arthritis. Mechanical factors such as malalignment, rather than inflammation, have been

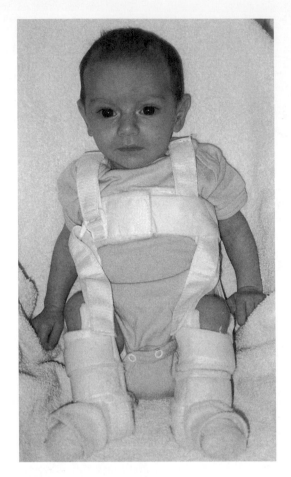

Figure 5-3 Pavlik harness is used to maintain the hip in flexion and abduction to promote acetabular development and prevent hip subluxation in infants with developmental hip dysplasia.

identified as the major destructive factor in degenerative arthritis (Radin et al., 1991). Malalignment alters the stress distribution across the joints of the lower extremity, especially the knee. Lower-extremity rotation abnormalities are common in ambulatory children with JRA or CP and dramatically increase the force across the knee (Tetsworth & Paley, 1994).

Conversely, if the limb is not used and subjected to the normal stresses of activity, it also does not develop properly. Nonuse can delay the appearance of secondary ossification centers or cause the bone to resorb. Therefore, children with significant movement impairments, such as those seen with severe CP, spina bifida, or arthrogryposis multiplex congenita, are at greater risk for fractures as a result of disuse atrophy, which can lead to demineralization of the bones.

Fortunately, bone mineral density in children can be increased with impact-loading exercise such as running and jumping. A group of typically developing children increased their hip-bone density by participating in a high-impact exercise program for 7 months and retained the increases after a 7-month period without exercise (Fuchs & Snow, 2002). Improvements in bone mineralization were not seen in children who participated in non–weight-bearing exercise such as swimming (Grimston, Willows, & Hanley, 1993).

Intervention programs to promote weight bearing has also been shown to increase bone mineral density and promote hip modeling in children with CP. These children were able to increase bone density by participating in 60 minutes of lower-extremity weight bearing 3 or more days per week (Stuberg, 1992). The benefits were not maintained when only 30 minutes of weight bearing was provided. It was also suggested that intermittent weight bearing with movement was most beneficial to hip joint modeling (Stuberg, 1992). Intermittent weight bearing with movement can be accomplished by partial weight-bearing ambulation through the use of a treadmill or gait trainer. Also, selecting an upright standing frame that allows some weight shifting would provide movement. Weight bearing is an important part of physical therapy intervention in young children with neuromuscular diseases that delay the development of stance.

Similar to its role in postnatal hip modeling, movement has been shown to be important for prenatal joint development in birds and is believed to be important in humans as well. It is believed that movement is more important than other mechanical factors, such as pressure, in forming initial prenatal joints. Inadequate in utero movement may impede the initial breakdown of the mesenchyme that forms the precursor to the joint space (Murray & Drachman 1969). The formation of human joints proceeds rapidly from onset of mesenchymal breakdown to formation of a structure resembling an adult joint. The process is generally completed within a 4- to 7-week period. This rapid progress is beneficial to the fetus as the joints are most susceptible to deformation from teratogens during this period (Walker, 1991). Arthrogryposis multiplex congenita is one disease in which a lack of movement may contribute to the deformation.

Arthrogryposis multiplex congenita is distinguished at birth by the presence of multiple congenital contractures (Table 5.3). In 90% of the cases, all four extremities are involved (Palmer, MacEwen, Bowen, & Mathews, 1985). Arthrogryposis is nonprogressive, but the child's functional abilities may change as the child grows. Despite the wide range of impairments that can accompany arthrogryposis, intelligence is not affected; therefore the children are adept at learning movement compensations or use of adaptive equipment. The prognosis of children with arthrogryposis is positive but depends on many factors, including severity of the disease, intelligence, and family support. In a study of 38 children with arthrogryposis, 85% were ambulatory by age 5 years and could complete all or most of their ADLs independently (Sells, Jaffe, & Hall, 1996).

An early, consistent physical therapy program can help promote a positive outcome for children with arthrogryposis. ROM is an integral intervention in arthrogryposis and should be initiated in the neonatal period (Palmer et al., 1985). The contractures are not inherently painful and present with a firm end feel. The chronic nature of arthrogryposis also makes a home-implemented program of ROM essential. The caregiver and the child should be instructed in methods to incorporate ROM exercises into the child's daily routine to optimize compliance. In addition to ROM exercises, more aggressive muscle-lengthening techniques are frequently used, including stretching, splinting, and casting. Night splints and periods of prone lying can provide a means to increase the amount of time the muscle spends in a lengthened state. Surgical methods may also be used to release contractures, improve bony alignment, or enhance function through tendon transfers.

The congenital deformities present in arthrogryposis can impede early movement. This can lead to weakness and delayed motor skill acquisition. Motor delay can, in turn, lead to more weakness. For this reason, early intervention should include developmental stimulation in addition to ROM. As soon as the child is able, strengthening and fitness programs should be encouraged as lifelong goals.

Mechanical stress associated with obesity can also be deforming to immature bones. **Tibia vara** or **Blount disease** is a progressive deformity resulting from abnormal growth slowing at the medial aspect of the proximal tibia (see Table 5.3). Blount disease can have an infantile or juvenile onset. Obese children who walk before 1 year of age are most likely to have the infantile type. Children normally have some degree of bowlegs until age 2 years; however, if it persists beyond 3 years of age, Blount disease should be considered (Do, 2001). Late-onset Blount disease is most common in obese African-American teenagers (Henderson, Kemp, & Hayes, 1993). A knee-ankle-foot orthosis worn during ambulation can be prescribed to attempt correction of the angulation in children under the age of 3 years (Do, 2001). For older children, surgical correction through a tibial osteotomy or external fixation can be performed to correct the deformity (Laville, Chau, Willemen, Kohler, & Garin, 1999).

Legg-Calvé-Perthes syndrome is a bone abnormality that affects a child's hips. The proximal femur receives its blood supply from three sources: the extracapsular arterial ring made up of the medial and lateral femoral circumflex vessels, the ascending cervical vessels, and the vessel of the ligamentum teres. Interruption of the blood flow from the medial femoral circumflex artery is suspected to lead to aseptic avascular necrosis and to Legg-Calvé-Perthes syndrome (Weinstein, 1996). The onset of Legg-Calvé-Perthes syndrome is generally between the ages of 4 and 8 years, and boys are affected 4 times more often than girls (Barker & Hall, 1986). Children with Legg-Calvé-Perthes generally present with a limp of insidious onset but may not complain of much pain unless prompted (Weinstein, 1996). The pain is usually aggravated by activity and relieved by rest and may be referred to the anteromedial thigh or knee. Parents may initially dismiss the child's complaints because of the inconsistent presentation of pain.

Intervention options for Legg-Calvé-Perthes disease include observation only, ROM exercises, bilateral long leg casts with a fixed abduction bar called Petrie casts, braces, and surgery. The goal of intervention is to optimize containment of the femoral head within the acetabulum. Hip abduction puts the head of the femur deepest into the acetabulum, thus preventing further flattening of the femoral head and encouraging remodeling back into a spherical shape. The necrotic tissue is gradually replaced with new bone, and the compression encourages congruent shaping. An irregularly shaped femoral head can lead to long-term degenerative changes such as osteoarthritis. The best prognostic indicator of lifelong hip health is the shape of the femoral head at skeletal maturity (Lecuire, 2002). Normal or flattened heads present few problems. Irregularly shaped heads are chronic sources of problems (Lecuire, 2002).

The surgical treatment for Legg-Calvé-Perthes disease is a proximal varus derotational osteotomy of the femur to reposition the femoral head securely in the acetabulum. A pelvic osteotomy might also be used, alone or in conjunction with the femoral procedure, to deepen the acetabulum and optimize the position of the femoral head. Consensus on the best treatment, or even if treatment is needed, has not been reached. One study indicated that, regardless of ages of onset and method of treatment, those with mild disease improved (Grasemann, Nicolai, Patalis, & Hovel, 1997). Optimal treatment for children with more severe disease was dependent on the age of onset. Children who were younger than 8 years at onset improved with conservative treatment, whereas children who were older than 8 years at onset improved more satisfactorily with surgery (Grasemann et al., 1997).

Another study looked at 197 hips and found no outcome difference between bed rest with traction, Petrie cast,

Table 5.3 Bony Disorders

Diagnosis	Etiology	Pathology	Impairments of Body Functions and Structures	Potential Activity Limitations and Participation Restrictions	Potential Interventions
Arthrogryposis multiplex congenita	• Unclear • Congenital disorder • Suspect teratogens • Lack of in utero movements may contribute • In utero muscular atrophy caused by muscle disease, virus, or maternal fever • Insufficient room caused by lack of amniotic fluid or abnormally shaped uterus	• Deficit in the motor unit leads to severe fetal weakness • Fetal immobility leads to hypoplastic joint development and contractures	• Characteristic contractures: shoulder adduction and internal rotation, elbow extension, wrist flexion and ulnar deviation, finger flexion, thumb in palm, hip flexion, abduction and external rotation, knee extension, clubfeet • Hip dislocation/subluxation • Jaw and tongue ROM limitations • Limbs appear tubular and lack normal joint creases • Diminished muscle mass and strength • Atypical fibrotic and lipid deposits • Fewer anterior horn cells in spinal cord	• Mobility difficulties • Diminished ADL skills such as dressing • Poor grasp and handwriting • Feeding or speech difficulties	• Child and family education • ROM program • Strengthening and fitness programs • Splinting • Developmental stimulation • Functional skills training • Mobility aids and assistive device selection
Blount disease (Tibia vara)	Two onset patterns • Infantile: obese children who walked before 1 year of age • Juvenile: most common in obese African-American teenagers	Compression of medial portion of proximal tibial physes that inhibits normal endochondral growth	• Lateral bowing of the tibia • Medial knee instability	• Pain • Knee instability may limit physical activities • Progressive joint degeneration • Cosmesis	• Postsurgical ambulation training • Splinting as needed

Diagnosis	Etiology	Pathology	Impairments of Body Functions and Structures	Potential Activity Limitations and Participation Restrictions	Potential Interventions
Legg-Calvé-Perthes disease	• Unclear • Current theory: vascular disruption leading to aseptic necrosis (Weinstein, 1996) • Numerous associated factors include later birth order, abnormal birth presentation, increasing parental age, attention deficit hyperactivity disorder • Higher incidence in lower socioeconomic, urban areas leads to hypothesis of nutritional deficit	• Unclear • Systemic component suspected because epiphyseal changes have been noted in the nonproblematic joints; blood content abnormalities	• Limp caused by pain or weak abductor muscles • Frequently positive Trendelenburg sign • Limited ROM in hip abduction and internal rotation • Pain in hip or groin with activity • May be referred knee pain	• Pain can limit play and ADLs • Limp	• Child and family education • ROM program • Ambulation training following casting or surgery • Positioning devices
Slipped capital femoral epiphysis	• Unclear • 2.5:1 male-to-female ratio • Higher incidence in African-Americans • Local trauma associated with about 25% of cases • Decreased anteversion • Inflammation may weaken physeal plate • Endocrine imbalance • Delayed skeletal maturity • Obesity • Hormone levels; generally prepubescent onset (ages 10–15 years) • Hereditary contribution	Posterior displacement of the capital femoral epiphysis from femoral neck through a weakened physis	• Antalgic limp • Pain in groin or referred to anteromedial thigh and knee • External rotation posturing • Decreased hip flexion, abduction, and internal rotation • Leg moves into external rotation when flexed	• Pain may limit activities • Long-term degenerative changes	• Child and family education • ROM program • Positioning program • Postsurgical ambulation training
Scurvy	Dietary insufficiency of vitamin C (ascorbic acid)	• Decreased thickness of bone cortex and epiphyseal plates • Decreased bone available for calcification	Fragile bones predisposed to fractures	Propensity for fractures limits play	• Child and family education • Developmental stimulation/weight bearing • Splinting

(Continued)

Table 5.3 Bony Disorders *(Continued)*

Diagnosis	Etiology	Pathology	Impairments of Body Functions and Structures	Potential Activity Limitations and Participation Restrictions	Potential Interventions
Rickets	Deficiency of vitamin D/lack of exposure to sunlight (Sunlight converts body substance into vitamin D)	Deficiency interferes with bone calcification	Long bones bend under body weight resulting in abnormalities such as genu varum or valgum	• Cosmesis • May interfere with play and ADLs	• Child and family education • Developmental stimulation/weight bearing • Splinting
Osteogenesis Imperfecta (Zeitlin, Fassier, & Glorieux, 2003)	• Dominant heritable genetic disorder • Spontaneous genetic mutation	• Collagen mutation resulting in fragile bones • Increased bone turnover • Sequelae include short stature, scoliosis, poor tooth formation, deafness, blue sclera, translucent skin, osteoporosis, and ligamentous laxity	• Propensity for fractures and deformities • Severe scoliosis may impair cardiorespiratory status	• Fragility interferes with play and ADLs • Deformities may diminish ADL skills and mobility	• Child and family education • ROM program • Strengthening and fitness programs • Developmental stimulation • Functional training • Behavioral modification to reduce injury • Splinting and ambulation aid selection

abduction brace, or pelvic or femoral osteotomy (Grzegorzewski, Bowen, Guille, & Glutting, 2003). This same study reported that between 60% and 70% of the hips had a satisfactory spherical shape after treatment (Grzegorzewski et al., 2003).

Nutritional and metabolic factors can also influence bone development. Although not commonly seen in the United States today as a result of improved knowledge and dietary supplements, both **scurvy** and **rickets** are diseases caused by dietary insufficiency that can lead to bone abnormalities (see Table 5.3).

Osteogenesis imperfecta is a generic collagen mutation that also manifests with fragile bones (see Table 5.3). Multiple fractures at birth are seen in severe forms of the disease. Mild forms of osteogenesis imperfecta, however, may not be detected until later childhood or even adulthood. The milder presentations may be noticed after the child begins walking and presents to the emergency room with a fracture resulting from a nonsignificant injury. Milder presentations of osteogenesis imperfecta may need to be distinguished from multiple fractures sustained through child abuse (Zaleske, 1996).

The physical therapist plays an important role in the management of children with osteogenesis imperfecta. Child and caregiver information is necessary to minimize recurrent fractures. Although rough-house play and contact sports should be avoided, an aggressive yet safe exercise and standing program will help the child develop strength and endurance, maintain or increase ROM, and promote mineralization through weight bearing. In addition, the physical therapist provides consultation for bracing and adaptive equipment selection. Developmental stimulation may also be needed if the neonate had fractures because early immobilization may lead to weakness and delayed skill acquisition.

Growing bones also present special considerations for fractures. Although bone can generally repair itself without complications if the fractured pieces are approximated, an **epiphyseal fracture** can cause arrested bone growth. Although the epiphysis is the weakest area of an immature bone, this type of injury accounts for only about 20% of pediatric fractures, with boys in the early adolescent period being the most likely to sustain an epiphyseal fracture (Mahabir, Kazemi, Cannon, & Courtemanche, 2001). If the fracture is contained with the epiphysis, healing is generally good. If the fracture extends through the epiphyseal border, growth arrest can occur completely or asymmetrically (Wattenbarger, Gruber, & Phieffer, 2002). A complete arrest can lead to a significant limb length inequality, and asymmetrical arrest may result in angular deformities because one portion of the bone continues growing. The extent of the abnormality that develops depends on the type of fracture, age of the child, and stage of skeletal maturity (Figure 5–4).

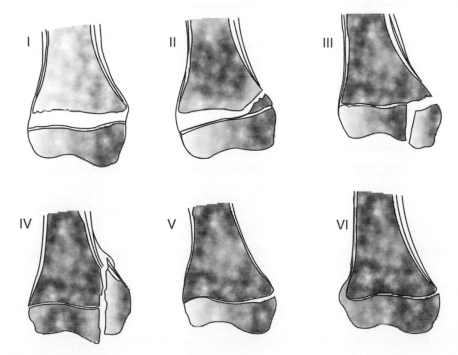

Figure 5-4 Types of epiphyseal fractures. *(I)* Transverse epiphyseal plate injury with separation of entire epiphysis. *(II)* Epiphyseal plate injury with fracture and separation of the metaphysis. *(III)* Epiphyseal plate injury with fracture of part of the epiphysis. *(IV)* Vertical; splitting of the epiphysis and epiphyseal plate. *(V)* Crushing injury to epiphyseal plate. *(VI)* Injury to peripheral perichondrial ring (not shown). (From Salter, R.B. (1999). *Textbook of disorders and injuries of the musculoskeletal system* [3rd ed., pp. 506–507]. Baltimore: Williams & Wilkins, with permission.)

Acquired Limb Length Discrepancy

Epiphyseal fractures are a potential cause of **acquired limb length discrepancy**. There are three general classifications of limb length discrepancy causes: direct, indirect though growth retardation, and indirect through growth stimulation. A direct discrepancy occurs when overriding segments of a fracture are not resolved. There are several mechanisms for growth stimulation or retardation (Table 5.4).

In addition to true bone length discrepancies, the examiner must consider "apparent" limb length discrepancies, which can be caused by many factors, including joint contractures, angular deformities, hip subluxation or dislocation, pelvic obliquity, or spinal alignment. A limb length examination, therefore, must incorporate examination of the muscle length, the joints above and below the bone in question, and the child's posture.

Intervention for limb length discrepancies is based on numerous factors, including the preferences of the child and family, age of the child, skeletal maturity, and neuromuscular status. The age and skeletal maturity of the child are important considerations because growth makes a limb length inequality a progressive problem. The plan must be tailored to achieve symmetry when the child is finished growing, and therefore is planned based on the expected discrepancy.

The first step in planning limb length correction is to analyze past growth of both limbs. The second step involves prediction of future growth, including the projected discrepancy. Predicting future growth involves determining a child's skeletal maturity level. Age is only a general indicator of skeletal maturity or growth. Skeletal maturity is determined by comparing a radiograph of the left hand and wrist with standards in either the *Greulich-Pyle Atlas* (Greulich & Pyle 1959) or the *Tanner-Whitehouse Atlas* (Tanner & Buckler, 1997). Estimating skeletal maturity

Table 5.4 Causes of Indirect Limb Length Discrepancy

Classification	By Growth Retardation	By Growth Stimulation
Congenital	• Congenital hemiatrophy • Developmental hip dysplasia • Clubfoot	• Syndromes associated with partial giantism such as Klippel-Trenaunay, Parkes-Weber • Hemophilia-induced hemarthrosis
Infection/ inflammation	Epiphyseal plate destruction caused by osteomyelitis, tuberculosis, or septic arthritis	• Increased blood flow associated with diaphyseal osteomyelitis, juvenile rheumatoid arthritis (particularly in children under age 3), and in chronic knee synovitis seen in children with hemophilia, may cause overgrowth • Metaphyseal tuberculosis • Septic arthritis
Mechanical	Long-term weight-relieving immobilization	Traumatic arteriovenous aneurysms
Neurological	Paralysis or movement dysfunction such as poliomyelitis, spina bifida, or cerebral palsy	
Trauma	• Damage to epiphyseal plate • Marked overriding of diaphyseal fragments • Severe burns	• Femur or tibia fractures can lead to osteosynthesis, particularly in young children • Diaphyseal operations; bone graft removal, osteotomy
Tumors	• Tumor may invade growth plate • Irradiation may damage growth plate • Tumor may originate in cartilage cells; Ollier disease, or enchondromatosis	• Tumors may cause vascular malformations and stimulate growth through excessive circulation; hemangiomatosis, Klippel-Trenaunay-Weber syndrome • Stimulation in nonvascular tumors; neurofibromatosis, Wilms' tumor
Others	• Legg-Calvé-Perthes disease • Slipped capital femoral epiphysis	

Source: Adapted from Moseley, C.F. (1996). Leg length discrepancy and angular deformity of the lower limbs. In R.T. Morrissy & S.L. Weinstein (Eds.), *Lovell & Winter's pediatric orthopedics* (4th ed.) (pp. 849–901). Philadelphia: Lippincott-Raven.

requires some subjective interpretation and is therefore susceptible to error, which contributes to the difficulty in accurately treating an inequality in leg length.

The last step is to estimate the effects of the planned corrective surgery. Longitudinal data will improve the accuracy of the estimation. Generally, children are followed for a minimum of 1 to 2 years before any decisions are made. Longer periods of monitoring will help minimize error.

The most obvious sequela of a moderate to severe limb length discrepancy is cosmesis. Activity limitations, pain, and secondary degenerative changes may also be present. The child will need to make gait pattern changes to accommodate the inequality that can result in secondary impairments. For example, if the child toe-walks on the short side, dorsiflexion ROM will be lost. In addition, the altered gait pattern may put atypical stress on the knees or back, resulting in pain or long-term degenerative changes. Even mild leg length discrepancies can increase energy expenditure, and a discrepancy as small as 1 cm alters the degree of postural sway (Mahar, Kirby, & MacLeod, 1985; Moseley, 1991). In the upper extremity, moderate or severe limb length discrepancies can interfere with bimanual activities.

There are general guidelines for the treatment of leg length inequality based on the magnitude of the discrepancy (Box 5.1). Treatment of a leg length inequality must also take into account many factors, including the child's general health, motivation, compliance, family support, intelligence, and emotional stability and the presence of additional pathology.

Shortening of the longer limb is generally accomplished through a timed epiphyseodesis. Growth can be slowed in the longer leg by surgically destroying the growth plate in the distal femur, proximal tibia/fibula, or both. An epiphyseodesis completely stops the growth at the epiphysis but only slows the growth of the leg because of the contributions of the other growth plates in the leg. The shorter leg continues to grow at its normal rate until it reaches skeletal maturity.

An epiphyseodesis shortens the longer leg. The shorter leg can also be lengthened, either alone or in combination with shortening of the opposite leg, and therefore can equalize greater discrepancies than epiphyseodesis alone. Leg lengthening, however, can be an expensive, prolonged process with risks of serious complications, including infection, malunion, scarring, and decreased bone strength. The procedure involves performing an osteotomy and then applying a device to distract the bone while providing external stability. Monolateral and circumferential devices are two main types of devices that can be used to distract the leg, provide stability, and correct angular deformities (Figures 5–5 and 5–6).

Regardless of the type of device, physical therapy is critical to ensure a functional outcome. Intervention goals include performing and instructing the family in pin site wound care to prevent infection, ROM, strengthening, and progressive ambulation.

ROM limitations can develop quickly during leg-lengthening procedures for several reasons. Initially, pain

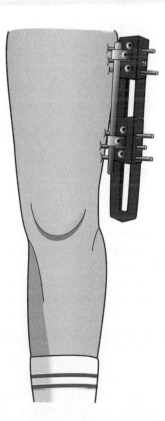

Figure 5-5 A monolateral lengthening device.

> **BOX 5.1** Leg Length Inequality General Treatment Guidelines
>
> - 0–2 cm: No treatment
> - 2–4 cm: Shoe lift
> - 2–6 cm: Epiphysiodesis, shortening
> - 6–20 cm: Lengthening that may or may not be combined with other procedures
> - >20 cm: Prosthetic fitting

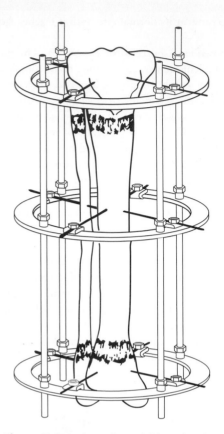

Figure 5-6 A circumferential lengthening device.

and anxiety associated with the surgery limit movement. In addition, the pins or wires that attach the fixator go through the muscle and can cause pain or physically limit movement. Finally, as the bone is lengthened, the muscles must also stretch to accommodate the new distance. ROM is commonly lost in hip extension, knee flexion and extension, and ankle dorsiflexion. Knee flexion limitations tend to resolve over time when the device is removed; however, knee extension deficits have been associated with more chronic limitations in activities (Moseley, 1991). The therapist should carefully monitor all joint motion because the type of apparatus, previous deformity, and the child's activities can all contribute to ROM complications.

Children who undergo leg lengthening are encouraged to be active. Typically, the child is encouraged to ambulate with weight bearing as tolerated. This promotes ROM, strength, and bone consolidation, as well as helping with the psychosocial aspects of the extended intervention. Temporary lifts for the child's short leg may need to be fabricated to allow weight bearing as the limb length changes.

Conditions Affecting Muscle

Muscle composition, including fiber type and size, fatty tissue, and connective tissue, influences muscle performance. Type I muscles perform sustained work, whereas type II muscles provide quick bursts of power.

Histological changes in muscle structure are seen in the muscular dystrophies. **Duchenne's muscular dystrophy (DMD)** is the most common muscular dystrophy and is a fatal disease causing progressive weakness of the skeletal and respiratory muscles (Table 5.5). DMD is caused by an X-linked recessive defect on the Xp21 portion of the X chromosome. The gene encodes the production of a protein called dystrophin that is linked to muscle function (Thompson, 1996). With X-linked recessive disease, males have the disease, whereas females are carriers and can pass on the disease but do not have symptoms. In addition to muscle changes, genetic and blood composition abnormalities are present. Elevated levels of serum creatinine phosphokinase (CPK) assist in achieving a differential diagnosis. Genetic testing is also used for diagnosis. A case study describing the evaluation and intervention of a child with DMD is presented in Chapter 22.

Boys with DMD are generally clumsy, may walk on their toes, and show gross motor regression over time. Pseudohypertrophy (enlargement without increased strength) of the calf muscles is present as a result of the accumulation of fat in the muscle. This may give the appearance of a strong muscle, but examination will reveal a pattern of weakness that affects proximal musculature greater than distal musculature. To compensate for the proximal weakness, a boy may use the upper extremities to manually assist knee extension by "walking" his hands up his lower extremities when moving from the floor to standing. This is referred to as **Gowers' sign** (Figure 5–7).

The initial proximal muscular weakness seen in DMD also results in other atypical movement patterns that can lead to soft tissue contractures. Boys adopt a wide base of support to maximize balance and use biomechanical alignment to maintain an upright position with the least muscular effort. For example, knee hyperextension and an increased lumbar lordosis move the child's center of gravity in front of the knee joint to reduce the need for active muscle contraction. Toe-walking is used to take advantage of joint end range as a means of stability. These alignment changes lead to equinus contractures of the ankles, hip flexion contractures, and iliotibial band contracture. As the disease progresses, ambulation abilities are lost, and both hip and knee flexion contractures and progressive scoliosis are accelerated.

Table 5.5 Muscular Disorders

Diagnosis	Etiology	Pathology	Impairments of Body Functions and Structures	Potential Activity Limitations and Participation Restrictions	Potential Interventions
Duchenne's muscular dystrophy	• X-linked recessive trait • Defect on the Xp21 portion of the X chromosome	• Muscle composition abnormalities • Progressive degeneration of the muscle fibers • Variation in fiber size • Connective and adipose tissue deposits	• Progressive muscle weakness; proximal >distal plantar flexion, hip flexion, and iliotibial band contractures • Progressive scoliosis	• Fatal in adolescence or early adulthood • Motor skill regression • Loss of ambulation	• Child and family education • ROM program • Strengthening and fitness programs • Ambulation and mobility aids as disease progresses • Aggressive postoperative care • Respiratory exercises and secretion elimination techniques • Adaptive equipment to ease caregiving as limitations progress • Referral to support systems
Spinal muscular atrophy (Nicole, Diaz, Frugier, & Melki, 2002) (see Table 5.6)	Autosomal recessive defect of chromosome 5	Unclear Includes nonprogressive loss of anterior horn cells	Muscular weakness	Progressive difficulty with physical activities, eventually ending in death	• Child and family education • ROM program • Strengthening and fitness programs • Ambulation and mobility aids as limitations progress • Aggressive postoperative care • Respiratory exercises and secretion elimination techniques • Adaptive equipment to ease caregiving • Referral to support systems
Muscular torticollis (Davids, Wenger, & Mubarak, 1993)	• Current theory is intrauterine or perinatal compartment syndrome for congenital • Acquired is positional	• Unilateral contracture of the sternocleidomastoid muscle • May lead to plagiocephaly (head asymmetry) if untreated	• Head is tilted toward involved side and chin is rotated toward opposite side • Limited ROM in lateral flexion toward uninvolved side and rotation toward involved side • Skewed vertical and midline orientation	• Cosmesis • Distorted orientation may interfere with play • Limited ROM may impede dressing • Developmental delay	• Parent education • Stretching program • Positioning to encourage head turning and prone propping • Developmental stimulation • Environmental modification to encourage head turning • Referral for plagiocephaly treatment

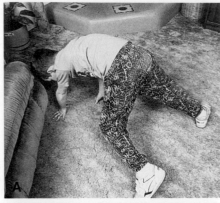

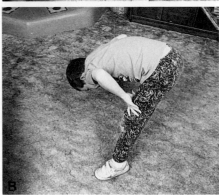

Figure 5-7 Gowers' sign used by children with muscular dystrophy to compensate for proximal weakness. (From Porr, S.M., & Rainville, E.B. [1999]. *Pediatric therapy: A systems approach.* Philadelphia: F.A. Davis, with permission. Photo courtesy of MDA, Tucson, AZ.)

Physical therapy intervention changes dramatically over the course of DMD because of the progressive, degenerative nature of the disease. Aggressive ROM early in the disease helps maintain optimal alignment so ambulation is efficient. Prolonged ambulation can help reduce further contractures, slow scoliosis, and promote cardiopulmonary fitness. Hip and knee flexion contractures are common but can be addressed through standing programs, prone lying, and night splints. Ankle-foot orthotics can aid in reducing plantar flexion contractures and provide stability as weakness progresses. End-stage ROM maintains sufficient flexibility to optimize caregiver handling and patient comfort. Despite ROM exercises, surgical intervention is also frequently needed (Biggar, Klamut, Demacio, Stevens, & Ray, (2002).

Aggressive postoperative physical therapy is important to minimize the debilitating effects of bed rest. Bedside ROM, strengthening, and spirometry may reduce rate of decline.

In addition, children with DMD are encouraged to resume ambulation quickly to avoid secondary complications, such as muscle atrophy or pneumonia. The progressive nature of DMD puts the child at increased risk for rapid decline with immobility.

Strengthening is also critical to optimizing the child's function. Strengthening should be started early in the disease process (Ansved, 2001; Fowler & Taylor, 1982; McCartney, Moroz, Garner, & McComas, 1988). To prevent overwork weakness, lower weights with more repetitions should be prescribed and the child closely monitored to avoid overfatigue (Ansved, 2001, Fowler & Taylor, 1982; McCartney et al., 1988). Strengthening of the respiratory muscles is also recommended and can be accomplished through the use of spirometers.

Equipment selection also helps prolong functional skills. Standing frames, orthotics, braces, and ambulation aids all help promote function. As the disease progresses, a wheelchair will be needed for mobility and positioning. In the final stages, equipment such as hospital beds and transfer lifts may be needed to aid in caregiving.

Spinal muscular atrophy (SMA) also manifests in muscular weakness. SMA consists of a group of disorders characterized by degeneration of the anterior horn cells of the spinal cord (Nicole, Diaz, Frugier, & Melki, 2002). The loss of anterior horn cells is not progressive, but the sequela of the disease process is progressive and fatal as the child outgrows the muscle's capacity. Some muscles are not involved; these include the diaphragm, sternothyroid, sternohyoid, and involuntary muscles of the intestine, bladder, and heart. Even though the primary muscles of respiration are spared, respiratory complications are still one of the main causes of death. Sensation and cognition are also not affected.

Three classifications of SMA are used; they reflect the severity, rate of decline, and age of onset of the disease (Nicole et al., 2002) (Table 5.6). Acute **Werdnig-Hoffman disease** (type 1) is the most severe form, with the earliest onset and most rapid death. The intermediate form of SMA is called Chronic Werdnig-Hoffman disease (type 2), and the form with the latest onset is Kugelberg-Welander disease (type 3). Clinical features of all three forms include limb and trunk weakness with muscle atrophy more pronounced proximally and in the lower extremities. Hypotonia and areflexia (absence of reflexes) are also present (Thompson, 1996). Orthopedic complications related to the muscle weakness include the development of soft tissue contractures, hip subluxation, and spinal deformity (Thompson, 1996) (see Table 5.5).

Table 5.6 Onset and Prognosis of Spinal Muscular Atrophy (SMA) Classifications

Type of SMA	Onset	Death	Motor Limits
1	0–6 mo	<2 yr	Does not sit
2	7–18 mo	>2 yr	Usually does not stand
3	>18 mo	Adult	Stands and walks alone

Congenital muscular torticollis is a nonprogressive unilateral contracture of the sternocleidomastoid muscle (see Table 5.5). Prognosis for correction with physical therapy is excellent if the intervention is initiated in the first 3 months of life and remains high if initiated in the first year of life (Cheng, Tang, Chen, Wong, & Wong, 2000; Demirbilek & Atayurt, 1999). Infants with mild contracture (<10°) respond well to active home exercises. This would include environmental changes, such as arranging the child's crib and changing table to promote turning the head to look at caregivers, and stimulating active head turning in response to toys or sounds. Towel rolls or small soft collars can be used to prevent the child's head from falling passively into the shortened direction. Encouraging symmetrical head lifting from a prone position can also stretch and strengthen muscles. This can be accomplished by placing the infant prone on the elbows over a small towel roll on the caregiver's chest and encouraging the infant to look up at the caregiver.

For children with more severe contracture, controlled manual stretching is added to ensure a good outcome (Cheng et al., 2001). The sternocleidomastoid muscle performs both lateral flexion toward the same side and rotation toward the opposite side. Stretching should be performed when the child is relaxed. Toys, sounds, music, or pictures can be used to distract the child. Stretching can be performed in two parts. For lateral flexion, stabilization is provided over the shoulder girdle to prevent elevation. Using an open flat hand and avoiding the ear, the caregiver moves the head into opposite side lateral flexion. For rotation, stabilization is moved anteriorly to prevent both elevation and protraction of the shoulder. Again using an open flat hand and avoiding the child's ear, the head is turned toward the involved muscle. Even with the addition of a stretching program, a small percentage of children (5%) will require surgical intervention, especially if physical therapy is not initiated early.

In addition to assessing ROM, the shape of the head, cervical vertebrae, and symmetry of facial features should be noted (Raco et al., 1999). Plagiocephaly (misshapen head) can be present at birth or may develop in response to untreated torticollis. Plagiocephaly may require the use of a custom-fitting helmet or surgical correction and should be evaluated by a physician (Raco et al., 1999).

Cerebral Palsy

Although CP is primarily seen as a neurological impairment, as discussed in Chapter 6, it is also accompanied by characteristic musculoskeletal impairments of varying severity. Children with CP can have bony deformities and muscle composition abnormalities. Individual muscle histology study results vary, but it is agreed that muscles of children with CP show more variability in the size of the muscle fibers, atrophy of fibers, and an increase in fatty and connective tissue deposits in the muscle (Castle, Reyman, & Schneider, 1979; Ito et al., 1996; Rose et al., 1994). Frequently, there is also a reversal in the expected fiber-type compositions. For example, Rose and colleagues (1994) found that in children with CP, the gastrocnemius did not have the usually higher ratio of type 2, fast-twitch, fibers but had more type 1, slow-twitch, fibers.

Research needs to be conducted to determine whether the fiber-type changes are present at birth and may be contributing to the abnormal movement patterns or whether the fiber types change over time as a result of demands placed by abnormal movement patterns. Additional information is necessary before clinical conclusions can be drawn from biopsy information; however, it is believed that this information will someday help direct specific strengthening and exercise programs for children with CP, designed to optimize muscle composition and force-generation capabilities.

The characteristic musculoskeletal abnormalities of CP will be presented for each body segment. For information on the neurological sequelae of CP, refer to Chapter 6.

Spine

Children with CP are more likely to develop scoliosis or other curvatures of the spine, such as a thoracic kyphosis. The overall incidence of scoliosis in children with CP is about 25%, but increases with increased severity (Renshaw,

Green, Griffin, & Root, 1996). The lack of stability combined with a decreased amount of movement places the child's spine in atypical postures for prolonged periods of time. Over time, this can result in either a flexible or fixed deformity. Additional contributing factors to spinal deformity can be atypical muscle pull or muscle imbalances. Finally, leg length inequality, which is frequently seen in children with hemiplegic CP, will disrupt pelvic symmetry and the spine compensates with a scoliosis.

Pelvis and Hip

Problems in the pelvis and hip occur in bone alignment and shape and in muscle length and function. The distribution of hypertonicity commonly seen in children with spastic types of CP can lead to poor posture and bone alignment. Limitations in ROM of the muscles around the hip are seen in the hip flexors, hamstrings, and adductors. The quadriceps may also have limited range in some children. A generalized decreased ability to generate force is also present, despite the false appearance of strength seen in muscles with hypertonicity. The pull on the pelvis from these muscular imbalances can result in pelvic alignment problems.

Pelvic alignment abnormalities include obliquity and posterior or anterior tilts. As mentioned previously, pelvic obliquity is most often associated with leg length discrepancy. A posterior pelvic tilt is typically attributable to limited hamstring range. The hamstrings are a two-joint muscle crossing both the hip and knee joints. In sitting, especially if the knees are extended, the hamstrings do not have sufficient range to accommodate a neutral pelvis. The pelvis rotates in a posterior direction to reduce the stretch on the hamstrings and the child will sit with the knees flexed, the pelvis rotated posteriorly, and the back rounded. Another way to reduce the pull on the hamstrings is to sit in a position called a **"W" sit position** (Figure 5–8). The child flexes both the hips and the knees and, in doing so, has placed the short hamstrings on slack. In standing position, hip flexor tightness will frequently pull the pelvis into an anterior pelvic tilt. If the hamstring length is significantly limited, the child will bend his or her knees to reduce the strain caused by the anterior pelvic tilt.

Another common problem in children with CP is **hip subluxation** or **dislocation**. Both bony and muscular factors contribute to hip instability. Neonates are born with a shallow acetabulum, flat femoral head, high femoral neck-shaft angle, and femoral antetorsion, all of which contribute to hip instability. In children who are developing typically, bony remodeling to deepen the acetabulum, make the femoral head more spherical, reduce anteversion, and decrease the femoral neck-shaft inclination occurs

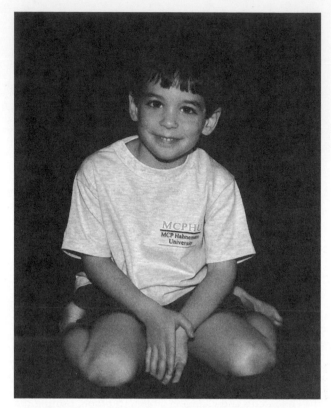

Figure 5-8 "W" sitting. The knees are flexed and the hips are flexed and internally rotated. Children with hip antetorsion, limited hamstring length, and/or limited hip external rotation use this position.

naturally through weight bearing and the normal pull of muscles. However, children with CP have delayed motor milestones; therefore they are not putting the normal weight-bearing forces through the joint at an early age.

The instability of the hip is compound by ROM limitations and atypical muscular pull/spasticity. Adequate ROM allows the hip to move into a stable well-covered position in the acetabulum. Children with CP tend to lose abduction range and develop hip flexion contractures, both of which are detrimental to hip stability. Critical ROM values for hip stability include maintaining at least 30° of abduction and avoiding a hip flexion contracture of 20° to 25° or more (Renshaw et al., 1996).

Foot and Ankle

The most common impairment of the foot and ankle is reduced dorsiflexion ROM attributable to a shortened gastrocnemius. Hypertonicity of the gastrocnemius, combined with an inability to generate sufficient stability around the ankle, results in the child assuming a plantar flexed position during weight bearing. Over time, this can result in severe limitations in dorsiflexion ROM. This will limit the child's ability to fit into orthotics or shoes and significantly reduces his or her base of support in standing.

The inability to maintain a stable foot also contributes to a breakdown of the longitudinal arch, resulting in an **equinovalgus** or "flatfoot" position. This further impairs the child's ability to perform balance reactions with the feet. Orthotics are used to control the plantar flexion as well as to maintain the longitudinal arch. When the child has reached skeletal maturity, a subtalar or triple arthrodesis procedure can be performed for a permanent correction. In a triple arthrodesis, the orthopedic surgeon will fuse the talocalcaneal, talonavicular, and calcaneocuboid joints, resulting in a rigid foot that is in a more anatomically correct position.

Posture

The musculoskeletal and neurological impairments seen in children with spastic CP culminate in characteristic postures. In standing, young children tend to stand on their toes with their knees extended, hips adducted and internally rotated, and the pelvis in an anterior tilt. As the child gets larger, the weight of the body, inadequate muscle power, and surgical lengthening of the muscles can result in the crouched posture of ankle dorsiflexion and knee flexion. The hips will generally remain in adduction, flexion, and internal rotation.

The hamstrings are one of the major influences in sitting posture of children with spastic CP. The limited range makes long sitting virtually impossible. When the child attempts this position, the knees are kept in partial flexion, and the pelvis rotates posteriorly to accommodate the shortened hamstrings. The pelvic tilt, in turn, results in compensating postures in the spine. The lumbar and thoracic spine is in a compensatory kyphotic position, and the child hyperextends the neck to maintain the head in a neutral position.

Intervention

CP is a complex manifestation of a brain injury resulting in a varied combination of impairments in body structures and functions and limitations in activities and participation. For a review of intervention options, refer also to Chapter 7 on neurological impairment. The interventions of the musculoskeletal manifestations are addressed in this chapter.

In children with CP, maintaining or increasing ROM is a high priority. ROM deficits change the normal skeletal alignment and often decrease fluency of movement. Stretching before and after exercise is a good way to warm up and may prevent injury in children with or without a disability. Unfortunately, simple ROM exercises are unlikely to remediate or prevent progressive contractures (Tardieu, Lespargot, Tabary, & Bret, 1988). The muscle needs to be in an elongated state for 6 hours or more to maintain range (Lespargot, Renaudin, Khouri, & Robert, 1994; Tardieu et al., 1988). Clearly, this cannot be done by a parental program of passive ROM. In a small study of adults with CP, passive ROM exercises had no effect on improving lower extremity ROM (Cadenhead, McEwen, & Thompson, 2002). If the child is not using the range during ADLs, splinting should be considered. Resting night splints can provide the required time without interfering with muscle exercise during the day. In addition, periods of prone lying while watching television, playing, reading, or sleeping can assist in maintaining hip extension. The decision to use braces, such as AFO (ankle-foot orthosis), should be carefully evaluated. The brace can help reduce gastrocnemius and soleus shortening and may provide a stable base of support, but it prevents the child from using ankle movements as a balance strategy and may lead to disuse atrophy. It is recommended that the child continue to spend time without the braces to determine if the braces are indeed beneficial (Kott & Held, 2003), to allow for continued unrestricted motor learning, and to promote ankle strength. If braces or splints are needed during the day, it is imperative that the problem of disuse atrophy be considered and a strengthening program be included in the child's intervention plan.

If ROM and splinting are not successful, the child may need tendon lengthening or transfers. A tendon lengthening is a surgical procedure that uses a cut in the tendon to allow it to elongate. Frequently several tendons are lengthened during the same procedure. The gastrocnemius, hamstrings, and hip adductors are the most commonly lengthened. A tendon transfer moves the tendon to a new attachment on the bone, allowing a more relaxed position, and may encourage a more efficient pull of the muscle. Selective dorsal rhizotomy and botulin are other methods of increasing ROM discussed in Chapter 7.

Children with CP also have a decreased ability to generate **force**. Despite the histological abnormalities seen in the muscles of children with CP, increases in the ability to generate force have been achieved through traditional strengthening protocols (Damiano, Kelly, & Vaugh, 1995) The child's ability to generate force has a strong relationship to both balance and functional skills; therefore, strengthening is an integral component of a comprehensive intervention program (Damiano & Abel, 1998; Lowes, Westcott, Palisano, Effgen, & Orlin, 2004). In general, an initial program of high repetitions with lower weights is advocated to minimize potential injury (American Academy of Pediatrics, 2001).

Down Syndrome

Children with Down syndrome have the potential for a number of health problems, such as cardiac, audiological, endocrine, developmental, dental, and other problems (Roizen, 2001). Growth deficiencies may also be present, along with the tendency for being overweight (Rubin, Rimmer, Chicoine, Braddock, & McGuire, 1998). People with Down syndrome often have low muscle tone (hypotonia) and lax ligaments, which may account for some of the orthopedic abnormalities (Roizen, 2001).

Children with Down syndrome may have a number of musculoskeletal disorders, such as hip dislocation (Greene, 1998), patellofemoral disorders, gait abnormalities such as a wide-based gait and external hip rotation (Shaw & Beals, 1992), mild scoliosis, pes planus, and rearfoot valgus. The most common orthopedic problem for children with Down syndrome, however, is a flexible flatfoot, or **pes planus** (Caselli, Sobel-Cohen, Thompson, Adler, & Gonzalez, 1991). Rigid flatfoot, or **pes valgus,** caused by a medially tilted superior aspect of the talus, may also be seen but is less common. There is little evidence of efficacy of orthoses in pes planus, although some authors suggest the use of straight-laced shoes and orthoses to improve and maintain skeletal alignment to assist with function (Caselli et al.,

1991). A recent study of the use of neutral position orthoses for children with Down syndrome demonstrated decreased rearfoot eversion when the children wore the orthoses. In addition, when they walked with orthoses, compared with walking without them, their angle of gait decreased, indicating more internal rotation, thus decreasing the more typical posture of hip external rotation common in children with Down syndrome (Selby-Silverstein, Hillstrom, & Palisano, 2001).

Another orthopedic anomaly of particular concern is **atlantoaxial instability.** This term describes an abnormally large space and excessive motion between the first and second cervical vertebrae, thought to be caused by ligamentous laxity, bony abnormalities, trauma, and upper respiratory infections (Gajdosik & Ostertag, 1996). Atlantoaxial instability exists in approximately 15% of all individuals with Down syndrome (Committee on Sports Medicine and Fitness, 1995). Most individuals with instability are asymptomatic; however, 1% to 2% have symptoms (Cohen, 1998; Gajdosik & Ostertag, 1996; Pueschel, 1998) of spinal cord compression because this enlarged space causes the cord to become compressed as a result of the excessive motion of the atlas on the axis. Symptoms may include walking difficulties, neck pain, limited neck motion, torticollis, spasticity, hyperreflexia, incoordination, clumsiness, and other signs of an upper motor neuron problem, such as loss of bowel or bladder control (Committee on Sports Medicine and Fitness, 1995). If these symptoms are noted, a physician should see the child immediately because these are all signs of spinal cord compression that may lead to paralysis if left untreated. A schematic drawing of atlantoaxial instability is shown in Figure 5–9.

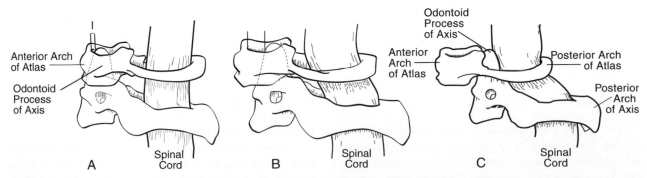

Figure 5-9 Atlantoaxial instability. *(A)* Normal relationship. *(B)* Atlantoaxial subluxation without spinal cord impingement. *(C)* Impingement on the spinal cord by the ondontoid process and posterior arch of the atlas. (Adapted from Gajdosik, C.G., & Ostertag, S. [1996]. Cervical instability and Down Syndrome: Review of the literature and implications for physical therapists. *Pediatric Physical Therapy,* 8, 31-36. Original source: Martich, V., Ben-Ami, T., Yousefzaden, D.K. & Roizen, N.J. (1992). Hypoplastic posterior of ach C-1 in children with Down Syndrome: A double jeopardy. *Radiology,* 183, [127].

Measurements from radiographs taken in three different lateral positions (flexion, extension, and neutral) are used to identify atlantoaxial instability. The measurement is taken between the anterior portion of the dens (also called the odontoid process) and the posterior portion of the anterior arch of the atlas. If this distance is greater than 4.5 mm, instability is considered to be present (Cohen, 1998). There is a great deal of controversy as to the screening and evaluation for atlantoaxial instability. In 1983, the Special Olympics issued a requirement that lateral neck radiographs be taken for all individuals with Down syndrome before they participated in their competitive programs. If there was evidence of instability, the individual was not permitted to participate in activities that placed undue stress on neck structures. At that time, the American Academy of Pediatrics agreed with that requirement. More recently, however, The Committee on Sports Medicine and Fitness of the American Academy of Pediatrics (1995) published an extensive review of the literature and identified several problems relative to routine screening. First, there are reliability problems with the radiographic screening technique; second, there is uncertainty whether *asymptomatic* atlantoaxial instability actually leads to *symptomatic* instability; and third, trauma such as a sports injury rarely causes the initial presentation or progression of symptoms. However, it is clear that an increased distance of 4.5 to 5 mm between the dens and the anterior arch is atypical, and at present, the only screening tools are lateral radiographs and neurological examinations. The Committee on Sports Medicine and Fitness concluded that lateral radiographs are "of potential but unproven value in detecting children at risk for developing spinal cord injury during sports participation" (1995, p. 153).

Today the Special Olympics continue to require radiographs before competition. The Down Syndrome Medical Special Interest Group suggests that initial radiographs be taken between 3 and 5 years of age but no longer suggests repeated routine screening radiographs other than those required for participation by the Special Olympics. However, they do strongly recommend ongoing neurological examination of individuals with Down syndrome. Any child with symptoms that indicate possible spinal cord compression should immediately be referred to a neurologist (Cohen, 1999). Symptoms can remain stable over time but may also progress to a more severe level, leading to catastrophic consequences (Committee on Sports Medicine and Fitness, 1995). Treatment for a child with symptomatic atlantoaxial instability is generally surgical fusion to halt the progression of cord compression (Cohen, 1998).

There are several clinical applications of this information for physical therapists. It is important to know the status of the child's neck, to act as a resource to the family regarding the risks, screening recommendations, and appropriate medical follow-up. Because neurological status is indicative of impending cord compression, the physical therapist who has routine contact with the child must monitor neurological status and report any abnormal neurological findings. Children with Down syndrome who have had documented normal neck radiographs do not need activity restrictions; however, those who have a demonstrated asymptomatic atlantoaxial instability should be restricted from any activity that places excessive stress on neck structures. Examples of these activities are gymnastics, swimming (butterfly stroke), diving, high jump, contact sports that could cause risk to the neck and head such as football and soccer, and any other exercises that place pressure on the head and neck (Cohen, 1999; Committee on Sports Medicine, 1984). In physical therapy, it is important to avoid exercises that may place excessive pressure on the head and neck, such as tumbling, and excessive neck flexion or extension in children who have asymptomatic atlantoaxial instability.

Idiopathic Scoliosis

Scoliosis is a lateral curvature of the spine that can be structural or nonstructural. A structural curve is fixed without the typical spinal flexibility, whereas a nonstructural curve is flexible (Lonstein, 1996). Scoliotic curves may be single or double. The Scoliosis Research Society defines *scoliosis* as a lateral curvature of greater than 10° using the Cobb method during a standing radiograph (Scoliosis Research Society, 2003). The **Cobb method** is the standard way to quantify curve size using an anteroposterior radiograph view. Figure 5–10 shows the Cobb method for measuring the amount of curvature.

The end vertebrae of the curve are identified. These are the vertebrae that are at the greatest tilt on either end of the curve. A line is drawn parallel to the top end plate of the top vertebra and the bottom end plate of the bottom vertebra. Perpendicular lines are then drawn from each of these. The angle formed where these two lines intersect is the amount of curvature (Tolo & Wood, 1993). The Cobb method is a good estimate of curvature magnitude but should not be used to quantify small changes because it can change according to the position of the patient during the radiographic procedure and the examiner lines. In addition, the Cobb method assesses only the lateral aspect of the curvature, and scoliosis is a three-dimensional problem. Along with the lateral curve, a rotation deformity is present and

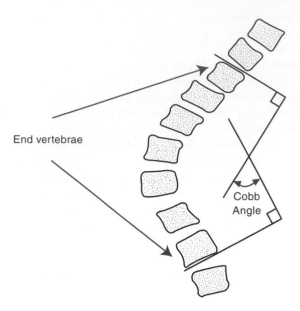

End vertebrae

Cobb
Angle

Figure 5-10 Cobb method of measuring scoliosis curve.

produces what is often termed a **"rib hump."** A rib hump is a prominence in the paravertebral area caused by trunk and rib rotation (Roach, 1999). It is most easily seen when the patient bends forward. The side with the rib hump will be elevated. Another component of scoliosis is a **lordosis** in the area of the apex of the curve (Dickson, 1999).

There are several types of idiopathic scoliosis that are classified by the age of appearance. **Infantile scoliosis** is seen in children younger than 3 years; **juvenile scoliosis** appears between the ages of 3 and 10 years; and **adolescent scoliosis** is diagnosed between age 10 years and skeletal maturity (Dobbs & Weinstein, 1999). **Idiopathic scoliosis** is differentiated from scoliosis that occurs in a neuromuscular disorder such as CP (discussed in the section on CP) in that it has no known cause. Adolescent idiopathic scoliosis is the most common type and occurs in 2% to 3% of children from 7 to 16 years of age (Bleck, 1991). This section will focus on structural adolescent idiopathic scoliosis, because it is more commonly seen than the other two types.

School screenings for scoliosis are commonly done in many states; however, there is some controversy regarding its value. A recent review of the scientific evidence enumerated the positive aspects of screening as well as the less positive ones and concluded that changes should be made in school scoliosis screenings (Morrissy, 1999). One area of concern is that at this time, it is not proved that early detection changes the natural history of the curve, so the usefulness of school scoliosis screenings is being questioned

(Karachalios et al., 1999). Along this line is the concern that some children are also incorrectly referred for unnecessary follow-up radiographs. Large radiographs expose the child to radiation, which in high amounts may result in a small but significant increase in cancer risk (Cote, Kreitz, Cassidy, Dzus, & Martel, 1998).

Although there is no consensus on the efficacy of routine school scoliosis screening, physical therapists who work with children must understand the elements of a scoliosis examination and be knowledgeable regarding how to perform the tests and when to make a referral. Scoliosis examination on an individual basis is extremely important so that children can be monitored for growth patterns and curve progression, which will allow better treatment planning. Scoliosis examination is also a vital component of an evaluation for children with low back pain, neurological impairment, and some genetic disorders.

Scoliosis can often be detected through the **Adam's forward-bend test** (described in Chapter 4), use of a scoliometer, or clinical examination of asymmetry. A leg length asymmetry can cause a nonstructural curve, and information on examination of leg length is provided earlier in this chapter. In addition, the therapist should look for other asymmetries, such as uneven hip or shoulder heights during standing, or an increased space between the elbow and the trunk on the concave side of the curve.

When an asymmetry is found, a scoliometer can be used to determine the angle of trunk rotation. A scoliometer is a level that is used with the individual in the same forward-bend position as the Adams forward-bend test (see Chapter 4). The scoliometer is placed on the back perpendicular to the long axis of the trunk at the apex of the curve with the center of the level placed on the most prominent spinous process. The angle of trunk rotation is measured, and anyone with a measurement of 7° or more should be referred to a physician (Bunnell, 1993).

A number of causes of idiopathic scoliosis have been, and continue to be, investigated, but there is still no clear etiology. One interesting line of research has been the role of muscle pathology and fiber type. Subjects with scoliosis have an increased number of type 1 muscle fibers in paraspinal muscles on the convex side of the curve compared with subjects without scoliosis (Gonyea, Moore-Woodard, Moseley, Hollman, & Wenger, 1985). Type 1 fibers are the slow-twitch tonic fibers; hence, if this imbalance in fiber type is a causative factor in the development of scoliosis, the preponderance of type 1 fibers would more likely be on the concave side because of their more constant tonic activity. However, the authors of this study concluded that the constant stretch placed on these fibers more likely caused a conversion to type 1 tonic fibers after the deforming process began. Therefore, the muscle fiber type changes found in this study would not be causative, but rather the result of a deforming factor that began as a result of other factors. Other factors that have been investigated are hormone system and growth mechanisms, subtle neurological abnormalities, and connective tissue disorders, but none have shown definitive causal evidence.

Adolescent idiopathic scoliosis has a hereditary component (Wynne-Davies, 1968). In cases of small curves of about 10°, the number of boys and girls is approximately equal, but among those with curves greater than 20° there are far more girls than boys, indicating that curve progression is greater in girls than in boys. An excellent review article by Machida (1999) examines several lines of research and suggests that the etiology of adolescent idiopathic scoliosis may be multifactorial.

Intervention and follow-up care for an adolescent with a structural scoliosis depend on the amount of the curve at diagnosis and how likely the curve is to continue to progress. In general, the curves that are most likely to progress are large double curves in skeletally immature children (Lonstein, 1996). As with many things in medicine, however, there are no absolute rules about curve progression, so estimates need to be made to predict future change. The physician will look at the curve magnitude over time at specific points during the process of skeletal maturity and the amount of potential growth left. In addition, the child's appearance and social factors play a role in decision making for intervention (Lonstein, 1996).

To predict the amount of growth a child has left, skeletal maturity is estimated. The **Risser sign** is one method of estimating skeletal maturity by using radiographs to grade the appearance of the secondary ossification center along the top of the iliac crest. It is graded from a 0 (no appearance) to a 4 (completed ossification). There are five stages, with different criteria for males and females.

Calculation of peak height velocities is another method for predicting growth patterns, and it has compared very favorably with the other maturity scales (Little, Song, Katz, & Herring, 2000). Using this method, height is measured over time, generally in 6-month intervals, and the height velocity is calculated as growth over time (Herring, 2002). This velocity calculation establishes the growth peak and predicts how much growth is left.

Intervention can be nonoperative or operative. Nonoperative intervention is aimed at controlling the curve progression so that the need for surgery may be avoided. Wearing an orthotic, electrical stimulation, and exercise are all nonoperative interventions. The most commonly used nonoperative intervention is bracing. Exercises are often part of an intervention program and are aimed at maintaining and/or improving spine flexibility and trunk strength (Herring, 2002). In children with large thoracic level curves, exercises for respiratory capability may be needed because the curve may impede thoracic expansion and limit breathing (Shepherd, 1995). Swimming can be used both preoperatively and postoperatively to improve general endurance and respiratory capacity (Shepherd, 1995). There is no evidence that exercise alone prevents curve progression or improves the curve itself (Negrini, Antonini, Carabalona, & Minozzi, 2003), nor is there evidence for the efficacy of electrical stimulation (Bowen, Keeler, & Pelegie, 2001; Bradford, Tanguy, & Vanselow, 1983; Sullivan, Davidson, Renshaw, Emans, Johnston, & Sussman, 1986).

Orthotic intervention is determined on an individual basis, but in general it is considered for children with a curve of greater than 30° (Lonstein, 1996). An orthotic may also be prescribed for a child with a smaller curve if it is progressing. In addition, an orthotic may be prescribed for a child with a curve in the 25°-to-30° range if the child has a low Risser sign and sexually immature physical characteristics because the child has considerable growth potential left (Lonstein & Winter, 1994).

Orthoses may include the **Milwaukee brace** or **Thoracolumbar Sacral Orthosis** (TLSO). The Milwaukee brace incorporates a cervical portion or neck ring attached to metal uprights, two posterior and one anterior. There are corrective pads connected to the uprights and a molded pelvic section. The TLSO is a molded orthotic having several different designs that may extend to just under the arms or end more distally low on the thorax. There are several of these, including the Boston brace and the Wilmington brace. Pads for pressure relief are also placed into the TLSO during its fitting and fabrication. Braces are chosen according to the type of curve, the age of the individual, and cosmesis. The Milwaukee brace is used for any type of curve but is the only appropriate choice for a curve with the apex above T8 (Lonstein, 1996). There are a number of studies that have looked at the effectiveness of various orthotics (Fernandez-Fieliberti, Flynn, Ramirez, Trautmann, & Alegria, 1995; Lonstein & Winter, 1994; Nachemson & Peterson, 1995). These have reported prevention of curve progression in some, but not in all, curves depending on factors such as the degree of curvature, age at initial diagnosis, gender, and pattern of curvature. Two review papers published recently have questioned the strength of the evidence for orthotic use (Dickson, 1999; Dickson & Weinstein, 1999).

The physical therapist working with children with scoliosis should provide information about treatment options to the child and family. If the child is fitted with an orthotic, the physical therapist should provide instruction on breathing exercises during orthotic wear and on trunk strengthening and trunk flexibility exercises in and out of the orthosis. In addition, and very important, the role of the physical therapist is to encourage the child to remain physically active during brace intervention and to provide ideas for activities that are stimulating and fun. Cardiopulmonary fitness is an important component of the child's health plan and can be achieved through specific exercises as well as community-based fitness activities, such as dancing, cycling, swimming, and various types of physical education classes.

Operative intervention is generally performed in three groups of children. These are children who are still growing and have a curve of more than 40° to 45°, children with curve progression of 40° to 45° despite nonoperative intervention, and mature adolescents with a curve of more than 50° to 60° (Lonstein, 1996). Surgical intervention is aimed at preventing curve progression through the achievement of a solid spinal fusion and placement of instrumentation into the spine. The fusion stops the curve progression and the placement of the instrumentation system helps to achieve maximal correction in all three planes with a balanced trunk (Drummond, 1991). Curve correction should occur in all three planes, not just the frontal plane. There have been several generations of procedures and instrumentation systems that have been used to achieve these goals. The Harrington rod was an earlier generation of distraction system applied to the concave side of the curve. The second-generation systems were called segmental spinal instrumentation, in which two rods were linked together and wired to the spine at multiple levels. A current example of a third-generation instrumentation system is the **Cotrel-Dubousset system**. This consists of at least two interlinked contoured rods with multiple hooks on each rod. The rods allow for distraction and compression to occur with one rod placed on each side of the spine through preplaced hooks. Several other systems similar to this one are also in use today. The surgical approach most often used is posterior, but an anterior approach may also be used depending on the location and complexity of the curve. Bone graft is placed into the disc spaces and facets as they are excised during the surgery (Lonstein, 1996). The child may need to wear an orthosis or plaster cast postsurgically while the spinal fusion heals.

During the postsurgical period, while the child is in the inpatient setting, the role of the physical therapist is to teach bed mobility, transfers, and other ADL skills. Log rolling is taught because spinal rotation should be avoided. The child can learn to don and doff the orthosis in bed while avoiding trunk rotation, and can also be taught general ROM exercises. Strengthening exercises without resistance, such as quadriceps and gluteal sets, can also be taught (Patrick, 2000).

Children are also seen for initial ambulation training after the fusion. When initiating ambulation training, the therapist must watch for orthostatic hypotension. Orthostatic hypotension is a rapid drop in blood pressure when moving into a standing position that can cause the child to become dizzy or faint. Postoperative bed rest after major surgery puts the child at risk for orthostatic hypotension. To avoid orthostatic hypotension, the child should be instructed to perform ankle pumps to promote blood circulation. To improve compliance, a gimmick such as asking the child to do 10 ankle pumps during each commercial while watching television can be used. When ambulation training is commenced, it is important to make the transition from lying to standing slowly. A tilt table is useful to raise the child to an upright position at tolerable increments.

Swimming is also helpful for strength, mobility, and cardiorespiratory function and can be started about 3 months after surgery (Patrick, 2000). Activity remains restricted, however, as the spinal fusion heals. The timing of return to athletic activity is based on radiographic evidence of spinal fusion.

Summary

The human body operates through a complex interaction of many body systems. The musculoskeletal system is an integral component of a healthy, efficient system. Interventions affecting the musculoskeletal system can improve a child's abilities. An understanding of the development and potential pathologies of children will allow the physical therapist to design effective interventions that meet the needs of the child and family. Compliance at home will be maximized if the activities are fun and incorporated into the family's normal routine and if the child and family are included in the planning. If the child and family have helped identify the problems and solutions, they will value the information and are more likely to comply with the program. Last, the therapist must remember that therapy interventions are only one component of the child's and family's life. Realistic expectations will allow the child and family to succeed and feel empowered.

DISCUSSION QUESTIONS

1. Discuss the implications for strength training in children with cerebral palsy.

2. Describe atlantoaxial instability and its symptoms of which you should be aware when working with children with Down syndrome. How would its presence change your therapy program?

3. What are the important components of a musculoskeletal examination for a child with Down syndrome?

4. List the components of a therapy intervention program for a child with polyarticular juvenile rheumatoid arthritis.

5. Discuss the factors that are considered when determining intervention for an adolescent with scoliosis.

6. What is the role of the physical therapist when working with an adolescent with scoliosis?

REFERENCES

American Academy of Pediatrics (2001). Policy Statement (RE0048): Strength training by children and adolescents. *Pediatrics, 107*(6), 1470–1472.

Ansved, T. (2001). The effects of strength training in patients with selected neuromuscular disorders. *Acta Physiologica Scandinavica, 171*(3), 359–366.

Bacon, M.C., Nicholson, C., Binder, H., & White, P.H. (1991). Juvenile rheumatoid arthritis. Aquatic exercise and lower-extremity function. *Arthritis Care and Research, 4*(2), 102–105.

Barker, D.J., & Hall, A.J. (1986). The epidemiology of Perthes' disease. *Clinical Orthopedics, 209*, 89–94.

Biggar, W.D., Klamut, H.J., Demacio, P.C., Stevens, D.J., & Ray, P.N. (2002). Duchenne muscular dystrophy: Current knowledge, treatment, and future prospects. *Clinical Orthopedics, 401*, 88–106.

Bleck, E.E. (1991). Adolescent idiopathic scoliosis. *Developmental Medicine and Child Neurology, 33*(2), 167–173.

Bowen, J.R., Keeler, K.A., Pelegie, S. (2001). Adolescent idiopathic scoliosis managed by a nighttime bending brace. *Orthopedics, 24*(10), 967–970.

Bradford, D.S., Tanguy, A., & Vanselow, J. (1983). Surface electrical stimulation in the treatment of idiopathic scoliosis: Preliminary results in 30 patients. *Spine, 8*, 757–764.

Bunnell, W.P. (1993). Outcome of spinal screening. *Spine, 18*(12), 1572–1580.

Cadenhead, S.L., McEwen, I.R., & Thompson, D.M. (2002). Effect of passive range of motion exercises on lower-extremity goniometric measurements of adults with cerebral palsy: A single-subject design. *Physical Therapy, 82*(7), 658–669.

Caselli, M.A., Sobel-Cohen, E., Thompson, J., Adler, J., & Gonzalez, L. (1991). Biomechanical management of children and adolescents with Down syndrome. *Journal of the American Podiatric Medical Society, 81*, 119–127.

Cashman, J.P., Round, J., Taylor, G., & Clarke, N.M. (2002). The natural history of developmental dysplasia of the hip after early supervised treatment in the Pavlik harness. A prospective, longitudinal follow-up. *The Journal of Bone and Joint Surgery, British Volume, 84*(3), 418–425.

Castle, M.E., Reyman, T.A., & Schneider, M. (1979). Pathology of spastic muscle in cerebral palsy. *Clinical Orthopedics, 142*, 223–232.

Cheng, J.C., Tang, S.P., Chen, T.M., Wong, M.W., & Wong, E.M. (2000). The clinical presentation and outcome of treatment of congenital muscular torticollis in infants—A study of 1,086 cases. *Journal of Pediatric Surgery, 35*(7), 1091–1096.

Cheng, J.C., Wong, M.W., Tang, S.P., Chen, T.M., Shum, S.L., & Wong, E.M. (2001). Clinical determinants of the outcome of manual stretching in the treatment of congenital muscular torticollis in infants. A prospective study of eight hundred and twenty-one cases. *Journal of Bone and Joint Surgery, American Volume, 83-A*(5), 679–687.

Cohen, W.I. (1999). Health care guidelines for individuals with Down syndrome: 1999 Revision. *Down Syndrome Quarterly, 3*(4), 1–15.

Cohen, W.I. (1998). Atlantoaxial instability. What's next? *Archives of Pediatric and Adolescent Medicine, 152*, 119–121.

Committee on Sports Medicine (1984). Atlantoaxial instability in Down syndrome. *Pediatrics, 74*(1), 152–154.

Committee on Sports Medicine and Fitness (1995). Atlantoaxial instability in Down syndrome: Subject review. *Pediatrics, 96*(1), 151–154.

Cote, P., Kreitz, B.G., Cassidy, J.D., Dzus, A.K., & Martel, J. (1998). A study of the diagnostic accuracy and reliability of the Scoliometer and Adam's forward bend test. *Spine, 23*(7), 796–802.

Damiano, D.L., & Abel, M.F. (1998). Functional outcomes of strength training in spastic cerebral palsy. *Archives of Physical Medicine and Rehabilitation, 79*(2), 119–125.

Damiano, D.L., Kelly, L.E., & Vaugh, C.L., (1995). Effects of quadriceps femoris muscle strengthening on crouch gait in children with spastic diplegia. *Physical Therapy, 75*, 658–667.

Davids, J.R., Wenger, D.R., & Mubarak, S.J. (1993). Congenital muscular torticollis: Sequelae of intrauterine or perinatal compartment syndrome. *Journal of Pediatric Orthopedics, 13*(2), 141–147.

Demirbilek, S., & Atayurt, H.F. (1999). Congenital muscular

torticollis and sternomastoid tumor: Results of nonoperative treatment. *Journal of Pediatric Surgery, 34*(4), 549–551.

Dhanendran, M., Hutton, W.C., Klennerman, L., Witemeyer, S., & Ansell, B.M. (1980). Foot function in juvenile chronic arthritis. *Rheumatology and Rehabilitation, 19*, 20–24.

Dickson, R.A. (1999). Spinal deformity—Adolescent idiopathic scoliosis. Nonoperative treatment. *Spine, 24*, 2601–2606.

Dickson, R.A., & Weinstein S.L. (1999). Bracing (and screening)—Yes or no? *The Journal of Bone and Joint Surgery, British Volume, 81*, 193–198.

Do, T.T. (2001). Clinical and radiographic evaluation of bowlegs. *Current Opinions in Pediatrics, 13*(1), 424–426.

Dobbs, M.B., Weinstein, S.L. (1999). Infantile and juvenile scoliosis. *Orthopedic Clinics of North America, 30*(3), 331–341.

Drummond, D.S. (1991) A perspective on recent trends for scoliosis correction. *Clinical Orthopaedics and Related Research, 264*, 90–102.

Fernandez-Feliberti, R., Flynn, J., Ramirez, N., Trautmann, M., & Alegria, M. (1995). Effectiveness of TLSO bracing in the conservative treatment of idiopathic scoliosis. *Journal of Pediatric Orthopedics, 15*, 176–181.

Fowler, W., & Taylor, M. (1982). Rehabilitation management of muscular dystrophy and related disorders: I. The role of exercise. *Archives of Physical Medicine and Rehabilitation, 63*(7), 319–321.

Fuchs, R.K., & Snow, C.M. (2002). Gains in hip bone mass from high-impact training are maintained: A randomized controlled trial in children. *Journal of Pediatrics, 141*(3), 357–362.

Gajdosik, C.G., & Ostertag, S. (1996). Cervical instability and Down syndrome: Review of the literature and implications for physical therapists. *Pediatric Physical Therapy, 8*, 31–36.

Giannini, M.J., & Protas, E.J. (1993) Comparison of peak isometric knee extensor torque in children with and without juvenile rheumatoid arthritis. *Arthritis Care and Research, 6*(2), 82–88.

Goldberg, M.J. (2001). Early detection of developmental hip dysplasia: Synopsis of the AAP Clinical Practice Guideline. *Pediatric Review, 22*(4), 131–134.

Gonyea, W.J., Moore-Woodard, C., Moseley, B., Hollmann, M., & Wenger D.(1985). An evaluation of muscle pathology in idiopathic scoliosis. *Journal of Pediatric Orthopedics, 5*(3), 323–329.

Grahame, R. (2000). Hypermobility—Not a circus act. *International Journal of Clinical Practice, 54*(5), 314–315.

Grasemann, H., Nicolai, R.D., Patalis, T., & Hovel, M. (1997). The treatment of Legg-Calvé-Perthes disease. To contain or not to contain. *Archives of Orthopaedic and Trauma Surgery, 116*(1–2), 50–54.

Greene, W.B. (1998). Closed treatment of hip dislocation in Down syndrome. *Journal of Pediatric Orthopedics, 18*, 643–647.

Greulich, W., & Pyle S. (1959). *Radiographic atlas of the skeletal development of the hand and wrist* (2nd ed.). Stanford, CA: Stanford University Press.

Grimston, S.K., Willows, N.D., & Hanley, D.A. (1993). Mechanical loading regime and its relationship to bone mineral density in children. *Medicine and Science in Sports and Exercise, 25*(11), 1203–1207.

Grzegorzewski, A., Bowen, J.R., Guille, J.T., & Glutting, J. (2003). Treatment of the collapsed femoral head by containment in Legg-Calvé-Perthes disease. *Journal of Pediatric Orthopedics, 23*(1), 15–19.

Guille, J.T., Pizzutillo, P.D., & MacEwen, G.D. (2000). Development dysplasia of the hip from birth to six months. *Journal of American Academy of Orthopedic Surgeons, 8*(4), 232–242.

Henderson, R.C., Kemp, G.J., & Hayes, P.R. (1993). Prevalence of late-onset tibia vara. *Journal of Pediatric Orthopedics, 13*(2), 255–258.

Heikkilä, E., Ryoppy, S., & Laihimo, I. (1985). The management of primary acetabular dysplasia. Its association with habitual side-lying. *The Journal of Bone and Joint Surgery, British Volume, 67*(1), 25–28.

Herring, J.A. (2002). Scoliosis. In J.S. Herring (Ed.), *Tachdjian's pediatric orthopedics* (3rd ed., pp. 213–321). Philadelphia: W.B. Saunders.

Ito, J., Araki, A, Tanaka, H., Tasaki, T., Cho, K., & Yamazaki, R. (1996). Muscle histopathology in spastic cerebral palsy. *Brain Development, 8*(4), 299–303.

Karachalios, T., Sofianos, J., Roidis, N., Sapkas, G,, Korres. D., & Nikolopoulos, K. (1999). Ten-year follow-up evaluation of a school screening program for scoliosis. Is the forward-bending test an accurate diagnostic criterion for the screening of scoliosis? *Spine, 15, 24*(22), 2318–2324.

Klepper, S.E. (1999). Effects of an eight-week physical conditioning program on disease signs and symptoms in children with chronic arthritis. *Arthritis Care and Research, 12*(1), 52–60.

Klepper, S.E., & Giannini, M.J. (1994). Physical conditioning in children with arthritis: Assessment and guidelines for exercise prescription. *Arthritis, Care and Research, 7*(4), 226–236.

Kott, K.M., & Held, S.L. (2003). Effects of orthoses on upright functional skills of children and adolescents with cerebral palsy. *Pediatric Physical Therapy, 14*(4), 199–207.

Laville, J.M., Chau, E., Willemen, L., Kohler, R., & Garin, C. (1999). Blount's disease: Classification and treatment. *Journal of Pediatric Orthopedics B, 8*(1), 19–25.

Lecuire, F. (2002). The long-term outcome of primary osteochondritis of the hip (Legg-Calvé-Perthes' disease). *The Journal of Bone and Joint Surgery. British Volume, 84*(5), 636–640.

Lespargot, A., Renaudin, E., Khouri, N., & Robert, M. (1994). Extensibility of hip adductors in children with cerebral palsy. *Developmental Medicine and Child Neurology, 36*(11), 980–988.

Little, D.G., Song, K.M., Katz, D., & Herring, J.A. (2000). Relationship of peak height velocity to other maturity indicators in idiopathic scoliosis in girls. *The Journal of Bone and Joint Surgery, American Volume, 82*(5), 685–693.

Lonstein, J. (1996). Idiopathic scoliosis. In R.T. Morrissy & S.L. Weinstein (Eds.), *Lovell & Winter's pediatric orthopedics* (4th ed., pp. 625–685). Philadelphia: Lippincott-Raven.

Lonstein, J.E., & Winter, R.B. (1994). The Milwaukee brace for the treatment of adolescent idiopathic scoliosis. *The Journal of Bone and Joint Surgery, American Volume, 76*(8), 1207–1221.

Lovell, D.J., Passo, M., Giannini, E., & Brunner, H. (2001). Systemic onset juvenile idiopathic arthritis: A retrospective study of 80 consecutive patients followed for 10 years. *Journal of Rheumatology, 28*(1), 220.

Lowes, L.P., Westcott, S.L., Palisano, R.J., Effgen, S.K., & Orlin, M.N. (2004). Muscle force and range of motion as determinants of standing balance in children with cerebral palsy. *Physical and Occupational Therapy in Pediatrics, 24*(1), 57–77.

Machida, M. (1999). Cause of idiopathic scoliosis. *Spine, 24,* 2576–2583.

Mahabir, R.C., Kazemi, A.R., Cannon, W.G., & Courtemanche, D.J. (2001). Pediatric hand fractures: A review. *Pediatric Emergency Care, 17*(3), 153–156.

Mahar, R.K., Kirby, R.L., & MacLeod, D.A. (1985). Simulated leg-length discrepancy: Its effect on mean center-of-pressure position and postural sway. *Archives of Physical Medicine and Rehabilitation, 66,* 822–824.

McCartney, N., Moroz, D., Garner, S.H., & McComas, A.J. (1988). The effects of strength training in patients with selected neuromuscular disorders. *Medical Science of Sport and Exercise, 20*(4), 362–368.

Miller, M.L., Kress, A.M., & Berry, C.A. (1999). Decreased physical function in juvenile rheumatoid arthritis. *Arthritis Care and Research, 12*(5), 309–313.

Morrissy, R.T. (1999). School screening for scoliosis. *Spine, 24,* 2584–2591.

Moseley, C.F. (1991). Leg lengthening: The historical perspective. *Orthopedic Clinics of North America, 22*(4), 555–561.

Moseley, C.F. (1996). Leg length discrepancy and angular deformity of the lower limbs. In R.T. Morrissy & S.L. Weinstein (Eds.), *Lovell & Winter's pediatric orthopedics* (4th ed. pp. 849–901). Philadelphia: Lippincott-Raven.

Murray, P.D., & Drachman, D.B. (1969). The role of movement in the development of joints and related structures: The head and neck in the chick embryo. *Journal of Embryology and Experimental Morphology, 22*(3), 349–371.

Nachemson, A.L., & Peterson, L.-E. (1995). Effectiveness of treatment with a brace in girls who have adolescent idiopathic scoliosis. *The Journal of Bone and Joint Surgery, American Volume, 77*(6), 815–822.

Negrini, S., Antonini, G., Carabalona, R., & Minozzi, S. (2003). Physical exercises as a treatment for adolescent idiopathic scoliosis. A systematic review. *Pediatric Rehabilitation, 6*(3–4), 227–235.

Nicole, S., Diaz, C., Frugier, T., & Melki, J. (2002). Spinal muscular atrophy: Recent advances and future prospects. *Muscle and Nerve, 26*(1), 4–13.

Oen, K., Malleson, P.N., Cabral, D.A., Rosenberg, A.M., Petty, R.E., & Cheang, M. (2002). Disease course and outcome of juvenile rheumatoid arthritis in a multicenter cohort. *Journal of Rheumatology, 29*(9), 1989–1999.

Palmer, P.M., MacEwen, G.D., Bowen, J.R., & Mathews, P.A. (1985). Passive motion therapy for infants with arthrogryposis. *Clinics in Orthopedics, 194,* 54–59.

Patrick, C. (2000). Spinal conditions. In S.K. Campbell, D.W. Vander Linden, & R.J. Palisano (Eds.), *Physical therapy for children* (2nd ed., pp. 260–281). Philadelphia: W.B. Saunders.

Pueschel, S.M. (1998). Should children with Down syndrome be screened for atlantoaxial instability? *Archives of Pediatric and Adolescent Medicine, 152,* 123–125.

Raco, A., Raimondi, A.J., De Ponte, F.S., Brunelli, A., Bristot, R., Bottini, D.J., & Ianetti, G. (1999). Congenital torticollis in association with craniosynostosis. *Childs Nervous System, 15*(4), 163–168.

Radin, E.L., Burr, D.B., Caterson, B., Fyhrie, D., Brown, T.D., & Boyd, R.D. (1991). Mechanical determinants of osteoarthrosis. *Seminars in Arthritis and Rheumatology, 21*(3 Suppl 2), 12–21.

Renshaw, T.S., Green, N.E., Griffin, P.P., & Root, L. (1996). Cerebral palsy: Orthopaedic management. *Instructional Course Lecture, 45,* 475–490.

Rhodes, V.J. (1991). Physical therapy management of patients with juvenile rheumatoid arthritis. *Physical Therapy, 71,* 910–919.

Roach, J.W. (1999). Adolescent idiopathic scoliosis. *Orthopedic Clinics of North America, 30*(3), 353–365.

Roizen, N.J. (2001). Down syndrome: Progress in research. *Mental Retardation Developmental Disabilities Research Review, 7*(1), 38–44.

Rose, J., Haskell, W.L., Gamble, J.G., Hamilton, R.L., Brown, D.A., & Rinsky, L. (1994). Muscle pathology and clinical measures of disability in children with cerebral palsy. *Journal of Orthopedic Research, 12*(6), 758–768.

Rubin, S.S., Rimmer, J.H., Chicoine, B., Braddock, D., & McGuire, D.E. (1998). Overweight prevalence in persons with Down syndrome. *Mental Retardation, 36*(3), 175–181.

Sacheti, A., Szemere, J., Bernstein, B., Tafas, T., Schechter, N., & Tsipouras, P. (1997). Chronic pain is a manifestation of the Ehlers-Danlos syndrome. *Journal of Pain Symptom Management, 14*(2), 88–93.

Schaller, J.G. (1997). Juvenile rheumatoid arthritis. *Pediatric Review, 18*(10), 337–349.

Scoliosis Research Society (March 31, 2003). Available at: *www.srs.org.*

Selby-Silverstein, L., Hillstrom, H.J., & Palisano, R.J. (2001). The effect of foot orthoses on standing foot posture and gait of young children with Down syndrome. *Neurorehabilitation, 16*(3), 183–193.

Sells, J.M., Jaffe, K.M., & Hall, J.G. (1996). Amyoplasia, the most common type of arthrogryposis: The potential for good outcome. *Pediatrics, 97*(2), 225–231.

Shaw, E.D., & Beals, R.K. (1992). The hip joint in Down's syndrome. A study of its structure and associated disease. *Clinical Orthopedics, 278,* 101–107.

Shepherd, R.B. (1995). Structural scoliosis. In R.B. Shepherd, *Physiotherapy in paediatrics* (3rd ed., pp. 303–310). Oxford, England: Butterworth-Heinemann Ltd.

Sherry, D.D., & Mosca, V.S. (1996). Juvenile rheumatoid arthritis and seronegative spondyloarthropathies. In R.T. Morrissy & S.L. Weinstein (Eds.), *Lovell & Winter's pediatric orthopedics* (4th ed., pp. 537–577). Philadelphia: Lippincott-Raven.

Simon, S., Whiffen, J., & Shapiro, F. (1981). Leg-length discrepancy in monarticular and pauciarticular juvenile rheumatoid arthritis. *The Journal of Bone and Joint Surgery, American Volume, 63,* 209.

Spraul, G., & Koenning, G. (1994). A descriptive study of foot problems in children with juvenile rheumatoid arthritis (JRA). *Arthritis Care and Research, 7*(3), 144–150.

Staheli, L.T. (1992). *Fundamentals of pediatric orthopedics.* New York: Raven Press.

Stuberg, W.A. (1992). Considerations related to weight bearing programs in children with developmental disabilities. *Physical Therapy, 72,* 35–40.

Sullivan, J.A., Davidson, R., Renshaw, T.S., Emans, J.B., Johnston, C., & Sussman, M. (1986). Further evaluation of the Scolitron treatment of idiopathic adolescent scoliosis. *Spine, 1,* 903–906.

Tanner, J.M., & Buckler, J.M. (1997). Revision and update of Tanner-Whitehouse clinical longitudinal charts for height and weight. *European Journal of Pediatrics, 156*(3), 248–249.

Tardieu, C., Lespargot, A., Tabary, C., & Bret, M.D. (1988). For how long must the soleus muscle be stretched each day to prevent contracture? *Developmental Medicine and Child Neurology, 30*(1), 3–10.

Tetsworth, K., & Paley, D. (1994). Malalignment and degenerative arthropathy. *Orthopedic Clinics of North America, 25*(3), 367–377.

Thompson, G.H. (1996). Neuromuscular disorders. In R.T. Morrissy & S.L. Weinstein (Eds.), *Lovell & Winter's pediatric orthopaedics* (4th ed., pp. 537–577). Philadelphia: Lippincott-Raven.

Tolo, V.T., & Wood, B. (1993). *Pediatric orthopedics in primary care* (pp. 83–102). Baltimore: Williams & Wilkins.

Walker, J. (1991). Musculoskeletal development: A review. *Physical Therapy, 71*(12), 878–889.

Wattenbarger, J.M., Gruber, H.E., & Phieffer, L.S. (2002). Physeal fractures, part I: Histologic features of bone, cartilage and bar formation in a small animal model. *Journal of Pediatric Orthopedics, 22*(6), 703–709.

Wenger, D.R. (1993). Developmental dysplasia of the hip. In D.R. Wenger & M. Rang (Eds.), *The art and practice of children's orthopedics* (pp. 256–296). New York: Raven Press.

Weinstein, S.L. (1996). Developmental hip dysplasia and dislocation. In R.T. Morrissy & S.L. Weinstein (Eds.), *Lovell and Winter's pediatric orthopedics.* Philadelphia: Lippincott-Raven.

Wessel, J., Kaup, C., Fan, J., Ehalt, R., Ellsworth, J., Speer, C., Tenove, P., & Dombrosky, A. (1999). Isometric strength measurements in children with arthritis: Reliability and relation to function. *Arthritis Care and Research, 12*(4), 238–246.

Wynne-Davies, R. (1968). Familial (idiopathic) scoliosis. A family survey. *The Journal of Bone and Joint Surgery, British Volume, 50,* 24–30.

Zaleske, D.J. (1996). Metabolic and endocrine abnormalities. In R.T. Morrissy & S.L. Weinstein (Eds.), *Lovell and Winter's pediatric orthopedics.* Philadelphia: Lippincott-Raven.

Zeitlin, L., Fassier, F., & Glorieux, F.H. (2003). Modern approach to children with osteogenesis imperfecta. *Journal of Pediatric Orthopedics B, 12*(2), 77–87.

Chapter 6

Neuromuscular System: Structures, Functions, Diagnoses, and Evaluation

— Sarah L. Westcott, PT, PhD
— Caroline Goulet, PT, PhD

The human nervous system is a fascinating system that includes all the neural and support cells located within the central nervous system (CNS) and the neural axons that enter or exit the brain and spinal cord. This complex system has a built-in innate organization that simplifies the control of movement. Redundancy exists at most levels within the system to allow a safety net when there is damage of neural structures. The capacity for neural plasticity can assist with recovery from injury or disease, with the most recovery occurring based on how the individual uses the system. Evidence in the fields of neuroscience, psychology, education, and sports has contributed to our current knowledge of how movement is controlled by the interaction of the neuromuscular system with the other systems and within the constraints of the task environment. Physical therapists need a functional knowledge of these neuroscience essentials to apply clinical reasoning skills to the evaluation and intervention of children with neuromuscular disorders.

This chapter will first review the essentials of neuroscience related to common pediatric neuromuscular conditions and recovery. A historical perspective of the theoretical framework for motor control as it relates to the development of neurorehabilitation models will follow. Finally, a task-oriented approach to examination of children with neuromuscular dysfunctions will be discussed.

Neuroscience Related to Common Pediatric Neuromuscular Disorders

Impairment of body structures and functions within diagnoses vary greatly, dependent on the location and severity of injury, age at the time of injury, motor behaviors that the child learns to use and practice in his or her regular environment, and available supports. One commonality among diagnoses is that the neuromuscular system is disrupted, causing the child to have difficulty with movement that often, in the long term, leads to low fitness levels. Although examination and intervention need to be individualized to the child's specific motor disability, a focus should be made on developing meaningful functional movement and promoting general long-term health and fitness. To do so, physical therapists need to fully understand the neural components involved in motor control, to facilitate optimal functional recovery of movement.

Children with neuromuscular disability will likely fall into one of the three Preferred Practice Patterns discussed in the *Guide to physical therapist practice* (2nd ed.) (American Physical Therapy Association [APTA], 2001): 5B: Impaired Neuromotor Development; 5C: Impaired

Motor Function and Sensory Integrity Associated with Nonprogressive Disorders of the Central Nervous System—Acquired in Infancy or Childhood; or 5D: Impaired Motor Function and Sensory Integrity Associated with Nonprogressive Disorders of the Central Nervous System—Acquired in Adolescence or Adulthood. A concise review of the neuroscience of the motor system will be presented in relation to common pediatric disorders included in those practice patterns. The most common pediatric diagnoses have been selected to demonstrate the major neuromuscular issues encountered in pediatric practice.

A review of specific issues related to neuromotor development should help you understand the origins of some impairments in body structures and functions and predict, with some accuracy, restrictions in activities and participation that may develop. The knowledge of what type of motor disability may develop allows the therapist to modify examination and intervention approaches to improve effectiveness and prevention of further disability. For example, based on knowledge of the specific CNS injury, you could predict that a child would develop hemiplegia, and then early intervention could begin with a specific focus on encouraging bilateral movement. However, it is important to be fully aware that our ability to predict a specific outcome based on the original CNS insult is in its infancy and is not absolutely accurate (Unanue & Westcott, 2001). This is a result of several factors: (1) current imaging techniques do not provide completely clear pictures of the CNS; (2) plasticity of the nervous system cannot currently be fully predicted; and (3) motor and cognitive outcomes are based on a combination of "nature and nurture" issues, the individual's genetic make-up, and the effects of environmental experience, which cannot always be predicted or controlled.

Growth of the CNS begins early in the embryonic stages of development and can be broken down into several processes: (1) neurulation, (2) ventral induction, (3) neuronal proliferation, (4) neuronal migration, (5) neural organization, and (6) myelination (Capone, 1996; England, 1988; Jacob & Sarnat, 1989; Sarnat, 1984; Volpe, 1995). Each process and examples of the outcome of the infant if neuromuscular development is disturbed during these stages are summarized in Table 6.1.

Table 6.1 Neurological System Development and Injury Consequences

Developmental Process	Timing from Conception	Definition of Process	Disorders Associated with Insult During Process	Definition of Disorder	Outcome of Disorders
Neurulation	3 to 4 weeks	Formation of neural tube	Encephalocele	Defects in neural tube closure in brain	Dependent on the extent and level of lesion, motor and/or cognitive impairments
			Meningomyelocele (MM)	Defects in neural tube closure in spinal cord	
Ventral induction	5 to 6 weeks	Formation of basic structures and brain subdivisions	Holoprosencephaly	Failure of cleavage of prosencephalon leaving deficit in midline facial development	Facial structure, feeding, and cognitive impairment, ranging from mild developmental delay to severe mental retardation (MR) and cerebral palsy (CP)
			Agenesis of the corpus callosum	Lack of development of corpus callosum (where fibers cross between left and right side of brain)	Bilateral coordination, visual perception, motor control, motor learning, and cognitive impairments, ranging from mild developmental delay to severe MR and CP

Developmental Process	Timing from Conception	Definition of Process	Disorders Associated with Insult During Process	Definition of Disorder	Outcome of Disorders
Neuronal proliferation	8 to 16 weeks	Neural and glial cells form and proliferate	Microencephaly Macroencephaly	Reduced brain size and weight Increased brain size and weight	Cognitive and motor impairments including abnormal muscle tone, postural control, and motor coordination, ranging from mild developmental delay to severe MR and CP
Neuronal migration	12 to 20 weeks	Neurons move from ventricular and subventricular zones to final destination	Generalized or focal seizures Lissencephaly Schizencephaly Focal cerebral dysgenesis	Abnormal excessive electrical activity in the brain Abnormalities in gyral development and cortical surface area Abnormal cavities or cysts in the brain Lack of development of specific cortical sites	Dependent on size and location of seizures, gyral abnormality, cysts, and lack of brain development; cognitive, sensory, and motor control impairments, ranging from mild to severe developmental delay to CP
Neuronal organization	24 weeks to 2–3 years	Establishment and differentiation of subplate neurons Alignment, orientation, and layering of neurons Growth of axons and dendrites Synaptogenesis Selective elimination of neurons, neuronal processes, and synapses Glial cell proliferation and differentiation	Frequently associated with other earlier neural development abnormalities	Lack of organization and extensive network of circuits intrinsic and extrinsic to cerebral cortex	Dependent on extent and presence or absence of other CNS defects, cognitive, sensory or motor control impairment ranging from mild coordination and learning disorders (DCD) to CP
Myelination	23 weeks to adulthood	Development of myelin membrane around axons	Cerebral white matter hypoplasia	Deficient or absent myelin production, decreased number of tracts between brain and spinal cord, slow transmission along tracts	Mild to severe postural and motor control and coordination problems; difficulty producing quick movements

Source: Unanue, R., & Westcott, S.L. (2001). Neonatal asphyxia. *Infants and Young Children, 13*(3), 13–24, with permission.

Impaired Neuromotor Development (Pattern 5B)

Down Syndrome

Down syndrome (DS) is a genetic disorder in which the majority (approximately 90%) of individuals shows an extra chromosome on chromosome pair 21. This usually occurs because of the nondysjunction of two homologous chromosomes during the first or second meiotic division. In a small percentage (3% to 4%), a translocation occurs in which, after breakage of homologous chromosomes the pieces reattach to other intact chromosome pairs. The remaining individuals (2% to 4%) with DS have a mosaic disorder, in which some cells are normal and others are trisomy 21 (Stoll, Alembik, Dott, & Roth, 1998). Neuropathological differences as a result of the chromosomal abnormality include small smooth (less convolutions) brain (similar to 76% of normal), especially in the frontal lobes; small (similar to 66%) cerebellum and brainstem (Aylward et al., 1997); structural differences in the dendritic spines of the pyramidal neurons; lack of myelin-ization of neurons in the cortex and cerebellum; and decrease of neurons in the hippocampus and an increase in Alzheimer neurofibrillary tangles with age (Harris & Shea, 1991).

Impairments of Body Structures and Functions Related to Motor Performance

Children with DS usually present with overall hypotonicity (Cioni et al., 1994), muscle weakness, and hyperflexible joints (Dichter, 1994; Shea, 1991) (Figure 6–1). Because of the joint laxity, some children (about 15%) with DS show specific joint instability in the cervical atlantoaxial joint (Ferguson, Putney, & Allen, 1997). This is verified by radiography, and the warning signs include gait changes, urinary retention, torticollis, reluctance to move the neck, and increased deep tendon reflexes. If instability exists, the therapist must be careful to not hyperflex the child's neck during any activity because slippage of this joint could cause a spinal cord injury. Contact sports and tumbling should be avoided. Precautions should be understood by the family and others who engage the child in physical activity.

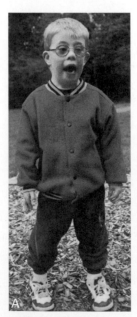 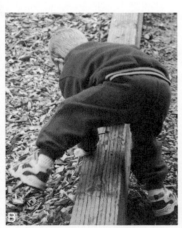 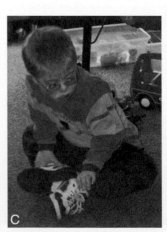 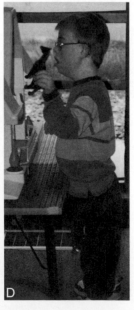

Figure 6-1 Child with Down syndrome. *(A)* When looking at the child's posture from the front, note his open mouth, sloping shoulders, and wide base of support, depicting lower muscle tone and poor postural control. *(B)* When asked to step over the low (4 inch) beam to enter the playground, he squats to support himself with his arms and sidesteps over the obstacle. *(C)* Note the wide base of support in sitting and the need to lean forward on his arms for assisted support to stay upright. *(D)* When looking at the child's posture from the side, note the open mouth, the choice to lean on the table for postural support, and the positioning of the legs locked into full knee extension, again to help maintain postural control and decrease the need for strength to maintain the position.

Because of the hypotonia, ligamentous laxity, and cognitive disorder, reaction times and movements of children with DS are generally slow and lack coordination (Inui, Yamanishi, & Tada, 1995). These findings have been demonstrated by studies of electromyographic (EMG) activity patterns during reaching in adults with DS. Individuals with DS tend to use more co-contraction of antagonistic muscle pairs than do individuals without DS (Aruin, Almeida, & Latash, 1996). This is thought to develop as a compensatory pattern for improved control of the movement and protection from external perturbations. There are four lines of defense to maintain a reaching movement to a target during a perturbation (Gottlieb, Corcos, & Agarwal, 1989; Houk, 1979; Latash, 1998a). In individuals with DS, the connective tissue is hypoextensible so the rebound effect of the connective tissue, the first line of defense, is reduced. The proprioceptors are not at a high state of readiness to respond (low muscle tone), and the brainstem areas may be slow to respond because of differences in cerebellum development. Therefore the effectiveness of the second (stretch reflex) and third lines of defense (long-latency reflex) is reduced. The fourth line of defense, voluntary redirection, must then be used. Fast voluntary responses to incoming feedback are generally not seen in individuals with DS, leaving the accuracy of the movement at great risk for not being redirected quickly enough to hit the target. To combat these problems, it is hypothesized that the individual co-contracts to produce better sensory feedback and limb stability. Excessive co-contraction causes movements to be slow. Moving slower also allows more time to receive and integrate feedback from proprioceptors.

The infant or child with DS takes a longer time to develop antigravity postures, and the postural alignment is different from typically developing children, because the child tends to "hang" on his or her ligaments (Haley, 1986; Kokubun et al., 1997; Lauteslager, Vermeer, & Helders 1998; Shumway-Cook & Woollacott, 1985). As a result of the delay in postural development and hypotonicity, the child will also widen the base of support and co-contract agonists and antagonists, or decrease the degrees of freedom for movement to develop stability (Aruin & Almeida, 1997). Therefore the movement experiences of a child with DS become limited, which causes further delay of the development of feedforward postural control and variable free movements. The small cerebellum of an individual with DS may have implications related to poor proprioception, difficulty using sensory input to learn motor behaviors, and problems using the vestibular system for postural control. This may explain why these children are visually dependent for postural control (Shumway-Cook & Woollacott, 1985).

The presence of hypotonicity, joint laxity, and decreased muscle strength will, over time, cause excessive wear and tear on the joints. Adults with DS develop early musculoskeletal changes including patellofemoral instability, genu valgus, pes planus, and hip instability (Hresko, McCarthy, & Goldberg, 1993; Merrick et al., 2000; Prasher, Robinson, Krishnan, & Chung, 1995).

Restrictions in Activities and Participation

The child with DS shows a delay in early motor and cognitive development. Development of antigravity postures of sitting and standing and of the early mobility skills of crawling and walking can be quite delayed. Use of treadmill training to facilitate earlier walking ability has demonstrated some success (Ulrich, Ulrich, Collier, & Cole, 1995; Ulrich, Ulrich, Angulo-Kinzler, & Yun, 2001). Once independent walking is achieved, the child will continue to have difficulty with eye-hand control and speed of movement required for ball skills, with the strength and speed needed for ballistic movements, such as jumping; and with the postural control needed for one-foot functional movement to negotiate stairs and kick a ball (Palisano et al., 2001; Spano et al., 1999). Unless there are other medical issues, these higher motor behaviors can eventually be addressed through adapted physical education or community recreation programs such as the Special Olympics.

Associated Medical Issues

Children with DS have varying degrees of mental retardation that lower their cognitive ability, their drive or curiosity about the world, and their motivation to try new things (Hayes & Batshaw, 1993; Pueschel, 1990). The therapist is challenged to find ways to communicate with the child, to understand his or her expressive communication, and to determine what will motivate the child to try different movements (Kokubun, 1999). Often this is the missing link in motor learning; the child may not be motivated to practice movement because it is difficult.

Congenital heart defects are a commonly (about 40% to 60%) associated medical disorder with DS that can affect exercise (Freeman et al., 1998). The most common defects are atrioventricular canal and ventriculoseptal defects, which usually can be surgically repaired. The therapist should understand the cardiac disorder and whether exercise needs to be modified to control effects on the heart.

Binaural hearing loss also is common in children with DS (Roizen, Wolters, Nicol, & Blondis, 1993). This is compounded by frequent otitis media. In addition to decreased response to sounds, there may be associated problems in the vestibular apparatus, which is located next to the sensory end organ for hearing. Vestibular impairment and cerebellar changes may combine to be the etiology of the muscle tone abnormalities. Eye conditions, including nearsightedness and farsightedness, lazy eye, astigmatism, nystagmus, and cataracts, are also common (Tsiaras, Pueschel, Keller, Curran, & Giesswein, 1999). Both the visual and vestibular deficits may account for part of the etiology of the postural control problems.

Potential Interventions

The physical therapist must coordinate and communicate with all other service providers as a member of an interdisciplinary team serving the needs of the child with DS and the family. Collaboration is beneficial to learn ways to structure communication and the play environment for better participation by the child. Generally, a structured environment, a small number of choices, and practice followed by rewards are successful strategies (McEwen, 2000). Special behavior management plans should be formulated, agreed on by the family and other professionals, and integrated into the plans of the entire team involved with the child.

A vital part of the intervention program is family education. The family is instructed in how to encourage appropriate developmental activities using the intervention strategies discussed in Chapter 7. Practice in different environments, which forces a change of critical factors about the movement, may teach the child new methods of postural and prime movement control (Dichter, DeCicco, Flanagan, Hyun, & Mongrain, 2000). The options for movement can be varied, which allows for greater exploration and learning. For example, in an attempt to change the co-contracted EMG activation patterns during reaching, researchers asked adults with DS to practice a reaching movement repetitively (1100 times per subject) at increasingly faster paces. The results showed that the subjects began to reach using a typical triphasic reaching pattern rather than the co-contraction pattern (Almeida, Corcos, & Latash, 1994). Use of variations in the environment, the components of the task, and practice are discussed in greater detail in Chapter 7.

Regular exercise programs should be incorporated into the child's routine for the health and fitness benefits because it is common for children with DS to become sedentary and obese as they age (Luke, Roizen, Sutton, & Schoellar, 1994; Rubin, Rimmer, Chicoine, Braddock, & McGuire, 1998). Intervention to improve strength and coordination and to decrease wear and tear on the weight-bearing joint structures should be implemented as preventive practice. For more information on Down syndrome, see the case study from birth to young adulthood of an individual with Down syndrome presented in Chapter 20.

Developmental Coordination Disorder

The *DSM-IV* defines **developmental coordination disorder (DCD)** as a motor skills disorder in which a child shows "marked impairment in the development of motor coordination that significantly interferes with academic achievement or activities of daily living" and that is not caused by a general medical condition or pervasive developmental disorder (PDD) (American Psychiatric Association, 1994). Children with DCD do not show specific signs of neuropathology or neurological insults, as are seen in children with DS. Furthermore, clumsiness may also be present in children with attention-deficit/hyperactivity disorder (ADHD) and specific learning disability (SLD). Imaging performed during activity (positron emission tomography [PET] scans and functional magnetic resonance imaging [MRI]) can now be used to diagnose ADHD and SLD. Current findings suggest problems in the basal ganglia and cerebellum (Born & Lou, 1999; Krageloh-Mann et al., 1999). Based on the function of these areas for motor control, problems with appropriate force production, timing of muscle activity, forming perceptions based on sensory input, and motor learning could be expected. Studies of children born prematurely suggest that damage to the CNS leading to DCD most likely occurs in the last trimester. Problems may occur with the final "wiring" during the neural migration and organization of the CNS, and may be accentuated by other environmental issues after birth (Hadders-Algra & Lindahl, 1999). The children with DCD are varied in terms of the specific motor skill problems they manifest and the severity of the disorder. Motor performance in daily activities is clumsy and below age expectations (Dewey & Wilson, 2001). Often there is poor performance in sports and handwriting. Many other labels have been given to children presenting with this disorder, such as apraxia, minimal brain dysfunction, clumsy child, developmental dyspraxia, motor coordination or learning problems, motor-perception dysfunction, physically awkward child, sensory integrative dysfunction, deficits in attention–motor control–perception (DAMP), and visuo-motor disabilities (Christiansen, 2000; Missiuna & Polatajko, 1995). These motor skill differences need to be differentiated from the maturational delay and normal variance that exist in the development of children's motor skill ability, which would not lead to a diagnosis of DCD

(Davies & Rose, 2000). Identifying children with DCD can be difficult, and the therapist needs to use clinical reasoning in conjunction with results from standardized tests (Crawford, Wilson, & Dewey, 2001). A diagnosis of DCD suggests that there is a specific motor disorder and professional intervention may be of assistance to the child (Dewey & Wilson, 2001). Sometimes the motor problems are accompanied by SLD and/or ADHD. Comorbidity of DCD with SLD is reported to be as high as 70%, and 75% of children with SLD also have ADHD. A number of children show symptoms of all three disorders (Polatajko, 1999).

Impairments of Body Structures and Functions Related to Motor Performance

Children with DCD show "soft" signs of neurological impairments, such as associated movements (unwanted movements that occur in unison with the desired primary movement); mild hypotonia and muscle weakness, especially in the hands; poor postural control; problems with motor coordination; and delayed acquisition of motor milestones (Christiansen, 2000; Cratty, 1994; David, 2000; Hadders Algra & Lindahl, 1999; Polatajko, 1999; Schoemaker, Hijlkema & Kalverboer, 1994; Sugden & Keogh, 1990) (Figure 6–2). Identification of the underlying neurological processes purportedly involved has been inconclusive. Theories for the postural and motor coordination problems have revolved around (1) poor processing of sensory systems, specifically the visual, somatosensory (proprioceptive and cutaneous), and vestibular systems (Horak, Shumway-Cook, Crowe, & Black, 1988; Rosblad & Von Hofsten, 1994; Willoughby & Polatajko, 1995); (2) poor integration and modulation of these sensory inputs for coordinating motor output (Mangeot et al., 2001; Willoughby & Polatajko, 1995); (3) less precise (force control) and consistent (timing control) motor output (Henderson, Rose, & Henderson, 1992; Missiuna, 1994); and (4) other CNS information-processing problems related to motor planning and memory (Horak et al., 1988; Skorji & McKenzie, 1997; van Dellen & Geuze, 1988; Wilson & McKenzie, 1998). The limited support from research studies for these theories may be because the diagnosis and etiology of DCD are poorly understood and appear so variable.

Restrictions in Activities and Participation

Functionally, children with DCD reach all of the typical motor milestones and complete most activities independently. However, tasks that are sometimes delayed in acquisition include (1) fine motor sequencing tasks, such as handwriting and tying shoelaces; (2) complex coordination tasks, such as skipping, and performing two different gross motor tasks in close succession, such as dribbling a soccer ball and then transitioning to kick for the goal; and (3) learning new tasks that require integration of sensory input and motor planning, such as climbing on playground structures. Longitudinal studies of children with DCD suggest some problems may decrease, although they usually do not disappear totally (Cantell, Smith, & Ahonen, 1994; Christiansen, 2000; Fox & Lent, 1996; Gillberg, 1988, 1999). Some adolescents with DCD continue to have low academic achievement, few hobbies, poor self-esteem, poor athletic competence, less participation in community sports, and low aspirations for future endeavors (Cantell et al., 1994).

Associated Medical Issues

Hyperactivity and problems focusing attention are common in children with DCD. Stimulant medications, such as Ritalin and Concerta, are often prescribed to increase attention span and thus improve learning. These medications can influence motor behavior by increasing the awareness of obstacles, therefore decreasing tripping and falling. Abnormalities in sensory modulation capability have been found in a subgroup of children with ADHD, and these sensory problems correlated with problems in emotional and attentional behavior (Mangeot et al., 2001). Specifically, children might have problems following directions and with behavioral control, leading to excessive frustration, low self-esteem, and depression (David, 2000; Gubbay, 1975; Hulme & Lord, 1986). As the child ages, these emotional issues may become more apparent and interfere with learning and function (Cantell et al., 1994; Christiansen, 2000; Gillberg, 1988; Rasmussen & Gillberg, 1999).

Potential Interventions

Interventions from a motor-learning perspective, which accentuate the use of augmented feedback for learning, memory cues, and practice in varied environments, may assist with improving functional and sports motor behaviors (David, 2000; Mandich, Polatajko, Macnab, & Miller, 2001; Mandich, Polatajko, Missiuna, & Miller, 2001; Missiuna, 2001; Polatajko, Mandich, Miller, & Macnab, 2001; Schoemaker et al., 1994). Assistance to make the child more successful and happy should include collaboration and consultation with the child, family, and other team members to (1) explain the nature of the disorder, (2) provide strategies for controlling sensory input to make learning more successful, and (3) devise appropriate consis-

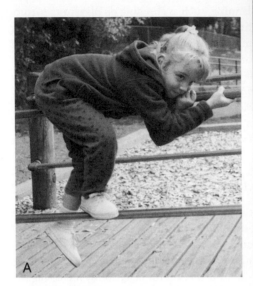
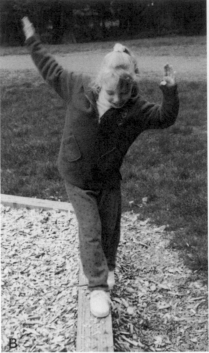
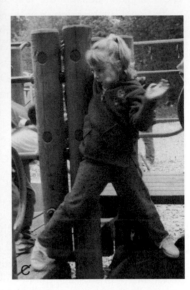

Figure 6-2 Child with a developmental coordination disorder. *(A)* This 5-year-old child was asked to climb up on the railing and take sidesteps along it. Note that the child stays as low as possible and wraps herself around the bar because of poor postural control and perceptual problems affecting motor planning for achieving the task. *(B)* When asked to walk along a 6-inch-wide board that is approximately 4 inches off the ground, she has problems maintaining her balance. *(C)* When the child is attempting to move from one level of the climber to another over the tire, a task requiring motor planning and postural control, you note an awkward position because of her need to continue to hold onto the structure for balance, and a protruding tongue in her cheek.

tent behavioral consequences to support the child in trying activities (Fisher, Murray, & Bundy, 1991; Gubbay, 1975; Harris, 1995).

Acquired Nonprogressive Disorders of the Central Nervous System (Patterns 5C and 5D)

Insults to the fetus' CNS can preferentially damage different structures based on the timing of the injury (Nickel, 1992). From 22 to 25 weeks' gestation is described as approximately the youngest survival age in babies born prematurely (Chan et al., 2001). By 24 weeks' gestation, the major structures of the brain are present. Infants who are born prematurely as a result of maternal problems versus a previous insult to the fetus are also at great risk for postbirth brain damage attributable to an immature cardiopulmonary system. A lack of oxygen to tissue in the brain can easily occur from relatively minor stress to the infant's system; therefore, the neonatal intensive care unit environment needs to be carefully controlled. Several terms are used to describe changes in oxygen to the brain. **Hypoxemia** is a decrease in the amount of oxygen in the blood. **Ischemia** is decreased perfusion to a tissue bed such as the brain. Often, hypoxemia and ischemia occur simultaneously or follow one another in premature infants. **Asphyxia** is the most severe lack of oxygen and by definition means "without pulse" (Rivkin, 1997; Volpe, 1995). Prolonged or sustained asphyxia generally results in hypotension and ischemia causing cellular death, which usually leads to permanent disability (Barkovich & Truit, 1990).

Selective neuronal necrosis in the full-term infant is a neuronal injury with a characteristic pattern in the CNS (Rivkin, 1997; Volpe, 1995). Early neuronal changes occur within 24 to 36 hours, with signs of cell necrosis within several days. Over the next several weeks, macrophages consume the necrotic cells. With severe lesions, a cavity may form in the cerebral cortex that becomes a fluid-filled cyst. The neurons in the cerebral cortex and the hippocampus are vulnerable to hypoxic ischemic insults. With severe injury, there is diffuse involvement of the cerebral cortex. Additional areas of the CNS commonly affected by selective neuronal necrosis are the basal ganglia, thalamus, brainstem, cerebellum, and spinal cord. All of these lead to motor disorders, dependent on the exact location of the lesion. Long-term neurological sequelae include cognitive impairments, spastic motor deficits, seizure disorders, visual impairments, and impairments of sucking, swallowing, and facial movements (Volpe, 1995).

Abnormal development of brain structures, lack of oxygen during early development, unknown genetic alterations causing neurological malformations or insults and trauma to the head, or lack of oxygen at or around birth can all lead to a diagnosis of cerebral palsy (Mutch, Alberman, Hagberg, Kodama, & Perat, 1992). Lesions are generally not well defined. The cortex, subcortical nuclei, cerebellum, and basal ganglia are the major areas of the brain involved in movement generation and control. The importance of these areas is summarized in Table 6.2.

Periventricular leukomalacia (PVL) is the primary ischemic lesion of the preterm infant (Rivkin, 1997; Volpe,

Table 6.2 Major Motor Control Functions of the Cerebellum, Basal Ganglia, and Cerebral Cortex

Area of the Brain	Inputs to Area	Outputs to Other Areas	Disorders in Humans with Lesions/Diseases	Motor Control and Learning Function

Cerebellum
Vestibulocerebellum:
  fastigial nuclei
Spinocerebellum:
  interpositus nuclei
  and dentate nuclei
	Vestibular nuclei
	Mossy fibers—
	  ascending and
	  descending
	  information
	Climbing fibers—
	  inferior olive
	  nuclei
		Via Purkinje cell to
		  cerebellar nuclei to:
		• *Vestibular nuclei* to
		  vestibulospinal tract
		  and vestibuloocular
		  tract
		• *Reticular formation*
		  to reticulospinal tract
		• *Red nucleus* to
		  rubrospinal tract and
		  olive
		• *VPL thalamus* to
		  cortex to corti-
		  cospinal tract
			Dysmetria (over/under-
			  shoot target)
			Dysdiadochokinesia
			  (inability to move with
			  a constant rhythm)
			Hypotonia
			Asynergia (impairment in
			  interjoint coordination)
			Kinetic tremors (during
			  voluntary movement)
			Intentional tremors (on
			  approach to target)
			Postural tremors (in
			  maintaining constant
			  position)
				Postural control
				Eye-head and eye-body
				  control
				Integration of sensory
				  input to affect
				  descending systems
				  for smooth volitional
				  multijoint movements
				Planning and
				  preparation for
				  movement
				Possible role in motor
				  learning and storage
				  of motor programs

Basal Ganglia
Paleostriatum:
  globus pallidus
Striatum:
  caudate and
  putamen
Subthalamic:
  substantia nigra
	Cerebral cortex:
	  primary motor,
	  premotor,
	  supplementary
	  motor, superior
	  parietal,
	  somatosensory
	Limbic structures:
	  hypothalamus,
	  fornix,
	  hippocampus,
	  amygdaloid,
	  cingulate gyrus
	  of cerebral
	  cortex
		Inhibition from globus
		  pallidus and excita-
		  tion from substantia
		  nigra to *VL of thala-*
		  mus to premotor and
		  supplementary motor
		  cerebral cortex to
		  motor cortex to
		  corticospinal tract
		  and other descend-
		  ing tracts
		Superior colliculi to
		  ocular areas
			Thalamic output to
			  cortex reduced, leads
			  to:
			• *Hypokinesias*: bradyki-
			  nesia (slow movement,
			  prolonged reaction
			  time); involuntary
			  tremor; rigidity;
			  postural deficits
			• *Dystonia*: sustained
			  postures of neck,
			  trunk, and limbs
			Thalamic output to
			  cortex increased, leads
			  to:
			• *Hyperkinesias*: chorea,
			  ballism (excessive
			  movement)
				Oculomotor control
				Movement initiation:
				  disinhibit areas of
				  motor cortex and
				  turn off postural
				  activity allowing
				  movement to occur
				Movement
				  coordination:
				  sequencing move-
				  ment fragments;
				  coordinate move-
				  ments in
				  parallel

(Continued)

Table 6.2 Major Motor Control Functions of the Cerebellum, Basal Ganglia, and Cerebral Cortex *(Continued)*

Area of the Brain	Inputs to Area	Outputs to Other Areas	Disorders in Humans with Lesions/Diseases	Motor Control and Learning Function
Cerebral Cortex Primary motor cortex (Brodmann's area 4) Somatosensory cortex (area 3) Premotor cortex (area 6): premotor and supplementary motor areas	Via thalamus from: *Spinal cord; basal ganglia; cerebellum* *Other cerebral cortex areas:* (particularly parietal and frontal)	*Cerebral cortex:* ipsilateral and contralateral sensory, motor, and other cortical areas *Basal ganglia* *Cerebellum* via pons *Red nuclei* *Reticular formation* *Spinal cord* via corticospinal tract	*Paralysis* *Spasticity*	*Perceiving and interpreting sensory information* *Making conscious decisions and generation of movements* *Controlling voluntary movement;* encoding direction of movement; control of movements in opposite directions, control of co-contraction (joint stiffness)

Source: Condensed from Cohen, H. (1999). *Neuroscience for rehabilitation* (2nd ed.). Philadelphia: Lippincott Williams & Wilkins; Latash, M.L. (1998c). *Neurophysiological basis of movement* (pp. 98–105). Champaign, IL: Human Kinetics; Leonard, C.T. (1998). *The neuroscience of human movement* (pp. 124–128). St. Louis: Mosby-Year Book; Lundy-Ekman, L. (1998). *Neuroscience: Fundamentals for rehabilitation* (pp. 69–84). Philadelphia: W.B. Saunders.

1995; Zupan et al., 1996). The highest incidence of cystic PVL (cysts form where neural tissue should be) occurs in infants born at 27 to 30 weeks' gestational age. PVL is located in the white matter and is usually more likely to injure the motor tracts of the lower extremities than those of the upper extremities at the border zones, or the watershed areas of the arterial circulation (Volpe, 1997). *Watershed regions* or *border zones* are terms used to describe the location between the end fields of the anterior, middle, and posterior cerebral arteries. The degree of ischemia needed to cause PVL varies as a function of gestational age and the development of the arterial circulation. The most common long-term motor outcome of PVL is spastic (hypertonic) diplegic (primarily lower extremities) cerebral palsy (Volpe, 1997).

Cerebral Palsy

Children with cerebral palsy (CP) have motor disability related to early damage of the brain in areas controlling motor behaviors. Different patterns of dyscontrol can be observed dependent on the etiology, location, and extent of the insult. Although the lesion does not progress, the sequelae may vary as the child ages as a result of the devel-

opment of atypical motor habits used by the children to compensate for poor motor and postural control, and motor learning deficits. Because movement is difficult, these children also tend to move less and develop poor cardiovascular fitness.

Classification of children with CP is very difficult. Historically, children with CP were classified by the *distribution* of the motor disability. Quadriplegia signified that all limbs were involved; hemiplegia, one side was involved; and diplegia, when primarily the lower extremities were involved, as seen in Figure 6–3. The figure legend notes the subtle differences that can be observed even from a still photograph. Differences in the body areas affected by CP become more apparent when the child is moving or stressed. The distributions can indicate the location of the lesion and sometimes the time the lesion occurred. This is based on the changing vulnerability of tissues in the developing fetus and infant. Although this classification system sounds simple, the actual determination of classification is controversial. Frequently there are subtle motor problems in all extremities and definite asymmetrical distributions of movement dysfunction.

A second classification method indicates the *type of muscle* tone or motor control disorder. Categories include

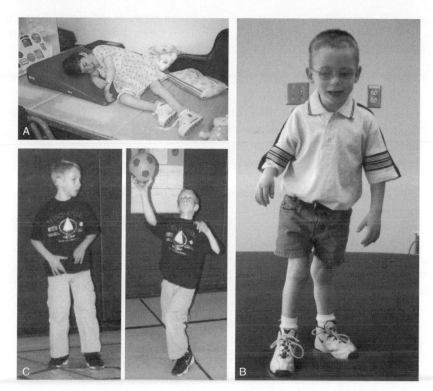

Figure 6-3 Children with cerebral palsy. *(A)* Child with spastic quadriplegia. Note the flexion at the head, shoulders, elbows, wrists, fingers, and trunk, and the positioning of the legs into extension on one side and flexion on the other. The child recently had adductor and hamstring muscle release surgery. This child has no voluntary movement. Bilateral ankle-foot orthoses (AFOs) hold her feet in a neutral position. *(B)* Child with spastic diplegia. Although the legs are more involved than the arms, the right upper extremity is also involved. Note the slight arm flexion greater on the right, the slight forward lean of the trunk, the hyperextension in both legs, and increased weight bearing on the left. Feet are flat on the surface with the use of AFOs. Another typical posture of a child with spastic diplegia would be with bilateral knee flexion, hip internal rotation, and weight bearing on toes bilaterally. *(C left)* Child with a mild left spastic hemiplegia. Left arm and leg show increased muscle tone through posturing of the left arm in greater elbow flexion than the right, and the thumb abducted into the palm of the hand; the left leg is also slightly flexed at the knee; and weight is borne on the ball of the foot only, the heel held off the surface. *(C right)* This weight-bearing posture is exaggerated when he exerts himself to catch a ball.

(1) hypertonia with subclassifications of rigidity (very stiff, minimal movement) and spasticity (high muscle tone but able to move), (2) hypotonia, (3) athetosis, and (4) ataxia (Olney & Wright, 2000). Children with CP have also been classified based on the *degree of movement disorder*, such as mild, moderate, or severe.

The reliability of these classifications is thought to be poor. Fluctuations in the behavioral state of the child (i.e., whether happy or sad, excited or disinterested) can affect muscle tone. Children also generally present with a mixture of tonal symptoms depending on the location of the original neurological insult. It is very common to find children with hypotonic trunk muscles and hypertonic extremity muscles. Muscle tone in different body areas can vary

depending on the position in which the child is tested; for example, generally there is higher extensor tone when the child is in supine compared with prone, perhaps because of the additional muscle activation caused by one of the primitive reflex pathways (tonic labyrinthine reflex). Research has also shown that measurements of muscle tone through examination of passive movement do not necessarily reflect what is observed during active movement by the child (Crenna, 1998, 1999; Holt, Butcher, & Fonseca, 2000). This difference is hypothesized to be caused by neurological differences and to the child actively co-contracting or "fixing" muscles to compensate for muscle weakness and poor postural control. This compensatory technique, "fixing," is also used by the typically developing child when learning new movements. A child will co-contract agonist and antagonist muscles to freeze or decrease the degrees of freedom to be controlled during early attempts to perform a motor skill (Damiano, 1993; Vereijken, van Emmerick, Whiting, & Newell, 1992). After practice, the child will learn to release the co-contractions to allow more free or variable, and thus more adaptive, movement. The child with CP may learn to use this technique exclusively and become fixed at this learning stage. Adaptive changes from only using this movement method can further exacerbate muscle weakness, joint contractures, and poor postural and prime movement control. New ways to document active muscle tone are currently being developed and are described under the Examination Section.

Another system to classify children with CP who are 3 to 12 years old is the *Gross Motor Classification System for Children with Cerebral Palsy* (Palisano et al., 1997). The severity of motor disability is rated on a 5-point scale that designates the functional mobility of the child (Table 6.3). This system may be more reliable and valid than other systems because the rater is making a judgment on functional ability rather than trying to classify by neurological symptoms (Beckung & Hagberg, 2000; Wood & Rosenbaum, 2000).

Table 6.3 Gross Motor Function Classification System for Cerebral Palsy

Level	Definition
I	Walks without restrictions; limitations in more advanced gross motor skills
II	Walks without assistive devices; limitations walking outdoors and in the community
III	Walks with assistive devices; limitations walking outdoors and in the community
IV	Self-mobility with limitations; children are transported or use power mobility outdoors and in the community
V	Self-mobility is severely limited, even with the use of assistive technology

Source: Palisano, R., Rosenbaum, P., Walter, S., Russell, D., Wood, E., & Galuppi, B. (1997). The development and reliability of a system to classify gross motor function in children with cerebral palsy. *Developmental Medicine and Child Neurology, 39,* 214–223, with permission.

Impairments of Body Structures and Functions Related to Motor Performance

The specific motor control impairments of children with CP are variable. The child may show paresis or less-than-normal EMG activity in muscles during movement (Dietz, Ketelson, Berger, & Quintern, 1986). The child could present with hypertonia as evidenced by greater EMG activity, higher spikes, and prolonged muscle activation, causing a decrease in passive range of movement (ROM) (Berger, Quintern, & Dietz, 1982; Dietz & Berger, 1983; Dietz, Quintern, & Berger, 1981; Lin, Brown, & Brotherstone, 1994). The child could show increased muscle co-contractions ("fixing") as evidenced by a temporary excessive simultaneous EMG activity in the agonist and antagonist muscles. These co-contractions can also be accompanied by an increased activation of adjacent agonists that are not necessary to complete the specific movement (El-Abd, Ibrahim, & Dietz, 1993; Fellows, Kaus, Ross, & Thilmann, 1994; Leonard, Moritani, Hirschfeld, & Forssberg, 1990). This hinders free variable movement. Finally, the child could show spasticity as evidenced by increased EMG activity during muscle stretch (Leonard, 1994). Because of some or all of these differences in motor control, the child with CP has abnormal timing and muscle activation patterns. This can cause the (1) initiation of movement to be delayed, (2) rate of force development to be slowed down, (3) muscle contraction time to be prolonged, and (4) timing of agonist to antagonist activation to be disrupted. Extremity movements appear slow and stiff and are coarse. That is, when trying to perform the primary movement, the child moves in mass flexion or extension patterns without being able to dissociate individual limb or joint movements. Development and use of reactive and anticipatory postural control also appear to be delayed and not integrated with the prime movement (Hadders-Algra, Brogen, Katz-Salamon, & Forssberg, 1999; Nashner, Shumway-Cook, & Marin, 1983; Woollacott et al., 1998). In standing, children with CP may lower their center of gravity by flexing the knees, with the feet in either excessive dorsiflexion or plantar flexion (Lowes, 1996). Co-contraction or immature activation of the lower extremity muscles is used for stability when perturbed by an externally or internally (the child's own movement) generated stimulus (Woollacott et al., 1998; Liu, 2001; Westcott et al. 1998a, 1998b; Zaino, 1999). The use of ankle and hip strategies depends on the environmental situation, with a preponderance to use proximal muscles first or just show mass co-contraction when perturbed (Hadders-Algra et al., 1999; Nashner et al., 1983). The biomechanical position, alone, also has been shown to influence the postural control activity of the child. Children without disability who position themselves in the crouched position will show postural muscle activity similar to that of children with CP when perturbed (Potter, Kirby, & MacLeod, 1990; Woollacott et al., 1998). Use of ankle-foot orthoses that control the foot position but allow some movement at the ankle seems to help the child with CP to establish more adaptable coordination patterns for postural control (Burtner, Woollacott, & Qualls, 1999; Woollacott et al., 1998).

Besides these neurological control issues, the child might eventually show musculoskeletal changes, such as weakness or inability to produce adequate muscle force, loss of type 2 high force–producing motor units, and tightness in the collagen tissue of the muscles, joints, and ligaments caused by limited movement (Booth, Cortina-Borja, & Theologis, 2001; Dietz & Berger, 1983; Dietz et al., 1981, 1986; Lin, Brown, & Walsh, 1994). These secondary changes further limit movement ability and endurance for activity. Also, less movement sets up the child for problems with osteoporosis caused by less weight bearing and decreased endurance caused by little activity (Chad et al., 2000).

These motor issues can be compounded by problems with sensory systems. Proprioception, vision, and vestibular information and the integration of this information to guide movement are often compromised in the child with CP. Therefore, the feedback the child is getting from the movement may be inaccurate, delayed, and/or insufficient for assisting with learning more coordinated movement.

Restrictions in Activities and Participation

Functionally, children with CP have difficulty with maintaining postural control in stationary postures, such as sitting and standing; transitional movements between supine, prone, sit, and stand; functional mobility; and more complex movement and athletic skills. They may have oral motor control problems resulting in feeding and speech disorders. Lack of practice with movement can decrease the child's movement experiences and learning opportunities. Because of the diffuse nature of the original lesion, difficulty with motor development may be compounded by the coexistence of cognitive impairment and sensory disorders (visual and/or hearing impairments). Cognitive impairments may affect the child's ability to understand the purpose of intervention and motivation to practice movement. Visual and hearing impairments limit the avenues for communication and community participation.

Associated Medical Issues

Because of the brain insult, children with CP often have a range of seizure disorders. Therapists need to monitor the occurrences of seizures, protect the child from external injury caused by the involuntary movement associated with the seizure, and watch for respiratory or cardiac problems during the seizure. If seizures are increasing, the child's family and physician should be contacted because increased brain damage might occur with every seizure. Most seizure disorders are pharmacologically controlled by medications such as Dilantin and Tegretol. Some medications cause the child to appear sedated. Caution should be taken with vestibular stimulation (swinging, spinning, and so on) in children with seizure disorders as this movement might trigger a seizure.

Potential Interventions

The limitations and restrictions that a child with CP might have include the mildest of minor gait deviations to the total inability to perform any activity of daily living (ADLs). Therefore, the range of interventions is equally diverse. As always, the physical therapist must coordinate and communicate with all other service providers as a member of an interdisciplinary team serving the needs of the child and family. The therapist will document that communication and the results of interventions. The parents and child will be instructed in an intervention program as appropriate. The family will frequently be instructed in how to maintain range of motion (ROM), increase strength, and encourage activities and participation within the child's ability levels. The specific procedural interventions to alter the child's motor control, to prevent or improve secondary impairments, to provide adequate sensory feedback to enhance motor learning, and to teach more flexible and functional motor patterns and skills are discussed in Chapter 7. Because many children with CP also have musculoskeletal and cardiopulmonary limitations, these areas must also be addressed, as presented in Chapters 4, 5, and 8. Many children with CP need to use assistive devices for mobility and other aids for ADLs, which are included in Chapters 16 and 17. A case study of a child with CP from birth to young adulthood is presented in Chapter 18.

Traumatic Brain Injury

Traumatic brain injury (TBI) occurs in more than 1.5 million people every year in the United States. Based on a

National Institutes of Health consensus statement (1998), the highest incidence is among persons aged 15 to 24 years, with another peak in incidence in children aged 5 years or younger. An analysis of U.S. emergency department data from 1992 to 1994 showed the highest overall incidence of TBI—1019 per 100,000—to have occurred in the younger-than-5-years age group (Jager, Weiss, Coben, & Pepe, 2000). Males were also more likely to be injured than were females. The injuries can be caused by falls, motor vehicle accidents, sports injuries, and other accidental or intentional blows to the head. The child can receive many musculoskeletal and vital organ injuries concomitant with the blow to the head. No head injury is exactly the same as another. Thus, examination and intervention for children with TBI are variable and complex.

Damage to the brain in closed head TBI occurs focally, from the point of impact, and diffusely, through the reverberations that occur to the brain within the cranium or shearing forces caused after the initial blow (Blaskey & Jennings, 1999; Geddes et al., 2001). Ischemic damage can also occur after the initial trauma if the child stops breathing (Geddes et al., 2001). Cerebral edema occurs after damage to brain cells and can destroy remaining unharmed brain tissue if left uncontrolled. Shunting procedures to relieve intracranial pressure can be used to improve outcomes for the child (DeLuca et al., 2000; Downard et al., 2000; Munch et al., 2000). Pharmacological agents are also used to control postinjury trauma caused by increased intracranial pressure, and later inflammation of tissues (Fulop, Wright, & Stein, 1998).

Impairments of Body Structures and Functions Related to Motor Performance

As a result of the injury, the child is generally comatose for a period of time. In general, the longer the child is comatose, the worse is the final outcome. Two measures are used frequently to rate coma state: the Glasgow Coma Scale (Teasdale & Jennett, 1974) and the Rancho Los Amigos Pediatric Levels of Consciousness for Infants, Preschoolers, and School-Age Children Scale adapted from the adult Rancho Levels of Cognitive Functioning Scale (Table 6.4) (Professional Staff Rancho Los Amigos Hospital, 1982). Both scales are used to rate the child's responses to sensory stimuli from pain to verbal commands, as well as to examine the child's understanding of time and circumstances. Directions for rating on the Rancho Children's Scale vary based on expectations as a result of age and normal cogni-

tive levels. A child is classified into one of five levels, with greater arousal and orientation described by the higher levels. An adult version of the scale can be used for older children (Hagan, 1998).

After the child gains consciousness, varying signs of motor and cognitive problems will be present, depending on the location of focal or diffuse brain damage. Within a relatively short period of time, on average 3 weeks, most, but not all, children with TBI can recover to preinjury functional motor status (Chaplin, Deitz, & Jaffe, 1993). However, cognitive and behavioral differences from the preinjury state often persist throughout the child's life (Coster, Haley, & Baryza, 1994; Jaffe, Polissar, Fay, & Liao, 1995; Whitlock & Hamilton, 1995).

Common impairments of body structures and functions related to movements that the child with TBI may show include spasticity, ataxia, musculoskeletal contractures, paralysis or muscle weakness, and difficulty with increasing speed of movement. These problems affect speech movements as well as other general movements (Chaplin et al., 1993; Haley, Cioffi, Lewin, & Baryza, 1990). Examination and intervention for these impairments can be the same as those used for similar impairments in children with DS and CP.

Postural control problems, specifically ataxia, are common in children with TBI (Haley et al., 1990). The children demonstrate difficulty grading their postural control to the task and environmental constraints. Both sensory and motor systems for postural control are compromised. Specifically, children with TBI who show ataxia generally have slow responses to perturbations, which are potentially caused by vestibular and sensory organization problems (Vatovec, Velikovic, Smid, Brenk, & Zargi, 2001) and the use of too much force (higher amplitude of EMG activity) when they respond. They also show abnormal spatial and temporal coordination of the postural synergies. These coordination problems are hypothesized to be caused by damage of the stored synergy motor programs, possibly in the cerebellum, and secondary musculoskeletal constraints, such as contractures that change the biomechanics of the child's movements.

Restrictions in Activities and Participation

Children with TBI can have a variety of limitations in movement that influence activities. These are dependent on concomitant injuries, but in general, they show relatively rapid improvements in ambulation and motor ability to

Table 6.4 Rancho Los Amigos Pediatric Levels of Consciousness Scale for Infants, Preschoolers, and School-Age Children

Level	Definition		
	Infants (6 Months to 2 Years)	Preschoolers (2 to 5 Years)	School-Age Children (5 Years and Older)
I	Interacts with environment a. Shows active interest in toys; manipulates or examines before mouthing or discarding b. Watches other children at play; may move toward them purposefully c. Initiates social contact with adults; enjoys socializing d. Shows active interest in bottle e. Reaches or moves toward person or object	Oriented to self and surroundings a. Provides accurate information about self b. Knows he or she is away from home c. Knows where toys, clothes, and so on, are kept d. Actively participates in treatment program e. Recognizes own room, knows way to bathroom, nursing station, and so on f. Is potty trained g. Initiates social contact with adults; enjoys socializing	Oriented to time and place; records ongoing events a. Provides accurate, detailed information about self and present situation b. Knows way to and from daily activities c. Knows sequence of daily routine d. Knows way around unit; recognizes own room e. Finds own bed; knows where personal belongings are kept f. Is bowel and bladder trained
II	Demonstrates awareness of environment a. Responds to name b. Recognizes mother or other family members c. Enjoys imitative vocal play d. Giggles or smiles when talked to or played with e. Fussing is quieted by soft voice or touch	Is responsive to environment a. Follows simple commands b. Refuses to follow commands by shaking head or saying "no" c. Imitates examiner's gestures or facial expressions d. Responds to name e. Recognizes mother or other family members f. Enjoys imitative vocal play	Is responsive to environment a. Follows simple verbal or gestured requests b. Initiates purposeful activity c. Actively participates in therapy program d. Refuses to follow request by shaking head or saying "no" e. Imitates examiner's gestures or facial expressions
III	Gives localized response to sensory stimuli a. Blinks when strong light crosses field of vision b. Follows moving object passed within field of vision c. Turns toward or away from loud sound d. Gives localized response to painful stimuli		
IV	Gives generalized response to sensory stimuli a. Gives generalized startle to loud sound b. Responds to repeated auditory stimulation with increased or decreased activity c. Gives generalized reflex response to painful stimuli		
V	No response to stimuli a. Complete absence of observable change in behavior to visual, auditory, or painful stimuli		

Source: Blaskey, J., & Jennings, M.C. (1999). Traumatic brain injury. In S.K. Campbell (Ed.), *Decision making in pediatric neurologic physical therapy* (pp. 84–139). Philadelphia: Churchill Livingstone, with permission.

complete ADLs (Chaplin et al., 1993; Haley et al., 1990). Subtle problems with functional movement may be affected by sensory and cognitive problems. Specifically, the child may have difficulty with the cognitive components related to movement, such as focussing attention, understanding verbal directions, and planning motor responses. For example, you might invoke an automatic motor response of arm movement by throwing a ball to the child, causing a functional catching response. The same movement can not be invoked with a verbal command to reach out. Hypothetically, this occurs because the cognitive planning of the volitional movement is disrupted as a result of frontal lobe damage. However, the lower motor centers (rubrospinal, reticulospinal, and vestibulospinal) can still invoke a normal motor reaction. Higher-level sports-related activities requiring complex motor planning, coordination, and postural control, such as jump-rope games or basketball, may continue to be difficult. Children with TBI also run the risk of becoming sedentary, causing lower levels of fitness. Encouragement to find an activity that the child enjoys will assist in maintenance and improvement of fitness levels.

Associated Medical Issues

Because of inactivity during the initial comatose state after the injury, children with TBI can show problems with hypertension. The blood pressure level generally will return to normal with neurological improvement. Once the child is mobile, problems with circulatory and ventilatory efficiency may also be seen. These are hypothesized to be caused by brainstem disturbances from the injury (Becker, Bar-Or, Mendelson, & Najenson, 1978; Sullivan, Richer, & Laurent 1990). These cardiopulmonary issues should be monitored and controlled for during examination and intervention.

Most children with TBI show some cognitive, emotional, and behavioral control problems during rehabilitation, attributed to the susceptibility of the frontal and temporal lobes to shearing force damage (Kirkwood et al., 2000; Vargha-Khadem, 2001). These problems can include hyperactivity, distractibility involving poor ability to filter out unimportant sensory stimuli in the environment, and difficulty with auditory and visual perception (Fay et al., 1994; Telzrow, 1987). Personality changes may include poor control of frustration and anger and difficulty with social judgment. Some of these problems may be reduced with drug therapies (Hornyak, Nelson, & Hurvitz, 1997). Overall, intellectual levels and memory ability of the child may also decrease from preinjury status (Bowen et al.,

1997; Ewing-Cobs et al., 1997; Jaffe et al., 1995), and the child often requires referral for special education programs on return to school.

Potential Interventions

Physical therapy interventions when the child is comatose include maintenance of ROM and stimulation of the senses through sensory inputs: cutaneous (brushing and tapping), auditory (talking and music), visual (use of lights and bright-colored objects), gustatory (introduction of different tastes—bitter, sweet—to the tongue), and olfactory (introduction of different odors—spices, flower scents—to the nose). The stimulation of the senses might trigger the child to come out of the coma. As the child is coming out of the coma, the therapist should request active movement by the child in response to the passive ROM and sensory stimuli.

Although intervention for children after TBI can be rewarding because of the changes in functional ability, the challenges are great, reflecting the complexity of neurological problems related to cognitive ability and behavioral control. We must work as a team with the child and family to determine and employ appropriate behavior management strategies. A structured environment, cues for improving functional memory, and consistency in responses to behavioral outbursts all facilitate the rehabilitation process (Sullivan, 1998). For example, a consistent daily routine should be developed that can be learned by the child. The younger child can have a schedule of activities depicted via pictures. The older child who can read can be given, or be taught to create, a written schedule to improve independent adherence to daily activities. When the child becomes frustrated or angry, consistent consequences should be used by everyone involved with the child. The consequences may range from warnings and then loss of rewards (such as recess or television privileges) to removal of the child from the activity in a "time-out" for recomposure and then completion of the task that initially provoked the child.

The social and emotional trauma to the family related to the suddenness and cause of the injury can be a challenge for the therapist in providing family-centered care. The children and their families may suffer from depression and guilt over the accident, making motivation for functional progress difficult. A family's behavior may range from ignoring the differences in the child's ability by requesting behaviors that are too difficult for the child, to overprotecting the child and not allowing him or her to work toward independence. These attitudes can vary day to day as acceptance of the child's new situation develops. Counselors and psychologists can assist when the children or families have continued difficulty moving through the stages of acceptance.

The specific procedural interventions used with the child will depend on the extent of limitations in body structures and functions and restrictions in activities and participation. The interventions might be similar to those used for children with CP or DS. Interventions using motor-learning concepts, detailed in Chapter 7, may assist the child to develop better coordination patterns.

Understanding the spinal circuitry is important because common therapeutic interventions are professed to change motor activity by altering sensory input to effect motor output from the spinal cord (Bobath & Bobath, 1984; Stockmeyer, 1967, 1972). For example, tapping or brushing muscles is thought to cause activation of the stimulated muscle. Positioning joint structures, such as stretching the shoulder into external rotation and flexion, has been demonstrated to decrease muscle activation around the joint; and compression of joint structures has been shown to increase contraction of muscles around the joint. These techniques are commonly used interventions for children. Some of these techniques are reviewed in Chapter 7. The primary ascending (dorsal column, spinothalamic, spinocerebellar, and spinoreticular) and descending (reticulospinal, vestibulospinal, rubrospinal, and corticospinal) pathways between the brain and the spinal cord that are involved in the control of movement are shown synthesized in Table 6.5. To understand the neurological reasons for these changes in motor output, readers are encouraged to review neurology texts for the information on circuitry of the stretch reflex, Golgi tendon organ reflex, Renshaw cell loop, flexor reflex afferents (FRA) reflex, reciprocal inhibition, and reciprocal contraction (sometimes referred to as co-contraction).

Intervention based on the use of standard simple input-output relationships of known reflexes to influence motor behavior may not always produce a constant response. The spinal cord circuitry is far more complex than the simple circuitry of the reflexes noted above. The pools of sensory afferents and motor neurons are intricately woven together and are always in some state of excitation or inhibition (Ornstein & Thompson, 1984). Most connections to motor neurons, both alpha and gamma, occur through numerous interneurons. Multiple inputs from the peripheral sensory afferents, descending systems from higher CNS levels, or special senses are always in a state of flux, raising or lowering the likelihood of activation of the interneurons and pools of motor neurons. Variable control of alpha and gamma motor neurons occurs during different types of movements (Hulliger, Durmuller, Prochazka, & Trend, 1989). *Irradiation,* which is the spreading out of input to neighboring neurons, also occurs via propriospinal interneurons that carry input to multiple levels of the spinal cord. Modulation of reflex activity occurs normally during movements, such as gait, depending on the environmental conditions (Stein, Yang, Belanger, & Pearson, 1993). Recent research on the spinal cord circuitry has also shown that the spinal cord may be able to learn (Cheung & Broman, 2000; Hutton, 1984; Little, Burns, James, & Stiens, 2000; Rossignol, 2000; Wolpaw & Tennissen, 2001).

Myelodysplasia

Spina bifida, or "split spine," indicates that bony structures of the spine fail to close over the posterior aspect of the spinal cord at some level or levels during neurulation, around week 3 or 4 of gestation. *Spina bifida*, also referred to as myelodysplasia, is defined as a displacement of some tissue in a sac that protrudes through the posterior opening of the spine. The degree to which neural elements are involved in this protrusion and the level of the spinal cord affected define the severity of the loss of motor and sensory function around and below that level. In **meningocele**, a sac protrudes at the spinal opening containing spinal fluid and meninges but no neural tissues; thus, lower motor neuron damage is unlikely. **Myelomeningocele** (MM) is a condition in which the protruding sac contains spinal fluid, meninges, and neural tissue (Figure 6–4). Either in utero, or very shortly after birth, the protruding tissue is excised and the spinal opening is surgically closed. The etiology of these defects is unknown but is thought to be a combination of genetics and environment. There appears to be a relationship between inadequate vitamin and folic acid intake and neural tube defects such as MM. The open lesions of MM in the fetus can be detected before birth, by measurement of the mother's serum alpha-fetoprotein levels, and by ultrasound, or more invasively by amniocentesis. This information is used to counsel families. The use of cesarean section for delivery is recommended to limit further damage.

Children with MM have a mixture of lower motor neuron and brain dysfunction that affects motor control, learning, and functional motor ability. The severity of these neuromuscular deficits varies depending on the type and amount of tissue involved in the congenital lesion and on complications such as hydrocephalus.

Table 6.5 Central Nervous System Connecting Pathways Between the Brain and Spinal Cord

Pathway	Origin	Destination	Type of Sensory Information	Motor Control and Learning Function
Ascending Central Nervous System Pathways				
Dorsal column	Sensory receptors in skin, joints, and muscles to spinal ganglia	Cuneate and gracile nuclei to cross to opposite ventral posterior lateral nucleus (VPL) of thalamus to cortex; small contribution to the olives to the cerebellum	Touch, pressure, proprioception	Primary and secondary (already processed in the spinal cord) sensory information to cortex for influence on descending cortical system
Spinothalamic	Sensory receptors in skin, joints, and muscles to dorsal and intermediate parts of spinal gray matter	Crosses in spinal cord to VPL of thalamus to cortex; small contribution to reticular formation	Touch, pressure, temperature, pain	Primary and secondary (already processed in the spinal cord) sensory information to cortex for influence on descending cortical system
Spinocerebellar	Sensory receptors in skin, joints, and muscles	Crossed and uncrossed paths to Clarke's column, cuneate nuclei (mossy fibers), olives (climbing fibers) to cerebellar nuclei and cortex	Touch, pressure, proprioception	Primary and secondary sensory information to cerebellum for influencing descending pathways and motor learning
Spinoreticular	Sensory receptors in skin, joints, and muscles	Reticular formation and cerebellar nuclei and cortex (mossy fibers)	Touch, pressure, proprioception	Primary and secondary sensory information to cerebellum for influencing descending pathways and motor learning
Descending Central Nervous System Pathways				
Reticulospinal	Reticular formation	Lateral component—axial and proximal limb extensor muscle excitation Medial component—inhibition extensors, excitation flexors	Diffuse input from all sensory systems, cerebellum, cortex	Postural control, adaptation of postural control to varied environments
Vestibulospinal	Vestibular nuclei	Inhibit flexors and excite axial and limb extensors	Diffuse and specific input from cerebellum and cortex	Postural control and orientation to environment

Pathway	Origin	Destination	Type of Sensory Information	Motor Control and Learning Function
Rubrospinal	Red nucleus	Distal musculature excitation of both flexion and extension	Modulated by input from sensory processing in cortex, cerebellum, and basal ganglia	Prime movement control
Corticospinal	Sensory, motor, premotor cerebral cortex	Distal musculature excitation of both flexion and extension	Modulated by input from sensory processing in cortex and cerebellum	Prime movement control, especially fine movement in hands

Source: Condensed from Cohen, H. (1999). *Neuroscience for rehabilitation* (2nd ed.). Philadelphia: Lippincott Williams & Wilkins; Latash, M.L. (1998c). *Neurophysiological basis of movement* (pp. 98–105). Champaign, IL: Human Kinetics; Leonard, C.T. (1998). *The neuroscience of human movement* (pp. 124–128). St. Louis: Mosby–Year Book; Lundy-Ekman, L. (1998). *Neuroscience: Fundamentals for rehabilitation* (pp. 69–84). Philadelphia: W.B. Saunders.

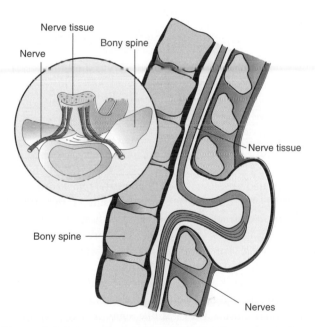

Figure 6-4 Schematic drawing of the myelomeningocele deformity. In this form of myelodysplasia, the sac protruding from the spinal cord contains meninges, spinal fluid, and neural elements, resulting in loss of neural innervation of structures below the level of the sac. (Redrawn from Gram M.C. [1999]. Myelodysplasia (spina bifida). In S.K. Campbell [Ed.], *Decision making in pediatric neurologic physical therapy* [p. 201]. Philadelphia: Churchill Livingstone. Redrawn from Meyers, G.J., Cerone, S.B., & Olson, A.L. [1981]. *A guide for helping the child with spina bifida* [p. 115]. Springfield, IL: Charles C Thomas.)

Labels in figure: Nerve tissue; Nerve; Bony spine; Nerve tissue; Bony spine; Nerves

Impairments of Body Structures and Functions Related to Motor Performance

Impairments of motor control, depending on the area and extent of neural damage, include partial to full paralysis of leg muscles, loss of trunk and leg sensation, orthopedic malalignment caused by muscle imbalances, postural control problems, and impairment of bowel and bladder control (Hinderer, Hinderer, & Shurtleff, 2000). Possible muscle function, common secondary impairments of body structures and functions for children with MM are provided in Table 6.6.

Restrictions in Activities and Participation

Functional motor limitations include problems with development of independent mobility. The degree of limitations is dependent on the spinal lesion level, cognitive ability of the child, and presence of associated medical issues.

Associated Medical Issues

In addition to the impairments of the spinal cord, the brain and other internal structures can also be affected in MM. Approximately 80% of children with myelodysplasia develop hydrocephalus after the primary spinal site is closed. The main cause of hydrocephalus is a congenital

Table 6.6 Muscle Function, Secondary Impairments, and Recommended Orthoses by Lesion Level for Children with Myelomeningocele

	Possible Muscle Function*	Possible Secondary Impairments	Orthoses Needed
T6–12	Upper trunk Non–lower-extremity muscles	Kyphoscoliosis Contractures: hip abduction; hip external rotation Clubfeet	Thoracolumbosacral orthosis (TLSO) Ankle-foot orthosis (AFO) Night splint (leg wraps) Parapodium
L1–3	Hip flexors Hip adductors Minimal knee extensors	Hip flexor contractures Hip dislocation Wind drift Scoliosis	Abduction splint Parapodium, early Hip-knee-ankle-foot orthosis (HKAFO), later
L4 L5	Knee extensors Ankle invertors/dorsiflexors Hip abductors Minimal knee flexors and extensors	Hip flexor contractures Hip dislocation Lumbar lordosis Calcaneovarus	Night splint (abduction) HKAFO Knee-ankle-foot-orthosis or AFO, later
S1–2	Knee flexors Hip extensors Ankle evertors/plantar flexors Toe flexors	Calcaneovarus Toe clawing Heel ulcers	AFO Supramalleolar orthosis (SMO), shoe inserts, or nothing
S3–5	All muscle activity normal	None	None

*Each lesion level has all the muscle power described in the category or categories above it, in addition to that described in the lesion-level box.

Source: Badell, A. (1992). Myelodysplasia. In G.E. Molnar (Ed.), *Pediatric rehabilitation* (2nd ed., p. 222). Baltimore: Williams & Wilkins.

brain malformation known as Arnold-Chiari or Chiari II malformation where the brainstem is displaced inferiorly beyond the foramen magnum, causing partial blockage of the passage of cerebrospinal fluid (CSF) from the brain to the spinal cord. Excessive CSF then builds up in the ventricles, causing pressure on the CNS tissue that can further compromise brain tissue and development. Hydrocephalus needs to be monitored closely and, if noticed, controlled. This is done via placement of a ventricular-peritoneal (V-P) shunt, which is a plastic catheter that routes the excess CSF from the ventricles into the peritoneal cavity where it is harmlessly reabsorbed (Hinderer et al., 2000). The V-P shunt can become clogged, shift, or become dysfunctional because of growth of the child. Children must be monitored closely for shunt failure and, if it is noted, referred immediately to their physician. Signs of shunt failure include headache, nausea, fever not related to a normal illness, increased spasticity in innervated muscles, and increased problems with vision, speech, postural control, or school performance.

Increased pressure of the CSF over the spinal cord, called hydromyelia, can also occur as a result of the Arnold-Chiari malformation. Increased weakness in the upper extremity muscles, particularly the hands, is common in hydromyelia. For example, the child will not have the strength to button and unbutton clothes. Also, as the child grows and develops, the spinal cord may tether as a result of the development of adhesions or bony spurs at the lesion closure site. Possible signs of tethering might include a change in sensation or continence, inability to perform or difficulty performing tasks that the child was previously capable of performing, and reduced activity level tolerance. Both of these conditions can cause changes in muscle tone and further paralysis of previously innervated muscles. Therefore, innervation levels and other signs of changes in status must be routinely monitored, and the child's physician informed so that surgical treatment can be instituted to prevent further damage and impairment.

Impairments in bowel and bladder control are common

because the innervations to these areas are at the sacral level of the spinal cord. Kidney problems may arise caused by difficulty emptying the bladder. Hydronephrosis occurs as a result of a spastic bladder wall and/or a spastic urethral sphincter. The pressure from this spasticity causes urine to reflux toward the kidney. Earlier in the 20th century, this damage was a major cause of death. Management of bowel and bladder secretions is critical to prevent the social problems associated with incontinence. Therapists need to assist the child and family with functional motor skills related to transfers and fine motor skills needed to manage daily bowel and bladder care.

Cognitive and visual perceptual deficits occur often in children with MM, especially in children with hydrocephalus. These deficits usually become apparent as the children are challenged with school work. Some children with MM will also show different verbal abilities in which they tend to "chatter," giving the appearance of understanding; however, when their words are analyzed, they lack meaning. This has been called the "cocktail party syndrome" (Tew, 1979). Therapists need to be aware of these issues to best modify the environment for better learning of motor skills and to provide appropriate exercise programs based on the child's abilities.

Potential Interventions

Children with MM will have a number of complex surgeries during their first few years of life. During this time, the physical therapist will collaborate with the team of professionals serving the child and family. Based on the extent of neural damage, overall goals for intervention would focus on (1) strengthening innervated muscles and teaching the compensatory patterns of movements and postural control necessary for the child to achieve functional movement; (2) prevention of further musculoskeletal problems (lower extremity contractures, osteoarthritis, scoliosis, kyphosis) or pain; and (3) prevention of skin breakdown (decubitus ulcers) caused by excessive pressure over bony protuberances as a result of loss of sensation below the level of the lesion.

The type of mobility encouraged must be individualized according to the child's and/or family's desires, social issues, the child's energy consumption for different types of mobility, and the child's cognitive development (Franks, Palisano, & Darbee, 1991; Knutson & Clark, 1991; Liptak, Shurtleff, Bloss, Baltus-Hebert, & Manitta, 1992; McDonald, Jaffe, Mosca, & Shurtleff, 1991; Park, Song, Vankoski, Moore, & Dias, 1997). Assistance with early mobility should be encouraged as studies of children have linked early mobility to development of some cognitive abilities. Studies including children with MM have shown that certain cognitive abilities, such as depth perception, cause-and-effect links, and object permanence (in which objects are understood to continue to exist even when out of sight), are learned by infants only if they are able to move around in their environment (Campos, Bertenthal, & Kermoian, 1992).

Based on experience and knowledge of the spinal levels of muscle innervation, basic rules for the type of mobility to recommend for children with MM have been developed (Gram, 1999; Sousa, Telzrow, Holm, McCartin, & Shurtleff, 1983) (see Table 6.6). Generally, children with lumbar level lesions should be encouraged to ambulate with appropriate orthoses and assistive devices. Children with higher-level lesions may find this very difficult and rely on wheelchair mobility. Changes in body size, energy expenditure for mobility, postural control, and other needs of children, as they grow, may also affect the type of mobility needed (Bartonek & Saraste, 2001; Cuddeford et al., 1997). For instance, a child who was able to ambulate with crutches may opt to use a wheelchair when moving into high school to negotiate quickly between classes. Because of the difficulty with mobility, children with MM have a tendency toward being sedentary, becoming obese, and having poor physical fitness. These issues should be addressed by the therapist through general counseling and planning for lifelong fitness programs.

Many movements may be controlled by the spinal cord without the need for higher-level CNS input. Cyclical movements, such as walking, are thought to be organized and controlled within the spinal cord to a great extent by networks of sensory and motor neurons called **central pattern generators (CPGs)** (Duysens & Van de Crommert, 1998; Grillner et al., 1995; Grillner & Wallen, 1985). When activated by centers in the brainstem, these complex circuits in the spinal cord can reverberate and continue the activation of the appropriate muscle contractions to perform a cyclical movement such as walking (Figure 6–5). This would then lead to reciprocal movement of the legs without requiring higher CNS input (Clarac, 1991). Although there is controversy about whether CPGs function in humans, the circuitry to run a perpetuating gait movement pattern is known to exist in the spinal cord (Calancie et al., 1995; Dietz, Colombo, & Jensen, 1994). To further support the existence of CPGs in humans, relationships have also been found between reflexive newborn stepping patterns and later walking (Thelen & Whitely-Cooke, 1987).

Activation of these CPGs for walking may be an effective

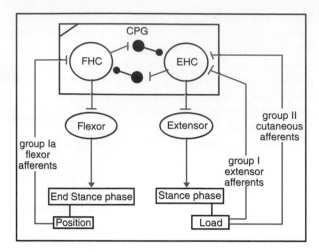

Figure 6-5 Central pattern generator (CPG) proposed circuitry for locomotion. The CPG neurons in the spinal cord consist of an extensor half center (EHC) and flexor half center (FHC) that can inhibit each other. During the stance phase of gait, the loading of the limb excites the EHC, which inhibits the FHC. At the end of the stance phase, excitation of the FHC occurs via afferents, which causes inhibition of the EHC. This back and forth excitation and inhibition is self-stimulating at the spinal cord for production of the locomotion cycle. (Reprinted from *Gait and Posture*, 7, Van de Crommert, H., Mulder, T., & Duysens, J. [1998]. Neural control of locomotion: Sensory control of the central pattern generator and its relation to treadmill training, page 254, Copyright 1998, with permission from Elsevier.)

intervention for children with neuromuscular disability to promote earlier and more coordinated walking. A reciprocal "gait pattern" could be stimulated by setting up the environment to trigger the full gait cycle in a repetitious manner, such as by simply having the child practice walking down a slope so that gravity and inertia assist the walking pattern. Children with spinal cord lesions also may be assisted to relearn to ambulate by external stimulation of the innate circuitry of the CPG located below the level of the lesion. Research using treadmills as an intervention technique, where the moving surface would potentially force the activation of the gait CPGs, is being explored. Positive effects of this intervention have been reported for children with DS and CP (Forssberg & Dietz, 1997; McNevin, Coraci, & Schafer, 2000; Richards et al., 1997; Schindl, Forstner, Kern, & Hesse, 2000; Ulrich et al., 1995, 2001; Van de Crommert, Mulder, & Duysens, 1998; Vereijken & Thelen, 1997; Visintin, Barbeau, Korner-Bitensky, & Mayo, 1998; Wirz, Colombo, & Dietz, 2001).

Abnormal Muscle Tone

Even when we are not voluntarily moving, there is an active "underlying movement" state of muscle contraction, a resting "readiness to move." This state is often referred to as *muscle tone*. Children with Impaired Neuromotor Development (Pattern 5B), or with Acquired Nonprogressive Neuromuscular Disorders (Patterns 5C and 5D) will frequently show aberrant states of resting and active muscle tone, from too high, **hypertonicity**, to too low, **hypotonicity**, and fluctuating varieties, **athetosis** and **ataxia**. Many interventions have been designed to alter aberrant muscle tone to help children with neuromuscular disability produce more typical motor behaviors.

Hypertonicity

Hypertonicity is a term used to describe an increased stiffness in a body part at either rest or during active movement. It can appear after damage to supraspinal areas of the brain, such as occur in CP and TBI, or after spinal cord injury and various other neurological damage. Neurological and musculoskeletal changes occur as hypertonicity develops.

Spasticity

The only definition of **spasticity** supported by research is "a velocity dependent resistance to passive movement" (Craik, 1991; Rothwell, 1994). Spasticity is thought to be caused by a lack of normal presynaptic inhibition. The basic circuitry is diagrammed in Figure 6–6. Increased afferent activation (attributable to decreased inhibition) of interneurons causes increased activation of both alpha and gamma motor neurons. Irradiation of this excessive input also causes overactivation of neighboring agonists and antagonists (i.e., co-contraction of muscles). As a result, the child appears stiff and unable to relax to move. Normal modulation of reflex activity that should occur during movements such as gait can also be disrupted (Stein et al., 1993).

A child may, however, show stiffness and not have exaggerated stretch reflex activity (Berger, Horstman, & Dietz, 1984). Weakness and paresis have been observed during movement in individuals with hypertonicity (Damiano & Abel, 1998; Wiley & Damiano, 1998). This is hypothesized to be caused by a reduced facilitation of the polysynaptic reflexes (Dietz, 1999; Dietz & Berger, 1995). This weakness can cause the child to voluntarily co-contract to

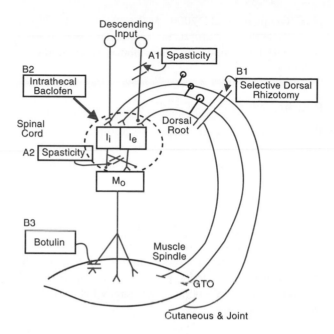

Figure 6-6 Schema of the spinal cord circuitry to demonstrate spasticity mechanisms and treatment. Sensory neurons from the muscle, skin, and joints traverse through the dorsal roots into the spinal cord to synapse on inhibitory interneurons (I_i) excitatory interneurons (I_e), and motor neurons (M_n). Descending input from higher levels of the spinal cord and brain also synapse on interneurons and motor neurons in the spinal cord. A balance of inhibitory and excitatory input regulates activation of motor neurons, which in turn activate muscle fibers. Spasticity is hypothesized to be caused by (A1) a reduction in descending inhibitory input or (A2) a reduction in presynaptic inhibitory input. Methods to reduce spasticity include (B1) selective dorsal rhizotomy or cutting some of the sensory afferents to decrease excitatory input into the spinal cord; (B2) intrathecal pump titrations of baclofen, a chemical that acts as an inhibitory neurotransmitter similar to gamma-aminobutyric acid, into the spinal cord to increase the inhibitory influence on the interneurons and motor neurons; and (B3) botulin (Botox) injections into the muscle to temporarily block transmission of the motor neuron to the muscles at the neuromuscular synapse. GTO = Golgi tendon organ.

create sufficient tension for postural control and movement. Musculoskeletal changes (contractures in the collagen tissue, decreases in the viscoelastic properties of the muscle tissue, collagen accumulation in the muscles, changes in muscle fibers [atrophy especially of type 2 fibers, predominance of type 1 fibers], and decreased force production of muscle cells) also occur and appear to account for a large amount of the stiffness and inability to

move (Booth et al., 2001; Dietz, 1999; Dietz & Berger, 1995; Thilmann, Fellows, & Ross 1991). Joint contractures can also develop as a result of the limited movement across joints.

The relationship between hypertonicity and motor function continues to be debated. Some professionals argue that intervention to reduce hypertonicity will improve motor function (Bly 1991; Bobath & Bobath, 1984). Therapists have made alteration of muscle tone a main focus of some types of therapy, such as neurodevelopmental therapy (NDT), for children with hypertonicity (Bobath & Bobath, 1984). The theory was that if the abnormal muscle tone could be prevented or normalized, then the child would move appropriately and the subsequent musculoskeletal changes would not occur to further hinder movement. This theory makes sense in that we know that there are secondary musculoskeletal and neurological changes that do occur that make "normal" movement impossible. However, this particular type of therapy (NDT) has not been shown to be able to change long-term motor learning (Barry, 1996; Butler & Darrah, 2001; Ottenbacher et al., 1986). New physical therapy intervention programs, such as the use of electrical stimulation and treadmill training, which incorporate long-term motor learning techniques, need to be developed and tested to determine their effectiveness in altering motor patterns, and possibly reducing secondary effects of hypertonicity (Barry, 1996; Dietz, 1999; Richards et al., 1997).

Other professionals argue that the development of hypertonicity is optimal for the best motor function available to the individual who has been injured (Landau, 1974; Sahrmann & Norton, 1977). There is evidence that during movement, such as gait, a given level of tension developed by a spastic muscle during stretch results in less EMG activity than in a healthy muscle. Consequently, the regulation of muscle tension at the spinal level may need to be increased to have optimal ability for independent ambulation (Dietz, 1999; Latash & Anson, 1996). This pattern for development of muscle tension (controlled completely at the spinal level versus from the supraspinal level) and an increased use of co-contraction of agonist and antagonist muscles may be the most efficient way for these individuals to move (Crenna, 1998; Damiano, 1993). The co-contraction may be a useful strategy to increase joint stability, to limit the degrees of freedom while learning a movement, or to allow the motor system to respond with more stability to perturbations (Damiano, Martellotta, Sullivan, Granata, & Abel, 2000; Vereijken et al., 1992; Latash & Anson, 1996). Recent research in a small number of children with CP (n = 10; mean age, 9.2 years) has shown that those who use more co-contraction muscle activity show better energy efficiency for overground ambulation (Damiano et al., 2000). So there may come a time where the use of hypertonic patterns of movement, to a certain extent, is optimal for functional movement and that therapy to reduce it may be detrimental to the individual (Latash & Nicholas, 1996).

Today there are also effective surgical and drug interventions aimed at decreasing spasticity by lowering excitation into the motor neuron pools (**selective dorsal rhizotomy**) (Graubert, Song, McLaughlin, & Bjornson, 2000; McLaughlin et al., 1998, 2002; Sacco, Tylkowski, & Warf, 2000; Steinbok et al., 1997; Steinbok, 2001), increasing inhibition in the motor neuron pools (**intrathecal baclofen**) (Albright, 1996; Albright, Barry, Shafton, & Ferson, 2001; Almeida, Campbell, Girolami, Penn, & Corcos, 1997; Armstrong et al., 1997; Barry, Albright, & Shultz, 2000; Butler & Campbell, 2000), or interrupting muscle contraction (**botulin injections**) (Boyd, Pliatsios, Starr, Wolfe, & Graham, 2000; Forssberg & Tedroff, 1997; Graham, 2000; Ubhi, Bhakta, Ives, Allgar, & Roussounis, 2000). Figure 6–6B demonstrates the activation site for each of these interventions to decrease spasticity. These therapies may be used for nonambulatory children with severe involvement to reduce muscle tone so that adequate personal care, ROM, and position changes can be performed. They also may be used for the child who is ambulatory, to improve the child's gait and functional mobility. Although studies have definitely reported reductions in spasticity with use of these three techniques, it is clear that once spasticity is altered through medication or surgery, normal movement does not just emerge (Giuliani, 1991). The underlying secondary musculoskeletal changes, that is, weakness and contractures, can still impede movement. The child also has learned motor patterns that are different because of the previous presence of spasticity. When the spasticity is decreased, those learned motor patterns do not just disappear, and they are potentially not effective for the new lower tone situation (Olree, Engsberg, Ross, & Park, 2000). For example, the child with hypertonicity in his or her legs may walk with excessive hip adduction, hip internal rotation, knee flexion, and plantar flexion. Once muscle tone is reduced, he or she may be unable to walk because he or she still attempts to use all or part of this pattern. Functional movement improvements demonstrated through research studies vary and have not always been shown to be better than aggressive strength and exercise programs routinely administered by physical therapists (Graubert et al., 2000; McLaughlin et al., 2002). Research on the ideal criteria under which to use these drug and surgical techniques in the ambulatory child should continue.

Rigidity

Rigidity is a more extreme type of hypertonicity (Rothwell, 1994). There is strong resistance to passive movement in muscles on all sides of the joint. There is no apparent increase in the stretch reflex activity; however, there is some postulation that transcortical long latency reflex activity may be responsible for the increased muscle tone. Another hypothesis is that the basal ganglia's normal interaction with the motor cortex anterior to the central sulcus may be disrupted. This rigidity can be uniform throughout the ROM or may cause a series of jerks, termed *cogwheel rigidity* (Iyer, Mitz, & Winstein, 1999; Lundy-Eckman, 1998; Rothwell, 1994).

Hypotonicity

Hypotonicity is excessively low resistance to passive stretch. Although there have not been numerous studies of hypotonicity, in clinical practice, more children receiving physical therapy services probably demonstrate lower muscle tone, especially in the trunk and neck, than show high muscle tone. Hypotonicity is hypothesized to occur because of a loss of efferent or afferent activity to lower motor neurons, and subsequent changes in the musculoskeletal tissue. This can be caused by injuries to lower motor neurons, muscular or connective tissue diseases (e.g., spinal muscular atrophy and congenital malformation of connective tissue), or reduction in descending input from the brain to activate the alpha and gamma motor neurons (Lundy-Eckman, 1998). Hypotonicity stemming from decreased descending input can be found in neuromuscular disabilities such as CP and DS. Some infants born at full term, without birth trauma or specific diagnoses, have also been shown to demonstrate hypotonicity. Although this may have some effect on early development, it has not been related to long-term delay in motor development (Paine, 1963; Parush et al., 1998; Pilon, Sadler, & Bartlett, 2000). The rest of our discussion on hypotonicity focuses on possible neurological etiologies.

Often with the loss of descending excitatory input, as is thought to occur in hypotonicity, there may be an associated cerebellar or vestibular disorder. The vestibulospinal descending pathway is important in the regulation of muscle tone, particularly in relation to control of posture and balance (Nashner, 1982; Lundy-Eckman, 1998; Westcott, 1993). Input from the vestibular apparatus, which provides us with information about gravitational forces, exerts excitatory influences on the extensor motor neurons, particularly those innervating postural muscles. With lower muscle tone, the child tends to hold stationary postures by extending the joints completely and "hanging" on ligaments. The shoulders may slope forward and the arms hang, excessive kyphosis or lordosis may be apparent, and the legs may be locked into full extension to hyperextension. Children with hypotonicity tend to have large ROMs in their joints, perhaps caused by lower muscle tone (Pilon et al., 2000). However, the continual strategy of "hanging" on the ligaments may further stretch the joint structures to extremes.

Reduction of gamma input will upset the regulation of the state of the muscle spindle. This sensor specifically gives us information on the length of the muscle and the velocity of change in length (Latash, 1998b; Rothwell, 1994). More important, the spindle afferent activity provides the primary information for our kinesthetic sense (Goodwin, McCloskey, & Matthews, 1972; Hulliger, Noth, & Vallbo, 1982). Knowing the position of your body in space has a powerful effect on movement ability. Coordinated movement is difficult without adequately sensing your changing position in space. Accordingly, children with low muscle tone tend to move less and demonstrate less coordination in the mid ranges of movement. For example, when standing still, the child with hypotonicity may appear to be steady, but when asked to lower to the floor, he or she will just drop down, going from one static position to another without smooth control. For movement transitions, we want to control the speed of movement, and we do not want the antagonist to completely relax. Instead, we want the antagonist to be maintained in a state of controlled co-contraction with the agonist. The balance between the activation of the agonist and antagonist may also be disrupted in children with hypotonicity.

Fluctuating Tone

Two other tonal disorders, which involve a combination of hypertonicity and hypotonicity, are **athetosis** and **ataxia**. Athetosis, sometimes termed dystonia, includes fluctuations between hypertonicity and hypotonicity in the prime movement muscles with overall hypotonicity between fluctuations (Yokochi, Hosoe, Shimabukuro, & Kodama, 1989). It can be characterized by uncontrolled slow and continuous writhing movements (Lundy-Eckman, 1998). However, chorea—rapid jerky involuntary movements—is also sometimes found with athetosis. This tonal disorder is associated with a basal ganglia lesion, specifically cell loss in the striatum (Hayashi, Satoh, Sakamoto, & Morimatsu, 1991). Because of the extra movement that occurs, persons with athetoid CP have been shown to have a higher than normal resting metabolic rate (Johnson, Goran, Ferrara, & Poehlman, 1996). The use of pharmacological agents to help control this tonal disorder has had varied success, and further research is necessary (Albright et al., 2001; Barry et al., 2000; Fahn, 1999; Gooch & Sandell, 1996).

Ataxia is a muscle control disorder that generally follows from cerebellar damage; it also causes fluctuations in muscle activity (Bastian, 1997). A child with ataxia has movements of normal strength with no hypertonia; however, the movements are jerky and inaccurate (Montgomery, 2000). Dependent on where the cerebellar lesion occurs, the child may have limb ataxia, truncal ataxia, or gait ataxia (Lundy-Eckman, 1998). Children with gait ataxia have poor balance and can be described as demonstrating movement similar to that of a person who is intoxicated.

Central Nervous System Plasticity in the Child

Neural tissue does not regenerate after injury, causing cell death. The nervous system has accommodated by building some redundancy found in both sensory and motor pathways. Loss of a few neurons usually will not significantly change the functional ability of the system. From birth through adulthood, there are usually several sensory and motor pathways to record similar sensations and generate similar movements. The fetus initially has an overabundance of neurons. As these neurons synapse with other neurons, there is an exuberance of neuronal projections that are later pruned for increased specificity of neuronal activity (Leonard, 1998). Part of the normal CNS development includes periods of cellular death that occur early, before cell migration, and then to a lesser extent again during the third trimester after neurons have extended their axons to synapse with the "correct" area of the CNS (Cabana, 1999; Oppenheim, 1991). If a CNS injury occurs before these normal cellular death periods, structural remodeling may occur to make up for the potentially deficient area (Hicks & D'Amato, 1970). The development of the nervous system might be modified to maintain cells that normally would have been allowed to die. Those cells could then be extended to areas of the brain where they might not have gone typically. Therefore, during fetal periods of cellular overabundance, damage from an injury to the nervous system may be reduced.

As physical therapists, we try to capitalize on neural plasticity to improve motor function. There is a plethora of information from scientific studies about **neural plasticity,** defined as any change in the nervous system that is not periodic and lasts more than a few seconds (Bach-y-Rita, 1990; Burleigh-Jacobs, 1998; Cabana, 1999; Held, 1998; Leonard, 1998). **Habituation** is a very short-term change in neurotransmitter release and postsynaptic receptor sensitivity causing a decreased response to a specific repetitive stimulus. In physical therapy intervention, therapists provide continued activation of sensory pathways to cause habituation. For example, if a child is overly sensitive to touch, the therapist may use a brushing program (continued pressure and light touch activation) to decrease touch sensitivity. **Long-term potentiation** (LTP) includes a synthesis of proteins to improve synaptic transmission and growth of new synaptic connections. It results in a more easily activated and maintained response of the neural pathways potentiated and is thought to explain learning and memory at the neural level. Therapists try to provoke LTP in children with neuromuscular dysfunction by using practice of motor skills. The potential for recovery of the neural system after injury is the underpinnings of intervention for children with neuromuscular dysfunction.

After neural injury, edema, caused by biological products leaking from the dead cells and normal immune system products sent by the body to combat the damage, aggregates at the area of injury. This suppresses remaining neural function in the area and may cause more neural cell death from pressure and chemical actions. Drug therapies given soon after the injury may reduce swelling and accumulation of toxic products, thus reducing cell damage and ultimately the functional deficit (Fulop et al., 1998; Held & Pay, 1999). To date, these drug therapies have primarily been used in adults after stroke and TBI (Burleigh-Jacobs, 1998; Fulop et al., 1998), but use in children is being explored. Careful monitoring to keep cranial pressure at a normal level after CNS injury in the premature infant or after TBI in a child is also being shown to promote better functional motor and cognitive outcomes (Johnston, 1995; Sharples, Stuart, Matthews, Aynsley-Green, & Eyre, 1995).

Recovery of the neural system after injury occurs by (1) recovery of synaptic effectiveness caused by decreased edema, (2) denervation hypersensitivity (increased sensitivity in postsynaptic membranes), (3) synaptic hypereffec-

tiveness (increased neurotransmitter in surviving synaptic connections), (4) unmasking of silent synapses (previously unused synapses called into use), and (5) cortical map reorganization (other cortical areas taking over the damaged area's function) (Held & Pay, 1999; Jenkins & Merzinich, 1992; Merzenich & Jenkins, 1993; Nudo, Wise, SiFuentes, & Milliken, 1996; Nudo & Milliken, 1996). Denervation hypersensitivity, synaptic hypereffectiveness, unmasking of silent synapses, and cortical map reorganization seem to be related to use after the original damage (Dobkin, 1998; Edgerton, 1997; Liepert, Bauder, Miltner, Taub, & Weiller, 2000; Morris, Crago, DeLuca, Pidikiti, & Taub, 1997; Segal, 1998), and experience in a variety of environments (Held, 1998). In simple words, the person needs to practice movement in varied environments after the neurological insult to enhance the positive changes. This finding can be summarized in the saying "use it or lose it." Researchers have been examining forced-use paradigms or constraint-induced therapy to improve movement control of the affected limbs in adults after strokes (Morris et al., 1997; Ostendorf & Wolf, 1981; Taub & Wolf, 1997; Wolf, Lecraw, Barton, & Jann, 1989). Some early research using a similar approach has been examined in children with some success (Charles, Lavinder, & Gordon, 2001; Crocker, Mackay-Lyons, & McDonnell, 1997; Freed, Catlin, Bobo, Fagan, & Moebes, 1999; DeLuca, Echols, Ramey, & Taub, 2003). The "use" hypothesis also becomes very important for children who have early insults and represents the basis for early intervention. Children may not be relearning a motor skill but instead are learning it for the first time. Therefore, the earliest assistance, guidance, and encouragement to move and experience a variety of environments may be very important for shaping the quality and quantity of later movements (Achenbach, Howell, Aoki, & Rauh, 1993; Guralnick, 1998; Harris, 1998; Majnemer, 1998; Pakula & Palmer, 1998). Early work on the use of virtual environment stimulation to specifically match the sensory and motor capacities of the child to provide the best environmental stimulation is under way (Latash, 1998a; Rose, Johnson, & Attree, 1997).

Although it is not the general rule that early brain damage necessarily results in greater recovery (Rose et al., 1997), damage to neural tissues during uterine development may have an advantage over similar damage in the infant or adult (Kolb, 1999; Kolb, Forgie, Gibb, Gorny, & Rowntree, 1998; Kolb, Gibb, & Gorny, 2000; Kolb & Whishaw, 1998; Kujala, Alho, & Naatanen, 2000). However, even though initial sparing may occur in early damage, other deficits may appear later in development related to decreased normal function of the areas that assisted with the early recovery. Further, secondary changes in the musculoskeletal tissues may also occur over time. Lack of movement or repetition of specific patterns of movement can alter the developing muscle and skeletal tissue. These changes can affect further development of movement, as discussed in Chapter 4.

Motor Control

Theories of Motor Control

Rehabilitation practices develop in parallel with scientific theories. From new knowledge in basic sciences emerge new theories or new viewpoints about how the brain controls movement and about the relative influence of, and organization between, the different systems involved. A theory of motor control provides clinicians with a set of assumptions about how movement is controlled. These assumptions are then translated into the clinical applications. Theories of motor control are used as the conceptual framework for hypothesis-oriented clinical practice. The theories endorsed by a therapist will influence the clinical decision-making process through the sets of assumptions underlying the hypotheses formulated from the examination findings, and through the prioritizing of problems to be addressed.

With this brief introduction to motor control theories, it is hoped that you can begin to understand how physical therapy practice has been shaped in the past and how acceptance of one or more of these theories would lead the therapist to different examinations and interventions. This is important for a beginning understanding of the nature of problems in some children with neuromuscular deficits and to comprehend current research on motor control. None of these theories hold the complete theoretical position to explain how we control and learn movement. Each theory builds on, and borrows from, the previous ones, as it should, based on support or lack thereof from scientific evidence. The process will continue as we all learn more, and you will need to periodically update your basis for examination and intervention.

Reflex Theory

The **Reflex Theory** of motor control proposed that sensory inputs are responsible for triggering all movement. At the turn of the 20th century, Sir Charles Sherrington,

an English neurophysiologist, mapped basic spinal cord reflexes in animal models (Sherrington, 1906, 1947). The reflex loop (sensory receptor–afferent sensory input–efferent motor output–muscle effector) was thought to be the basic unit of movement (Figure 6–7). Sherrington suggested that activation of one reflex triggered the activation of another reflex and that movement was the result of a series of reflex-triggered events. Based on this theory, sensory inputs are essential to movement generation. This was the time of poliomyelitis epidemics. Polio selectively destroys alpha motor neurons, decreasing the number of healthy motor units. Facilitation of reflexes was used to generate movement and compensate for the muscle weakness observed in individuals with poliomyelitis.

Much has been learned about spinal cord circuitry from Sherrington's work. However, it is clear that movement is possible in the absence of sensory inputs. For example, sensory deprived animals can still learn and develop functional movements (Taub, 1976), although deafferented monkeys (no sensory inputs from skin, joints, or muscle after dorsal roots lesion) deprived of visual inputs (eyes sewn shut) from birth took much longer to learn new movements than did intact animals, and movements were not as smooth or coordinated (Taub, Goldberg & Taub,

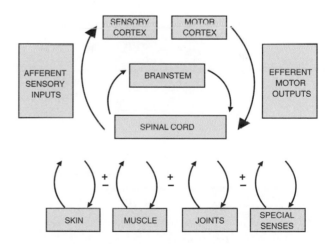

Figure 6-7 Reflex theory of motor control. Sensory (afferent) input causes motor (efferent) output between the peripheral nervous system and the spinal cord, as well as between the spinal cord and the brainstem and cortex. (Redrawn from Horak, F.B. [1991]. Assumptions underlying motor control for neurological rehabilitation. In M.J. Lister [Ed.], *Contemporary management of motor problems: Proceedings of the II STEP Conference* [p. 13]. Alexandria, VA: Foundation for Physical Therapy.)

1975). Another example are ballistic movements that occur so quickly there is probably insufficient time for transmission of sensory input into the CNS to activate the movement. Although sensory inputs are undeniably important for motor learning and motor control, they are not obligatory as originally suggested by Sherrington.

Hierarchical Theory

The **Hierarchical Theory** considered the reflex a "primitive behavior" rather than the basic unit of movement as suggested by the Reflex Theory. It proposed that motor control was achieved in a top-down fashion from the cerebral cortex to the spinal cord (Jackson & Taylor, 1932; Phillips & Porter, 1977; Reed, 1982; Walsche, 1961).

Reflexes triggered by specific sensory input were described as the simplest form of movement, whereas voluntary movements were more complex movements (Figure 6–8). Behaviors such as sucking, grasping, or neonatal walking observed in infants were described as primitive reflexes occurring at the spinal level. It was believed that as the infant matured, further neural differentiation and myelination of neurons occurred, leading to the emergence of head- and trunk-righting abilities. The cortex

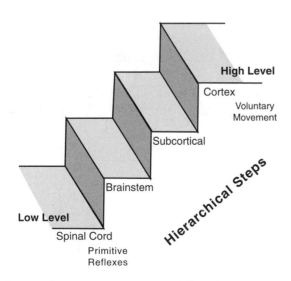

Figure 6-8 Hierarchical theory of motor control. Via stepwise levels of motor control, the cortex controls all lower levels of the neural system. (Adapted from Horak, F.B. [1991]. Assumptions underlying motor control for neurological rehabilitation. In M.J. Lister [Ed.], *Contemporary management of motor problems: Proceedings of the II STEP Conference* [p. 15]. Alexandria, VA: Foundation for Physical Therapy.)

eventually matured to initiate and control all lower levels, allowing the development of more complex and skillful movements, such as reaching to grasp an object, or crawling. The so-called primitive reflexes were thought to be suppressed with the development of higher control. Reflex testing was therefore used to detect problems with the development of the nervous system. Motor control was thought of as a relatively fixed predefined series of steps. Correlations were drawn with the reappearance of certain "primitive" behaviors after brain damage such as in stroke and head injury.

Arguments against the Hierarchical Theory include the fact that reflex responses are not simple stereotyped movements but can vary based on the person's internal state and on the external environment without any influence from cortical input (Wolpaw, 1985). Some lower-level reflexes such as the withdrawal reflex to a painful stimulus sometimes appropriately dominate movement. Automatic postural movements, which are not under cortical control, are also influenced by the task and environment (Burleigh, Horak, & Malouin, 1994; Burleigh & Horak, 1996). Furthermore, development does not occur in the stepwise manner described in the Hierarchical Theory. Reaching and walking have been shown to be self-generated movements responsive to ongoing sensory feedback and not requiring cortical control (Lee, von Hofsten, & Cotton, 1997; Thelen, Kelso, & Fogel, 1987; Ulrich, Ulrich, Angulo-Kinzler, & Chapman, 1997; von Hofsten, 1980). The Hierarchical Theory also suggested that the brain controlled and generated muscle activation for every movement. This would be a most inefficient method of control and would not account for our ability to execute complex movements in the absence of feedback. Finally, recent evidence suggests that reflex testing may not correlate as highly as previously thought with the degree of motor disorder (Bartlett, 1997).

These early theories of motor control had a major impact on physical therapy practice in the late 1950s and early 1960s. From these assumptions originated the main neuro-facilitation approaches such as Bobath's NDT (Bobath, 1964, 1985; Bobath & Bobath, 1984), Brunnstrom's and Rood's approaches (Brunnstrom, 1992; Stockmeyer, 1967), Kabat and Knott's Proprioceptive Neuromuscular Facilitation (PNF) (Knott & Voss, 1968), and Ayres' Sensory Integration Therapy (SI) (Ayres, 1979). The abnormal reflexes and muscle tone observed after damage to the cortex in children with CP, or in individuals after a cerebrovascular accident or a TBI, were believed to be the origin of abnormal movements. Consequently, therapists thought that if they could inhibit primitive reflexes and normalize tone, neural plasticity could be induced through facilitation of residual higher brain regions to assume functions of damaged brain regions. Although effective to improve quality of movement, the treatment effects were not long lasting, and did not appear to transfer from one setting or environment to another (Harris, 1990; Horak, 1992; Ottenbacher et al., 1986; Shumway-Cook & Woollacott, 2001). Over the last 30 years, new theories of motor control have gradually emerged from advances in neuroscience as well as from an overture to look at other disciplines' perspective on movement (Sweeney, Heriza, & Markowitz, 1994).

Motor Programming Theory

A contemporary version of the Hierarchical Theory, the **Motor Programming Theory**, suggested that the cortex would generate the desired motor outcome as opposed to the details for how this outcome was achieved. It viewed reflexes as less flexible, more rapid response programs, rather than primitive behaviors. Within the spinal cord, networks of neurons cooperate as a whole to produce rhythmic, patterned motor commands, such as the commands for repetitive stepping (locomotion). As discussed previously under myelomeningocele, CPGs are the neural structures generating rhythmic, stereotypic programs. As a result of motor learning, more complex programs developed at the cortex level are used to simplify the production of movement. Given a specific task, environment, and expected sensory consequences for evaluating the accuracy of response, the motor programs specify the relationships between past movement experiences (conditions, execution parameters, outcomes, and sensory consequences) and the required movement parameters, such as force, velocity, and amplitude among others. Whether you sign your name on a piece of paper in small script using finger movement or on a blackboard in large script using the whole arm and shoulder, your signature pattern is similar, with the motor program being the same. The specific muscle activations would be coordinated at lower levels (Rothwell, 1994).

Systems-Oriented Theories

Systems Theory

The **Systems Theory**, originally known as the Distributive Theory, was first introduced in the 1930s by Nicolai Bernstein, a Russian physiologist (Bernstein, 1967; Latash, 1998c). His research was not translated until 1967.

Bernstein hypothesized that movements, rather than being either peripherally or centrally driven as previously suggested, emerge from the interaction of many systems (musculoskeletal, sensorimotor, comparing, environmental, regulation, and commanding), each contributing to different aspects of motor control (Figure 6–9). There is no single focus of control; the control can shift among systems depending on the individual's internal state, the specific motor task, and the environmental conditions. The Distributive Theory label originated from the sharing of control among the different systems (Latash, Latash, & Meijer, 1999, 2000).

Bernstein (1967) described a "degrees of freedom" problem caused by the availability of too many neurons, muscles, and joint motions to allow for conscious control over every action. He suggested that the interaction between systems to produce patterns or synergies of movement solved the degrees of freedom problem. Specific neurons and muscles worked together as units to create specific movements. Given a specific environment and task, humans have been shown to share similar coordinated patterns. For example, we use consistent movement strate-

SYSTEMS THEORY OF MOTOR CONTROL

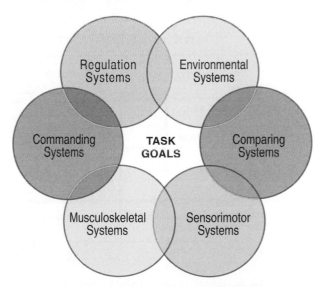

Figure 6-9 Systems theory of motor control. The interlocking circles depict the circular motor control with the task goals as the central outcome desired. (Redrawn from Horak, F.B. [1991]. Assumptions underlying motor control for neurological rehabilitation. In M.J. Lister [Ed.], *Contemporary management of motor problems: Proceedings of the II STEP Conference* [pp. 11–28]. Alexandria, VA: Foundation for Physical Therapy.)

gies to maintain our balance in standing (Horak & Nashner, 1986; Nashner, 1982). When standing on a platform, a sudden backward motion of the surface will result in the sequential activation of the gastroc/soleus, hamstrings, and paraspinal muscles in a coordinated distal to proximal pattern named the **ankle strategy** (Figure 6–10A). If the environmental conditions are changed, a different and more adaptive response will appear; for example, when standing crosswise on a narrow balance beam, a more challenging task, the strategies used to maintain balance change. A proximal to distal sequential activation of the abdominals, quadriceps, and tibialis anterior muscles will be used (Figure 6–10B). This **hip strategy** is used in response to bigger threats to balance. The timing and amplitude of these postural responses to perturbation have been shown to vary with the amplitude and speed of the perturbation (Horak, 1991; Inglis, Horak, Shupert, & Jones-Rycewicz, 1994; Shumway-Cook & Woollacott, 2001). These responses occur within 80 to 100 milliseconds from the perturbation as opposed to a simple spinal reflex response that would occur within 30 milliseconds of the stimulus, or a consciously driven movement where transmission to and from the cortex requires greater than 100 milliseconds. Terms such as *long latency reflex responses* (transmission to and from the brainstem), *automatic*

postural responses, motor programs, or *synergies* have been used to describe these strategies believed to be ways to simplify the control of standing balance.

Bernstein (1967) also emphasized the constraints of the musculoskeletal system and environment (e.g., inertia and gravity) on movement. These could influence physical therapy interventions designed to improve movement. For example, if joint contracture impeded movement, the therapist would focus on interventions to increase ROM.

From the Systems Theory evolved the **Task-Oriented Theory** of motor control, in which all systems interact to control movement in the context of a functional task in a meaningful environment (Gordon, 1987; Horak, 1991). For instance, when we want a drink at the dinner table, we do not activate a specific reaching movement but instead complete the task of getting a drink so we can assuage our thirst. Implications for examination and intervention focussing on functional movement, rather than movements without a purpose, follow from this variation of the theory. With this in mind, therapists first identify the critical systems involved in carrying out a task (e.g., the visual, somatosensory, and vestibular systems are all involved in balance), evaluate and treat those impairments amenable to modification (ROM, muscle weakness, and cardiopulmonary deconditioning), and identify tasks and activities

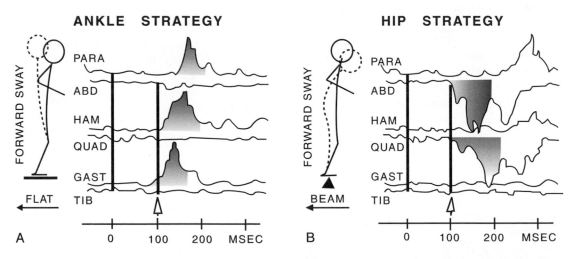

Figure 6-10 Automatic postural muscle responses to backwards perturbations of the floor surface. *(A)* An "ankle strategy" is used when falling forwards on the flat surface. A finely sequenced group of contractions begins around 80 to 100 msec after the floor moves, in the posterior muscles as shown by the onset of the gastrocnemius, followed by hamstrings, followed by paraspinals. *(B)* When the threat to balance is greater, a different strategy to control posture is triggered. A "hip strategy," abdominals first, followed by the quadriceps and anterior tibialis muscles, is selected to maintain postural control. (Adapted from Horak, F.B., & Nashner, L.M. [1986]. Central programming of postural movements: Adaptation to altered support configurations. *Journal of Neurophysiology, 55,* 1372. Copyright 1986 by American Physiology Society. Reprinted with permission.)

important to the child. These activities or tasks may be used to structure the physical therapy examination and intervention.

Dynamic Systems Theory

The **Dynamic Systems Theory** supports a systems-like theory of motor control that assumes that control of movement by a specific system is short lived and that control shifts among systems following a principle of self-organization between the components that make up the individual and the surrounding environment (Kelso et al., 1980; Kelso & Tuller, 1984; Kugler, Kelso, & Turvey, 1980; Schoner & Kelso, 1988; Thelen, Kelso, & Fogel, 1987). In a simplistic interpretation, this principle states that order will occur naturally in an environment made up of charged particles. A common example in the inanimate world is the organization that occurs in flowing water particles when the speed of the stream of water is increased. At first, if the flow of water is slow, the water organizes into drops. As the flow increases, the water forms into a stream. This "organization" is dependent on the controlling variable of the velocity/volume of water flow. A common example given in the animate world related to movement is the switch a horse makes from a walking gait pattern to a canter and then to a gallop, which occurs simply as a result of an increased speed of movement and a greater change in the angle of hip extension (Bernstein, 1967; Heriza, 1991a). Experiments involving oscillating finger movements have shown that the mathematical methods, as well as principles of change from one pattern to another, can be applied to transitions in movement behavior in humans. If you start moving your right and left index fingers in alternate abduction-adduction pattern at a slow speed, you can accomplish the task. But if you keep speeding up the movements, at a certain speed, the movements of the two fingers will automatically become that of simultaneous adduction-abduction. This experiment is demonstrated by EMG recordings of finger muscles shown in Figure 6–11 (Kelso, 1984, 1986, 1995; Kelso, Buchanan, & Wallace, 1991; Schoner & Kelso, 1988).

Scholz (1990) describes concepts from the Dynamic Systems Theory by applying them to the case of a young child with CP creeping on its hands and knees. Under certain conditions, the child is able to use a reciprocal creeping pattern (opposite side arm and leg moving together). Under other conditions, however, the organization of the motor behavior changes or transitions to another pattern, moving both legs together symmetrically

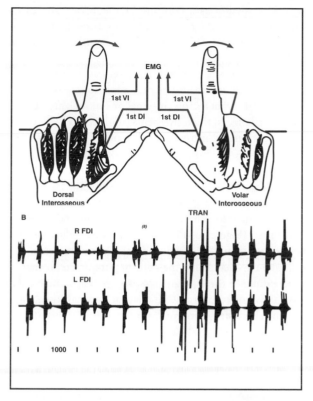

Figure 6-11 Dynamic systems theory of motor control. In this experiment, internal EMG recordings were made of the first dorsal interosseus (FDI) and the first volar interosseus (FVI). The subjects were asked to move their index fingers in phase back and forth to the right and left. Alternating EMG activity between both fingers depicts that movement. As the subject increases the frequency of the movement, a phase shift occurs in the coordination pattern. This transition (TRAN) is noted in the EMG traces when both FDI muscles have shifted to contracting at the same time. (From Schoner, G., & Kelso, J.A.S. [1988]. Dynamic pattern generation in behavioral and neural systems. *Science, 239,* 1514, with permission.)

to advance forward (referred to as bunny hopping). He discusses the critical concept of a **control parameter**, which is any variable internal or external to the child that influences the system to transition. In the case of creeping, one control parameter is the speed of the quadruped movement, or the frequency of the oscillations of the hip movements. This could qualify as a control parameter because, as the rate of hip movements increases, the tendency to keep a controlled reciprocal pattern becomes unstable (likely to change), and the locomotor pattern transitions to a bunny hop. The degree of stiffness at the hip and pelvic girdle could also qualify as a control parameter because, as the stiffness increases, the reciprocal pattern becomes less stable (likely to change) until eventually the pattern changes to the bunny hop.

The concept of a control parameter can be very important for clinical interventions because it suggests that therapists identify what factors, internal or external, are likely to promote change in the movements produced. These control parameters can be intrinsic to the individual, or extrinsic such as in the environment or motor task to be accomplished. This idea of a triad of constraints consisting of the person, the environment, and the task—and the spontaneous interaction of systems affecting motor control—has greatly influenced our current examination and intervention ideas (Figure 6–12). For example, following this theory, we would observe and take measurements of a movement to determine the control parameters so that we could influence these parameters, and perhaps cause a shift of the movement to a more efficient or optimal coordinated pattern. Use of this concept for intervention is discussed in Chapter 7.

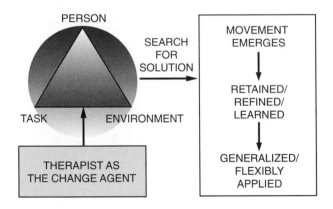

Figure 6-12 Triad of constraints to movement. Considering the individual, the environment, and the task to be accomplished, a movement solution is initiated. A first movement attempt emerges. After practice, the movement can be retained, refined, and learned. Once the movement plan is learned, it is stored in memory. This theory suggests that it can be generalized and applied to other similar tasks and/or environments. The therapist can act as a change agent in this process by altering the person's state or experience level, the task, and/or the environment, causing the solution and learning process to lead to a different outcome. (Adapted from Newell, K.M., & Valvano, J. [1998]. Therapeutic intervention as a constraint in learning and relearning movement skills. *Scandinavian Journal of Occupational Therapy*, *5*, 53, with permission.)

Neuronal Group Selection Theory

One of the problems therapists have had in accepting the Systems Theory or Dynamic Systems Theory is that the theories place little emphasis on the CNS. A new theory, the **Neuronal Group Selection Theory (NGST)**, offers a balance between a pure systems approach and one that recognizes the powerful role that the CNS plays in movement (Hadders-Algra, 2000). According to this theory, cortical and subcortical systems dynamically organize into variable neural networks (Edelman, 1989, 1993; Sporns & Edelman, 1993; Sporns, Edelman, & Meijer, 1998). The neural networks are collections of interconnected neurons that act as functional units dealing with a specific type of motor behavior or information from a specific sensory system. The structure and function of these groups are created by the infant's development (genetic coding) and behavioral experience (environmental exposure and active movement). In the beginning of development, there is a set of developmentally crude or variable primary neuronal groups determined by evolution, which has been termed the *primary repertoire*. For example, in the development of postural stability in sitting, 4- to-6-month-old infants show crude anterior and posterior trunk muscle contraction patterns to maintain the sitting position (Hadders-Algra, Brogren, & Forssberg, 1996). After environmental experiences, the afferent information induces modifications in the strength of synaptic connections within and between some of the neuronal groups. In this way, some neuronal groups are selected over others as more adaptable to the environmental situation and a secondary repertoire of neuronal groups is created. These secondary groups allow for situation-specific selection of neuronal groups, for example, to invoke the most efficient postural adjustment in sitting (Diener, Bootz, Dichgans, & Bruzek, 1983; Hadders-Algra, Brogren, & Forssberg, 1998) or a well-coordinated reaching pattern (Konczak, Borutta, & Dichgans, 1997; Konczak, Borutta, Topka, & Dichgans, 1995; Konczak & Dichgans, 1997) based on the environment and task.

During the primary phase, motor activity is variable and not strictly tuned to the environmental conditions. This variable movement gives rise to self-generated, variable afferent information. The afferent information gives rise to motor behaviors that are functional in a diverse set of situations. After the transient phase of selection, variability of movement responses are reduced at first and then increased because of the barrage of sensory input from continued experience. The phase of secondary or adaptive variability starts, leading to a variable movement repertoire, with efficient motor function for each specific situation. Individuals can adapt movements to task-specific constraints or generate a repertoire of motor solutions for a single motor task.

Therapists would try to judge the stage of development that the child is in—primary versus secondary variability—and then design intervention to assist the child in developing success with efficient and variable movement for a motor skill. For example, a child with severe motor disability related to CNS damage may not have basic primary neuronal networks. To increase the child's primary repertoire for movement, you might provide the child with variable practice in different postures: supine, prone, sitting, and so on. You would then provide frequent experience with trial and error movement to facilitate selection of the secondary repertoire of neuronal groups. To date, there is still a lack of evidence supporting these intervention methods (Hadders-Algra et al., 1996; Vereijken & Thelen, 1997).

Movement Classifications

Motor scientists generally agree that not all movements are controlled in the same manner. Different classifications of movement have been proposed over the years. Although these different classifications are described separately, none of these systems are mutually exclusive. Overlap of hypotheses occurs among the systems. Also, some of the examination and intervention strategies that follow from adherence to a particular classification system are similar.

Reflex to Voluntary Movement

One classification of movements comes from the early literature that followed the Reflex Theory and Hierarchical Theory of motor control. These theories describe movements on a continuum from least voluntary to most voluntary, or simple short latency spinal reflexes to more complex long latency reflexes, which are transmitted through midbrain and brainstem structures, to complex individual voluntary movements involving cortical control (Fuchs, Anderson, Binder, & Fetz, 1989). Perturbations during reaching movements illustrate this classification system. Typically developing individuals primarily use a triphasic muscle activation pattern when reaching for a target. Activation of the agonist muscle moves the limb to the target; activation of the antagonist slows the movement down; and finally, another burst of agonist activation occurs for final contact with the target (Corcos, Gottlieb, & Agarwal, 1989). If the intended movement is perturbed

unexpectedly, the typically developing individual has four response levels: (1) instantaneous rebound provided by the elasticity of the connective tissue (Rothwell, 1994); (2) stretch reflex triggered by the muscle spindles, causing an increase in EMG activity in the stretched muscle within approximately 30 milliseconds; (3) longer latency reflex response of approximately 100 milliseconds, which is hypothesized to transmit through the brainstem, and causes an increase in EMG activity in the stretched muscle; and (4) voluntary contraction to change the trajectory of the arm (Gottlieb, Corcos, & Agarwal, 1989; Houk, 1979; Latash, 1998a; Rothwell, 1994). Therapists using this classification of movement would determine whether reflexes or voluntary movements were impaired in the child. Depending on the type of deficit, facilitation of movement via sensory stimulation for reflex behavior or manipulation of the environment for activation of voluntary movements would be used during intervention.

Feedback and Feedforward Movement

Another classification of movement originates from the use of sensory information to trigger a "feedback" or closed-loop movement as opposed to a "feedforward" or open-loop movement, triggered by a motor command from the cerebral cortex or brainstem structures (Horak, 1991). Figure 6–13 depicts the pathways for both feedback and feedforward movements. With the exception of the monosynaptic reflexes, feedback movements are generally slower than feedforward movements because of the added transmission time for the sensory information to initially trigger or modify the motor output.

Most movements are probably a combination of feedforward and feedback mechanisms. The individual decides to do a motor activity and feeds forward a prestructured set of motor commands based on past learning and experience. In feedforward movements, two things happen simultaneously. A motor plan to produce the appropriate muscle activations for the motor task is sent to the spinal cord. Also, a copy of the plan, the so-called **efference copy** or corollary discharge, is hypothesized to be stored elsewhere in the brain. As the person moves, the sensory systems provide feedback information, an **afference copy**, on how the movement is progressing and the potential success of the movement (Burleigh & Horak, 1996; Burleigh et al., 1994; Fuchs et al., 1989). This allows for alterations to occur during the movement to improve the final outcome. Based on the final outcome, the feedforward plan can also be

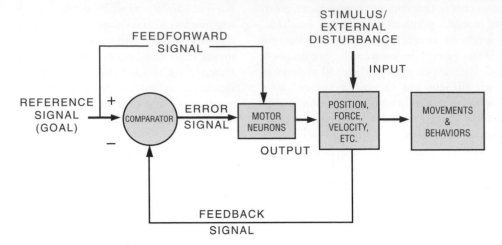

Figure 6-13 Feedback and feedforward movment. A closed-loop negative feedback system for control of movements (lighter arrows) is depicted for slower movements with ongoing adjustment caused by feedback. Feedforward signals (darker arrows) allow quicker and preplanned movement in anticipation of sensory input. (From Horak, F.B. [1991]. Assumptions underlying motor control for neurological rehabilitation. In M.J. Lister [Ed.], *Contemporary management of motor problems: Proceedings of the II STEP Conference* [p. 14]. Alexandria, VA: Foundation for Physical Therapy.)

modified for future use by comparing the afference copy with the efference copy, and making the necessary modifications. These learned or stored plans for movement have been called *motor programs* (Schmidt, 1991; Shumway-Cook & Woollacott, 2001). The motor programs that relate to the control of posture have been called the *central set* (Hay & Redon, 1999; Horak & Diener, 1994; Horak, Deiner, & Nashner, 1989). If the therapist classified movements in this fashion, he or she would examine the child to see if there were problems with movement when sensory feedback drove the movement or when the child had to call up previously learned programs for fast movements. Based on the conclusions of this examination, intervention may focus on triggering movements via sensory input or designing the therapy to practice movements that require use of previously learned motor programs.

Prime and Postural Movement

Attempts have also been made to classify movements as either **postural** or **primary movements**. It is proposed that there would be different areas of the brain exerting control over posture versus primary movements; these two control systems interact and overlap, as do all areas of the brain (Cordo & Nashner, 1982; Frank & Earl, 1990; Massion, 1992, 1998; Slijper, Latash, & Mordkoff, 2002). Postural activity can precede (i.e., anticipatory) the desired primary movement so that posture is adequately controlled before the coordinated movement starts. For example, when you

reach out for an object, before the arm muscles contract and the arm begins to move, muscles in your legs contract to stabilize your balance in anticipation of the balance perturbation with arm movement. This contributes to smooth and coordinated movements. This classification is still controversial, and it has been argued that there really are no clear differences between postural and prime movement control (Aruin & Latash, 1995; Thelen & Spencer, 1998). Using this classification system, if you believed there were separate control systems for postural control and prime movement control, the therapist would examine the postural control ability separately from prime movement ability. Based on the findings, intervention could be directed specifically toward improving postural control without a prime movement focus, or improving prime movement without a postural control focus, in a feedback or feedforward mode. If the therapist subscribed to the lack of separation of postural and prime movement control, then the examination and intervention would focus on practice of both together rather than trying to isolate each.

Motor Development

Normal motor development has always influenced neurological physical therapy for children. Normal development of motor skills is fascinating and beautiful. With motivation and persistence, typically developing children seem to flow through acquisition, fluency, and generalization of motor behaviors. Without struggle, new motor skills emerge. Most examination and intervention techniques for children were based on a developmental model. Historically, it was hypothesized that children must be taken through a normal developmental sequence to appropriately learn basic motor skills (Bobath, 1964; Domain et al., 1960; Stockmeyer, 1967; Voss, 1972). For example, a child must learn to crawl before walking. Based on new hypotheses related to normal motor development and theories on motor control and motor learning, this model has largely been replaced by the idea that intervention should focus on teaching age-appropriate functional motor behaviors. A child of 12 years should not have an intervention goal of developing crawling; rather, if mobility is the objective, the child should be encouraged to either walk with assistive devices or learn to propel a wheelchair. For a child with milder neurological deficits, the typical patterns seen in children with normal development may function as the gold standard for the most effective and efficient movements (Atwater, 1991).

Therapists need to understand the typical developmental progression of postural control to comprehend problems in development versus those caused by disease or insult. This allows for adjustment of examination and intervention. The control of posture is hypothesized to be a "missing link" in the ability to produce coordinated and efficient functional movements in many children with neuromuscular disability. If one cannot maintain or regain balance, then it becomes very difficult to move with purposeful intent.

Postural and movement control has been historically described as developing in a cephalocaudal manner, meaning that head control develops before trunk and lower extremity control. Also, proximal control (at the trunk) was thought to develop before distal motor control (at the hand and feet). However, more recently, motor development has been described as having regional and intertwining circles of development with no areas of the body developing in isolation from other areas (Adolph & Eppler, 2002; Atwater, 1991; Thelen & Spencer, 1998). The infant is always developing movements and postural control throughout the body. As the infant moves up against gravity in sitting, and then in standing, the postural control components become more important because they balance more mass farther from a smaller base of support (BOS). Interventions to improve postural control are commonly used when working with children with neuromuscular dysfunction because problems with postural control can potentially limit further development of movement and exploration.

Table 6.7 summarizes the development of postural control system by system, including the musculoskeletal system (muscles, connective tissue, and joints for actual movement), the sensory system (visual, vestibular, and somatosensory cues for postural adjustments), and the neuromuscular system (neural coordination and activation of motor neurons). Development of the **musculoskeletal system** is important primarily in the first year of life as the development of muscle strength can limit postural control ability. After the first year, adequate muscle strength and joint ROM are available for control of stationary postures, such as sitting and standing, and during movement. This system does affect postural control during growth spurts where the child needs to adjust muscle activations for changes in body size. The **sensory system organization** for postural control proceeds from being primarily visually dependent to one where somatosensory inputs can trigger motor output to control balance. At transition stages (e.g., beginning to sit, beginning to stand), visual dependence reemerges until the child learns more stability. The ability to resolve sensory conflicts (mismatched input from the three senses) matures gradually to an adultlike state by 7 to 10 years of age. For **reactive postural control** (when responding to an external sensory cue) within the **neuromuscular system**, there appear to be innate patterns of muscle coordination (postural strategies), loosely organized for sitting balance and, perhaps, more tightly organized for standing balance. These patterns show a stagelike development with disorganization in standing postural motor coordination patterns at 4 to 6 years of age, which may be attributed to growth spurts or lack of maturation of the sensory organization necessary for postural control. Adultlike postural control in this system again appears evident at 7 to 10 years of age. Development of **anticipatory postural control** (feedforward postural plans that actually precede the prime movement) seems to follow a similar sequence to reactive control; however, the patterns of motor coordination depend more on practice and learning of different tasks and activities in different environments. There also appear to be periods in development when infants and children use co-contraction to reduce the degrees of freedom to be controlled. With practice, the use of these co-contraction strategies gradually decreases, which allows more flexible and adaptable control of posture.

Examination and Evaluation

This section provides information that augments that presented in Chapter 1 regarding a Pediatric Physical Therapy Examination and Plan of Care (see Table 1.3).

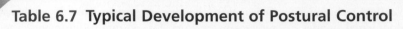

Table 6.7 Typical Development of Postural Control

System	Components	Age of Maturation to Adultlike Capacity and Related Issues
Musculoskeletal	Force production	Developing through life • Under 1 year of age, low force production capability is a constraint for sitting and standing • After 1 year of age, this should not be a constraint
	Range of motion	Developing through the teen years Should not be a constraint until elderly
	Body geometry	Changes rapidly during growth spurts at different ages dependent on gender and hormonal development Infants have large heads in relation to body size
Sensory	Vision	Sensory receptor mature at birth, acuity improves for distance vision over first year Preference for reliance on visual input for postural orientation corrections from birth to 1 year for sitting balance, and to about 3 years for standing balance From birth to death, vision used as primary information when first learning a task or in a novel environment
	Somatosensory (cutaneous and proprioceptive)	Sensory receptor mature at birth • Infants 6 months or older can use somatosensory inputs for maintenance of sitting balance • Children 4 to 6 years of age show beginning ability to use somatosensory input for sensory conflict resolution • Children 7 to 10 years of age show adultlike ability to use somatosensory input for sensory conflict resolution
	Vestibular	Sensory receptor mature at birth • Children 7 to 10 years of age can use vestibular input as the reference system in an adultlike manner for resolution of sensory conflict
	Sensory integration	• Children 7 to 10 years of age can choose and select sensory information accurately for maintenance of postural control.
Neuromuscular	Sitting: reactive postural control (muscle coordination patterns [MCPs])	Presitting infant (5 to 6 months): activation of directionally specific MCPs (agonists opposite to the side to which the child is falling), but variable timing (co-contractions and reversals of proximal to distal patterns), and poor adaptation to task-specific conditions Sitting infant (7 to 10 months): decreased timing variability of directionally specific MCPs (activations of leg, trunk, neck muscles) Transient toddling phase (9 months to 3 years): invariant use of directionally specific MCPs, some use of co-contractions; good modulation of pelvic muscles at BOS for adaptations to task-specific conditions About 3 years to adulthood: variability in directionally specific MCPs, less co-contraction and use of neck muscles to improve variability of postural control

System	Components	Age of Maturation to Adultlike Capacity and Related Issues
Neuromuscular (continued)	Standing reactive MCPs	As soon as standing independently (about 1 year of age): grossly directionally specific (distal to proximal) MCPs • $1\frac{1}{2}$ to 3 years of age: directionally specific MCPs consistent • 4 to 6 years of age: variability of MCPs occurs (perhaps because of growth spurts or sensory integration changes) • 7 to 10 years of age: adultlike use of directionally specific MCPs Other determinants of reactive MCP choice for maintenance of postural control: type of surface standing on; availability of sensory cues; instructions for task, regularity for perturbations
	Anticipatory postural activations (APAs)	About 1 year of age, APAs in some tasks observed 4 to 6 years of age, APAs in lever pull task 6 to 8 years of age, variable APAs in stand and reach task 9 to 12 years of age, more consistent APAs in stand and reach task Dependent on the task; mature after reactive MCPs in a particular posture and after practice/experience with movement in the posture First APA response in a new movement is usually a co-contraction (freezing the degrees of freedom); then after practice, more variability in postural control and movement occurs (Vereijken et al., 1992)

Details of testing procedures and standardized tests of function and development commonly used for children with neuromuscular disabilities are described in this chapter. In Chapter 2, the use of reliable and valid tests and measures is presented, as well as a more extensive list of tests and measures (see Table 2.12 and Appendix 2.B). A discussion of issues to consider in developing the examination of motor problems in children with neuromuscular disease or disability appears in this chapter.

The major goal of interventions for a child should be to improve the child's motor ability for activity and participation in the home, school, and community. Therefore, functional movements required for activities and community participation (e.g., gait and locomotion, balance, reach and grasp, transfers) that are important to the child and caregiver must be evaluated first. After observation and testing of how the child moves and the quality of movement, then the causes of the restrictions in activity and participation can be determined by assessing impairments of body structures and functions (e.g., ROM, strength, coordination).

Examination of children with neuromuscular disabilities is complex and requires testing of different domains. The therapist might be required to refer children to designated testing centers for complex measurement if specific and complicated decisions are necessary (e.g., gait laboratory assessments to make surgery determinations). It is important, however, not to get lost in high-technology information and lose sight of improving the outcome of personal functional activity and participation in the home, school, and community. There is a need for the development of new reliable, valid tests and measures for many areas related to children with neuromuscular disease or disability, including satisfaction with services and quality of life measures. Therapists should be diligent in following research that describes new tests and measures.

The *Guide* (APTA, 2001), Parts One and Two, list many constructs that we should evaluate through use of tests and measures, the basic tools for gathering this data, and the type of data that can be generated for documentation of motor behaviors in children who have neuromuscular disability. Table 6.8 lists the most commonly used tests and measures specific to children with neuromuscular disability (Patterns 5B, 5C, and 5D) organized by the *Guide*'s testing categories. The age range for the tests and their recommended use based on the three major testing purposes (discriminative, predictive, evaluative) can also be found in Table 6.8. Specific testing considerations and descriptions of some of these tests follow. Readers are referred to the references and other chapters for more details related to all tests.

Testing Considerations

Testing can be difficult in children with neuromuscular disability because of the variable nature of their motor

Table 6.8 Common Tests and Measures for Children with Neuromuscular Disability

Guide to Physical Therapist Practice Tests and Measures Categories	Tests and Measures	Age	Level of Measurement	Recommended Use
Gait, Locomotion, and Balance	Laboratory analysis/posturography (kinematic, kinetic, EMG)	Any age	Body function	Discriminative Predictive Evaluative
	Infant Tests			
	• Test of Infant Motor Performance (TIMP)	32 weeks preterm to 13 weeks post-term	Body function Activity	Discriminative Predictive Evaluative
	• Movement Assessment of Infant (MAI)	0–12 months		
	• Harris Infant Neuromotor Test (HINT)	3–12 months		
	• Alberta Infant Motor Scale (AIMS)	0–18 months		
	Developmental Tests			
	• Bayley Scales of Infant Development, 2nd ed. (BSID2)	0–2 years	Activity	Discriminative Predictive Evaluative
	• Peabody Developmental Motor Scales, 2nd ed. (PDMS2)	0–6 years		
	• Bruininks-Oseretsky Test of Motor Proficiency (BOTMP)	4.5–14.5 years		
	Single-Item Tests			
	• Functional Reach Test (FRT)			
	• Timed Up-and-Go (TUG)			
	• Timed Up and Down Stairs (TUDS)	4–12 years	Activity	Discriminative
	• Timed Obstacle Ambulation Test (TOAT)			
	• Fisher Reach Test			
	• Pediatric Clinical Test for Sensory Interaction in Balance (P-CTSIB)	4–12 years	Body function	Discriminative
	• Clinical Observation of Motor and Postural Skills (COMPS)	5–9 years	Body function	Discriminative Evaluative
Neuromotor and Sensory Integration	• Miller Assessment of Preschoolers (MAP)	2–5 years	Body function Activity	Discriminative Evaluative
	• Southern California Sensory Integration Tests (SCSIT)	6–16 years	Body function	
	Developmental Tests			
	• BSID2	0–2 years	Activity	
	• PDMS2	0–5 years		
	• BOTMP	5–14 years		

Category	Objectives	Age	ICF Domain	Purpose
	• Goal Attainment Scaling (GAS)	Any age		Evaluative
	• Gross Motor Function Measure (GMFM)	2–5 years	Activity	Discriminative, Evaluative
Motor Function (motor control and learning)	• MAI • TIMP • HINT • AIMS	Infants	Body function, Activity	Discriminative, Predictive, Evaluative
	• GMFM	2–5 years		
	• Gross Motor Performance Measure (GMPM)			
	• Videography	Any age		
	• Laboratory tests (kinematics, kinetics, EMG, endurance)	Any age	Body function	Discriminative, Evaluative
	• Pediatric Evaluation of Disability Inventory (PEDI)	6 months –7.5 years		
	• School Function Assessment (SFA)	5–14 years	Activity	
	• Childhood Health Assessment Questionnaire (CHAQ)	1–19 years	Participation	
	• Pediatric PT Outcome Measure System (PT-OMS)	0–21 years		
Reflex Integrity	• MAI • TIMP	Infants	Body function, Activity	Discriminative, Predictive, Evaluative
Muscle Tone	• Modified Ashworth Scale			Discriminative
	• Spasticity Measurement System (SMS)	Any age	Body function	Discriminative, Evaluative

For further information on these tests and measures, go to Chapter 2, Appendix 2B, and Finch, E., Brooks, D., Stratford, P.W., & Mayo, N.E. (2002). *Physical rehabilitation outcome measures—A guide to enhanced clinical decision making, 2nd ed.* Philadelphia: Lippincott Williams & Wilkins and American Physical Therapy Association (2002). *Interactive guide to physical therapist practice—With catalog of tests and measures, Version 1.0.* Alexandria, VA: Author.

behaviors. Tests and measures of, for example, ROM, muscle strength, and postural control have demonstrated variability of the child's performance by the low reliability of results across time. The variability can be attributed to fluctuating abnormal muscle tone, poor motor coordination, medications or factors related to fatigue, age, behavior, pain, and attention, among others. Variability in motor coordination can occur because of immaturity of development, where the child is trying different patterns of motor activity in an attempt to arrive at the most efficient pattern. Variability could be a result of specific neuromuscular differences causing impaired control of descending input to the motor neuronal pools or integration of sensory inputs. Most likely, it is a combination of many factors. The important point is that test items may need to be repeated across time in a single session, and again at a later session to determine both the best and most common behavior.

The setting for the examination is important because children perform differently in different environments. Some tests are completed by observation in the child's natural environment or by interview of the parent or child about the child's abilities in natural settings . These evaluations may provide a more accurate view of the child's ability to use his or her motor capabilities within the day-to-day environment.

The child with neuromuscular disorders may have concomitant cognitive deficits and/or emotional/behavioral problems. Although it is difficult to determine how much these affect the child's motor performance, these issues should be monitored and measured in simple but reliable ways so that their extraneous effect on motor outcomes may be estimated. For example, short behavioral checklists have been created to accompany some developmental tests. Alternatively, you can use a standard three-point behavioral rating indicating simply that the child (1) appears to understand and comply to best of ability, (2) appears to understand and comply some of the time with testing procedures, and (3) frequently appears to not understand or comply with testing. By using this scale to estimate the validity of your examination results, you can interpret your findings in a more consistent manner.

Tests and measures that rely more heavily on observation of typical motor behaviors, rather than on asking the child to perform specific motor skills, may reduce the child's problems with understanding and complying with testing procedures. Observational measurements also help with evaluation of infants or young children who are not developmentally ready to follow directions. Observations at different times of the day and in different settings also provide insight into either internal biorhythms or environmental effects on motor behaviors.

Examination of Neuromotor and Sensory Integration and Motor Function

There are several standardized screening and developmental tests for infants and young children that are based on the typical sequence of motor skill acquisition. Each presents a scheme for observational and handling examination of children's motor function, reflexes, and postural patterns. Rating of the quality of postural control, presence of reflex movements, and coordination in static positions of lying, sitting, and standing, and during movements is described. Examples of these tests include the Harris Infant Neuromotor Test (HINT) (Harris & Daniels, 2001), Test of Infant Motor Performance (TIMP) (Campbell, Kolobe, Wright, & Linacre, 2002), Movement Assessment of Infant (MAI) (Chandler, Andrews, & Swanson, 1980), Gross Motor Performance Measure (GMPM) (Boyce et al., 1995), and the Alberta Infant Motor Scale (AIMS) (Piper & Darrah, 1994). Developmental tests for young children include items related to complex balance and coordination, such as balance on one foot, hopping, galloping, jumping patterns, and skipping. Examples of these are the Bayley Scales of Infant Development (2nd ed.) (BSID2) (Bayley, 1993), the Gross Motor Function Measure (Russell et al., 1993), and the Peabody Developmental Motor Scales (2nd ed.) (PDMS2) (Fewell & Folio, 2000). The Bruininks-Oseretsky Test of Motor Proficiency (BOTMP) (Bruininks, 1978) is one of the few tests of motor performance for children aged 4 to 14 years. These tests have moderate to good reliability and validity and therefore might be used for discriminative, evaluative, and predictive purposes.

The Pediatric Evaluation of Disability Inventory (PEDI) (Haley et al., 1992; Coster et al., 1994), the Childhood Health Assessment Questionnaire (CHAQ) (Singh, Athreya, Fries, & Goldsmith, 1994; Feldman et al., 1995), the School Function Assessment (SFA) (Coster et al., 1998), and a test under development, the Pediatric Physical Therapy Outcome Management System (PPT-OMS) (Palisano, Haley, Westcott, & Hess, 1999), are examples of tools to measure children's participation in home, school, and community activities and their personal activity and participation in society. Reliability and validity have been shown to be appropriate for the PEDI and the SFA (Coster et al., 1994, 1998; Haley et al., 1992), but further research is necessary for the CHAQ and PPT-OMS. These developmental and functionally based tests measure many aspects of movement. By focusing on specific items within the scales, the physical therapist can use them as discriminative tests to document general problems with postural stability or coordination. They are also useful as evaluative measures to document functional movement outcomes related to intervention to improve postural control or other impairments.

Care should be taken regarding the test used and population being examined because of problems with the responsivity (ability of a test to reflect meaningful change across time) of some of these tests (Coster et al., 1994; Palisano, Kolobe, Haley, Lowes, & Jones, 1995). These tests were designed specifically to document development of motor behaviors. Many of these tests are normed on large groups of children, allowing the tests to function well in a discriminative manner. Appropriate reliability and validity have also been established for most, so the tests can also be used for evaluative purposes. In children with severe neuromuscular disability, or when examining very specific motor behaviors, use of a developmental motor test is often not responsive to the small changes the child may make with time or procedural interventions. Tests that are individualized and sensitive to the specific motor objectives of your intervention may be unavailable. Also, in children with neuromuscular involvement, sometimes the intervention is focused on educating the caregiver to influence the child's motor skill and practice. Standardized tests that document specific caregiver positioning and handling behaviors are currently nonexistent, with the exception of the PEDI, which includes a scale to rate the amount of caregiver assistance needed for several activities of daily living. New tests need to be developed in this area.

Examination of Gait, Locomotion, and Balance

Testing procedures for gait and locomotion are discussed in Chapter 4. Postural control or the ability to maintain balance may be measured by examining the systems that contribute to our ability to balance (musculoskeletal, sensory, and neuromuscular) or by examining motor behaviors that stress one's ability to maintain balance (Westcott, Lowes, & Richardson, 1997). Several tests are described here.

Musculoskeletal System

Examination of the musculoskeletal system's contribution to postural control, for example, ROM and muscle force production, can be completed following the methods discussed in Chapter 4 and elsewhere. Adaptations of these tests for use with children with neuromuscular disability may be necessary because of the presence of contractures, abnormal muscle tone, sensory deficits, and cognitive disorders. The therapist should try to follow the standardized procedures and, if changes in procedures are made, record the changes. Retesting, using the same procedures, will ensure better reliability.

Sensory System

To examine the sensory system's contribution to postural control, the visual and somatosensory information available to the child can be systematically altered, and the effect on balance observed and measured. This can be accomplished by computer-driven equipment that varies the visual environment and the support surface (floor) that the child stands on to determine the effectiveness of the child's use of vision, somatosensation (cutaneous and proprioceptive information), and vestibular information. For the posturography test, the child stands on a computer-controlled, movable force platform facing the center of a three-sided movable visual enclosure. The support surface and visual surroundings can be rotated in proportion to body sway, thus providing inaccurate visual and somatosensory inputs regarding the orientation of the body's center of mass. Body sway in standing is measured under six sensory conditions, as detailed in Table 6.9. By testing under these different conditions, a particular sensory system or combinations of systems causing problems with postural control in standing can be estimated. Platform posturography measurement of sensory organization is being used with increasing frequency in clinics, despite the high cost of the apparatus (Rine, Rubish, & Feeney, 1998). Procedural interventions focused on practice using the deficit sensory system, or safety precaution instructions for when the child is in an environment requiring the deficit sensory system, can be prescribed based on the test results.

The Pediatric Clinical Test of Sensory Interaction for Balance (P-CTSIB) was developed as a low-cost clinical method to test sensory organization for maintenance of standing balance (Crowe, Deitz, Richardson, & Atwater, 1990); it is an inexpensive clinical alternative to platform posturography (Figure 6–14). The P-CTSIB uses the same

Table 6.9 Sensory Organization Test

Condition	Sensory Systems Available and Providing Accurate Information
1: Eyes open, normal surface	All sensory systems; vision, somatosensory, and vestibular available and providing accurate information about body position
2: Eyes closed, normal surface	No vision, must use accurate somatosensory and vestibular information
3: Visual conflict, normal surface	Sensory conflict caused by inaccurate visual information from visual surround moving in synchrony with the body sway, must ignore vision and use accurate somatosensory and vestibular information
4: Eyes open, somatosensory conflict	Sensory conflict caused by inaccurate somatosensory information from platform rotating in synchrony with the body sway, must ignore somatosensory and use accurate visual and vestibular information
5: Eyes closed, somatosensory conflict	No vision, sensory conflict caused by inaccurate somatosensory, must ignore somatosensory and use accurate vestibular information
6: Visual conflict, somatosensory conflict	Sensory conflict caused by inaccurate somatosensory and visual information, must ignore both and use accurate vestibular information

Source: Forssberg, H., & Nashner, L.M. (1982). Ontogenetic development of postural control in man: Adaptation to altered support and visual conditions during stance. *Journal of Neuroscience, 2*, 545–552; Shumway-Cook, A., & Woollacott, M.H. (1985). Dynamics of postural control in the child with Down syndrome. *Physical Therapy, 65*, 1315–1322, with permission.

six sensory conditions as platform posturography. Visual conflict is provided by use of a hatlike apparatus made up of a lightweight dome that, although allowing some diffuse light to come through, impedes the peripheral vision. As the child sways, the dome moves in synchrony with the head to simulate the moving visual surround of the platform posturography tests. Somatosensory conflict is provided by having the child stand on a piece of medium-density closed-cell foam, which dampens somatosensory input during somatosensory conflict conditions. Both the amount of time the child can stand in a feet-together position, and an observational measurement of anterior-posterior sway is recorded. These raw measurements are then combined for each of the six conditions and transformed into an ordinal scale spanning the inability to balance in the condition to the ability to balance for a maximum of 30 seconds with less than 5° of sway. These ordinal scores are then summed across sensory conditions to yield sensory system scores, which are thought to provide the tester with information about whether the child can process and use each of the three sensory systems: vision, somatosensory, and vestibular (Deitz, Richardson, Westcott, & Crowe, 1996).

Interrater reliability (Crowe et al., 1990) and test-retest reliability (Pelligrino, Buelow, Krause, Loucks, & Westcott, 1995; Westcott, Crowe, Deitz, & Richardson, 1994) of the P-CTSIB have been established for both children with and without disability. Although interrater reliability for sway measurements is moderate, test-retest reliability is lower. Pilot norms have been established for typically developing children (Deitz, Richardson, Atwater, & Crowe, 1991; Richardson, Atwater, Crowe, & Deitz, 1992). This was an easy test for children with typical development, ages 4 to 9 years. The children were able to stand for 30 seconds with less than 5° of sway in all conditions except the last two, where the time dropped by a few seconds, and the sway increased by several degrees, especially in the younger children. The P-CTSIB has been used to identify sensory organization differences between children who are typically developing and subsets of children with learning disability (Deitz et al., 1996), CP (Lowes, 1996), and DS (Westcott, Lowes, Richardson, Crowe, & Deitz, 1997), which demonstrates some construct validity for the test. Scores on the P-CTSIB also correlate with functional activities related to postural stability; therefore, performance on the test to some extent reflects functional ability (Lowes, 1996). Because of the level of interrater reliability, the beginning normative, and validity information, this test

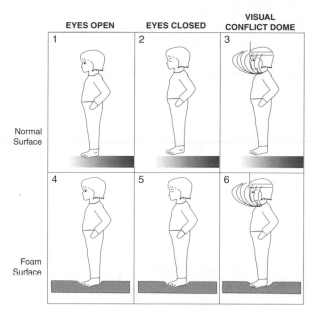

Figure 6-14 Pediatric clinical test of sensory interaction for balance (P-CTSIB). Testing conditions for the P-CTSIB include (1) eyes open, normal surface: vision, somatosensory and vestibular available; (2) eyes closed, normal surface: no vision, somatosensory, and vestibular available; (3) dome, normal surface: vision compromised, somatosensory and vestibular available; (4) eyes open, foam surface: somatosensory compromised, vision and vestibular available; (5) eyes closed, foam surface: no vision, somatosensory compromised, vestibular available; and (6) dome, foam surface: vision and somatosensory compromised, vestibular available. (From Crowe, T.K., Deitz, J.C., Richardson, P.K., & Atwater, S.W. [1990]. Interrater reliability of the Clinical Test of Sensory Interaction for Balance. *Physical and Occupational Therapy in Pediatrics, 10,* 9, with permission.)

could be useful for discriminative purposes. However, because of the moderate test-retest reliability, it is less appropriate for evaluative purposes without further research.

Neuromuscular System

Coordination

Testing of impairments in movement coordination, agility, initiation, modification, and control is difficult and generally requires a laboratory with complex computerized equipment that measures kinematics, kinetics, and EMG during movements such as gait (Graubert et al., 2000) and reaching (Fetters & Kluzik, 1996). In a slightly less compli-

cated manner, single joints during movement can be characterized using only kinematic data. An example of this testing method is the quantification of leg-kicking coordination (Geerdink, Hopkins, Beek, & Heriza, 1996; Heriza, 1991b). Markers were placed on the lower extremity joints of infants to allow recording of kinematics during spontaneous voluntary leg kicking. The joint angle data were then plotted in angle-time diagrams. Differences in the amount and velocity of movement in the joint of a full-term infant at 40 weeks' gestational age and a high-risk premature infant at the same gestational age is illustrated in Figure 6–15. Differences in coordination can be noted visually or quantified via measurements, such as maximal joint angle movement or velocity. Using this technique, subtle coordination differences can be used in a discriminative manner to compare across children with typical and atypical movement capability, and in an evaluative manner for examining intervention effectiveness.

To specifically examine the neuromuscular system for motor coordination problems during balancing, EMG recording of muscle activity, ground force reaction recordings via use of force plates to calculate center of pressure (COP) movement, and recording of three-dimensional (3-D) kinematics to either document movement at the joints or to calculate center of mass (COM) movement have been used in laboratory settings (Horak & Diener, 1994; Liu, 2001; Moe-Nilssen, 1998; Westcott & Zaino 1997; Zaino, 1999). This type of examination allows determination of actual selection, timing, sequencing, and amplitude of muscle activity; estimations of the COP (under the feet); and COM (whole body) movement and control during the motor activity. These sophisticated, labor-intensive, and expensive types of testing may be necessary for children when important decisions are being made regarding invasive surgical procedures or during research studies of procedural interventions. This equipment will probably not be available for routine use; however, the ability to interpret results from this testing is necessary because of its widespread use in hospitals and in research studies.

Clinical testing of the neuromuscular system usually involves methods of observational analysis of motor coordination during balancing. For example, therapists can place the child on a moveable surface (e.g., tilt boards, balls), move the surface under the child, and subjectively grade the motor response caused by the perturbation. This information is reported as "clinical observations" and is intended to document whether the child has the appropriate balancing motor strategies of head and trunk righting, arm and leg

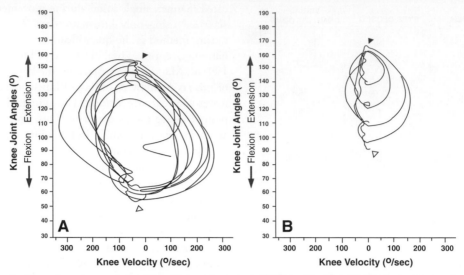

Figure 6-15 Evaluation of motor coordination. Phase-plane trajectories of knee joint angle to knee velocity during spontaneous kicking behavior of two infants: *(A)* Low-risk premature infant at 40 weeks gestation; *(B)* High-risk infant at 40 weeks gestation. Note that the low-risk infant shows greater range of knee joint movement at a greater variety of velocities compared to the high-risk infant. The difference in the coordination pattern can be visualized and quantified. (From Heriza, C.B. [1991b]. Implications of a dynamical systems approach to understanding infant kicking behavior. *Physical Therapy, 71*[3], 117. Reprinted with permission.)

counterbalancing, and protective extension. Although these tests are informative, their reliability is questionable. A more reliable method was developed by Fisher and Bundy (1982) using a flat board and tilt board reach test to measure motor coordination during balancing. In the test, children are photographed standing either on a flat board or tilt board with feet slightly apart and reaching as far laterally as they can for a toy held by the examiner. A standardized method for scoring head and trunk position, and arm and leg counterbalancing was developed and found to have good interrater reliability when photographed images were scored (Fisher, 1984). The test-retest reliability has not been examined. Construct validity for the test has been supported, as the test discriminates between children with learning disability and children who are developing typically (Fisher & Bundy, 1982). This test is unique because it provides a measurement of a feedforward postural response during the relatively functional task of reaching laterally. With the results, identification of motor coordination problems may be localized to head, trunk, or arms and legs, so appropriate procedural interventions can focus on the missing behaviors. This test can be used for discriminative purposes, but because of the current lack of test-retest reliability studies, it should not be used to evaluate progress.

Videotapes have been made of the children's balancing behavior during testing on the P-CTSIB (Lowes, 1996). These videotapes were later coded for the child's predominant motor coordination pattern used to balance during the testing, for example, use of ankle strategy, hip strategy, or crouching strategy. The interrater and intrarater reliabilities were moderate among three raters (Luyt et al., 1996). These researchers noted that repeated viewing of the videotapes may improve their reliability, but a more detailed analysis of the strategy through use of EMG may be necessary. Further modification and testing of this system of coding motor coordination responses need to be done before this can be a viable measurement system.

Reflex Integrity Including Muscle Tone

Reflex testing is included in many of the developmental tests described in the *Guide* (APTA, 2001) categories of Neuromotor and Sensory Integration, and Motor Function as noted in Table 6.8. Measurement of muscle tone, classified under this category, is described in more detail as related to children with neurological disabilities.

Objectively assessing muscle tone is difficult because of the variety of factors (spasticity, muscle weakness or poor power production, morphological changes in muscle and

Table 6.10 Modified Ashworth Scale

Score	Definition
0	No increase in muscle tone (MT)
1	Slight increase in MT, catch/release, increase at end of range
2	Slight increase in MT, catch and minimal resistance through rest of range
3	More marked increase in MT through most of range
4	Considerable increase in MT, passive movement difficult
5	Affected parts rigid in flexion or extension

Source: Bohannon, R.W., & Smith, M.B. (1987). Interrater reliability of a modified Ashworth scale of muscle spasticity: Suggestion from the field. *Physical Therapy, 65,* 46–47, with permission.

connective tissue, and co-contraction of antagonistic muscle groups) influencing muscle tone. The most commonly used way to quantify muscle tone is to evaluate resistance to passive movement at different speeds of movement using a *mild, moderate, severe* scale or the more descriptive modified Ashworth scale (Table 6.10) (Bohannon & Smith, 1987). The modified Ashworth scale is a structured method for assessing passive resistance to movement limitations (Pandyan et al., 1999). Although acceptable interrater reliability was found between testers in upper extremity muscles of adults with muscle tone differences (Sloan, Sinclair, Thompson, Taylor, & Pentland, 1992), studies in other adult populations showed varied reliability scores from moderately acceptable to good, especially in grading the plantar-dorsiflexion range through the ankle (Allison, Abraham, & Petersen, 1996; Gregson et al., 1999, 2000; Haas, Bergstrom, Jamous, & Bennie, 1996). No study reports specific reliability of scores in children; however, the modified Ashworth scale has been used in numerous studies involving children in which authors reported good reliability as part of their studies (Graubert et al., 2000; Hays et al., 1998). When using the modified Ashworth scale, care should be taken to document the methods to improve reliability on retesting. Rating levels of spasticity using the Ashworth scale show little correlation with functional ability (Fellows, Kaus, & Thilmann, 1994).

This is hypothesized to be caused by the complex nature of muscle tone, which varies during volitional movement. Finally, the sensitivity of the modified Ashworth scale to differentiate children with mild to moderate quadriceps spasticity has been shown to be low but can be improved by using a drop pendulum test (Fowler, Nwigwe, & Ho, 2000). In this test, an electric goniometer is placed on the knee to record the excursion of the first swing when the leg was dropped from full knee extension to knee flexion. Clinical use of this type of testing can improve the ability to show subtle change in spasticity across time or with intervention.

For highest sensitivity, there is the high-tech Spasticity Measurement System (SMS) (Lehmann, Price, deLateur, Hinderer, & Traynor, 1989; Price, Bjornson, Lehmann, McLaughlin, & Hays, 1991). The SMS requires complex mathematical computations and special computer-driven equipment (Lehmann et al., 1989). The ankle is strapped into a motor-driven rotating joint apparatus, and resistance to the movement, torque, is recorded at various speeds. The child is not to contract the muscles or resist the movement. A peripheral nerve block is used, if necessary, to ensure there is no voluntary muscle activation. The resistance to the movement is broken down into its sinusoidal components to calculate elastic stiffness and viscous stiffness. The relation between the stiffness and the speed of movement about a joint is calculated into a path length, which is reported to reflect reflex gain or spasticity. Test-retest reliability was found to be high (Lehmann et al., 1989). This test is valuable, especially for examination of the efficacy of invasive surgical or drug therapies on spasticity. Therapists need to be able to interpret these results to understand and evaluate studies designed to change spasticity.

Measurements of muscle tone during passive movement have not been shown to be valid estimates of the influence of muscle tone on active movement (Crenna, 1999; Dietz, 1999; Holt et al., 2000; Rothwell, 1994). Therefore, changes in tone as reflected on passive tests may not relate to changes in active functional movement. New techniques to assess muscle tone or stiffness during voluntary movement are currently under development for laboratory (Crenna, 1999) and clinical use (Holt et al., 2000). Clinical measurements of leg length, body weight, and swing cycle (seconds) during leg swinging in supported standing can be used to quantify stiffness based on the motion for a hybrid mass-spring pendulum. This measure was shown to correlate highly with a high-technology motion systems analysis of the leg swinging, and to show validity and reliability in a small group of children with and without CP (Holt et al.,

2000). Muscle tone tests of this nature will likely become the preferred measure in the future.

Although it is important to recognize and be able to describe muscle tone, emphasis on altering tone with physical therapy intervention may not be appropriate or effective. Emphasizing intervention to change motor coordination through practice and use of additional sensory cues may be more appropriate and long lasting, as discussed in Chapter 7.

Examination of Activities and Participation

Several functional tests that either directly or indirectly examine the child's activity and participation levels have already been discussed (e.g., SFA and PEDI). In addition, there are a few functional tests related to postural control developed for older adults that have now been studied in children. These tests are relatively simple to administer and score; thus they are easily used in clinical practice. The Berg Balance Scale is a functional balance test composed of movements and positions used by people throughout the day, such as moving from sit to stand, picking up objects from the floor, reaching, and turning in standing (Berg & Norman, 1996). Although originally developed for older adults, the directions, encouragement given, and safety procedures have recently been modified for use in pediatrics and renamed the Pediatric Balance Scale (Blair, 1999; Franjoine, Gunther, & Taylor, 2003). Test-retest and interrater reliability were high when reviewing videotapes of children performing the items, so this test could be used for evaluative purposes.

Several single-item tests also exist. The Functional Reach Test (FRT) (Duncan, Weiner, Chandler, & Studenski, 1990) quantifies the distance an individual can reach forward in standing (Donahoe, Turner, & Worrell, 1994; Wheeler, Shall, Lewis, & Shepherd, 1996). The "Timed Up-and-Go" (TUG) Test (Podsiadlo & Richardson, 1991) consists of recording the amount of time required to rise from a chair, walk 3 m, turn around, return to the chair, and sit down again (Habib & Westcott, 1998; Habib, Westcott, & Valvano, 1999). The Timed Obstacle Ambulation Test (TOAT) is currently being developed. It consists of an obstacle course that requires the child to move across different floor surfaces; step up, down, and over; duck under obstacles; and negotiate through turns and a narrow path (Benedetto et al., 1999). Interrater, intrarater, and test-retest reliability on these single-item tests, as examined in small research studies, are generally high, making them good tests for evaluative purposes. However, more research is needed using larger pediatric populations to determine if they can also be used for discriminative or predictive purposes.

Diagnosis and Prognosis

After the chosen tests and measures are completed, the therapist needs to formulate the evaluation of the child, which weighs all examination issues related to the child as well as the family, school, and community. This evaluation will lead to a diagnostic classification as delineated in the *Guide* (APTA, 2001). The therapist also must hypothesize a prognosis for the child in terms of motor function. The evaluation, diagnosis, and prognosis should lead to the plan of care and the components of the intervention.

Because functional changes in activities and participation are the overall goal of intervention, the intervention should be child-centered and reflect meaningful functional activities for the child or caregiver (Randall & McEwen, 2000). Goal Attainment Scaling (GAS) (Brown, Effgen, & Palisano, 1998; King, McDougall, Palisano, Gritzan, & Tucker, 1999; Maloney, 1993; Palisano, 1993) is a system that allows the therapist to write specific objectives for an individual child and then code progress related to those objectives using a point system. The therapist develops the individual standard for each level of improvement or decline on the objective. An example of GAS for the specific objective to ascend and descend four steps on a ramp without assistance or holding is described in Table 6.11. Strategies to develop the plan of care for children with neuromuscular disorders are described in Chapter 7.

Summary

The neurological system, from conception, includes some redundancy of neurons and pathways to decrease the effect of injury. Although the neural tissue does not regenerate after injury, there are many ways that functional recovery can occur through maintaining or expanding the capacity of the uninjured neurons and support cells. The primary way to influence the recovery of motor behaviors appears to be through continued use and practice of movements. This represents the basis for early intervention with infants and children immediately after injury or at high risk for later disability. It is recommended that therapists think through the rationale for their examination and intervention and be clear about the perspective that is driving the techniques selected.

Table 6.11 Goal Attainment Scaling Example

Objective: Bill will be able to ascend and descend the 4 steps into his school without assistance or holding the railing, 3 out of 3 times by December 1. (Bill's current ability is to ascend and descend 2 steps into his school, slowly and safely while holding the railing, 3 out of 3 times.)

Score	Objective Level
+2	Bill will be able to ascend and descend the 4 steps into his school, safely without assistance or holding the railing, *quickly enough to walk to and from his classroom within 1 minute,* * 3 out of 3 times by December 1.
+1	Bill will be able to ascend and descend the 4 steps into his school safely without assistance or holding the railing, *quickly enough to walk to and from his classroom within 5 minutes,* 3 out of 3 times by December 1.
0	Bill will be able to ascend and descend the 4 steps into his school *safely without assistance or holding the railing,* 3 out of 3 times by December 1.
–1	Bill will be able to ascend and descend the 4 steps into his school *safely while holding the railing,* 3 out of 3 times by December 1.
–2	Bill will be able to ascend and descend the 4 steps into his school *safely with stand-by assistance while holding the railing,* 3 out of 3 times by December 1.

* The italicized portions represent the criteria change of the objective across the different score levels.

DISCUSSION QUESTIONS

1. Construct a table using the headings below for each pediatric neuromuscular disorder presented in this chapter (DS, DCD, CP, TBI, and MM).

Diagnosis	Impairments of Body Functions	Potential Activity Limitations and Participation Restrictions

Now, using the information from the table, compare and contrast impairments in body functions, potential activity limitations, and participation restrictions.

2. What criteria would you use to help you decide if and when spasticity is a concern for rehabilitation?

3. Explain how theories of motor control influence rehabilitation practice.

4. Which motor control theory is more likely to influence your examination approach to a 3-year-old with a traumatic brain injury? Explain why.

5. How would your physical therapy examination of a 2-year-old boy with spastic diplegic CP differ from your examination of a 7-year-old girl with DCD?

6. Discuss the benefits and disadvantages of several methods of testing postural control.

REFERENCES

Achenbach, T.M., Howell, C.T., Aoki, M.F., & Rauh, V.A. (1993). Nine-year outcome of the Vermont intervention program for low birth weight infants. *Pediatrics, 91*(1), 45–55.

Adolph, K.E., & Eppler, M.A. (2002). Flexibility and specificity in infant motor skill acquisition. *Progress in Infancy Research, 2,* 121–167.

Albright, A.L. (1996). Intrathecal baclofen in cerebral palsy movement disorders. *Journal of Child Neurology, 11,* (Suppl. 1), 29–35.

Albright, A.L., Barry, M.J., Shafton, D.H., & Ferson, S.S. (2001). Intrathecal baclofen for generalized dystonia. *Developmental Medicine and Child Neurology, 43*(10), 652–657.

Allison, S.C., Abraham, L.D., & Petersen, C.L. (1996). Reliability of the Modified Ashworth Scale in the assessment of plantar flexor muscle spasticity in patients with traumatic brain injury. *International Journal of Rehabilitation Research, 19*(1), 67–78.

Almeida, G.L., Campbell, S.K., Girolami, G.L., Penn, R.D., & Corcos, D.M. (1997). Multidimensional assessment of motor function in a child with cerebral palsy following intrathecal administration of baclofen. *Physical Therapy, 77,* 751–764.

Almeida, G., Corcos, D.M., & Latash, M.L. (1994). Practice and transfer effects during fast single-joint elbow movements in individuals with Down syndrome. *Physical Therapy, 74,* 1000–1016.

American Physical Therapy Association (APTA) (2001). Guide to physical therapist practice (2nd ed). *Physical Therapy, 81,* 1–768.

American Psychiatric Association (1994). *Diagnostic and statistical manual of mental disorders (DSM-IV).* Washington, DC: Author.

Armstrong, R.W., Steinbok, P., Cochrane, D.D., Kube, S.D., Fife, S.E., & Farrell, K. (1997). Intrathecally administered baclofen for treatment of children with spasticity of cerebral origin. *Journal of Neurosurgery, 87*(3), 409–414.

Aruin, A.S., Almeida, G.L., & Latash, M.L. (1996). Organization of a simple two-joint synergy in individuals with Down syndrome. *American Journal of Mental Retardation, 101*, 256–268.

Aruin, A.S., & Almeida, G.L. (1997). A coactivation strategy in anticipatory postural adjustments in persons with Down syndrome. *Motor Control, 1*, 178–191.

Aruin, A.S., & Latash, M.L. (1995). The role of motor action in anticipatory postural adjustments studied with self-induced and externally triggered perturbations. *Experimental Brain Research, 106*, 291–300.

Atwater, S.W. (1991). Should the normal motor developmental sequence be used as a theoretical model in pediatric physical therapy? In M.J. Lister (Ed.), *Contemporary management of motor problems: Proceedings of the II STEP Conference* (pp. 89–93). Alexandria, VA: Foundation for Physical Therapy.

Aylward, E.H., Habbak, R., Warren, A.C., Pulsifer, M.B., Barta, P.E., Jerram, M., & Pearlson, G.D. (1997). Cerebellar volume in adults with Down syndrome. *Archives of Neurology, 54*, 209–212.

Ayres, A.J. (1979). *Sensory integration and the child*. Los Angeles, CA: Western Psychological Services.

Bach-y-Rita, P. (1990). Brain plasticity as a basis for recovery of function in humans. *Neuropsychologia, 28*(6), 547–554.

Badell, A. (1992). Myelodysplasia. In G.E. Molnar (Ed.), *Pediatric rehabilitation* (2nd ed., pp. 222). Baltimore: Williams & Wilkins.

Barkovich, A.J., & Truit, C.L. (1990). Brain damage from perinatal asphyxia: Correlation of MR findings with gestational age. *American Journal of Neuroradiology, 11*, 1087–1096.

Barry, M.J. (1996). Physical therapy interventions for patients with movement disorders due to cerebral palsy. *Journal of Child Neurology, 11,* (Suppl. 1), S51–S60.

Barry, M.J., Albright, A.L., & Shultz, B.L. (2000). Intrathecal baclofen and the role of the physical therapist. *Pediatric Physical Therapy, 12*, 77–86.

Bartlett, D. (1997). Primitive reflexes and early motor development. *Developmental and Behavioral Pediatrics, 18*, 151–157.

Bartonek, A., & Saraste, H. (2001). Factors influencing ambulation in myelomeningocele: A cross-sectional study. *Developmental Medicine and Child Neurology, 43*, 253–260.

Bastian, A.J. (1997). Mechanisms of ataxia. *Physical Therapy, 77*, 672–675.

Bayley, N. (1993). *Bayley Scales of Infant Development* (2nd ed). San Antonio, TX: Psychological Corporation.

Becker, E., Bar-Or, O., Mendelson, L., & Najenson, T. (1978). Pulmonary functions and responses to exercise of patients following craniocerebral injury. *Scandinavian Journal of Rehabilitation Medicine, 10*, 47.

Beckung, E., & Hagberg, G. (2000). Correlation between ICIDH handicap code and Gross Motor Classification System in children with cerebral palsy. *Developmental Medicine and Child Neurology, 42*, 669–673.

Benedetto, M., Thawinchai, N., Prasertsukdee, S., Tieman, B., O'Brien, M., & Westcott, S. (1999). Reliability and validity of a new assessment tool to measure pediatric functional mobility: A pilot study. *Pediatric Physical Therapy, 11*, 214–215.

Berg, K.O., & Norman, K.E. (1996). Functional assessment of balance and gait. *Clinics in Geriatric Medicine, 12*, 705–723.

Berger, W., Horstmann, G., & Dietz, V. (1984). Tension development and muscle activation in the leg during gait in spastic hemiparesis: Independence of muscle hypertonia and exaggerated stretch reflexes. *Journal of Neurology, Neurosurgery, and Psychiatry, 47,* 1029–1033.

Berger, W., Quintern, J., & Dietz, V. (1982). Pathophysiology of gait in children with cerebral palsy. *Electroencephalography and Clinical Neurophysiology, 53*, 538–548.

Bernstein, N. (1967). *The coordination and regulation of movement*. London, England: Pergamon Press Ltd.

Blair, L.C. (1999). Assessment of functional balance of a pediatric client using the Berg Balance Test. *Pediatric Physical Therapy, 11*, 225.

Blaskey, J., & Jennings, M.C. (1999). Traumatic brain injury. In S.K. Campbell (Ed.), *Decision making in pediatric neurologic physical therapy* (pp. 84–139). Philadelphia: Churchill Livingstone.

Bly, L. (1991). A historical and current view of the basis of neurodevelopmental therapy. *Pediatric Physical Therapy, 3*, 131–135.

Bobath, B. (1964). Facilitation of normal postural reactions and movement in the treatment of cerebral palsy. *Physiotherapy, 50*, 246–262.

Bobath, B. (1985). *Abnormal postural reflex activity caused by brain lesions*. Rockville, MD: Aspen Publishers Inc.

Bobath, K., & Bobath, B. (1984). The neuro-developmental treatment. In D. Scrutton (Ed.), *Management of the motor disorders of children with cerebral palsy* (pp. 6–17*)*. Philadelphia: Lippincott.

Bohannon, R.W., & Smith, M.B. (1987). Interrater reliability of a modified Ashworth scale of muscle spasticity: Suggestion from the field. *Physical Therapy, 65,* 46–47.

Booth, C.M., Cortina-Borja, M.J.F., & Theologis, T.N. (2001). Collagen accumulation in muscles of children with cerebral palsy and correlation with severity of spasticity. *Developmental Medicine and Child Neurology, 43*, 314–320.

Born, P., & Lou, H.C. (1999). Imaging in learning disorders. In K. Whitmore, H. Hart, & G. Willems (Eds.), *A neurodevelopmental approach to specific learning disorders* (pp. 247–258). London: MacKeith Press.

Bowen, J.M., Clark, E., Bigler, E.D., Gardner, M., Nilsson, D., Gooch, J., & Pompa, J. (1997). Childhood traumatic brain injury: Neuropsychological status at the time of hospital discharge. *Developmental Medicine and Child Neurology, 39*(1), 17–25.

Boyce, W.F., Gowland, C., Rosenbaum, P.L., Lane, M., Plews, N., Goldsmith, C.H., Russell, D.J., Wright, V., Potter, S., & Harding, D. (1995). The Gross Motor Performance Measure: Validity and responsiveness of a measure of quality of movement. *Physical Therapy, 75*(7), 603–13.

Boyd, R.N., Pliatsios, V., Starr, R., Wolfe, R., & Graham, H.K. (2000). Biomechanical transformation of the gastroc-soleus muscle with botulinum toxin A in children with cerebral palsy. *Developmental Medicine and Child Neurology, 42*(1), 32–41.

Brown, D.A., Effgen, S.K., & Palisano, R.J. (1998). Performance following ability-focused physical therapy intervention in individuals with severely limited physical and cognitive abilities. *Physical Therapy, 78*(9), 934–947.

Bruininks, R. (1978). *Bruininks-Oseretsky test of motor proficiency.* Circle Pines, MN: American Guidance Service.

Brunnstrom, S. (1992). *Movement therapy in hemiplegia* (2nd ed.). Philadelphia: Lippincott.

Burleigh, A., & Horak, F. (1996). Influence of instruction, prediction, and afferent sensory information on the postural organization of step initiation. *Journal of Neurophysiology, 75,* 1619–1627.

Burleigh, A.L., Horak, F.B., & Malouin, F. (1994). Modification of postural responses and step initiation: Evidence for goal-directed postural interactions. *Journal of Neurophysiology, 72,* 2892–2902.

Burleigh-Jacobs, A. (1998). Neuroplasticity. In: L. Lundy-Ekman (Ed.), *Neuroscience: Fundamentals for rehabilitation* (pp. 58–68). Philadelphia: W.B. Saunders.

Burtner, P.A., Woollacott, M.H., & Qualls, C. (1999). Stance balance control with orthoses in a group of children with spastic cerebral palsy. *Developmental Medicine and Child Neurology, 41,* 748–757.

Butler, C., & Campbell, S. (2000). Evidence of the effects of intrathecal baclofen for spastic and dystonic cerebral palsy. *Developmental Medicine and Child Neurology, 42,* 634–645.

Butler, C., & Darrah, J. (2001). Effects of neurodevelopmental treatment (NDT) for cerebral palsy: An AACPDM evidence report. *Developmental Medicine and Child Neurology, 43,* 778–790.

Cabana, T. (1999). Development of the nervous system. In H. Cohen (Ed.), *Neuroscience for rehabilitation* (2nd ed., pp. 369–399). Philadelphia: Lippincott Williams & Wilkins.

Calancie, B., Needham-Shropshire, B., Jacobs, P., Willer, K., Zych, G., & Green, B.A. (1995). Involuntary stepping after chronic spinal cord injury: Evidence for a central rhythm generator for locomotion in man. *Brain, 117,* 1143–1159.

Campbell, S.K., Kolobe, T.H.A., Wright, B., & Linacre, J.M. (2002). Validity of the Test of Infant Motor Performance for prediction of 6-, 9-, and 12-month scores on the Alberta Infant Motor Scale. *Developmental Medicine and Child Neurology, 44,* 263–272.

Campos, J.J., Bertenthal, B.I., & Kermoian, R. (1992). Early experience and emotional development: The emergence of wariness of heights. *Psychological Science, 3,* 61–64.

Cantell, M.H., Smith, M.M., & Ahonen, T.P. (1994). Clumsiness in adolescence: Educational, motor, and social outcomes of motor delay detected at 5 years. *Adapted Physical Activity Quarterly, 13,* 61–73.

Capone, G.T. (1996). Human brain development. In A.J. Capute & P.J. Accardo (Eds.), *Developmental disabilities in infancy and childhood: Vol. I. Neurodevelopmental diagnosis and treatment* (2nd ed., pp. 25–75). Baltimore: Paul H. Brookes Publishing Co.

Chad, K.E., McKay, H.A., Zello, G.A., Bailey, D.A., Faulkner, R.A., & Snyder, R.E. (2000). Body composition in nutritionally adequate ambulatory and non-ambulatory children with cerebral palsy and a healthy reference group. *Developmental Medicine and Child Neurology, 42,* 334–339.

Chan, K., Ohlsson, A., Synnes, A., Lee D.S., Chien, L.Y., & Lee, S.K. (2001). Survival, morbidity, and resource use of infants of 25 weeks' gestational age or less. *American Journal of Obstetrics and Gynecology, 185*(1), 220–226.

Chandler, L., Andrews, M., & Swanson, M. (1980). *Movement assessment of infants.* Rolling Bay, WA: Rolling Bay Press.

Chaplin, D., Deitz, J., & Jaffe, K.M. (1993). Motor performance in children after traumatic brain injury. *Archives of Physical Medicine and Rehabilitation, 74,* 161–164.

Charles, J., Lavinder, G., & Gordon, A.M. (2001). Effects of constraint-induced therapy on hand function in children with hemiplegic cerebral palsy. *Pediatric Physical Therapy, 13,* 68–76.

Christiansen, A.S. (2000). Persisting motor control problems in 11- to 12-year-old boys previously diagnosed with deficits in attention, motor control, and perception (DAMP). *Developmental Medicine and Child Neurology, 42,* 4–7.

Cheung, M.E., & Broman, S.H. (2000). Adaptive learning: Interventions for verbal and motor deficits. *Neurorehabilitation and Neural Repair, 14*(3), 159–169.

Cioni, M., Cocilovo, A., Di Pasquale, F., Araujo, M.B., Siqueira, C.R., & Bianco, M. (1994). Strength deficit of knee extensor muscles of individuals with Down syndrome from childhood to adolescence. *American Journal of Mental Retardation, 99*(2), 166–174.

Clarac, F. (1991). How do sensory and motor signals interact during locomotion? In D.R. Humphrey & H.J. Freund (Eds.), *Motor control: Concepts and issues* (pp. 199–221). New York: John Wiley & Sons.

Cohen, H. (1999). *Neuroscience for rehabilitation* (2nd ed.). Philadelphia: Lippincott Williams & Wilkins.

Corcos, D.M., Gottlieb, G.L., & Agarwal, G.C. (1989). Organizing principles for single joint movements: II. A speed-sensitive strategy. *Journal of Neurophysiology, 62,* 358–368.

Cordo, P.J., & Nashner, L.M. (1982). Properties of postural adjustments associated with rapid arm movements. *Journal of Neurophysiology, 47,* 287–302.

Coster, W., Deeney, T., Haltiwanger, J., & Haley, S. (1998). *School function assessment.* San Antonio, TX: Psychological Corporation.

Coster, W.J., Haley, S., & Baryza, J. (1994). Functional performance of young children after traumatic brain injury: A 6-month follow-up study. *American Journal of Occupational Therapy, 48,* 211–218.

Craik, R.L. (1991). Abnormalities of motor behavior. In M.J. Lister (Ed.), *Contemporary management of motor problems: Proceedings of the II STEP Conference* (pp. 155–164). Alexandria, VA: Foundation for Physical Therapy.

Cratty, B.J. (1994). *Clumsy child syndrome: Descriptions, evaluation, and remediation.* Chur, Switzerland: Harwood Academic Publishers.

Crawford, S.G., Wilson, B.N., & Dewey, D. (2001). Identifying developmental coordination disorder: Consistency between tests. *Physical and Occupational Therapy in Pediatrics, 20*(2–3), 29–50.

Crenna, P. (1998). Spasticity and spastic gait in children with cerebral palsy. *Neuroscience Biobehavioral Review, 22,* 571–578.

Crenna, P. (1999). Pathophysiology of lengthening contractions in human spasticity: A study of the hamstring muscles during locomotion. *Pathophysiology, 5,* 283–297.

Crocker, M., Mackay-Lyons, M., & McDonnell, E. (1997). Forced use of the upper extremity in cerebral palsy: A single case design. *American Journal of Occupational Therapy, 51,* 824–833.

Crowe, T.K., Deitz, J.C., Richardson, P.K., & Atwater, S.W. (1990). Interrater reliability of the Clinical Test of Sensory Interaction for Balance. *Physical and Occupational Therapy in Pediatrics, 10,* 1–27.

Cuddeford, T.J., Freeling, R.P., Thomas, S.S., Aiona, M.D., Rex, D., Sirolli, H., Elliott, J., & Magnusson, M. (1997). Energy consumption in children with myelomeningocele: A comparison between reciprocating gait orthosis and hip-knee-ankle-foot orthosis ambulators *Developmental Medicine and Child Neurology, 39,* 239– 242.

Damiano, D.L. (1993). Reviewing muscle cocontraction: Is it a developmental, pathological, or motor control issue? *Physical and Occupational Therapy in Pediatrics, 12,* 3–20.

Damiano, D.L., & Abel, M.F. (1998). Functional outcomes of strength training in spastic cerebral palsy. *Archives of Physical Medicine and Rehabilitation, 79,* 119–125.

Damiano, D.L., Martellotta, M.S., Sullivan, D.J., Granata, K.P., & Abel, M.F. (2000). Muscle force production and functional performance in spastic cerebral palsy: Relationship of cocontraction. *Archives of Physical Medicine and Rehabilitation, 81,* 895–900.

David, K.S. (2000). Developmental coordination disorders. In S.K. Campbell, D.W. Vander Linden, & R.J. Palisano (Eds.), *Physical therapy for children* (2nd ed., pp. 471–501). Philadelphia: W.B. Saunders.

Davies, P.L., & Rose, J.D. (2000). Motor skills of typically developing adolescents: Awkwardness or improvement? *Physical and Occupational Therapy in Pediatrics, 20*(1), 19–42.

Deitz, J.C., Richardson, P.K., Atwater, S.W., & Crowe, T.K. (1991). Performance of normal children on the Pediatric Clinical Test of Sensory Interaction for Balance. *Occupational Therapy Journal of Research, 11,* 336–356.

Deitz, J., Richardson, P.K., Westcott, S.L., & Crowe, T.K. (1996). Performance of children with learning disabilities on the Pediatric Clinical Test of Sensory Interaction for Balance. *Physical and Occupational Therapy in Pediatrics, 16,* 1-21.

DeLuca, S.C., Echols, K., Ramey, S.L. & Taub, E. (2003). Pediatric constraint-induced movement therapy for a young child with cerebral palsy: Two episodes of care. *Physical Therapy, 83,* 1003–1013.

De Luca, G.P., Volpin, L., Fornezza, U., Cervellini, P., Zanusso, M., Casentini, L., et al., (2000). The role of decompressive craniectomy in the treatment of uncontrollable post-traumatic intracranial hypertension. *Acta Neurochirurgica, Supplementum, 76,* 401–404.

Dewey, D., & Wilson, B.N. (2001). Developmental coordination disorder: What is it? *Physical and Occupational Therapy in Pediatrics, 20*(2-3), 5-27.

Dichter, C.G. (1994). Relationship of muscle strength and joint range of motion to gross motor abilities in school-aged children with Down syndrome. Unpublished doctoral dissertation, Hahnemann University, Philadelphia, PA.

Dichter, C.G., DeCicco, J., Flanagan, S., Hyun, J., & Mongrain, C. (2000). Acquiring skill through intervention in adolescents with Down syndrome. *Pediatric Physical Therapy, 12,* 209.

Diener, H.C., Bootz, F., Dichgans, J., & Bruzek, W. (1983). Variability of postural "reflexes" in humans. *Experimental Brain Research, 52*(3), 423–428.

Dietz, V. (1999). Supraspinal pathways and the development of muscle-tone dysregulation. *Developmental Medicine and Child Neurology, 41,* 708–715.

Dietz, V., & Berger, W. (1995). Cerebral palsy and muscle transformation. *Developmental Medicine and Child Neurology, 37,* 180–184.

Dietz, V., & Berger, W. (1983). Normal and impaired regulation of muscle stiffness in gait: A new hypothesis about muscle hypertonia. *Experimental Neurology, 79,* 680–687.

Dietz, V., Colombo, G., & Jensen, L. (1994). Locomotor activity in spinal man. *Lancet, 344,* 1260–1262.

Dietz, V., Ketelsen, U.P., Berger, W., & Quintern, J. (1986). Motor unit involvement in spastic paresis: Relationship between leg muscle activation and histochemistry. *Journal of the Neurological Sciences, 75,* 89–103.

Dietz, V., Quintern, J., & Berger, W. (1981). Electrophysiological studies of gait in spasticity and rigidity: Evidence that altered mechanical properties of muscle contribute to hypertonia. *Brain, 104,* 431–449.

Dobkin, B.H. (1998). Activity-dependent learning contributes to motor recovery. *Annals of Neurology, 44,* 158–160.

Domain, R.J., Spitz, E.B., Zucman, E., et al. (1960). Children with severe brain injuries: Neurological organization in terms of mobility. *Journal of the American Medical Association, 17,* 257–262.

Donahoe, B., Turner, D., & Worrell, T. (1994). The use of functional reach as a measurement of balance in boys and girls without disabilities ages 5 to 15 years. *Pediatric Physical Therapy, 6,* 189–193.

Downard, C., Hulka, F., Mullins, R.J., Piatt, J., Chesnut,

R., Quint, P., & Mann, N.C. (2000). Relationship of cerebral perfusion pressure and survival in pediatric brain-injured patients. *Journal of Trauma, 49*(4), 654–658.

Duncan, P.W., Weiner, D.K., Chandler, J., & Studenski, S. (1990). Functional reach: A new clinical measure of balance. *Journal of Gerontology, 45*, M192–M197.

Duysens, J., & Van de Crommert, H.W.A.A. (1998). Neural control of locomotion: Part 1: The central pattern generator from cats to humans. *Gait and Posture, 7*, 131–141.

Edelman, G.M. (1989). *The remembered present: A biological theory of consciousness.* New York: Basic Books.

Edelman, G.M. (1993). Neural Darwinism: Selection and reentrant signaling in higher brain function. *Neuron, 10*, 115–125.

Edgerton, V.R. (1997). Use-dependent plasticity in spinal stepping and standing. *Advances in Neurology: Neuronal Regeneration, Reorganization, and Repair, 72*, 233–247.

El-Abd, M.A.R., Ibrahim, I.K., & Dietz, V. (1993). Impaired activation pattern in antagonistic elbow muscles of patients with spastic hemiparesis: Contribution to movement disorder. *Electromyography and Clinical Neurophysiology, 33*, 247–255.

England, M.A. (1988). Normal development of the central nervous system. In M.I. Levene, M.J. Bennett, & J. Punt (Eds.), *Fetal and neonatal neurology and neurosurgery* (pp. 3–27). New York: Churchill Livingstone.

Ewing-Cobbs, L., Fletcher, J.M., Levin, H.S., Francis, D.J., Davidson, K., & Miner, M.E. (1997). Longitudinal neuropsychological outcome in infants and preschoolers with traumatic brain injury. *Journal of the International Neuropsychological Society, 3*, 581–591.

Fahn, S. (1999). Generalized dystonia: Concept and treatment. *Clinical Neuropharmacology, 9* (Suppl. 2), S37–S48.

Fay, G.C., Jaffe, K.M., Polissar, N.L., Liao, S., Rivara, J.B., & Martin, K.M. (1994). Outcome of pediatric traumatic brain injury at three years: A cohort study. *Archives of Physical Medicine and Rehabilitation, 75*, 733–741.

Feldman, B.M., Ayling-Campos, A., Luy, L., Stevens, D., Silverman, E.D., & Laxer, R.M. (1995). Measuring disability in juvenile dermatomyositis: Validity of the Childhood Health Assessment Questionnaire. *Journal of Rheumatology, 22*, 326–331.

Fellows, S.J., Kaus, C., & Thilmann, A.F. (1994). Voluntary movement at the elbow in spastic hemiparesis. *Annals of Neurology, 36*, 397–407.

Fellows, S.J., Kaus, C., Ross, H.F., & Thilmann, A.F. (1994). Agonist and antagonist EMG activation during isometric torque development at the elbow in spastic hemiparesis. *Electroencephalography and Clinical Neurophysiology, 93*, 106–112.

Ferguson, R.L., Putney, M.E., & Allen, B.L., Jr. (1997). Comparison of neurologic deficits with atlanto-dens intervals in patients with Down syndrome. *Journal of Spinal Disorders, 10*(3), 246–252.

Fetters, L., & Kluzik, J. (1996). The effects of neurodevelopmental treatment versus practice on the reaching of children with spastic cerebral palsy. *Physical Therapy, 76*(4), 346–358.

Fewell, R., & Folio, R. (2000). *Peabody developmental motor scales* (2nd ed.). Austin, TX: Pro-Ed.

Fisher, A.G. (1984). Equilibrium: Development and clinical assessment. Unpublished doctoral dissertation, Boston University, Boston.

Fisher, A.G., & Bundy, A.C. (1982). Equilibrium reactions in normal children and in boys with sensory integrative dysfunctions. *Occupational Therapy Journal of Research, 2*, 171–183.

Fisher, A.G., Murray, E.A., & Bundy, A.C. (1991). *Sensory integration: Theory and practice.* Philadelphia: F.A. Davis.

Forssberg, H., & Dietz, V. (1997). Neurobiology of normal and impaired locomotor development. In K.J. Connolly & H. Forssberg (Eds.), *Neurophysiology and neuropsychology of motor development* (pp. 78-100). London: MacKeith Press.

Forssberg, H., & Nashner, L.M. (1982). Ontogenetic development of postural control in man: Adaptation to altered support and visual conditions during stance. *Journal of Neuroscience, 2*, 545–552.

Forssberg, H., & Tedroff, K.B. (1997). Botulinum toxin treatment in cerebral palsy: Intervention with poor evaluation? *Developmental Medicine and Child Neurology, 39*(9), 635–640.

Fowler, E.G., Nwigwe, A.I., & Ho, T.W. (2000). Sensitivity of the pendulum test for assessing spasticity in persons with cerebral palsy. *Developmental Medicine and Child Neurology, 42*(3), 182–189.

Fox, A.M., & Lent, B. (1996). Clumsy children. Primer on developmental coordination disorder. *Canadian Family Physician, 42*, 1965–1971.

Franjoine, M.R., Gunther, J.S., & Taylor, M.J. (2003). The pediatric balance scale: A modified version of the Berg Scale for children with mild to moderate motor impairment. *Pediatric Physical Therapy, 15*(2), 114–128.

Frank, J.S., & Earl, M. (1990). Coordination of posture and movement. *Physical Therapy, 12*, 855–863.

Franks, C.A., Palisano, R.J., & Darbee, J.C. (1991). The effect of walking with an assistive device and using a wheelchair on school performance in students with myelomeningocele. *Physical Therapy, 71*, 570–578.

Freed, S.S., Catlin, P.A., Bobo, L.M., Fagan, E.L., & Moebes, M.N. (1999). The effect of constraint-induced movement on upper extremity function in children with hemiplegia. *Pediatric Physical Therapy, 11*, 226–227.

Freeman, S.B., Taft, L.F., Dooley, K.J., Allran, K., Sherman, S.L., Hassold, T.J., Khoury, M.J., & Saker, D.M. (1998). Population-based study of congenital heart defects in Down syndrome. *American Journal of Medical Genetics, 80*(3), 213–217.

Fuchs, A.F., Anderson, M.E., Binder, M.D., & Fetz, E.E. (1989). The neural control of movement. In Patton, H.D., Fuchs, A.F., Hille, B., Scher, A.M., & Steiner, R. (Eds.), *Textbook of physiol-*

ogy: *Excitable cells and neurophysiology,* Vol. 1 (pp. 503–509). Philadelphia: W.B. Saunders.

Fulop, Z.L., Wright, D.W., & Stein, D.G. (1998). Pharmacology of traumatic brain injury: Experimental models and clinical implications. *Neurology Report of Neurology Section of American Physical Therapy Association, 22,* 100–109.

Geddes, J.F., Hackshaw, A.K., Vowles, G.H., Nickols, C.D., & Whitwell, H.L. (2001). Neuropathology of inflicted head injury in children. I. Patterns of brain damage. *Brain, 124*(7), 1290–1298.

Geddes, J.F., Vowles, G.H., Hackshaw, A.K., Nickols, C.D., Scott, I.S., & Whitwell, H.L. (2001). Neuropathology of inflicted head injury in children. II. Microscopic brain injury in infants. *Brain, 124*(7), 1299–1306.

Geerdink, J.J., Hopkins, B., Beek, W.J., & Heriza, C.B. (1996). The organization of leg movements in preterm and full-term infants after term age. *Developmental Psychobiology, 29*(4), 335–351.

Gillberg, C. (1999). Management of behavioral problems in specific learning disorders. In K. Whitmore, H. Hart, & G. Willems (Eds). *A neurodevelopmental approach to specific learning disorders* (pp. 270–279). London: MacKeith Press.

Gillberg, I.C. (1988). Generalized hyperkinesis: Follow-up study from 7 to 13 years. *Journal of the American Academy of Child and Adolescent Psychiatry, 27,* 55–59.

Giuliani, C.A. (1991). Dorsal rhizotomy for children with cerebral palsy: Support for concepts of motor control. *Physical Therapy, 71,* 248–259.

Gooch, J.L., & Sandell, T.V. (1996). Botulinum toxin for spasticity and athetosis in children with cerebral palsy. *Archives of Physical Medicine and Rehabilitation, 77*(5), 508–511.

Goodwin, G.M., McCloskey, D.J., & Matthews, P.B.C. (1972). The contribution of muscle afferents to kinaesthesia shown by vibration-induced illusions of movement and by effects of paralysing joint afferents. *Brain, 95,* 705–748.

Gordon, J.H. (1987). Assumptions underlying physical therapy intervention: Theoretical and historical perspectives. In J.S. Carr & R.B. Shepherd (Eds.), *Movement science: Foundation for physical therapy in rehabilitation* (pp. 1–30). Rockville, MD: Aspen Publishers.

Gottlieb, G.L., Corcos, D.M., & Agarwal, G.C. (1989). Strategies for the control of voluntary movements with one mechanical degree of freedom. *Behavior and Brain Science, 12,* 189–250.

Graham, H.K. (2000). Botulinum toxin A in cerebral palsy: Functional outcomes. *Journal of Pediatrics, 137,* 300–303.

Gram, M.C. (1999). Myelodysplasia (spina bifida). In S.K. Campbell (Ed.), *Decision making in pediatric neurologic physical therapy* (pp. 198–234). Philadelphia: Churchill Livingstone.

Graubert, C., Song, K.M., McLaughlin, J.F., & Bjornson, K.F. (2000). Changes in gait at 1 year post-selective dorsal rhizotomy: Results of a prospective randomized study. *Journal of Pediatric Orthopaedics, 20*(4), 496–500.

Gregson, J.M., Leathley, M., Moore, A.P., Sharma, A.K., Smith, T.L., & Watkins C.L. (1999). Reliability of the Tone Assessment Scale and the modified Ashworth scale as clinical tools for assessing poststroke spasticity. *Archives of Physical Medicine and Rehabilitation, 80*(9), 1013–1016.

Gregson, J.M., Leathley, M.J., Moore, A.P., Smith, T.L., Sharma, A.K., & Watkins, C.L. (2000). Reliability of measurements of muscle tone and muscle power in stroke patients. *Age and Ageing, 29*(3), 223–228.

Grillner, S., Deliagina, T., Ekeberg, A., El Manira, A., Hill, R.H., Lansner, A., Orlovsky, G.N., & Wallen, P. (1995). Neural networks that co-ordinate locomotion and body orientation in lamprey. *Trends in Neuroscience, 18,* 270–279.

Grillner, S., & Wallen, P. (1985). Central pattern generators for locomotion, with special reference to vertebrates. *Annual Review of Neuroscience, 8,* 233–261.

Gubbay, S.S. (1975). *The clumsy child. A study of developmental apraxia and agnosticataxia.* London: W.B. Saunders.

Guralnick, M.J. (1998). Effectiveness of early intervention for vulnerable children: A developmental perspective. *American Journal of Mental Retardation, 102*(4), 319–345.

Haas, B.M., Bergstrom, E., Jamous, A., & Bennie, A. (1996). The interrater reliability of the original and of the modified Ashworth scale for the assessment of spasticity in patients with spinal cord injury. *Spinal Cord, 34*(9), 560–564.

Habib, Z., & Westcott, S. (1998). Assessment of anthropometric factors on balance tests in children. *Pediatric Physical Therapy, 10,* 101–109.

Habib, Z., Westcott, S.L., & Valvano, J. (1999). Assessment of dynamic balance abilities in Pakistani children age 5–13 years. *Pediatric Physical Therapy, 11,* 73–82.

Hadders-Algra, M. (2000). The neuronal group selection theory: Promising principles for understanding and treating developmental motor disorders. *Developmental Medicine and Child Neurology, 42,* 707–715.

Hadders-Algra, M., Brogren, E., & Forssberg, H. (1996). Ontogeny of postural adjustments during sitting in infancy: Variation, selection, and modulation. *Journal of Physiology (London), 493,* 273–288.

Hadders-Algra, M., Brogren, E., & Forssberg, H. (1998). Postural adjustments during sitting at preschool age: Presence of a transient toddling phase. *Developmental Medicine and Child Neurology, 40,* 436–447.

Hadders-Algra, M., Brogren, E., Katz-Salamon, M., & Forssberg, H. (1999). Periventricular leucomalacia and preterm birth have different detrimental effects on postural adjustments. *Brain, 122,* 727–740.

Hadders-Algra, M., & Lindahl, E. (1999). Pre- and perinatal precursors of specific learning disorders. In K. Whitmore, H. Hart, & G. Willems (Eds), *A neurodevelopmental approach to specific learning disorders* (pp. 166–190). London. MacKeith Press.

Hagan, C. (1998). *Revised Rancho Levels of Cognitive Functioning.* Rancho Los Amigos National Rehabilitation Center, Department of Communication Disorders, Harriman Building, 7601 E. Imperial Highway, Downey, CA.

Haley, S.M. (1986). Postural reactions in infants with Down syndrome: Relationship to motor milestone development and age. *Physical Therapy, 66,* 17–22.

Haley, S.M., Cioffi, M.I., Lewin, J.E., & Baryza, M.J. (1990). Motor dysfunction in children and adolescents after traumatic brain injury. *Journal of Head Trauma Rehabilitation, 5,* 77–90.

Haley, S.M., Coster, W.J., Ludlow, L.H., Haltiwanger, J.T., & Andrellas, P.J. (1992). *Pediatric evaluation of disability inventory.* Boston: PEDI Research Group.

Harris, J.C. (1995). *Developmental neuropsychiatry. volume 1, The fundamentals.* New York: Oxford University Press.

Harris, S.R. (1990). Therapeutic exercise for children with neurodevelopmental disabilities. In J.V. Basmajian & S.L. Wolf (Eds.), *Therapeutic exercise* (pp. 163–176). Baltimore: Williams and Wilkins.

Harris, S.R. (1998). The effectiveness of early intervention for children with cerebral palsy and related motor disorders. In M.J. Guralnick (Ed.), *The effectiveness of early intervention.* (pp. 327–347). Baltimore: Paul H. Brookes.

Harris, S.R., & Daniels, L.E. (2001). Reliability and validity of the Harris Infant Neuromotor Test. *Journal of Pediatrics, 139*(2), 249–253.

Harris, S.R., & Shea, A.M. (1991), Down syndrome. In S.K. Campbell (Ed.), *Pediatric neurologic physical therapy* (2nd ed.) (pp. 131–168). New York: Churchill Livingstone.

Hay, L., & Redon, C. (1999). Feedforward versus feedback control in children and adults subjected to a postural disturbance. *Experimental Brain Research, 125,* 153–162.

Hayashi, M., Satoh, J., Sakamoto, K., & Morimatsu, Y. (1991). Clinical and neuropathological findings in severe athetoid cerebral palsy: A comparative study of globo-luysian and thalamo-putaminal groups. *Brain Development, 13*(1), 47–51.

Hayes, A., & Batshaw, M.L. (1993). Down syndrome. *Pediatric Clinics of North America, 40*(3), 523–535.

Hays, R.M., McLaughlin, J.F., Bjornson, K.F., Stephens, K., Roberts, T.S., & Price R. (1998). Electrophysiological monitoring during selective dorsal rhizotomy, and spasticity and GMFM performance. *Developmental Medicine and Child Neurology, 40*(4), 233–238.

Held, J.M. (1998). Environmental enrichment enhances sparing and recovery of function following brain damage. *Neurology Report, 22,* 74–78.

Held, J.M., & Pay, T. (1999). Recovery of function after brain damage. In H. Cohen (Ed.), *Neuroscience for rehabilitation* (2nd ed., pp. 419–439). Philadelphia: Lippincott Williams & Wilkins.

Henderson, S.E., Rose, P., & Henderson, S. (1992). Reaction time and movement time in children with developmental coordination disorder. *Journal of Child Psychology and Psychiatry, 33,* 895–905.

Heriza, C. (1991a). Motor development: Traditional and contemporary theories. In M.J. Lister (Ed.), *Contemporary management of motor problems: Proceedings of the II STEP Conference*

(pp. 99–126). Alexandria, VA: Foundation for Physical Therapy.

Heriza, C.B. (1991b). Implications of a dynamical systems approach to understanding infant kicking behavior. *Physical Therapy, 71*(3), 222–235.

Heriza, C.B., & Sweeney, J.K. (1994). Pediatric physical therapy: Part I, Practice scope, scientific basis, and theoretical foundation. *Infants and Young Children, 7*(2), 20–32.

Hicks, S.P., & D'Amato, C.J. (1970). Motor-sensory and visual behavior after hemispherectomy in newborn and mature rats. *Experimental Neurology, 29*(3), 416–438.

Hinderer, K.A., Hinderer, S.R., & Shurtleff, D.B. (2000). Myelodysplasia. In S.K. Campbell, D.W. Vander Linden, & R.J. Palisano (Eds.), *Physical therapy for children* (2nd ed.) (pp. 621–670). Philadelphia: W.B. Saunders.

Holt, K.G., Butcher, R., & Fonseca, S. (2000). Limb stiffness in active leg swinging of children with spastic hemiplegic cerebral palsy. *Pediatric Physical Therapy, 12,* 50–61.

Horak, F.B. (1991). Assumptions underlying motor control for neurological rehabilitation. In M.J. Lister (Ed.), *Contemporary management of motor problems: Proceedings of the II STEP Conference* (pp. 11–28). Alexandria, VA: Foundation for Physical Therapy.

Horak, F.B., & Diener, H.C. (1994). Cerebellar control of postural scaling and central set in stance. *Journal of Neurophysiology, 72,* 479–493.

Horak, F.B. (1992). Motor control models underlying neurologic rehabilitation of posture in children. In H. Forssberg & H. Hirschfeld (Eds.), *Movement disorders in children* (pp. 21–30). Basel: Karger.

Horak, F.B., Diener, H.C., & Nashner, L.M. (1989). Influence of central set on human postural responses. *Journal of Neurophysiology, 62,* 841–853.

Horak, F.B., & Nashner, L.M. (1986). Central programming of postural movements: Adaptation to altered support configurations. *Journal of Neurophysiology, 55,* 1369–1381.

Horak, F.B., Shumway-Cook, A., Crowe, T.K., & Black, F.O. (1988). Vestibular function and motor proficiency of children with impaired hearing, or with learning disability and motor impairments. *Developmental Medicine and Child Neurology, 30,* 64–79.

Hornyak, J.E., Nelson, V.S., & Hurvitz, E.A. (1997). The use of methylphenidate in paediatric traumatic brain injury. *Pediatric Rehabilitation, 1,* 15–17.

Houk, J.C. (1979). Regulation of stiffness by skeletomotor reflexes. *Annual Reviews in Physiology, 41,* 99–114.

Hresko, M.T., McCarthy, J.C., & Goldberg, M.J. (1993). Hip disease in adults with Down syndrome. *Journal of Bone and Joint Surgery, British Volume, 75*(4), 604–607.

Hulliger, M., Durmuller, N., Prochazka, A., & Trend, P. (1989). Flexible fusimotor control of muscle spindle feedback during a variety of natural movement. *Progress in Brain Research, 80,* 87–100.

Hulliger, M., Noth, E., & Vallbo, A.B. (1982). The absence of position response in spindle afferent units from human finger muscles during accurate position holding. *Journal of Physiology*, *322*, 167–179.

Hulme, C., & Lord, R. (1986). Clumsy children—A review of recent research. *Child: Care, Health, and Development*, *12*, 257–269.

Hutton, R.S. (1984). Acute plasticity in spinal segmental pathways with use: Implications for training. In M. Kumamoto (Ed.), *Neural and mechanical control of movement*. Kyoto: Yamaguchi Shoten.

Inglis, J.T., Horak, F.B., Shupert, C.L., & Jones-Rycewicz, C. (1994). The importance of somatosensory information in triggering and scaling automatic postural responses in humans. *Experimental Brain Research*, *101*(1), 159–164.

Inui, N., Yamanishi, M., & Tada, S. (1995). Simple reaction times and timing of serial reactions of adolescents with mental retardation, autism, and Down syndrome. *Perceptual Motor Skills*, *81*(3 Pt 1), 739–745.

Iyer, M.B., Mitz, A.R., & Winstein, C. (1999). Motor 1: Lower centers. In H. Cohen (Ed.), *Neuroscience for rehabilitation* (2nd ed.) (pp. 209–242). Philadelphia: Lippincott Williams & Wilkins.

Jackson, J.H., & Taylor J. (1932). *Selected writings of John B. Hughlings, I and II*. London: Hodder & Stoughter.

Jacob, P., & Sarnat, H.B. (1989). Influences of the brain on normal and abnormal muscle development. In A. Hill & J.J. Volpe (Eds.), *Fetal neurology* (pp. 269–292). New York: Raven Press.

Jaffe, K.M., Polissar, N.L., Fay, G.C., & Liao, S. (1995). Recovery trends over three years following pediatric traumatic brain injury. *Archives of Physical Medicine and Rehabilitation*, *76*, 17–26.

Jager, T.E., Weiss, H.B., Coben, J.H., & Pepe, P.E. (2000). Traumatic brain injuries evaluated in U.S. emergency departments, 1992–1994. *Academy of Emergency Medicine, 7*(2), 134–140.

Jenkins, W.M., & Merzinich, M.M. (1992). Cortical representational plasticity: Some implications for the bases of recovery from brain damage. In N. von Steinibuchel, D. Y. von Cramon, & E. Poppel (Eds.), *Neuropsychological rehabilitation* (pp. 20–35). Berlin: Springer-Verlag.

Johnson, R.K., Goran, M.I., Ferrara, M.S., & Poehlman, E.T. (1996). Athetosis increases resting metabolic rate in adults with cerebral palsy. *Journal of the American Diet Association*, *96*(2), 145–148.

Johnston, M.V. (1995). Neurotransmitters and vulnerability of the developing brain. *Brain Development, 17*(5), 301–306.

Kelso, J.A.S. (1984). Phase transitions and critical behavior in human bimanual coordination. *American Journal of Physiology: Regulatory, Integrative and Comparative Physiology, 15*, R1000–R1004.

Kelso, J.A.S. (1986). Pattern formation in multidegree of freedom speech and limb movements. *Experimental Brain Research Supplement, 15*, 105–128.

Kelso, J.A.S. (1995). *Dynamic patterns: The self-organization of brain and behavior*. Cambridge, MA: MIT Press.

Kelso, J.A.S., Buchanan, J.J., Wallace, S.A. (1991). Order parameters for the neural organization of single, mutijoint limb movement patterns. *Experimental Brain Research, 85*, 432–444.

Kelso, J.A.S., Holt, K.G., Kugler, P.N., et al. (1980). On the concept of coordinative structures as dissipative structures: II. Empirical lines of convergence. In G.E. Stelmach & J. Requin (Eds), *Tutorials in motor behavior* (pp. 49–70). New York: Elsevier Science.

Kelso, J.A.S., & Tuller B. (1984). A dynamical basis for action systems. In M. Gassaniga (Ed.), *Handbook of cognitive neuroscience* (pp. 321–356). New York: Plenum.

King, G.A., McDougall, J., Palisano, R.J., Gritzan, J., & Tucker, M.A. (1999). Goal attainment scaling: Its use in evaluating pediatric therapy programs. *Physical and Occupational Therapy in Pediatrics, 19*(2), 31–52.

Kirkwood, M., Janusz, J., Yeates, K.O., Taylor, H.G., Wade, S.L., Stancin, T., & Drotar, D. (2000). Prevalence and correlates of depressive symptoms following traumatic brain injuries in children. *Neuropsychological Developmental Cognition Section C Child Neuropsychology, 6*(3), 195–208.

Knott, M., & Voss, D. (1968). *Proprioceptive neuromuscular facilitation*. New York: Harper & Row.

Knutson, L.M., & Clark, D.E. (1991). Orthotic devices for ambulation in children with cerebral palsy and myelomeningocele. *Physical Therapy, 71*, 947–960.

Kokubun, M. (1999). The relationship between the effect of setting a goal on standing broad jump performance and behaviour regulation ability in children with intellectual disability. *Journal of Intellectual and Disability Research, 43*(Pt 1), 13–18.

Kokubun, M., Shinmyo, T., Ogita, M., Morita, K., Furuta, M., Haishi, K., Okuzumi, H., & Koike, T. (1997). Comparison of postural control of children with Down syndrome and those with other forms of mental retardation. *Perceptual Motor Skills, 84*(2), 499–504.

Kolb, B. (1999). Synaptic plasticity and the organization of behaviour after early and late brain injury. *Canadian Journal of Experimental Psychology, 53*(1), 62–76.

Kolb, B., Forgie, M., Gibb, R., Gorny, G., & Rowntree, S. (1998). Age, experience and the changing brain. *Neuroscience and Biobehavior Review, 22*(2), 143–159.

Kolb, B., Gibb, R., & Gorny, G. (2000). Cortical plasticity and the development of behavior after early frontal cortical injury. *Developmental Neuropsychology, 18*(3), 423–444.

Kolb, B., & Whishaw, I.Q. (1998). Brain plasticity and behavior. *Annual Review of Psychology, 49*, 43 64.

Konczak, J., Borutta, M., & Dichgans, J. (1997). The development of goal-directed reaching in infants. II. Learning to produce task-adequate patterns of joint torque. *Experimental Brain Research, 113*(3), 465–474.

Konczak, J., Borutta, M., Topka, H., & Dichgans, J. (1995). The development of goal-directed reaching in infants: Hand trajectory formation and joint torque control. *Experimental Brain Research, 106*(1), 156–168.

Konczak, J., & Dichgans, J. (1997). The development toward stereotypic arm kinematics during reaching in the first 3 years of life. *Experimental Brain Research, 117*(2), 346–354.

Krageloh-Mann, I., Toft, P., Lunding, J., Andresen, J., Pryds, O., & Lou, H.C. (1999). Brain lesions in preterms: Origin, consequences and compensation. *Acta Paediatrica, 88*(8), 897–908.

Kugler, P.N., Kelso, J.A.S., & Turvey, M.T. (1980). On the concept of coordinative structures as dissipative structures: I. Theoretical lines of convergence. In G.E. Stelmach & J. Requin (Eds), *Tutorials in motor behavior* (pp. 3–47). New York: Elsevier Science.

Kujala, T., Alho, K., & Naatanen, R. (2000). Cross-modal reorganization of human cortical functions. *Trends in Neuroscience, 23*(3), 115–120.

Landau, W.M. (1974). Spasticity: The fable of a neurological demon and the emperor's new therapy. *Archives of Neurology, 31*, 217–219.

Latash, M.L. (1998a). Virtual reality: A fascinating tool for motor rehabilitation (to be used with caution). *Disability Rehabilitation, 20*(3), 104–105.

Latash, M.L. (1998b). *Progress in motor control: Bernstein's traditions in movement studies.* Champaign, IL: Human Kinetics.

Latash, M.L. (1998c). *Neurophysiological basis of movement* (pp. 98–105). Champaign, IL: Human Kinetics.

Latash, M.L., & Anson, G. (1996). What are "normal" movements in atypical populations? *Behavioral and Brain Sciences, 19*, 55–106.

Latash, L.P., Latash, M.L., & Meijer, O.G. (1999). 30 years later: The relation between structure and function in the brain from a contemporary point of view (1996), part I. *Motor Control, 3*(4), 329–332, 342–345.

Latash, L.P., Latash, M.L., & Meijer, O.G. (2000). 30 years later: On the problem of the relation between structure and function in the brain from a contemporary viewpoint (1996), part II. *Motor Control, 4*(2), 125–149.

Latash, M.L., & Nicholas, J.J. (1996). Motor control research in rehabilitation medicine. *Disability Rehabilitation, 18*(6), 293–299.

Lauteslager, P.E.M., Vermeer, A., & Helders, P.J.M. (1998). Disturbances in the motor behavior of children with Down's syndrome: The need for a theoretical framework. *Physiotherapy, 84*, 5–13.

Lee, D.N., von Hofsten, C., & Cotton, E. (1997). Perception in action approach to cerebral palsy. In K.J. Connolly & H. Forssberg (Eds), *Neurophysiology and neuropsychology of motor development* (pp. 257–258). London: MacKeith Press.

Lehmann, J.F., Price, R., deLateur, B.J., Hinderer, S., & Traynor, C. (1989). Spasticity: Quantitative measurements as a basis for assessing effectiveness of therapeutic intervention. *Archives of Physical Medicine and Rehabilitation, 70*, 6–15.

Leonard, C.T. (1998). *The neuroscience of human movement* (pp. 124–128). St. Louis: Mosby–Year Book.

Leonard, C.T. (1994). Motor behavior and neuronal changes following perinatal and adult-onset brain damage: Implications for therapeutic interventions. *Physical Therapy, 74*, 753–767.

Leonard, C.T., Moritani, T., Hirschfeld, H., & Forssberg, H. (1990). Deficits in reciprocal inhibition of children with cerebral palsy as revealed by H reflex testing. *Developmental Medicine and Child Neurology, 32*, 974–984.

Liepert, J., Bauder, H., Miltner, W.H.R., Taub, E., & Weiller, C. (2000). Treatment-induced cortical reorganization after stroke in humans. *Stroke, 31*, 1210–1216.

Lin, J.P., Brown, J.K., & Brotherstone, R. (1994). Assessment of spasticity in hemiplegic I: Proximal lower-limb reflex excitability. *Developmental Medicine and Child Neurology, 36*, 116–129.

Lin, J.P., Brown, J.K., & Walsh, E.G. (1994). Physiological maturation of muscles in childhood. *Lancet, 343*, 1386–1389.

Liptak, G.S., Shurtleff, D.B., Bloss, J.W., Baltus-Hebert, E., & Manitta, P. (1992). Mobility aids for children with high-level myelomeningocele: Parapodium versus wheelchair. *Developmental Medicine and Child Neurology, 34*, 787–796.

Little, J.W., Burns, S.P., James, J.J., & Stiens, S.A. (2000). Neurologic recovery and neurologic decline after spinal cord injury. *Physical Medicine Rehabilitation Clinics of North America, 11*(1), 73–89.

Liu, W. (2001). Anticipatory postural adjustments in children with cerebral palsy and children with typical development during forward reach tasks in standing. Unpublished doctoral dissertation, MCP Hahnemann University, Philadelphia.

Lowes, L.P. (1996). An evaluation of the standing balance of children with cerebral palsy and the tools for assessment. Unpublished doctoral dissertation, MCP Hahnemann University, Philadelphia.

Luke, A, Roizen, N.J., Sutton, M., & Schoeller, D.A. (1994). Energy expenditure in children with Down syndrome: Correcting metabolic rate for movement. *Journal of Pediatrics, 125*(5 Pt 1), 829–838.

Lundy-Eckman, L. (1998). *Neuroscience: Fundamentals for rehabilitation* (pp. 69–84). Philadelphia: W.B. Saunders.

Luyt, L., Bodney, S., Keller, J., et al. (1996). Reliability of determining motor strategy used by children with cerebral palsy during the Pediatric Clinical Test of Sensory Interaction for Balance. *Pediatric Physical Therapy, 8*, 180.

Majnemer, A. (1998). Benefits of early intervention for children with developmental disabilities. *Seminars in Pediatric Neurology, 5*(1), 62–69.

Maloney, F.P. (1993). Goal attainment scaling. *Physical Therapy, 73*(2), 123.

Mandich, A.D., Polatajko, H.J., Macnab, J.J., & Miller, L.T. (2001). Treatment of children with developmental coordination disorder: What is the evidence? *Physical and Occupational Therapy in Pediatrics, 20*(2–3), 51–68.

Mandich, A.D., Polatajko, H.J., Missiuna, C., & Miller, L.T. (2001). Cognitive strategies and motor performance in children with developmental coordination disorder. *Physical and Occupational Therapy in Pediatrics, 20*(2–3), 125–143.

Mangeot, S.D., Miller, L.J., McIntosh, D.N., McGrath-Clarke, J., Simon, J., Hagerman, R.J., & Goldson, E. (2001). Sensory modulation in children with attention-deficit-hyperactivity disorder. *Developmental Medicine and Child Neurology, 43,* 399–406.

Massion J. (1992). Movement, posture, and equilibrium: Interaction and coordination. *Progressive Neurobiology, 38,* 35–56.

Massion, J. (1998). Postural control systems in developmental perspective. *Neuroscience Biobehavior Review, 22,* 465–472.

McDonald, C.M., Jaffe, K.M., Mosca, V.S., & Shurtleff, D.B. (1991). Ambulatory outcome of children with myelomeningocele: Effect of lower-extremity muscle strength. *Developmental Medicine and Child Neurology, 33,* 482–490.

McEwen, I. (2000). Children with cognitive impairments. In S.K. Campbell, D.W. Vander Linden, & R.J. Palisano (Eds.), *Physical therapy for children* (2nd ed.) (pp. 502–532). Philadelphia: W.B. Saunders.

McLaughlin, J.F., Bjornson, K.F., Astley, S.J., Graubert,C., Hays, R.M., Roberts, T.S., Price, R., & Temkin, N. (1998). Selective dorsal rhizotomy: Efficacy and safety in an investigator-masked randomized clinical trial. *Developmental Medicine and Child Neurology, 40*(4), 220–232.

McLaughlin, J.F., Bjornson, K., Temkin, N., Steinbok, P., Wright, V., Reiner, A., Roberts, T., Drake, J., O'Donnell, M., Rosenbaum, P., Barber, J., & Ferrel, A. (2002). Selective dorsal rhizotomy: Meta-analysis of three randomized controlled trials. *Developmental Medicine and Child Neurology, 44*(1), 17–25.

McNevin, N.H., Coraci, L., & Schafer, J. (2000). Gait in adolescent cerebral palsy: The effect of partial unweighting. *Archives of Physical Medicine and Rehabilitation, 81*(4), 525–528.

Merrick, J., Ezra, E., Josef, B., Hendel, D., Steinberg, D.M., & Wientroub, S. (2000). Musculoskeletal problems in Down syndrome. European Paediatric Orthopaedic Society survey: The Israeli sample. *Journal of Pediatric Orthopedics B, 9*(3), 185–192.

Merzenich, M.M., & Jenkins, W.M. (1993). Reorganization of cortical representations of the hand following alterations of skill inputs induced by nerve injury, skin island, transfers, and experience. *Journal of Hand Therapy, 18,* 89–104.

Meyers, G.J., Cerone, S.B., & Olson, A.L. [1981]. *A guide for helping the child with spina bifida.* Springfield, IL: Charles C. Thomas.

Missiuna, C. (1994). Motor skill acquisition in children with developmental coordination disorder. *Adapted Physical Activity Quarterly, 11,* 214–235.

Missiuna, C. (2001). Strategies for success: Working with children with developmental coordination disorder. *Physical and Occupational Therapy in Pediatrics, 20*(2–3), 1–4.

Missiuna, C., & Polatajko, H. (1995). Developmental dyspraxia by any other name: Are they all just clumsy children? *American Journal of Occupational Therapy, 49,* 619–627.

Moe-Nilssen, R. (1998). A new method for evaluating motor control in gait under real-life environmental conditions. Part 2: Gait analysis. *Clinical Biomechanics, 13,* 328–335.

Montgomery, P.C. (2000). Achievement of gross motor skills in two children with cerebellar hypoplasia: Longitudinal case reports. *Pediatric Physical Therapy, 12,* 68–76.

Morris, D., Crago, J., DeLuca, S., Pidikiti, R., & Taub, E. (1997). Constraint induced movement therapy for recovery after stroke. *Neurorehabilitation, 9,* 29–43.

Munch, E., Horn, P., Schurer, L., Piepgras, A., Paul, T., & Schmiedek, P. (2000). Management of severe traumatic brain injury by decompressive craniectomy. *Neurosurgery, 47*(2), 315–322.

Mutch, L., Alberman, E., Hagberg, B., Kodama, K., & Perat, M.V. (1992). Cerebral palsy epidemiology: Where are we now and where are we going? *Developmental Medicine and Child Neurology, 34,* 547–551.

Nashner, L.M. (1982). Adaptation of human movement to altered environments. *Trends in Neurosciences, 10,* 358–361.

Nashner, L.M., Shumway-Cook, A., & Marin, O. (1983). Stance posture control in select groups of children with cerebral palsy: Deficits in sensory organization and muscular coordination. *Experimental Brain Research, 49,* 393–409.

National Institute of Neurological Disorders and Stroke, National Institutes of Health (1990). *Interagency head injury task force reports.* Bethesda, MD: Author.

National Institutes of Health Consensus Statement (1998). Rehabilitation of persons with traumatic brain injury. *16*(1), 1–41.

Newell, K.M., & Valvano, J. (1998). Therapeutic intervention as a constraint in learning and relearning movement skills. *Scandinavian Journal of Occupational Therapy, 5,* 51–57.

Nickel, R.E. (1992). Disorders of brain development. *Infants and Young Children, 5*(1), 1–11.

Nudo, R.J., & Milliken, G.W. (1996). Reorganization of movement representations in primary motor cortex following focal ischemic infarcts in adult squirrel monkeys. *Journal of Neurophysiology, 75,* 2144–2149.

Nudo, R.J., Wise, B.M., SiFuentes, F., & Milliken, G.M. (1996). Neural substrates for the effects of rehabilitative training on motor recovery after ischemic infarct. *Science, 272,* 1791–1794.

Olney, S.J., & Wright, M.J. (2000). Cerebral palsy. In S.K. Campbell, D.W. Vander Linden, & R.J. Palisano (Eds.), *Physical therapy for children* (2nd ed.) (pp. 533–570). Philadelphia: W.B. Saunders.

Olree, K.S., Engsberg, J.R., Ross, S.A., & Park, T.S. (2000). Changes in synergistic movement patterns after selective dorsal rhizotomy. *Developmental Medicine and Child Neurology, 42,* 297–303.

Oppenheim, R.W. (1991). Cell death during development of the nervous system. *Annual Review of Neuroscience, 14,* 543–501.

Ornstein, R., & Thompson, R.F. (1984). *The amazing brain.* Boston: Houghton Mifflin.

Ostendorf, C., & Wolf, S. (1981). Effect of forced use of the upper extremity of a hemiplegic patient on changes in function. *Physical Therapy, 61,* 1022–1028.

Ottenbacher, K.J., Biocca, Z., DeCremer, G., Gevelinger, M., Jedlovec, K.B., & Johnson, M.B. (1986). Quantitative analysis of the effectiveness of pediatric therapy: Emphasis on the neurodevelopmental treatment approach. *Physical Therapy, 66,* 1095–1101.

Paine, R.S. (1963). The future of the "floppy infant": A follow-up study of 133 patients. *Developmental Medicine and Child Neurology, 5,* 115–124.

Pakula, A.L., & Palmer, F.B. (1998). Early intervention for children at risk for neuromotor problems. In M.J. Guralnick (Ed.), *The effectiveness of early intervention* (pp. 99–108). Baltimore: Paul H. Brookes.

Palisano, R.J. (1993). Validity of goal attainment scaling in infants with motor delays. *Physical Therapy, 73*(10), 651–658.

Palisano, R.J., Haley, S.M., Westcott, S., & Hess, A. (1999). Pediatric Physical Therapy Outcome Management System. *Pediatric Physical Therapy, 11,* 220.

Palisano, R.J., Kolobe, T.H., Haley, S.M., Lowes, L.P., & Jones, S.L. (1995). Validity of the Peabody Developmental Gross Motor Scale as an evaluative measure of infants receiving physical therapy. *Physical Therapy, 75,* 939–948.

Palisano, R., Rosenbaum, P., Walter, S., Russell, D., Wood, E., & Galuppi, B. (1997). The development and reliability of a system to classify gross motor function in children with cerebral palsy. *Developmental Medicine and Child Neurology, 39,* 214–223.

Palisano, R.J., Walter, S.D., Russell, D.J., Rosenbaum, P.L., Gemus, M., Galuppi, B.E., & Cunningham, L. (2001). Gross motor function of children with Down syndrome: Creation of motor growth curves. *Archives of Physical Medicine and Rehabilitation, 82*(4), 494–500.

Pandyan, A.D., Johnson, G.R., Price, C.I., Curless, R.H., Barnes, M.P., & Rodgers, H. (1999). A review of the properties and limitations of the Ashworth and Modified Ashworth Scales as measures of spasticity. *Clinical Rehabilitation, 13*(5), 373–383.

Park, B.K., Song, H.R., Vankoski, M.S., Moore, C.A., & Dias, L.S. (1997). Gait electromyography in children with myelomeningocele at the sacral level. *Archives of Physical Medicine and Rehabilitation, 78,* 471–475.

Parush, S., Yehezkehel, I., Tenenbaum, A., Tekuzener, E., Bar-Efrat/Hirsch, I., Jessel, A., & Ornoy, A. (1998). Developmental correlates of school-age children with a history of benign congenital hypotonia. *Developmental Medicine and Child Neurology, 40*(7), 448–452.

Pelligrino, T.T., Buelow, B., Krause, M., Loucks, L.C., &

Westcott, S.L. (1995). Test-retest reliability of the Pediatric Clinical Test of Sensory Interactions for Balance and the Functional Reach Test in children with standing balance dysfunction. *Pediatric Physical Therapy, 7,* 197.

Phillips, C.G., & Porter, R. (1977). *Corticospinal neurones: Their role in movement.* New York: Academic Press.

Pilon, J.M., Sadler, G.T., & Bartlett, D.J. (2000). Relationship of hypotonia and joint laxity to motor development during infancy. *Pediatric Physical Therapy, 12,* 10–15.

Piper, M., & Darrah, J. (1994). *Motor assessment of the developing infant.* Philadelphia: W.B. Saunders.

Podsiadlo, D., & Richardson, S. (1991). The timed "up and go": A basic functional mobility test for frail elderly persons. *Journal of the American Geriatric Society, 39,* 142–148.

Polatajko, H.J. (1999). Developmental coordination disorder (DCD): Alias the clumsy child syndrome. In K. Whitmore, H. Hart, & G. Willems (Eds.), *A neurodevelopmental approach to specific learning disorders* (pp. 119–133). London: MacKeith Press.

Polatajko, H.J., Mandich, A.D., Miller, L.T., & Macnab, J.J. (2001). Cognitive Orientation to Daily Occupational Performance (CO-OP): Part II—the evidence. *Physical and Occupational Therapy in Pediatrics, 20*(2–3), 83–106.

Potter, P.J., Kirby, R.L., & MacLeod, D.A. (1990). The effects of simulated knee-flexion contractures on standing balance. *American Journal of Physical Medicine and Rehabilitation, 69,* 144–147.

Prasher, V.P., Robinson, L., Krishnan, V.H., & Chung, M.C. (1995). Podiatric disorders among children with Down syndrome and learning disability. *Developmental Medicine and Child Neurology, 37*(2), 131–134.

Price, R., Bjornson, K.F., Lehmann, J.F., McLaughlin, J.F., & Hays, R.M. (1991). Quantitative measurement of spasticity in children with cerebral palsy. *Developmental Medicine and Child Neurology, 33,* 585–595.

Professional Staff Association of Rancho Los Amigos Hospital (1982). *Rancho Los Amigos Pediatric Levels of Consciousness for Infants, Preschoolers, and School-Age children scale. Rehabilitation of the head injured adult: Comprehensive physical management.* Downey, CA: Author.

Pueschel, S.M. (1990). Clinical aspects of Down syndrome from infancy to adulthood. *American Journal of Medical Genetics Suppl, 7,* 52–56.

Randall, K.E., & McEwen, I.R. (2000). Writing patient-centered functional goals. *Physical Therapy, 80,* 1197–1203.

Rasmussen, P., & Gillberg, C. (1999). AD(H)D, hyperkinetic disorders, DAMP, and related behavior disorders. In K. Whitmore, H. Hart, & G. Willems (Eds.), *A neurodevelopmental approach to specific learning disorders* (pp. 134–156). London: MacKeith Press.

Reed, E.S. (1982). An outline of a theory of action systems. *Journal of Motor Behavior, 14,* 98–134.

Richards, C.L., Malouin, F., Dumas, F., Marcoux, S., LePage, C., & Menier, C. (1997). Early and intensive treadmill locomotor training for young children with cerebral palsy: A feasibility study. *Pediatric Physical Therapy, 9*, 158–165.

Richardson, P.K., Atwater, S.W., Crowe, T.K., & Deitz, J.C. (1992). Performance of preschoolers on the Pediatric Clinical Test of Sensory Interaction for Balance. *American Journal of Occupational Therapy, 46*, 793–800.

Rine, R.M., Rubish, K., & Feeney, C. (1998). Measurement of sensory system effectiveness and maturational changes in postural control in young children. *Pediatric Physical Therapy, 10*, 16–22.

Rivkin, M.J. (1997). Hypoxic-ischemic brain injury in the term newborn: Neuropathology, clinical aspects, and neuroimaging. *Clinics in Perinatology, 24*, 607–625.

Roizen, N.J., Wolters, C., Nicol, T., & Blondis, T.A. (1993). Hearing loss in children with Down syndrome. *Journal of Pediatrics, 123*(1), S9–S12.

Rosblad, B., & Von Hofsten, C. (1994). Repetitive goal-directed arm movements in children with developmental coordination disorders: Role of visual information. *Adapted Physical Activity Quarterly, 11*, 190–202.

Rose, F.D., Johnson, D.A., & Attree, E.A. (1997). Rehabilitation of the head-injured child: Basic research and new technology. *Pediatric Rehabilitation, 1*, 3–7.

Rossignol, S. (2000). Locomotion and its recovery after spinal cord injury. *Current Opinion in Neurobiology, 10*, 708–716.

Rothwell, J. (1994). *Control of human voluntary movement.* Cambridge, England: Cambridge University Press.

Rubin, S.S., Rimmer, J.H., Chicoine, B., Braddock, D., & McGuire, D.E. (1998). Overweight prevalence in persons with Down syndrome. *Mental Retardation, 36*, 175–181.

Russell, D., Rosenbaum, P., Gowland, C., Hardy, S., Lane, M., Plews, N., McGavin, H., Cadman, D., & Jarvis, S. (1993). *Gross motor function measure* (2nd ed.). Hamilton, Ontario, Canada: Gross Motor Measure Group.

Sacco, D.J., Tylkowski, C.M., & Warf, B.C. (2000). Nonselective partial dorsal rhizotomy: A clinical experience with 1-year follow-up. *Pediatric Neurosurgery, 32*(3), 114–118.

Sahrmann, S.A., & Norton B.J. (1977). The relationship of voluntary movement to spasticity in the upper motor neuron syndrome. *Annals of Neurology, 2*, 460–465.

Sarnat, H.B. (1984). Anatomic and physiologic correlates of neurologic development in prematurity. In H.B. Sarnat (Ed.), *Topics in neonatal neurology* (pp. 1–25). Orlando: Grune & Stratton.

Schindl, M.R., Forstner, C., Kern, H., & Hesse, S. (2000). Treadmill training with partial body weight support in nonambulatory patients with cerebral palsy. *Archives of Physical Medicine and Rehabilitation, 81*, 301–306.

Schmidt, R.A. (1991). *Motor performance and learning: Principles for practitioners.* Champaign, IL: Human Kinetics.

Schoemaker, M.M., Hijlkema, M.G., & Kalverboer, A.F. (1994). Physiotherapy for clumsy children: An evaluation study. *Developmental Medicine and Child Neurology, 36*(2), 143–155.

Scholz, J.P. (1990). Dynamic pattern theory—Some implications for therapeutics. *Physical Therapy, 70*(12), 827–843.

Schoner, G., & Kelso, J.A.S. (1988). Dynamic pattern generation in behavioral and neural systems. *Science, 239*, 1513–1520.

Segal, R.L. (1998). Spinal cord plasticity is a possible tool for rehabilitation. *Neurology Report, 22*, 54–60.

Sharples, P.M., Stuart, A.G., Matthews, D.S., Aynsley-Green, A., & Eyre, J.A. (1995). Cerebral blood flow and metabolism in children with severe brain injury. Part 1: Relation to age, Glasgow Coma Scale, outcome, intracranial pressure, and time after injury. *Journal of Neurology, Neurosurgery, and Psychiatry, 58*(2), 145–152.

Shea, A.M. (1991). Motor attainments in Down syndrome. In M.L. Lister (Ed.), *Contemporary management of motor problems: Proceedings of the II STEP Conference* (pp. 225–236). Alexandria, VA: Foundation for Physical Therapy.

Sherrington, C.S. (1906). *The integrative action of the nervous system.* Silliman Lectures. New Haven, CT: Yale University Press.

Sherrington, C.S. (1947). *The integrative action of the nervous system.* Cambridge, MA: Cambridge University Press.

Shumway-Cook, A., & Woollacott, M.H. (1985). Dynamics of postural control in the child with Down syndrome. *Physical Therapy, 65*, 1315–1322.

Shumway-Cook, A., & Woollacott, M.H. (Eds.). (2001). *Motor control: Theory and practical applications* (2nd ed.). Philadelphia: Lippincott Williams & Wilkins.

Singh, G., Athreya, B.H., Fries, J.F., & Goldsmith, D.P. (1994). Measurement of health status in children with juvenile rheumatoid arthritis. *Arthritis and Rheumatology, 37*, 1761–1769.

Skorji, V., & McKenzie, B. (1997). How do children who are clumsy remember modeled movements? *Developmental Medicine and Child Neurology, 39*(6), 404–408.

Slijper, H., Latash, M.L., & Mordkoff, J.T. (2002). Anticipatory postural adjustments under simple and choice reaction time conditions. *Brain Research, 924*(2), 184–197.

Sloan, R.L., Sinclair, E., Thompson, J., Taylor, S., & Pentland, B. (1992). Inter-rater reliability of the modified Ashworth Scale for spasticity in hemiplegic patients. *International Journal of Rehabilitation Research, 15*(2), 158–161.

Sousa, J.C., Telzrow, R.W., Holm, R.A., McCartin, R., & Shurtleff, D.B. (1983). Developmental guidelines for children with myelodysplasia. *Physical Therapy, 63*, 21–29.

Spano, M., Mercuri, E., Rando, T., Panto, T., Gagliano, A., Henderson, S., & Guzzetta, F. (1999). Motor and perceptual-motor competence in children with Down syndrome: Variation in performance with age. *European Journal of Paediatric Neurology, 3*(1), 7–13.

Sporns, O., & Edelman, G.M. (1993). Solving Bernstein's problem: A proposal for the development of coordinated movement by selection. *Child Development, 64*(4), 960–981.

Sporns, O., Edelman, G.M., & Meijer, O.G. (1998). Bernstein's dynamic view of the brain: The current problems of modern neurophysiology. *Motor Control, 2*(4), 283–305.

Stein, R.B., Yang, J.F., Belanger, M., & Pearson, K.G. (1993). Modification of reflexes in normal and abnormal movements. *Progress in Brain Research, 97*, 189–196.

Steinbok P. (2001). Outcomes after selective dorsal rhizotomy for spastic cerebral palsy. *Child's Nervous System, 17*(1–2), 1–18.

Steinbok, P., Reiner, A.M., Beauchamp, R., Armstrong, R.W., Cochrane, D.D., & Kestle, J. (1997). A randomized clinical trial to compare selective posterior rhizotomy plus physiotherapy with physiotherapy alone in children with spastic diplegic cerebral palsy. *Developmental Medicine and Child Neurology, 39,* 178–184.

Stockmeyer, S.A. (1967). An interpretation of the approach of Rood to the treatment of neuromuscular dysfunction. *American Journal of Physical Medicine, 46,* 901–956.

Stockmeyer, S.A. (1972). A sensorimotor approach to treatment. In P.H. Pearson & C.E. Williams (Eds.), *Physical therapy services in the developmental disabilities* (pp. 186–222). Springfield, IL: Charles C Thomas.

Stoll, C., Alembik, Y., Dott, B., & Roth, M.P. (1998). Study of Down syndrome in 238,942 consecutive births. *Annals of Genetics, 41*(1), 44–51.

Sugden, D., & Keogh, J. (1990). *Problems in movement skill development.* Columbia, SC: University of South Carolina Press.

Sullivan, K.J. (1998). Functionally distinct learning systems of the brain: Implications for brain injury rehabilitation. *Neurology Report of Neurology Section of American Physical Therapy Association, 22,* 126–131.

Sullivan, S.J., Richer, E., & Laurent, F. (1990). The role of and possibilities for physical conditioning programmes in the rehabilitation of traumatically brain-injured persons. *Brain Injury, 4,* 407–414.

Sweeney, J.K., Heriza, C.B., & Markowitz, R. (1994). The changing profile of pediatric physical therapy: A 10-year analysis of clinical practice. *Pediatric Physical Therapy, 6,* 113–118.

Taub, E. (1976). Motor behavior following deafferentation in the developing and motorically mature monkey. *Advances in Behavioral Biology, 18,* 675–705.

Taub, E., Goldberg, I., & Taub, P. (1975). Deafferentation on monkeys: Pointing at a target without visual feedback. *Experimental Neurology, 46,* 178–186.

Taub, E., & Wolf, S. (1997). Constraint induced movement techniques to facilitate upper extremity use in stroke patients. *Topics in Stroke Rehabilitation, 3,* 38–61.

Teasdale, G., & Jennett, B. (1974). Assessment of coma and impaired consciousness: A practical scale. *Lancet, 2,* 81–84.

Telzrow, C.F. (1987). Management of academic and educational problems in head injury. *Journal of Learning Disabilities, 20*(9), 536–545.

Tew, B. (1979). The cocktail party syndrome in children with hydrocephalus and spina bifida. *British Journal of Disorder in Communication, 14*(2), 89–101.

Thelen, E., Kelso, J.A.S., & Fogel, A. (1987). Self-organizing systems and infant motor development. *Developmental Review, 7,* 30–65.

Thelen, E., & Spencer, J. (1998). Postural control during reaching in young infants: A dynamic systems approach. *Neuroscience and Biobehavioral Reviews, 22,* 507–514.

Thelen, E., & Whitely-Cooke, D. (1987). Relationship between newborn stepping and later walking: A new interpretation. *Developmental Medicine and Child Neurology, 29,* 380–393.

Thilmann, A.F., Fellows, S.J., & Ross, H.F. (1991). Biomechanical changes at the ankle joint after stroke. *Journal of Neurology, Neurosurgery, and Psychiatry, 54,* 134–139.

Tsiaras, W.G., Pueschel, S., Keller, C., Curran, R., & Giesswein, S. (1999). Amblyopia and visual acuity in children with Down's syndrome. *British Journal of Ophthalmology, 83*(10), 1112–1114.

Ubhi, T., Bhakta, B.B., Ives, H.L., Allgar, V., & Roussounis, S.H. (2000). Randomised double blind placebo controlled trial of the effect of botulinum toxin on walking in cerebral palsy. *Archives of Disorders in Children, 83,* 481–487.

Ulrich, B.D., Ulrich, D.A., Angulo-Kinzler, R., & Chapman, D.D. (1997). Sensitivity of infants with and without Down syndrome to intrinsic dynamics. *Research Quarterly in Exercise and Sport, 68*(1), 10–19.

Ulrich, D.A., Ulrich, B.D., Angulo-Kinzler, R.M., & Yun, J. (2001). Treadmill training of infants with Down syndrome: Evidence-based developmental outcomes. *Pediatrics, 108*(5), E84.

Ulrich, B.D., Ulrich, D.A., Collier, D., & Cole E.L. (1995). Developmental shifts in the ability of infants with Down syndrome to produce treadmill steps. *Physical Therapy, 75,* 20–29.

Unanue, R., & Westcott, S.L. (2001). Neonatal asphyxia. *Infants and Young Children, 13*(3), 13–24.

Van de Crommert, H., Mulder, T., & Duysens, J. (1998). Neural control of locomotion: Sensory control of the central pattern generator and its relation to treadmill training. *Gait and Posture, 7,* 251–263.

Van Dellen, T., & Geuze, R.H. (1988). Motor response processing in clumsy children. *Journal of Child Psychology and Psychiatry, 29,* 489–500.

Vargha-Khadem, F. (2001). Generalized versus selective cognitive impairments resulting from brain damage sustained in childhood. *Epilepsia, 42* (Suppl. 1), 37–40; discussion, 50–51.

Vatovec, J., Velikovic, M., Smid, L., Brenk, K., & Zargi, M. (2001). Impairments of vestibular system in infants at risk of early brain damage. *Scandinavian Audiology Supplement, 52,* 191–193.

Vereijken, B., & Thelen, E. (1997). Training infant treadmill stepping: The role of individual pattern stability. *Developmental Psychobiology, 30*(2), 89–102.

Vereijken, B., van Emmerick, R.E.A., Whiting, H.T.A., & Newell, K.M. (1992). Free(z)ing degrees of freedom in skill acquisition. *Journal of Motor Behavior, 24,* 133–142.

Visintin, M., Barbeau, H., Korner-Bitensky, N., & Mayo, N. (1998). A new approach to retrain gait in stroke patients through body weight support and treadmill stimulation. *Stroke, 29,* 1122–1128.

Volpe, J.J. (1995). *Neurology of the newborn* (3rd ed.). Philadelphia: W.B. Saunders.

Volpe, J.J. (1997). Brain injury in the premature infant: Neuropathology, clinical aspects, pathogenesis, and prevention. *Clinics in Perinatology, 24*, 567–587.

von Hofsten, C. (1980). Predictive reaching for moving objects by human infants. *Journal of Experimental Child Psychology, 30*, 383–388.

Voss, D.E. (1972). Proprioceptive neuromuscular facilitation: The PNF method. In P.H. Pearson & C.E. Williams (Eds.), *Physical therapy services in the developmental disabilities* (pp. 223–282). Springfield, IL: Charles C Thomas.

Walsche, F.M.P. (1961). Contribution of John Hughlings Jackson to neurology. *Archives of Neurology, 5*, 99–133.

Westcott, S.L. (1993). Comparison of vestibulospinal synaptic input and IA afferent synaptic input in cat triceps surae motoneurons. Unpublished doctoral dissertation, University of Washington, Seattle, WA.

Westcott, S.L., Crowe, T.K., Deitz, J.C., & Richardson, P.K. (1994). Test-retest reliability of the Pediatric Clinical Test of Sensory Interaction for Balance (P-CTSIB). *Physical and Occupational Therapy in Pediatrics, 14*, 1–22.

Westcott, S.L., Lowes, L.P., & Richardson, P.K. (1997). Evaluation of postural stability in children: Current theories and assessment tools. *Physical Therapy, 77*, 629–645.

Westcott, S.L., et al. (1998a). Comparison of anticipatory postural control and dynamic balance ability in children with and without cerebral palsy. Platform presentation at American Academy of Cerebral Palsy and Developmental Medicine, San Antonio, TX. *Developmental Medicine and Child Neurology, 40*(Suppl.).

Westcott, S.L., et al. (1998b). Anticipatory postural coordination and functional movement skills of children with cerebral palsy by severity level of disability. Poster presentation for Society for Neurosciences Annual Meeting, Los Angeles, CA. *Neuroscience Abstracts, 24*.

Westcott, S.L., Lowes, L.P., Richardson, P.K., Crowe, T.K., & Deitz, J. (1997). Difference in the use of sensory information for maintenance of standing balance in children with different motor disabilities. *Developmental Medicine and Child Neurology, 39*(Suppl. 75), 32–33.

Westcott, S.L., & Zaino, C.A. (1997). Comparison and development of postural muscle activity in children during stand and reach from firm and compliant surfaces. *Neuroscience Abstracts, 23*, 1565.

Wheeler, A., Shall, M., Lewis, A., & Shepherd, J. (1996). The reliability of measurements obtained using Functional Reach in children with cerebral palsy. *Pediatric Physical Therapy, 8*, 182.

Whitlock, J.A., & Hamilton, B.B. (1995). Functional outcome after rehabilitation for severe traumatic brain injury. *Archives of Physical Medicine and Rehabilitation, 76*, 1103–1112.

Wiley, M.E., & Damiano, D.L. (1998). Lower extremity strength profiles in spastic cerebral palsy. *Developmental Medicine and Child Neurology, 40*, 100–107.

Willoughby, C., & Polatajko, H.J. (1995). Motor problems in children with developmental coordination disorder: A review of the literature. *American Journal of Occupational Therapy, 49*, 787–797.

Wilson, P.H., & McKenzie, B.E. (1998). Information processing deficits associated with developmental coordination disorder: A meta-analysis of research findings. *Journal of Child Psychiatry, 6*, 829–840.

Wirz, M., Colombo, G., & Dietz, V. (2001). Long term effects of locomotor training in spinal humans. *Journal of Neurology, Neurosurgery, and Psychiatry, 71*(1), 93–96.

Wolf, S., Lecraw, D.E., Barton, L.A., & Jann, B.B. (1989). Forced use of hemiplegic upper extremities to reverse the effect of learned nonuse among chronic stroke and head injured patients. *Experimental Neurology, 104*, 125–132.

Wolpaw, J. (1985). Adaptive plasticity in the spinal stretch reflex: An accessible substitute of memory? *Cellular and Molecular Neurobiology, 5*, 147–165.

Wolpaw, J.R., & Tennissen, A.M. (2001). Activity-dependent spinal cord plasticity in health and disease. *Annual Review of Neuroscience, 24*, 807–843.

Wood, E., & Rosenbaum, P. (2000). The Gross Motor Function Classification System for Cerebral Palsy: A study of reliability and stability over time. *Developmental Medicine and Child Neurology, 42*, 292–296.

Woollacott, M.H., Burtner, P., Jensen, J., Jasiewicz, J., Roncesvalles, N., & Sveistrup, H. (1998). Development of postural responses during standing in healthy children and children with spastic diplegia. *Neuroscience and Biobehavioral Reviews, 22*, 583–589.

Yokochi, K., Hosoe, A., Shimabukuro, S., & Kodama, K. (1989). Motoscopic analysis of gross motor patterns in athetotic cerebral palsied children. *Brain Development, 11*(5), 317–321.

Zaino, C.A. (1999). Motor control of a functional reaching task in children with cerebral palsy and children with typical development: A comparison of electromyographic and kinetic measurements. Unpublished doctoral dissertation, MCP Hahnemann University, Philadelphia.

Zupan, V., Gonzalez, P., Lacaze-Masmonteil, T., Boithias, C., d'Allest, A.M., Dehan, M., & Gabilan, J.C. (1996). Periventricular leukomalacia: Risk factors revisited. *Developmental Medicine and Child Neurology, 38*, 1061–1067.

Chapter 7

Neuromuscular System: The Plan of Care

— Joanne Valvano, PT, PhD

Developing the *plan of care* is a very rewarding process. A thoughtful plan of care leads physical therapists to intervention strategies that will ultimately improve the quality of life for the children they work with. Developing the plan can be a challenging problem-solving activity. The physical therapist brings to the task multiple dimensions of knowledge and judgment, including basic knowledge of motor control, learning, and development; knowledge of body structures and functions and the limitations associated with specific diagnoses; knowledge of physical therapy interventions; problem-solving skills; and, most important, skills in communicating with children and their families. Therapists also rely on formal strategies of clinical decision making for developing a plan for intervention.

Heriza and Sweeney (1994) describe a process for developing an intervention plan for an infant or a child who presents with a problem concerning functional movement. Elements of this process are consistent with recommendations in the American Physical Therapy Association (APTA)'s *Guide to physical therapist practice* (2001), hereafter referred to as the *Guide* (2001). First, the physical therapist determines the family's concerns and priorities (or the concerns of the education team in the school environment). Through that collaboration, preliminary functional **goals and objectives** are established. Second, during the process of examination and evaluation, the therapist determines the child's or infant's developmental and functional status and identifies limitations in body structures and functions that affect functional activity and community participation. Third, the physical therapist arrives at a **diagnosis**, which determines how impairments and/or limitations in body structures and functions identified on examination interfere with functional activities and/or community participation. Fourth, the physical therapist arrives at a **prognosis**, or a prediction regarding the gains or improvement in function that might be expected as a result of the intervention. Finally, from the diagnosis and prognosis, the **plan for intervention** can be developed. These steps are consistent with a **top-down approach** (P. H. Campbell, 1991) in which desired outcomes are determined first, then components that limit these outcomes are assessed.

The following principles should enhance the intervention plan of care for infants, children, and adolescents with neurological disability:

1. The intervention plan should increase the child's participation in life's roles and improve the child's quality of life, through the preservation and enhancement of function as well as prevention. Every effort should be expended to determine the needs and priorities perceived by the child, family, and school personnel. All should be involved in planning the intervention activities.

2. The plan of care should meet the developmental needs of the child, with consideration of the current life roles of the child. The child's collaboration in developing the plan and setting goals should be encouraged, when developmentally appropriate.

245

3. Well-written, measurable goals and objectives should be the basis for the implementation of intervention. Efforts by physical therapists to refine this writing competency will be rewarded time and again in practice. They are necessary for fulfilling administrative requirements for the individualized education program (IEP) and the individualized family service plan (IFSP), or for reimbursement. Furthermore, the productivity of the intervention time will be enhanced by goals that are well thought out and clearly stated. There is evidence that the focus and integrity of the goals and objectives that guide intervention affect the success of the intervention for those with neurological dysfunction. Bower, McLellan, Arney, and Campbell (1996) evaluated the effects of the amount of physical therapy (conventional versus intensive) and the type of goals set by the therapist (general aims versus specific goals) with four randomized experimental groups. The outcome measures were dimensions of the Gross Motor Function Measure related to the subjects' goals or aims. After a 2-week period, the intensive physical therapy (1 hour per day) produced a slightly better effect than the conventional intensity, but the statistically significant factor more strongly associated with increased motor skill acquisition was the use of specific measurable goals.

4. To the greatest extent possible, the plan for physical therapy intervention should be integrated into an interdisciplinary plan for the child that is focused on the endpoint of enhanced performance in school, home, and community.

5. The plan of care should effectively integrate three components of intervention outlined by the *Guide* (2001). The first component includes communication and coordination with parents, other members of the interdisciplinary team, and community agencies. For example, a physical therapist might communicate with an orthotist regarding an ankle-foot orthosis or with an adaptive physical education teacher regarding a child's readiness for a particular gym activity. The second component involves instruction to family, classroom staff, and child in many areas, including safety, assistive technology, and adaptations to the home or classroom environment. The third component includes procedural interventions, which are "hands-on" interventions individualized to each child's plan of care.

6. When developing a plan of care, the physical therapist should develop a systematic method to evaluate the therapeutic effect of the intervention activities provided to each child.

7. For children with neurological impairments, it is important to reflect on the impact of impairments on function, not only for the short term but also for the lifetime of the child (Campbell, 1999). A thorough knowledge of the impairments in body structure and function and limitations in activities and participation associated with neurological impairments is critical to prevent secondary impairments as well as to preserve and enhance function.

8. To increase quality of life across the life span, intervention should foster the family's development as advocates and decision makers who can be proactive about their child's needs. It is also important to foster independence in the children with whom we work, so that they can learn to take responsibility and advocate for their own needs as they approach adulthood.

Intervention Strategies

Although all three components of intervention outlined in the *Guide* (2001) are fundamental to the plan of care, the discussion in this chapter will focus on direct therapeutic interventions, or procedural interventions, provided by the physical therapist, family members, or other members of the intervention team. With a plan of care established and goals and objectives delineated, the physical therapist is faced with the practical question: "What can I do to optimally support these functional goals and objectives?" Because of the complexity of neuromuscular impairments, there are many approaches or intervention strategies (Adams & Snyder, 1998; Barry, 1996). Optimally, we should have evidence to tell us the most effective strategies for intervention. Unfortunately, even after so many years of intervention with children having neurological impairments, there is insufficient evidence to tell us what is the optimal approach (Barry, 1996).

The paucity of evidence for intervention approaches, to some extent, may be related to methodological issues. The highest level of evidence for efficacy of medical interventions requires randomized controlled trials, in which subjects are randomly assigned to an intervention group or a control group. The individual expression of most neurological disabilities makes it difficult to have a control group. Also, ethical concerns make nontreatment control groups difficult to plan. Statistically significant differences between a treatment group receiving a particular intervention and a control group may not be reached because of small sample sizes, which limit statistical power. The measurements used in some studies may not be sensitive to change in children with neurological impairments, thereby making a significant difference difficult to identify. Furthermore, in the past, outcomes research has focused primarily on impairments, such as spasticity or postural control, rather than the functional outcomes that matter to children and families.

Currently, in pediatric physical therapy there is a strong commitment to evidence-based practice (Fetters, Harris, & Palisano, 2002) and clinical researchers are working to find creative solutions to methodological challenges to demonstrate efficacy. Clinical management guidelines (Section on Pediatrics, American Physical Therapy Association, 2004) are being developed to outline the sequence and timing of interventions that should achieve the best outcome for children with specific diagnoses. These guidelines rely on evidence about effectiveness of intervention strategies. The *Guide* (2001) facilitates study of the efficacy of interventions by systematically categorizing them. Given all of these efforts, there is optimism that pediatric physical therapy will make strides in the next decade in developing guidelines for optimal outcomes based on clinical evidence.

In the absence of an evidence-based consensus about intervention activities, physical therapists are challenged to make judgments about intervention strategies by seeking a broad base of knowledge about possible approaches to treatment and critically evaluating the evidence of scientific merit, as well as their practical merit in the clinic. Physical therapists should develop strategies for evaluating the efficacy of activities or procedures that we use in our practice and develop a network for sharing with colleagues. In this chapter, information on multiple intervention strategies for children with neurological impairments is presented. The author expects that the reader will contemplate them, seek additional information on preferred strategies, and develop personal guidelines for intervention.

Specific intervention activities or procedures that therapists use to improve functions such as ambulation are usually related to a recognized approach to treatment. Approaches to intervention for children with neurological impairments have historically gained popularity among therapists because their theoretical bases are consistent with contemporary beliefs about motor control and because of

clinical judgments about their efficacy. Current approaches to physical therapy intervention are based on the systems model of motor control, discussed in Chapter 6. The systems model of motor control presents a very rich perspective on how movement works because not only is it based in neuroscience, but it also integrates science from the domains of motor learning and control, kinesiology, and the behavioral sciences. The systems model of motor control is also a suitable framework for developing practice models because it emphasizes the multiple interacting systems working cooperatively to achieve a functional motor behavior.

Because of this focus on functional movement behavior, rather than on muscle activity or movement patterns, current approaches to interventions based on the system's model of motor control have been called "**task oriented**" (Horak, 1991; Shumway-Cook & Woollacott, 1995, 2001). In these task-oriented approaches, it is assumed that the child is an active participant in a learning process, motivated by the goal to accomplish a specific task. Changes in multiple systems, including motor and sensory, are driven by the active participation in the functional activity. Later in this chapter, characteristics of the "task-oriented" approaches will be applied to a category of interventions I will refer to as "activity focused." Current task-oriented approaches are different from traditional physical therapy approaches. Although the ultimate objective of the traditional approaches was to improve the function of the child, the means to that end was facilitation of normal patterns of movement through the skillful handling and sensory inputs provided by the therapist. Current approaches described in this chapter do not emphasize specific handling techniques or procedures, but they provide concepts or principles for how to support the infant's or child's learning of motor skills. The physical therapist is charged with interpreting and applying these concepts in the context of each child's individual needs.

Concept of Therapeutic Practice

As the infant or child engages in developmental movement activity or the practice of a skill, the therapist takes on the role of a change agent to facilitate or support the process of motor development or learning (Newell & Valvano, 1998). In doing so, the therapist adapts a child's goal-directed motor activity or structures practice sessions that are suited to the specific characteristics and needs of the child. These characteristics include those related to neurological diagnoses as well as attributes of the child that support learning. These task-oriented (or activity-focused) interventions may be referred to as **therapeutic practice.** The physical therapist's contributions are unique and important because of his or her thorough understanding of motor development and learning, as well as the impact of impairments in body functions on the process of learning motor skills. This special contribution of the physical therapist will be the basis for the model of intervention presented later in this chapter.

The concept of therapeutic practice might apply to a young infant at risk for cerebral palsy (CP) who is learning visually guided reach; a 5-year-old with myelomeningocele (MM) who is learning to walk with crutches; and a 10-year-old with developmental coordination disorder (DCD) who is learning to play soccer. Although the motor tasks and the processes of motor learning associated with them are unique, each situation involves the organization of systems around action- or goal-directed functional motor behaviors. The physical therapist's role in the therapeutic practice might be to increase the infant's readiness to participate in the reaching task, encourage attention to the task, modify the reaching task to increase the likelihood of success, or provide physical guidance to help introduce the infant to the basic coordination of the task. For crutch and soccer activities, the nature of the tasks requires more intentional practice by the children, who are developmentally capable of focused attention and verbally mediated problem solving. Therefore, the input from the therapist might include verbally mediated supports, which include instruction, verbal guidance, feedback, and motivating cues, in addition to task manipulations and physical guidance.

The motor learning program for adults after stroke developed by Carr and Shepherd (1987) illustrates the concept of therapeutic practice in adults. The motor learning program emphasizes relearning of real-life activities that have meaning for the individual by practicing specific tasks and generalizing their application. The therapist also addresses impairments associated with stroke for each individual, by working with components of movement that are missing or lacking because of the manifested impairments in body functions.

This chapter addresses strategies for conducting therapeutic practice. First, I review learning theories, which provide the framework for active motor learning strategies. Next, I discuss intervention strategies that emphasize active motor learning experiences but also address impairments in body structures and functions that place limits on motor performance and learning.

Active Process of Motor Learning: Theoretical Perspectives

Information-Processing Perspective

Two major perspectives that have guided the research on motor learning and development are the **information-processing perspective** and **dynamic systems perspectives.** Concepts from these perspectives are presented to give the reader an understanding of the theory that supports motor learning strategies. Then practical guidelines for conducting therapeutic practice for children will be suggested. Recommended readings on the conceptual framework of each of these perspectives are provided at the end of the chapter.

The information-processing perspective emphasizes the cognitive processes associated with learning motor skills. Understanding these cognitive processes, which are the basis for many motor learning principles, should help us apply these principles more effectively to practice by children with special needs. The information-processing perspective views the learner as an active processor of information. Information processing is essential to motor learning, which is defined as "a set of internal processes associated with practice or experience leading to a relatively permanent change in the capability for a motor skill" (Schmidt, 1988, p. 375). Repeated motor activity without active participation and information processing would yield very little gain in terms of motor learning. For example, how could a baseball player perfect his batting if he were passively moved through each hit in practice? Likewise, how could an infant learn visually guided reaching if his or her hand were passively directed to the object, or how could a child with CP learn to complete a transfer if he or she were passively moved on each repetitive trial?

Stages of Information Processing

The information processing that occurs before the actual production of the movement commences contributes to the process of motor learning (Light, 2003). According to a model proposed by Schmidt (1988), the processing that occurs before movement execution includes (1) stimulus identification, which involves selectively attending to and integrating relevant stimuli from the environment; (2) response selection, which involves choosing a suitable motor response; and (3) response programming, which structures or prepares the appropriate response in the central nervous system (CNS) (Figure 7–1). These processing steps affect **reaction time,** which is the duration in time

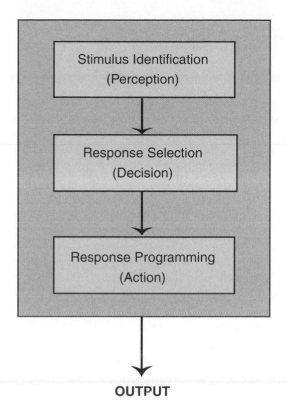

OUTPUT

Figure 7-1 Information-processing model. (Adapted by permission from Schmidt, R.A., & Lee, T.D. [1999]. *Motor control and learning* [3rd ed., p. 45]. Champaign, IL: Human Kinetics.)

between the presentation of an environmental stimulus, or the intent to move, and the actual initiation of the movement response. The stages of information processing interact with two other elements of the information-processing perspective: memory and attention. The slow, awkward quality of movement seen in children with neurological impairments may be accounted for by information-processing deficits in addition to limitations in the production of movement.

The inefficient movement characteristic of DCD has been explained in terms of deficits in the stages of information processing (David, 1995, 2000; Maruff, Wilson, Trebilcock, & Currie, 1998; Wilson & McKenzie, 1998). Deficits in selective attention, or the ability to maintain focus on relevant stimuli, are very common. David (2000) suggests that deficits in stimulus identification are apparent in children with visual perception deficits, who demonstrate difficulty with spatial organization or with judging distances. These children might bump into objects or have difficulty with spatial judgments on the playground.

Kinesthetic feedback may also be unreliable. David also describes how memory functions could affect the response selection in children with DCD. A child playing baseball might not recall the best orientation relative to the plate when hitting the baseball or the best way to hold the bat. In soccer, the child may not remember the best kick, based on the configuration of his opponents on the field. Moreover, David (2000) proposed that difficulties with timing of responses and with grading the level of force also relate to deficits in response selection. Response programming involves the retrieval of a plan of action. Therefore, impairments in response programming might affect the ability to remember the sequence of elements of a functional action. Children may depend heavily on feedback, especially visual, if they do not use anticipatory control, developed from prior experience (Missiuna, Rivard, & Bartlett, 2003). If the sequence of a movement response, such as tying a shoelace or getting onto a tricycle, cannot be taken from memory and executed, the child must rely on the feedback provided in the course of performance, thereby making the movement slow and laborious. Production deficits may also contribute to the inefficient movement.

Developmental aspects of information processing have been addressed in the literature. The time to process information is age related. It takes younger children longer to process feedback information, especially complex information. The precision of information that can be used for feedback also varies with age (Gallagher & Thomas, 1989; Newell & Carlton, 1980; Newell & Kennedy, 1978).

The stages of information processing have limitations in depicting the process of learning completely novel movements and may not address the complex learning issues for children with disability. However, the stages of information processing might help us grade the challenge for motor learning during therapeutic practice. To illustrate an application, we can apply the stages of information processing to the practice of walking with a cane by a child with traumatic brain injury (TBI). Because of perceptual, cognitive, and attention constraints, as well as frustration levels during the course of recovery, the child's physical therapist might grade the challenge in terms of the information-processing demands. The child's therapist might begin working in a very quiet part of a gym with very little equipment and no other children. This would reduce demands on attention and make it easier to identify and process relevant stimuli. The therapist might even help the child to focus on salient visual cues. Gradually a more complex stimulus array could be introduced. Selective attention is a critical element to motor learning, and attention processes should be a focus of effective learning interventions.

After the basic ability to walk with a cane is acquired, the therapist might decide to teach the child to walk around obstacles. To grade the challenge for stimulus identification, the obstacles should initially be large, brightly colored, and contrasting with the floor. Eventually the obstacles might be more subtle and challenging to detect. The placement of obstacles in the child's way could also be graded in terms of the complexity of their pattern. When the therapist conducts the practice in the hallway, the number of response options might also increase the challenge. In addition to obstacles to step around, the therapist might present additional movement challenges, such as a broom to step over, an unexpected person to walk around, or a small box that has to be moved out of the path.

Finally, the number of elements that have to be chained together to execute the response increases the challenge for response programming. The number of response elements would be minimal if the walking were initiated, on cue, from a standing position with the cane already placed in the child's hand. The programming requirements (and reaction time) would be increased if the child were required, on cue, to grasp the cane and move from sitting to standing and then initiate a step. Programming requirements could also be graded by the degree of accuracy required in the movement response. The programming requirements should be adjusted to the stage of learning, with the ultimate focus on the requirements in the child's functional environment.

A critical concept from the information-processing perspective is **memory**. Memory functions are important to enable the learner to benefit from prior experience. There are many elaborate models to depict the functions of memory in motor learning in the literature. The fundamental components of memory are depicted in Figure 7–2.

Two basic concepts relevant to therapeutic practice by children are **short-term** and **long-term memory** (Schmidt, 1988; Schmidt & Wrisberg, 2000). Children are constantly bombarded by environmental stimuli that are held very briefly in what is referred to as the short-term sensory store. Only relevant stimuli are selectively attended to and processed in a theoretical structure called short-term memory. This short-term memory is also called the working memory because it is the theoretical structure where information about the goal-oriented movement and the sensory cues associated with the movement are processed. Information resides in short-term memory only for seconds. If there is adequate active mental processing in the short-term memory, information can be encoded or packaged for storage into the long-term memory. Examples of an active mental processing are allocating attention to focus on the movement, mentally rehearsing a movement, evaluating the outcome of the movement, or making comparisons with previous movement trials. Encoding into long-term memory is critical in the information-processing perspective because information "stored" in the long-term memory can be retrieved when it is needed again for a functional movement response. Active practice and processing are very important for encoding information into long-term memory, or "making memories," that can be retrieved and adapted for future performance.

The memory representation of a movement that can be retrieved when needed for a functional action is called the **motor program**. A motor program can be viewed as a prestructured motor command, which defines and shapes the essential details of a skilled action (Schmidt & Wrisberg, 2000). The motor program is responsible for determining the major events in the movement pattern. However, there is often considerable interaction with sensory processes to refine the movement and adapt it to

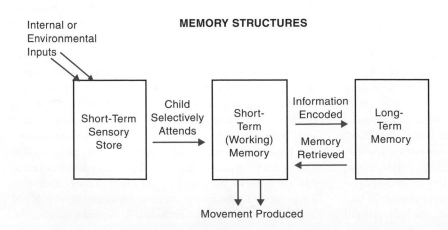

MEMORY STRUCTURES

Figure 7-2 Model of memory structures. (Adapted, by permission, from Schmidt, R.A. (1988). *Motor control and learning*, [2nd ed., p. 91]. Champaign, IL: Human Kinetics.)

environmental demands (Schmidt & Wrisberg, 2000). There cannot be a motor program for all of the possible variations of a movement class (e.g., throwing at different velocities, at different intensities, and in different directions). The concept of the **generalized motor program** is described by Schmidt (1988) to address this limitation. The generalized motor program has basic, invariant features related to the spatiotemporal structure of the movement, as well as changeable or variant features, which modify the movement to meet task requirements. (Schmidt & Wrisberg, 2000). For example, the generalized motor program for kicking a soccer ball has invariant features that define kicking, such as the relative time it takes to complete each component of the movement. Variant or changeable features of the motor program, such as the overall force with which the ball is kicked, or the direction of the kick are called **parameters** of the motor program. Practicing many variations of a movement class, like kicking, is called **variable practice.** Variable practice involves the practice of different parameters of the motor program, makes the mental representation more flexible, and therefore should help with retention and generalization of the skill to new situations (Schmidt & Wrisberg, 2000). A clinical example of a movement class is a transfer from sit to stand. A physical therapist might provide variable practice by working on the transition from chairs of varied heights and with different seat surfaces.

The difference between performance and learning is an important distinction for developing and refining motor programs. **Learning** is a relatively permanent effect of practice or experience. On the other hand, changes in **performance** that are immediately seen during the practice of a task may not be permanent (Schmidt, 1988; Winstein, 1991). Certain practice variables have different effects on performance and learning. For example, high amounts of guidance or feedback may encourage essentially error-free performance. However, the effect on long-term learning is quite the opposite. The memory representation, which accounts for retention and transfer, could not be adequately developed with so much guidance provided.

Motor programs are theoretically important for functional motor performance because, once the motor program, or mental representation, is firmly established, the performer does not have to direct as much attention to generating the movement response. If a movement is well learned and the motor program is established and refined, the child can execute the response quickly (e.g., kicking a soccer ball), with relatively little attention (automatically). For complex tasks, if certain parts are performed without attention demands, information-processing resources can

be available for other parts of the movement. For example, if the kicking action is automatic, the soccer player can direct his or her attention to the actions of the opponents and the configuration of the players on the field.

Motor programs typify **feedforward modes of motor control** described in Chapter 6. Limitations in feedforward control typical of children with neurological involvement are illustrated by a study of the control of precision grip forces (Eliasson, Gordon, & Forssberg, 1992). Children who are developing typically will, after grasping an object a few times, program the force in advance for subsequent grasping and lifting. That is, the amount of force required to grip and lift the object is determined before the grip force is exerted on the object. This mode of control is efficient because the child does not have to rely on feedback to generate the appropriate force to grip the object. Children with CP rely more on sensory feedback from the fingertips to develop the force required to grip the object. Therefore, they may generate the force with many pulses, use exaggerated grip forces, and take many more trials to develop the anticipatory control of grip force (Eliasson et al., 1992; Gordon & Duff, 1999).

These findings suggest that some children with neurological impairments (specifically CP) demonstrate difficulty in the development of motor programs or abstract representations of motor responses based on experience (Eliasson, Gordon, & Forssberg, 1995; Giuliani, 1991). Therefore, they may require additional practice (Gordon & Duff, 1999) or be more dependent on feedback during the execution of the movements than their typically developing peers. This requirement for feedback may make their movement slow and less smooth and efficient, especially with complex and demanding tasks. Another example of feedback versus feedforward modes of control is the child with CP who relies on visual and tactile feedback to judge the degree of flexion in the lower extremities required to ascend stairs. This reliance on feedback is in contrast to the child with typical development, who quickly ascends the whole flight of stairs, with the amount of flexion programmed in advance.

Through practice, the child must develop (1) the capability for producing the motor response skillfully and (2) a reference for the correct movement, which is required to evaluate performance and to detect errors. Feedback about the just-completed movement helps to develop this reference. Feedback or any information provided to the learner by a change agent is called **extrinsic or augmented information.** It is called augmented information because it augments or supplements the intrinsic information that is naturally available to the performer by executing the movement (Schmidt & Wrisberg, 2000). Feedback and other modes of augmented information are discussed later in the chapter.

The final construct of information processing that I discuss is attention. **Attention** can be defined as the allocation and focusing of information-processing resources. Selective attention involves focusing on the relevant stimuli for interaction with the environment. This concept has relevance for infants with neurological immaturity, who have difficulty focusing attention. It also has implications for motor learning by children who have attention deficit disorder, for whom filtering out irrelevant environmental stimuli is difficult. The construct of attention has applications to therapeutic practice, based on the assumption that there is a limited capacity of attention. Basically, children can concentrate on a limited amount of information at one time. We know that, in natural environments, such as the classroom, children are required to focus on many things at once.

Researchers have learned about attention limitations by using dual task or divided attention paradigms. In these paradigms, a competing, or dual, task is introduced as the child performs a primary task. The effects of performance on the primary and secondary tasks are observed. Basically, the interference that one task has with another depends on how well learned or automatic is the primary task. If it is well learned, it does not require much attention (Huang & Mercer, 2001; Schmidt & Wrisberg, 2000). The attention demands that are required to perform a motor skill are discussed in terms of the controlled versus automatic processing dichotomy. Controlled processing in the early phase of learning is slow, attention demanding, and effortful. On the other hand, automatic processing, which requires a lot of practice to achieve, is fast and does not demand many attention resources, thereby making resources available for another task presented simultaneously (Schmidt, 1988; Schmidt & Wrisberg, 2000). Recall that the motor program permits automatic performance.

Applications to therapeutic practice might include (1) taking the child to a high level of primary task performance before introducing interference of competing tasks; (2) using dual tasks to evaluate level of learning of a primary task; and (3) practicing functional tasks in the natural environment where attention is divided among competing tasks.

Constructs from the information-processing perspective, especially memory, have been applied to developmental research with young infants. However, they have not been formally applied to models of early intervention strategies for infants at risk for neurological impairments.

Information processing has been applied more directly to intentional motor skill learning that requires focused attention and verbally mediated processes. These constructs are relevant to therapeutic practice because they structure our appreciation of the cognitive aspects of learning.

In summary, the information-processing framework emphasizes the cognitive aspects of motor learning. It embodies constructs, such as attention, memory, and mental representations, that are established and refined through experience and practice. This framework has been the basis for much of the research on practice variables that enhance motor learning, including augmented information and structure of practice.

Dynamic Systems Perspective

Over the past two decades, the **dynamic systems perspective** has grown in emphasis in the field of motor learning. The theory for the dynamic systems perspective on motor learning parallels the dynamic systems perspective on motor control defined in Chapter 6. This section revisits and expands on selected concepts presented in Chapter 6 and suggests practical application of the concepts to therapeutic practice. Recommended readings at the end of the chapter offer a more complete understanding of the dynamic systems perspective.

There have been two major influences on the dynamic systems perspective: the writings of Nickolai Bernstein (1967) and the science of nonlinear dynamics applied to organization and nonlinear change in complex physical and biological systems. According to Bernstein, motor learning involves problem solving, or actively finding a coordination strategy that will enable a functional motor task to be executed. The process of learning does not merely involve repetition of the movement; it involves repeatedly going through the process of solving the problem again and again (Bernstein, 1967). This is apparent in the school-aged child who spends hours trying to master a computer game and in early walkers who practice upright balance. Adolph, Vereijken, & Shrout (2003) report that infant walkers practice balance walking for more than 6 accumulated hours per day and average between 500 and 1500 steps per hour!

Complex Movement Systems With Many Component Systems

Bernstein emphasized the multiple systems that cooperate in the performance of functional movement. According to the dynamic systems perspective, movement behavior does not occur because of a programmed or prepackaged response triggered in the brain. Rather, the **coordination** required to achieve a task emerges because it is preferred or "natural," given the interaction of all of the elements of the **complex movement system** under specific task and environmental conditions. Shumway-Cook and Woollacott (1995) compare the self-organization of the elements of the movement system with the cells in the heart, which work collectively to make the heart beat. The interaction of multiple systems, reiterated several times in Chapter 6, is the foundation for the systems model of motor control, which has had great influence on task-oriented models of intervention for adults and children with neurological impairments.

The concept of a complex self-organizing movement system is applied to the development of independent stepping by infants (Heriza & Sweeney, 1994; Thelen, 1986). Thelen proposed that each of the multiple systems associated with locomotion has its own developmental timetable, and progresses at its own rate. The process of stepping is self-organizing because progression in each of the component systems (including motivation, strength, tonus control, and body characteristics) alters the intrinsic coordination tendencies of the infant. If all of the subsystems are at a specific state or level of organization, walking merges as the preferred or "natural" pattern of locomotion. If one of the participating systems is not at the proper state (e.g., hip extension strength not developed), the organization of the subsystems would not support the coordination necessary for walking, and walking would not emerge as the preferred behavior. The self-organizing movement system

intrinsic to the infant also interacts with the task and the context of the action, which drive the motor behavior. Stepping behaviors will not emerge unless the infant perceives the action goal, such as moving toward a parent or favorite toy. Figure 7–3 depicts the interaction of multiple systems intrinsic to the child, with the task and the environment in the systems model of development adapted by Heriza and Sweeney (1994).

These notions about multiple systems challenge traditional perspectives on motor learning, which stress neurological maturation as the driving force for developmental change. Thelen and Fisher (1982) examined the stepping reflex in infants of about 4 months of age. According to traditional perspectives on motor development, the diminished activity in stepping is related to integration of the primitive reflex from higher centers of the CNS. Thelen and Fisher (1982) challenged this interpretation by demonstrating that increased leg mass relative to ability to generate force, as well as environmental context, contributed to the change in the preferred motor behavior (from automatic stepping to no stepping). Infants who did not demonstrate the stepping over ground demonstrated the stepping in the buoyant environment of water. In this case, the motor behavior reflected self-organization of the multiple systems, not just neurological, in the context of the stepping task, and a specific environmental context (over ground versus water). The reader is encouraged to read the dynamic systems interpretation to development and its contrast to more traditional theories by Heriza (1991).

From a dynamic systems perspective, external or physical

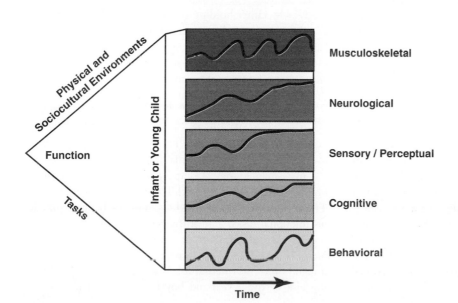

Figure 7-3 Systems model of development depicting the child, the task, and the characteristics of the physical and sociocultural environment, which contribute to functional behavior. (Reprinted with permission from Heriza, C.B., & Sweeney, J.K. [1994]. Pediatric physical therapy: Part I: Practice, scope, scientific basis, and theoretical foundation. *Infants and Young Children, 7*, 29.)

forces complement the internal forces generated by muscle activation patterns (theoretically directed by the motor program). Sources of physical forces are gravity, inertia, and motion-dependent forces. Motion-dependent forces are forces that act on one segment as a result of movement from adjacent segments in the body. Try shaking your hand vigorously and note that there are forces that are apparently acting on the humerus. Also, think of the forces generated by a countermovement, such as when a pitcher winds up and twists before pitching the baseball. The contribution of these physical forces to movement challenges the traditional notion of a motor program, which can, theoretically, be retrieved to execute a movement. Let us take the case of infant kicking. The organization of the kicking movement in young infants has fundamental properties that define kicking. However, the motor program that specifies a single muscle activation pattern for kicking would be an inadequate description. Additional non-neural forces such as gravity, inertia, and motion-dependent forces complement the forces that contribute to the kick from neural activation. The interaction of these forces is different when the baby kicks in supine position from when the baby kicks while supported in a semireclining position (Jensen, Ulrich, Thelen, Schneider, & Zernicke, 1994). We intuitively respect the effects of gravity in our basic therapeutic exercise. Additional considerations in motor behavior, such as speed of movement or use of countermovements, might be considered during therapeutic practice.

Movement Versus Action

In the dynamic systems perspective, the difference between action and movement is critical. **Action** involves the accomplishment of a task, the intention to realize a functional goal, and a strategy to achieve the goal (Gentile, 1987; Majsak, 1996; Newell & Valvano, 1998). Change at the movement level involves the coordination of movement patterns, which allows the action goal to be achieved. Change at the movement level is not sufficient for action. The emphasis on action in the dynamic systems perspective is compatible with current models of motor control, which focus on purposeful activity rather than the achievement of movement components for their own sake. Van der Weel, van der Meer, and Lee (1991) evaluated the component of forearm supination in children with CP. This movement is difficult for children who demonstrate an imbalance toward a flexion pattern in the upper extremity. The experiment demonstrated that increased active supination was achieved when the children used the limb to perform a functional action, beating on a drum, compared with when they prac-

ticed the movement of supination. The task gave meaning and a goal structure to the movement pattern.

Degrees of Freedom

Bernstein suggested that finding a coordination solution to a movement problem involved controlling all of the redundant **degrees of freedom** (**DFs**), or all the possible independent planes of motion in the joints in the body to coordinate an efficient movement (Newell & McDonald, 1994). The DFs are redundant in that there are more available options for movement than the child needs to perform the task. According to Bernstein, this coordination of the DFs of the joints, which exceed 100, is accomplished by organizing these DFs into functional groups or synergies that constrain the muscles or joints to act as functional units. The concept of DFs is explained in terms of the muscle activation patterns that are coordinated to control balance reactions in Chapter 6. The hip and knee in walking, or the elbow and shoulder in reaching, are linked together as functional units. That is, the movement of one segment can be easily predicted by the movement of the other. However, in the case of walking and reaching, the linkage of the distal segments may be more variable, to adapt the movement to the task demands.

During practice of more complex skills, which require discrete movement at all segments, basic synergies are differentiated and refined, so the movement can be more flexibly adapted to task demands. This process of differentiation is illustrated by the differences between novice and expert skiers. The novice skier appears "stiff" as he skis down the hill. The movement is stiff because he "freezes" the DFs by either holding the joints stiff in co-contraction or using simple, undifferentiated synergies of the trunk and leg segments. It is too challenging for the novice to control muscular forces of all of the segments and coordinate them with passive forces such as the force of gravity. Over time, the skier learns to differentiate the joints and adapt to subtle challenges on the hill. The advanced skier is able to use the physical effects of gravity and the motion-dependent forces from the leg and trunk movements to make smooth, fast movements down the hill.

This sequence may also apply to functional movements physical therapists teach to children. Children with CP and TBI may adaptively "freeze" DFs in the early phase practice of functional tasks. The stiffness can be mistakenly attributed to the impairments of spasticity affecting the movement (Bly, 1991). The flexible control of DFs and the integration of non-neural forces are depicted in the throwing task of the 7-year old boy in Figure 7–4A. Note the differentiation at the spine, the intuitive use of a counter-movement (which uses the elastic properties of muscle and connective tissue to contribute to the force generation), and the weight shift (motion-dependent forces) that character-ize this movement. Contrast this to the throwing behaviors of the child with CP in Figure 7–4B, who limits the DFs by holding the trunk stiffly, minimizing the motion-dependent forces and forces of gravity and inertia. The expected difference in functional outcome of the throwing movement between the two children is obvious.

The coordination of the DFs during functional activity is individual for each child, given the characteristics of the child's movement system. The individual quality of move-ment seen in children with neurological impairments reflects this individuality and may explain why it is often difficult to change the form or quality of the movement. Our work with control of grip forces by children with CP illustrates this point (Valvano & Newell, 1998). Children with CP practiced the control of isometric grip force production in two conditions, in one of which they had to control all of the DFs in the hand to grip a surface with thumb and index finger. In the other condition, the distal forearm and hand were supported in a posture that opti-mally placed their thumb and index finger at the grip surface. One would expect that the fingers of the supported hand would produce the best grip force, because the hand was positioned "optimally" for gripping and there was no proximal requirement to actively support the arm. On the contrary, grip force production was not better in the supported condition. In fact, there was a trend toward better control in the unsupported condition. This may have been attributable to the ability of the children to organize and use the DFs in the manner that had emerged over time. Latash and Anson (1996) propose that the atypical quality of movement of children with disability represents the best solution for achieving a functional goal, given the impair-ments in the component systems that contribute to the movement. However, we know that certain "preferred" patterns of movement may be inefficient or lead to second-ary impairments. For example, sitting in an asymmetrical manner might lead to scoliosis; sitting in a "W-sit" pattern may affect the integrity of the hip joint and soft tissue. The judgment of the physical therapist, as the change agent, is critical here in determining the efficacy of intervention goals at the movement level. When practicing functional tasks, such as ascending or descending stairs, the therapist might try to differentiate between components of move-ment that are critical for safely executing the task and those that relate more to style and aesthetics.

Concepts About Change

In the past decades, movement scientists have applied mathematical principles to develop a **dynamic pattern theory** that addresses Bernstein's questions about organiza-tion of movement and changes that occur during motor learning (Haken, Kelso, & Bunz, 1985; Kelso, 1984; Scholz, 1990). This section will focus on a few practical concepts from dynamic pattern theory that can be useful in conducting therapeutic practice.

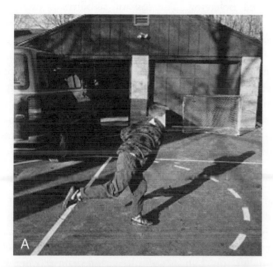

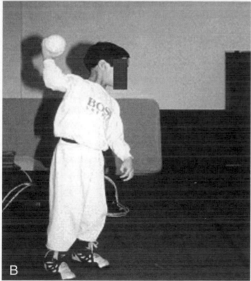

Figure 7-4 Coordination of the degrees of freedom during throwing tasks (*A*) for a boy with typical develop-ment and (*B*) for a boy with spastic diplegia.

Dynamic systems are systems that change. For motor behaviors to change, with intentional skill learning or during development, the intrinsic coordination tendencies of the child must change (Kelso, 1984; Newell, 1996; Newell & Valvano, 1998; Scholz, 1990; Zanone, Kelso, & Jeka, 1993). The term **coordination**, from a dynamic systems framework, refers to the organization of the body segments into a behavioral unit, which clinicians might call a pattern of movement. There can be qualitative change in the coordination, which defines the relationship of segments to one another (e.g., palmar grasp versus pincer grasp). There can also be quantitative change, such as changes in speed, timing, or magnitude of the movement. The latter refine or scale the basic pattern to meet task demands. According to dynamic pattern theory, changes in motor behavior are induced by variables called **control parameters.** Control parameters take on different values and, when they reach a critical value, they provide the necessary conditions to induce a change in motor behavior.

Although we cannot mathematically model motor behavior according to dynamic pattern theory, the metaphor of the control parameter can be applied to clinical interventions. The physical therapist, through careful task analysis and analysis of the child's movement characteristics, can identify factors that will support the desired change during the practice of functional tasks. Control parameters can reside in one or many of the multiple subsystems that contribute to the complex movement system. They can also be external to the performer. Let us take the common clinical example of toe-walking by a child with CP. Often, if the child walks very slowly, he or she demonstrates heel strike at initial contact. However, as the speed of the walking increases, the child contacts with the forefoot. External control parameters that influence the transition from heel contact to forefoot contact could be the requirement of increased velocity, the surface of the floor, or the physical forces associated with increased velocity. The control parameters internal to the child could be the degree of stiffness, selective muscle control, hip range of motion (ROM), anxiety, or the postural control abilities associated with the increased velocity. Transitions in preferred behavior of children may spontaneously occur because of change in the control parameters, relative to the task or context. For example, an ankle-foot orthosis may be a control parameter that changes the degree of stiffness in the ankle, resulting in heel contact during gait. Another example of transition is the systematic change in grip patterns used for functional grasp and release. Grip pattern changes in a systematic way so that the number of fingers

(2 to 10) used to grip can be predicted by the size of the object relative to the thumb span (Newell, Scully, McDonald, & Baillargeon, 1989). A final example is the predictable transition from walk to run by a child on a treadmill, as the speed of the treadmill is increased.

The concept of **stability** in the dynamic systems perspective describes the resistance to change or transition to another motor behavior. The stability of a certain movement pattern, or coordination, used to achieve an action is determined by the intrinsic characteristics of the child's movement system under certain task and environmental conditions. The behavior that is stable is called the **preferred behavior**. The loss of stability of one motor behavior supports a pattern switch or transition. Transitions or pattern shifts occur in development because change in the component systems of the infant makes the current pattern unstable or less "natural." These component systems self-organize, and new motor patterns emerge as the preferred ones to achieve an action (e.g., belly crawling transitions to creeping on hands and knees for locomotion).These periods of instability are critical for progression to new motor behaviors.

In the examples of transition given above, the new coordinations were available to the children, and the control parameters provided the necessary conditions for the systems to reorganize (or transition) to the new preferred behaviors. Often the coordination (or patterns of movement) required to perform functional activities, such as serving a tennis ball or walking with crutches, is not available to the child. In these cases, the acquisition of the coordination required to achieve the action requires focused, intentional effort with instruction, feedback, or other information provided by a change agent.

Experiments that examine the concept of stability suggest that, for intentional learning, the coordination of to-be-learned motor behavior is in competition with the intrinsic existing tendencies of the mover. If the existing pattern is very stable, practice may have diminished effect. If the existing pattern is not stable, goal-directed practice results in a destabilization of the existing movement pattern and a transition to the desired behavior. Also, the likelihood of change is affected by the degree to which the requirements of the to-be-learned behavior are different from those of the current behavior (Scholz & Kelso, 1990; Schoner, Zanone, & Kelso, 1992; Wenderoth, Bock, & Krohn, 2002; Zanone & Kelso, 1994). Concepts about stability and the likelihood of change can be applied to the process of prognosis in the *Guide*, which requires therapists to anticipate the potential for change in the child.

Constraints on Action

The idea of the control parameter has been applied to practical learning situations (Newell, 1986) through the construct of **constraints on action.** Constraints do not emphasize the mathematical quality of the control parameter but rather emphasize the metaphor of change. Constraints can be multiple factors related to the performer, the task, and the environment (or context of learning) that interact with each other to influence the preferred behavior that will emerge. This concept has been applied to interventions with varied clinical populations (Clark; 1995; Majak, 1996; Newell, 1986; Newell & Valvano, 1998). These factors are called constraints because they limit or constrain the possible movement outcomes that might emerge as the child attempts to achieve an action. Constraints can be enablers or positive influences to learning (because they restrict the possible outcomes to positive ones) or limiters to learning (because they inhibit change or support the outcome that is not desired). In the latter case, they are called rate limiters (Clark, 1995). **Task constraints** relate to the goal of the task or the rules of the activity, which may be implicit or explicit. The **environmental constraints** involve physical manipulations, such as the support medium as well as physical supports, such as adaptive equipment. The environment also includes the psychosocial environment and the performance environment. The performance environment includes augmented information, such as feedback and guidance that are provided to the child to enhance learning. These will be discussed in detail later in this section.

Newell and Valvano (1998) propose that the physical therapist, along with parents and other professionals on the intervention team, are change agents as the child learns functional motor activities. The change agents support and foster change to meet the action goals in the plan of care. The physical therapist interacts with constraints related to the task, the environment, and the characteristics of the infant or child to support the transition, which embodies the achievement of the action goal. In that way, the input from the physical therapist can be considered a constraint on the action that emerges with practice.

Guidelines for Conducting Activity-Focused Practice

This section discusses a model (Figure 7–5) that assigns primacy to improving functional motor activity to increase independence and participation. The physical therapist is a change agent who plans and adapts **activity-focused interventions,** which will lead to the desired functional change outlined in the plan of care. Activity-focused interventions involve structured practice and repetition of functional actions. The physical therapist, as a change agent, also integrates activity-focused interventions with **impairment-level interventions.** The latter address impairments in body functions and structures that affect the process of motor

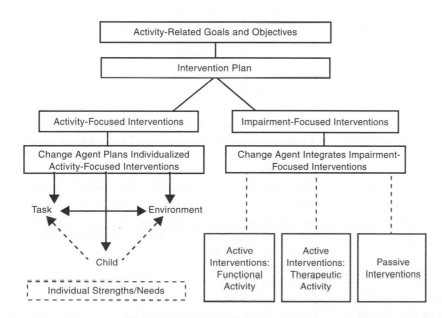

Figure 7-5 Model of interventions for children with neurological impairments, which integrates activity-focused interventions with impairment-focused interventions by physical therapist or occupational therapist as change agent. (Reprinted from Valvano, J. [2004] Activity-focused motor interventions for children with neurological conditions *Physical and Occupational Therapy in Pediatrics, 24,* with permission.)

learning and may cause secondary impairments (see Valvano, 2004 for details of the model for intervention).

Three practical steps for activity-focused interventions are:

1. Develop **activity-related goals and objectives** that will increase participation and quality of life, based on priorities of the child and family, in collaboration with the intervention team.

2. Plan **activity-focused interventions** by (1) using motor learning guidelines from the literature as a foundation for planning therapeutic practice, with focus on environment and task variables, and (2) adapting these practice guidelines, when necessary, to address the child's individual learning strengths and needs.

3. Integrate **impairment-focused interventions** with activity-focused interventions. These are optimally executed in the context of goal-related functional activity , but may also be executed outside the context of functional activity.

Developing Goals for Practice

Long-term goals of the intervention plan are developed in collaboration with the child and family or education team. The first part of this chapter discussed concepts that should be integrated into goals and objectives. From the long-term goals established in the intervention plan of care (usually every 6 months for an IFSP, every school year for an IEP, and more frequently in the hospital setting), **short-term objectives** are developed. Remember that short-term objectives can be directed toward (1) acquiring a new motor task, (2) increasing skill of a motor task or generalizing it to natural environments, or (3), in some cases, reducing an impairment to prevent secondary disability. I propose that the physical therapist also develop **practice objectives**, which guide the development of practice strategies for a single or group of practice sessions. These practice goals should eventually lead to the achievement of the long-term functional goal. The physical therapist should consider the stability of the current behavior to develop expectations for change or the prognosis.

Planning Activity-Focused Interventions

The model for intervention depicted in Figure 7–5 (Valvano, 2004) depicts the interaction of the constraints related to the task, environment, and the person. It suggests that the physical therapist intervene with practice strategies directed toward the task and the environment to promote learning. The broken lines from the child to the task and environment signify the importance of individualizing these task and environmental interventions to meet the special learning strengths and limitations of the child.

Many practice variables from the motor learning literature have been studied in adults or children with no disability. These practice variables provide an important foundation for conducting practice, based on processes of learning common to all learners. I refer the reader to elegant discussions of the application of motor learning variables to learning by children with disability (Duff & Quinn, 2002; Gentile, 1992; Larin, 2000). However, empirical data to verify that these motor-learning principles apply to children with neurological impairments are just emerging. Therefore, the physical therapist should personalize interventions for each learner and consider how developmental factors and characteristics of the child, including strengths and limitations, might affect the process of motor learning.

The process of motor learning may be affected by neurological impairments. Selective attention may be impaired (Hood & Atkinson, 1990) and the children also may have sensory deficits, including visual, perceptual, proprioceptive, and tactile deficits that affect judgments important for motor learning (Boehme, 1988; Lee & Cook, 1990; Stiers et al., 2002). These deficits in the perception and integration of sensory inputs may affect utilization of intrinsic and extrinsic sensory information during practice. Slow information processing has been documented in children with CP by Parks, Rose, and Dunn (1989). Because children with neurological diagnoses have limited experience, they have a limited repertoire of movements to draw on for development of a movement plan for novel tasks (Goodgold-Edwards & Gianutsos, 1991). They may have difficulty developing memory representations of movements and may rely on sensory feedback for performance (Eliasson et al., 1992, 1995). There are deficits in force production, in terms of strength (Damiano, Dodd, & Taylor, 2002) as well as in selective control. The latter impairs timing and coordination of movement (Campbell, 1991; Olney & Wright, 2000) and the ability to perform components of movement critical to a task (Bly, 1991; Bobath & Bobath, 1984). There is also greatly increased trial-to-trial variability when children with neurological impairments practice a skill (Eliasson et al., 1992; Thorpe & Valvano, 2002; Valvano & Newell, 1998). Limitations in motor control cause the process of motor learning to be more effortful and complex. The increased complexity increases the requirement for practice. These findings may also be relevant to the effects of augmented information and practice organization. (See Valvano, 2004, for details.)

In the following section, I review guidelines for practice that can increase the efficiency of practice. These guidelines are intuitive applications from the motor learning literature, and from discussions of pediatric applications provided by, but not limited to, Duff and Quinn (2002), Heriza (1991), Gentile (1992), and Larin (2000). Most of the proposed guidelines have not been empirically tested. I encourage the reader to reflect on the applications and test these guidelines in clinical settings.

Guideline No. 1: Practice! Practice! Practice!

Remember that, from a dynamic systems perspective, motor learning involves many trials for active problem solving. From an information-processing perspective, active learning and problem solving require many trials of practice to develop memory representations. As children practice, we should not expect error-free learning. The development of error detection and problem-solving capabilities is an important part of motor learning. Remember that active learning is not restricted to the practice session. Help the parents and classroom personnel to challenge the child with movement problems throughout the course of the day and to reinforce and generalize learning to different environments.

The literature does not provide us with optimal guidelines for the frequency, duration of practice, and timing of rests during practice sessions. The motor learning literature evaluates the relative benefits of **massed practice** (duration of practice greater than duration of rest) versus distributed practice (rest greater than practice) (Schmidt & Wrisberg, 2000). However, these findings are difficult to generalize to the type of practice, the learning context, and the characteristics of children during practice by children with neurological impairments. Issues of fatigue and attention in children, as well as external factors relating to type of setting, academic schedule, and travel by the therapist, set constraints on frequency and scheduling. Studies of the effectiveness of increased frequency of intervention in children with CP are equivocal. Optimally, the frequency and schedule of practice sessions should be focused around the learning goal, the phase of practice, and the rate of learning of the child. For example, a child may be scheduled for weekly sessions of physical therapy. For this child, short-term high-frequency sessions might support learning of the emergent skill. A reduced frequency might be adequate as the child solidifies and practices the new skill. Integrating the practice into the natural environment and the creativity and involvement of parents and school personnel may be contributing factors.

The stage of learning has implications for many practice strategies. Gentile proposed two very practical stages of learning: early and late. During the early stage of learning, the learner discovers (1) the conditions that must be met in order to be successful with the task and (2) a possible coordination strategy to achieve the task. In the later stage of practice, the learner develops skill, the coordination is refined, and the movement becomes efficient (Gentile, 1992). Remember that the sensory motor and motor production deficits demonstrated by children with neurological impairments may prolong the early phases of practice and have implications for variables discussed later in this section.

Planning Activity-Focused Interventions: Task

Task constraints are those that relate to the actual content of practice and the goal of the task or the rules of the activity, which may be implicit or explicit. Task constraints also include implements used during practice, including toys. There is much discussion of the task-related variables in the motor-learning literature, and the reader is encouraged to pursue the recommended readings.

Guideline No. 2: Make Practice Fun and Motivating

Because repeated trials are required to learn a motor skill, the challenge for the physical therapist is to balance the rigors of therapeutic practice with a learning environment that is fun and motivating. Remember that play is the work of children. Often motor learning goals can be incorporated into playful games. Physical therapists must be skillful in using motivational strategies to maximize performance and having the activity meet developmental abilities. Selective attention to the task should be obtained when the task is presented. Allowing children who are developmentally capable to set the goals in the intervention plan enhances the motivation to practice.

Guideline No. 3: Determine the Focus or Content of the Activity

The content of practice relates to the nature of the tasks that are practiced (What does the child do in the practice?).

The task practiced may be the identical task specified in the activity goal of the intervention plan, such as eating solids with a fork, ascending stairs with no railing, driving a power chair, or kicking a soccer ball. On the other hand, the activity structured for the practice session may be a related task or developmental play activity that addresses a component of movement that is required for the activity specified in the intervention plan of care. Impairments in body functions or structures can limit the performance of task-specific components of movement. Therapists often use developmental play activities related to the goal activity specified in the plan of care because of the practical challenges of having young children perform repeated practice trials of the same task. The therapist also flexibly structures tasks, to permit an appropriate degree of exploration and decision making by the child.

The therapist should always carefully evaluate whether the achievement of the component practiced in a related task will transfer to the activity outlined in the intervention plan of care. One goal for Katey, the kindergarten student in Figure 7–6, is to ascend or descend a standard staircase with one railing in less than 2 minutes, with supervision only. Impairments in antigravity force generation and impaired selective control of lower extremity muscles may limit the ability to advance the leg and accurately place the foot onto the step. Katey's physical therapist complements the practice of the target task of ascending the steps with an alternate task, climbing on the jungle gym, to address these components.

In general, motor learning theory predicts a small amount of transfer between tasks, so practice of the target skill is recommended (Schmidt & Wrisberg, 2000; Winstein, Gardner, McNeal, Barto, & Nicholson, 1989). However, practice of related tasks that focus on shared movement components may play an increased role in motor learning by children with neurological impairments, who must develop the movement patterns required for the targeted activity. The extent to which components of movement practiced in a related activity transfer to the targeted activity requires empirical study. Horne, Warren, and Jones (1995) reported on interventions that involved six or seven activities specifically designed to facilitate acquisition of

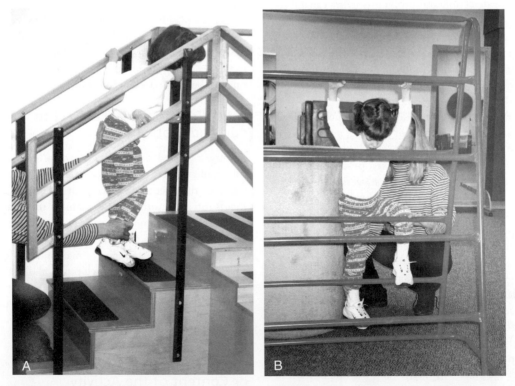

Figure 7-6 (*A*) Practice of a functional target task specified in the intervention Plan of Care. (*B*) Practice of a functional play task, which focuses on a component of movement required for performance of the target task.

specific movement components. Practice of these activities increased performance in children from 21 to 34 months of age. The children also demonstrated generalization of each movement component to untreated exemplar activities. For children with cognitive limitations, practice of prerequisite skills may not be advisable because of difficulty with transfer to the targeted activity (McEwen, 2000).

Guideline No. 4: Use Toys to Promote Desired Functional Outcomes

Toys are implements that can drive the motor behavior. The toys should meet the developmental needs of the child. The features of the objects drive the motor behavior that emerges, so the perceptual and physical features of the toys should be carefully evaluated. The toys may be used as motivators for a child to participate, but should not detract the child's selective attention from the primary focus of the practice.

Guideline No. 5: Adapt Tasks to Reduce Complexity and Difficulty

The **complexity of the task** is a way to judge difficulty for older children. The task should be at the appropriate level of difficulty and should be carefully individualized for the child. Physical therapists should try to plan activities with just the right amount of challenge relative to the child's skills (Campbell, 1999). They should develop a plan regarding where to start and where to progress with the course of practice. The complexity of the task can be graded on how many elements there are to achieve and whether it is an open or a closed task. Remember that additional elements increase the information-processing requirements as well as the production requirements. Children with neurological impairments have limitations in these areas. In a **closed task**, the task remains the same from one practice trial to another. In an **open task**, on the other hand, the conditions change on each trial, so there are many solutions to find (Schmidt & Wrisberg, 2000). Gentile (1987) developed a taxonomy of tasks that characterizes the nature of the task based on the spatial and temporal characteristics of the environment and the degree to which the task involves manipulation of an object or body transport. The difficulty of the task for each learner is individual because of the special learning characteristics of the learner.

Adaptations to practice may provide a less difficult version of the task so an optimal level of performance can be maintained. A gradual transition to a more difficult version of the task is made as the child progresses. Although

this strategy is not advisable in the typical motor learning literature, it may be applicable to children with limits in strength and endurance. Safety is another reason for grading the difficulty of the task. Adaptations can be made by reducing the task requirements or by giving physical support for safety. Assistive aids, such as walkers, crutches, or parapodium, can be used in functional mobility tasks. The optimal features of assistive aids can significantly affect function for children with disability. For example, posterior walkers enhance locomotor function of certain children with CP (Logan, Byers-Hinkley, & Ciccone, 1990). Guidelines for selecting assistive aids are covered in Chapters 5 and 17. An example of adapted practice is working on gait in the parallel bars, with the intention of progressing to independent walking. Repeated practice trials in the parallel bars may increase skill in the parallel bars but teaches a different dynamic and coordination than what is needed for independent walking. Sometimes, safety and skill level require task adaptations. However, the therapist should reflect on the transfer of learning to the goal in the plan of care.

Part-task training is another practice adaptation. It is generally defined as practice on some component of the whole task as pretraining for performance of the whole task. The motor learning literature suggests using part-task training for complex skills when practicing the whole task is too difficult for the learner (Schmidt & Wrisberg, 2000). One common type of part-practice is segmentation, in which one part is practiced and then another part is added; finally, the parts are all practiced together. An example of segmentation is starting with practice of dribbling a basketball and then combining it with passing to a team member or shooting it into the hoop. The effectiveness of part-practice depends on the nature of the target skill and how intricately the component parts are related (Schmidt & Wrisberg, 2000). Part-practice is not effective if separating the components changes the way in which the individual parts are performed. For example, practicing the back swing component of a golf swing separately from the forward swing would change the dynamics of the forward swing, because the sequence of muscle activity and the momentum for the forward swing depend on continuity with the backward swing. Also, for part-task practice to be effective, it must transfer to the whole task learning. Part-practice is especially effective with tasks having many parts, such as most activities of daily living. Part-practice is most useful when the practiced component is a subaction or small whole contained within the functional complex task (Lee, 1988; Schmidt & Wrisberg, 2000; Winstein, Pohl, &

Lewthwaite, 1994). This principle was demonstrated in a study by Winstein and colleagues (1994) that examined the effects of part-practice, which focused on shifting weight in standing onto the leg affected by a stroke. These adult subjects demonstrated improved weight shifting in standing with feet in line after part-practice, but there was no improvement in functional gait measures. In this case, the lateral weight shift was not a naturally occurring unit of the task of walking, which involves more forward shift of the center of mass. Part-task training may be required when children show sequencing deficits or difficulty with components of movement critical to performance of the task.

Guideline No. 6: Schedule Practice to Enhance Retention and Transfer

The motor learning literature provides research on two practice variables that apply here: **variable versus specific practice** and **random versus blocked practice**. According to motor programming theory, variable practice is important for enhancing the parameters of the motor program, which improves generalization of motor skills. It may also increase stability of the coordination strategy, across environmental and task changes, from a dynamic systems perspective. The advantages of variable practice in typically developing children have been demonstrated (Wulf, 1991) with an experimental task. The effects of variable practice have not been studied specifically in children with neurological physical impairments, but our clinical observation of the difficulty that some children have with transfer of skills to new situations may support this as a practice strategy.

When two or more tasks are performed in a practice session, they can be scheduled in a drill-like fashion where each variation is practiced until it is achieved. This is called *blocked practice*. Random practice involves practice of all of the variations in a random order. Research with adult subjects shows a very robust effect for random practice because random practice encourages more active processing that makes a more well-developed memory representation. However, the effect for children is somewhat equivocal. The decision to schedule practice according to a blocked or random fashion may relate to the characteristics of the task and the child learner. Taylor (1999) conducted a pilot study to evaluate the relative effects of blocked versus random practice on the learning of three variations of crutch tasks by 7-year-olds with no disability. The advantage of random practice was not demonstrated. The multiple effects of the child's learning style, the degree of difficulty of the task variations, and prior experience were noted. A combination

of blocked practice early on until the learner gets the basic idea of the movement, followed by random practice later has been suggested to be optimal for children for variations of certain tasks (Gentile, 1987, 1992; Pigott & Shapiro, 1984). It is possible that the increased trial-to-trial variability in children with neurological diagnoses may increase the requirement for blocked practice. Furthermore, the complexity of the movement may prolong the early stage of practice. Issues of memory and attention should also be considered. For some children, random practice may enhance learning because it reduces the boredom associated with drill practice of one task.

Planning Activity-Focused Interventions: Environment

The **environment-related interventions** will be discussed in terms of the **physical environment,** the **psychosocial environment,** and the **performance environment.** The performance environment involves the augmented information provided by the change agent.

Guideline No. 7: Adapt the Physical Environment to Support Desired Motor Behaviors

The physical environment includes objects (including assistive technology) and persons in the environment, as well as sensory features of the environment. Perception-action theory (Adolph, Eppler, & Gibson, 1993; Gibson, 1979), which has been integrated into dynamic systems approaches, stresses that the movement behaviors that emerge during activity are intricately tied to the features of environment, with reference to the physical characteristics and the movement capabilities of the child. This perception/action match is typified by the tendency of adults to select a strategy for executing a stairway, based on the ratio of the stair riser height to the leg length (Warren, 1984) and extensor strength in the legs (Konczak, 1990). There is some evidence that infants and young children also perceive actions according to their own movement capabilities. This concept is illustrated in Figure 7–7. The young boy, at 2 years of age, is challenged by the action goal of ascending the stairs. A four-point movement solution naturally emerged when the stair riser was high relative to his size and movement capabilities. The two-point solution (upright) naturally emerged when the riser height relative to his leg length decreased. Note that he instinctively sought assistance to descend the stairs because the task and the

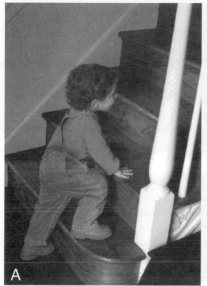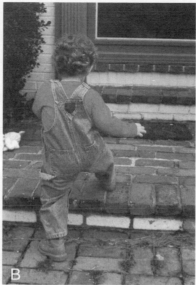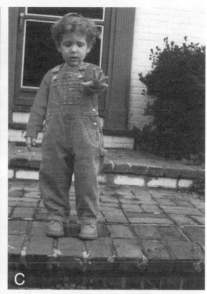

Figure 7-7 Variations of stair tasks by a 2-year-old boy with typical development, influenced by the features of the environment relative to his movement capabilities. (*A*) Four-point movement for high step; (*B*) two-point solution when riser height is reduced; and (*C*) seeking assistance to descend step.

environmental features did not match his perceived motor capabilities. Objects in the environment that provide opportunities for movement are called **affordances.** As we adapt tasks and the environment for therapeutic practice, we should evaluate the affordances available to the child for movement. The affordances, such as the steps in this case, can be control parameters or constraints that affect action.

For children with neurological impairments, sensory stimuli in the environment can influence the learning experience, especially if selective attention is impaired. Children who have difficulty with automatic performance of one task may find it difficult to perform when competing tasks or events are present. The physical environment is especially important for infants and children for whom sensory inputs can be disorganizing. Children with DCD may have associated sensory integration disorders. Factors such as ambient temperature, lighting, noise level, or even odors can significantly affect the ability to selectively attend to and participate in practice activities. The physical environment might be modified to reduce fear and increase security for the child. Knowing the child's special needs will help to maximize the sensory aspects of the physical environment.

Other features of the physical environment include equipment and the floor surface for locomotor activities. Therapeutic equipment, such as balls and bolsters, is often used during practice to support the emergence of a certain

movement skill. The physical therapist might use the movable surface of an exercise ball to elicit transition from prone to sit. The buoyancy of the water is an environmental adaptation that enhances motor behavior in aquatic therapy.

The success of activity-oriented behaviors is often dependent on appropriate use of adapted equipment. McEwen (1992) suggests that adaptive equipment could be a constraint (a control parameter) on the social interactions that a child performs in the classroom. Children perform better when they feel comfortable and secure in their environment. They do poorly when they perceive a threat to balance or posture, such as sitting in a chair, which is not optimal. Well-planned seating and mobility aids are "enabling technology" that enhance function (Wilson Howle, 1999). Adapted seats, sidelyers, and supportive standers can also improve participation in classroom and home. The issues relating to adaptive equipment are discussed in Chapter 16.

Guideline No. 8: Conduct Practice in the Functional Environment When Practical

There is evidence that optimal learning for children with neurological impairments occurs in the functional environment (Karnish, Bruder, & Rainforth, 1995). The natural environment provides constant opportunities for motor learning. Therefore it is the role of the change agent not only to teach motor activities but also to help families and classrooms to create environments that support and promote opportunities for learning and teach the family motor learning strategies that will support learning in the children. This is especially the case for children with cognitive limitations, for whom transfer from the clinical to natural environment is difficult (McEwen, 2000).

Guideline No. 9: Consider the Influence of the Psychosocial Environment

Therapists should support the psychosocial environment through sound family-centered practice and integration of physical therapy into the classroom and the community. This aspect of intervention is a critical element of current models of intervention. Strategies for supporting the family are elaborated in Chapter 3 and throughout the text. Strategies for early intervention are discussed in Chapter 10; for the classroom, in Chapter 11; and for other settings, in Chapters 12 to 15. The psychological environment in the intervention session is also critical to success, because of the motivational aspects of learning. The therapist should be in tune with the child's needs and flexibly adapt practice. Children should be given choices and participate in decision making (Larin, 2000).

Guideline No. 10: Thoughtfully Provide Augmented Information

The performance environment refers to the augmented information provided during the learning situation. Recall that augmented information involves information provided by an external source to complement the intrinsic information available to the learner through problem solving and performance of the task. According to the dynamic systems perspective, the change agent provides augmented information to guide the child's search for a coordination that will enable the functional action to be achieved. The change agent can dramatically affect the outcome of practice by carefully choosing and executing augmented information.

Recall that there are many sources of augmented information besides feedback. Although much of the literature focuses on feedback, in terms of the opportunities for augmented information, the options are numerous. The planning of augmented information involves three dimensions: the type of augmented information characterized by the mode of presentation, the content, and the timing. It is difficult to give hard and fast rules regarding augmented information during therapeutic practice because of the lack of empirical data. Theoretically, it is important to integrate the augmented information with modifications of the task and the environment and how they interact with the special learning needs of the child.

Knowledge of Results and Knowledge of Performance. **Knowledge of results** provides information about how well the outcome of the child's practice trial met the task goal (Schmidt & Wrisberg, 2000). Consider the child's developmental level, in terms of how much time the child needs to process the information and the complexity of the information. This would be especially pertinent for children with cognitive delays or impaired information processing. The requirement for feedback should be evaluated for each child, relative to the task that is practiced. Verbal feedback is often critical in adult motor learning studies, in which the goal is to improve accuracy or timing of a simple experimental task and the increments of change are not perceptible by the learner (Magill, 1992; Salmoni, Schmidt, & Walter, 1984). However, in the clinical environment, the outcome of a practice trial for many tasks (such as throwing a bean bag into a box) may be obvious to the child, making knowledge of results redundant and not necessary. On the other hand, for certain tasks, impaired proprioceptive or visual integration may increase the requirement for feedback about the outcome of the movement.

Knowledge of performance provides feedback information about the movement patterns that the child uses to perform movements. Intuitively, this would seem to be more valuable in teaching children with physical impairments. However, there is some evidence that the verbal information associated with feedback about patterns of movement may be difficult for some children with neurological deficits to process as they try to perform difficult movements (Thorpe & Valvano, 2002). A more external focus toward the task goal in the environment may be more appropriate (Thorpe et al., 2003) because, according to current models, motor control emerges in the context of functional activity.

Because children with neurological impairments may have difficulty with developing a plan of action, it may be more practical to provide cues about what to do on future trials to improve performance, based on prior performance (Kernodle & Carlton, 1992; Newell & Valvano, 1998). These cues may be especially important when the task is unfamiliar to the child and when the child must develop a new pattern of coordination to achieve the functional activity goal.

Cognitive Strategies. Another form of verbal support provided by the change agent that has been studied in children with CP is the reminder to use cognitive strategies. Cognitive strategies are learning tools or techniques that facilitate learning by addressing cognitive systems, such as attention and memory. They are tools that help the learner to organize, store, or retrieve information (Alley & Deshler, 1979). Examples of cognitive strategies are mental rehearsal of the movement, use of labels to enhance memory, use of rhymes or rhythms to remember a sequence, and strategies for comparing one trial with another for accuracy. Although children with typical development usually develop these cognitive strategies intuitively and use them to aid performance (David, 1985), children with learning disabilities or mental retardation often do not use cognitive strategies to improve memory during practice of a motor skill. There is some evidence that helping children to use strategies improves their learning (Dawson, Hallahan, Reeve, & Ball, 1980; Horgan, 1985). For children with neurological diagnoses, teaching them to mentally rehearse the skill might enhance skill acquisition (Thorpe & Valvano, 2002). Using imagery may also help some children with neurological impairments learn a motor skill more efficiently (Thorpe & Valvano, 2002).

Demonstration and Modeling. Augmented information provided through the visual mode is effective for young children, who rely heavily on the sense of vision (Shumway-Cook & Woollacott, 1985). Some children, like those with Down syndrome, demonstrate relatively less skill with verbal processing than visual processing (Iarocci & Burack, 1998). Modeling of the motor task, from a video or live model, can enhance motor learning and self-confidence in children (Larin, 2000). When providing live or video demonstrations, it is advisable to cue the child to the features of the movement to which they should attend (Kernodle & Carlton, 1992). There has not been any study of live or video demonstrations in children with neurological impairments, but the effects of video demonstration would be easy for therapists to examine.

Physical Guidance. An important mode for providing augmented information for the physical therapist is **physical guidance**. Physical guidance provides a general "feel" of the movement that will achieve a function (Wulf, Shea, & Whitacre, 1998). These physical cues are similar to those provided by a coach in guiding a golf swing or a gymnastic maneuver. Facilitation techniques from the neurodevelopmental treatment (NDT) approach, provide physical

guidance because they give information about the target movement pattern; they also have therapeutic goals such as muscle elongation, joint stability, and increased ROM (Bly & Whiteside, 1997; Bobath & Bobath, 1984). From a motor learning perspective, the informational properties of the guidance are emphasized.

In a series of single-case studies, physical guidance was found to be beneficial in the early phases of learning a novel, complex motor skill by children with CP for whom the task presented a reasonable challenge. After getting the general idea of the movement, these children continued to improve performance, even when the guidance was withdrawn (Valvano, Heriza, & Carollo, 2002). Furthermore, kinematic analysis provides preliminary evidence that the physical guidance encouraged the development of task-specific patterns of movement required to perform the task. Physical guidance, for some children, can be beneficial in the early phases of practice because it is difficult for the child with neurological impairments to develop a coordination plan.

Physical guidance may save effort and frustration in the early phase of learning for children with special needs. However, physical guidance should not be given on every trial and should be phased out or withdrawn after the child gets the general idea of the movement solution. Then, the child should be given the opportunity to problem solve and self-correct as he or she refines the movement strategy.

When teaching a motor skill, it is advisable to determine, for the individual child, the amount and type of information that will be useful for error detection and skill development. The amount of information should not allow the child to become overly dependent on it, which would limit the active processing important for learning. Children develop a reference for correctness through active exploration and trial and error. Discovery learning is associated with better retention than learning that is heavily guided in typical children.

The requirement for guidance may be increased for children with neurological impairments, who may require increased guidance, especially early in practice, to help develop a "feel for the goal movement" to achieve a task goal. Furthermore, it has been demonstrated that the complexity of a gross motor skill affects the requirement for augmented information. Wulf, Shea, and Matschiner (1998) demonstrated an advantage of high-frequency augmented feedback for adults practicing a complex ski slalom task. The need for augmented information may be increased for children with neurological impairments, especially in the early phases of learning, because of greatly increased inter-trial variability and the limited repertoire of movement patterns they may bring to the learning situation. The responsible clinician, therefore, should monitor the effects of augmented information and be sensitive to the learning style and personal characteristics of the learners engaging in therapeutic practice.

Guideline No. 11: Apply Behavioral Strategies for Children Unable to Benefit From Verbally Mediated Guidance and Feedback

The type of feedback, instruction, and guidance provided depends on the nature of the learning required for the skill. During explicit learning, the performer is aware of goals and features of the task critical for performance. In implicit learning, the focus is on specific aspects of performance, not on the rules or verbally mediated instruction. Implicit learning is not passive or unconscious. The learner attends to the task that is practiced, but the rules are not consciously attended to (Schmidt & Wrisberg, 2000). There may be a combination of implicit and explicit learning in all motor skills.

For children with mental retardation, learning may depend more on visual cues and repetition (McEwen, 2000). For some children, especially those with behavior disorders or TBI, **behavioral programming**, commonly referred to as *applied behavior analysis*, is an appropriate methodology to assist in achieving goals. Learning is believed to occur as a result of the consequences of behavior. Behavioral programming emphasizes manipulation of the environment through the use of positive reinforcement of desired behaviors and ignoring unwanted behaviors. Concepts about behavioral programming are discussed in Chapter 1.

Integrating Impairment-Focused Interventions With Activity-Focused Interventions

One way to individualize practice is to adapt task and environment to meet the special learning needs associated with impairments of body structures and functions. According to the model in Figure 7–5, focus on the characteristics of the child also involves integration of impairment-level interventions with the activity-focused interventions. According to P. Campbell (1991) and Heriza and Sweeney (1994), problem solving about impairments of body function and structures begins after the specified functional goals are established. Impairment-level interventions are

important, not only to support function but also to reduce the risk of secondary impairments. Impairments in body structures and functions associated with neurological diagnoses are numerous and have a unique expression in each child. Likewise, the interventions are numerous and should be individualized. According to Figure 7–5, impairment-focused interventions are divided into two major categories: active and passive.

Active Impairment-Focused Interventions That Involve Functional Activity

Active impairment-focused interventions attempt to ameliorate the effects of impairments, or limitations in body functions, through practice of a meaningful functional task or developmental activity. The theoretical support for addressing impairments in the context of activity is based on the assumption that motor control emerges in the context of purposeful activity. In these cases, the benefits of practicing the activity are twofold: improved performance of the functional activity and amelioration of impairments. The impairment-focused activity may be the target activity specified in the goal, or an alternate activity that addresses the impairment. Figures 7–6 and 7–8 demonstrate how impairments in neurological systems can be addressed in the context of functional play activities. Activities shown in Figure 7–6 focus on functional gains in stair skills, and also address impairments in force generation and selective control, which limit task-specific components of movement. Figure 7–8 depicts functional play activities enjoyed by Joey, a kindergarten student who demonstrates a pattern of increased flexion associated with hypertonicity in the right upper extremity. These impairments, which limit supporting on the hand and functional reach and grasp, are addressed in these activities.

The therapist should evaluate transfer of impairment-level gains to the target activity. Dichter, DeCicco, Flanagan, Hyun, and Mongrain (2001) demonstrated that play activities by children with Down syndrome geared toward impairments in balance, visual motor control, and strength did transfer to functional tasks for Special Olympics competition. In terms of impairments in strength, physical education programs, adapted swimming, modified aerobics, and dancing (including wheelchair dancing) are all activities that are helpful in increasing strength, as well as stamina and endurance (Eckersley & King, 1993).

Activities directed toward impairments in body functions and structures can be enhanced by motor learning strategies described previously in this chapter. A commonly

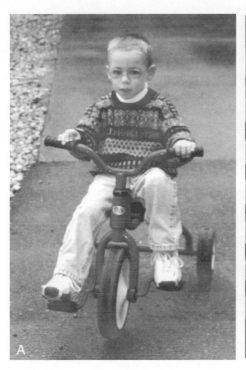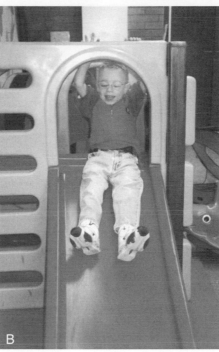

Figure 7-8 Functional activities that address impairments associated with flexor hypertonicity in the right upper extremity of a kindergarten student. *(A)* Riding tricycle. *(B)* Sliding down sliding board.

used strategy is physical guidance. In Figure 7–6A, the therapist provides physical guidance that is intended to give the young learner the "feel" of supporting himself on one leg and advancing with the other. The therapist constantly evaluates and modifies the nature of the physical guidance. On subsequent trials, the therapist might provide physical guidance more proximally, to address trunk and pelvis postures. On subsequent trials, the therapist might complement the physical guidance with verbal cues about the position of Katey's hands on the railings. Figure 7–9A depicts the use of physical guidance by Joey's physical therapist in the early phase of practice of a stepping task. The guidance gives him a "feel" for the flat foot placement and the advancement of the tibia over the right foot, which are limited by hypoextensible plantar flexor muscles and reduced selective control of lower extremity muscles. This reduction in impairments eventually carries over into performance of a stepping task in the context of play (Figure 7–9B).

Activities that address impairments can also be enhanced by therapeutic adaptations. These adaptations might include assistive technology or mechanical aids used to enhance the performance of the activity. These include application of tone-inhibiting casts, which are used as adjuncts to therapy to stabilize the foot and improve the alignment, and ankle foot orthoses to provide support (Knutson & Clark, 1991) and perhaps reduce energy expenditure in gait (Mossberg, Linton, & Friske, 1990).

Modifications of the task or environment also address impairments of body structure and function during activity. In aquatic therapy, the purposeful activities performed by children in the water might address impairments such as increased stiffness and weakness. The aquatic environment provides weight relief to the body, warmth, buoyancy, antigravity positioning, and increased resistance. This medium allows greater ease of movement, relaxation of spastic muscles, and strengthening (Dumas & Francesconi, 2002). There is no systematic line of evidence for the effectiveness of aquatic therapy, but empirical evidence of improvement, mostly case studies, is emerging.

Hippotherapy is an example of purposeful activity by the child, in which the task and environment are directed to reduce limitations in posture, balance, and mobility. While riding the horse, the child practices active postural and balance strategies under functional, motivating, and changing environmental conditions. There is evidence that facilitation of movement components in the context of hippotherapy is efficacious for children with CP. Gains in strength and postural control have been demonstrated, along with reduced energy expenditure during gait and

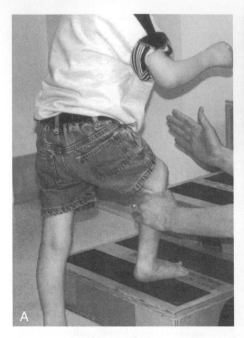
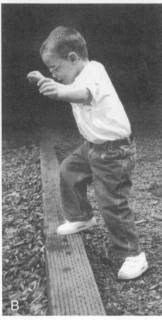

Figure 7-9 (*A*) Use of physical guidance during practice of a stepping task performed by a child with cerebral palsy, addressing impairments in lower extremity tone and selective control. (*B*) Carryover of impairment-level gains to a stepping task in the play environment.

improved scores on the Gross Motor Function Measure (McGibbon, Andrade, Widener, & Cintas, 1998). Favorable effects have also been documented for therapeutic horseback riding, which focuses more on gains in the recreational aspects of the riding. These gains may represent the importance of meaningful activity for children. The review by MacKinnon, Noh, Laliberte, Lariviere, and Allan (1995) identifies favorable effects of therapeutic riding for children with CP, learning disability (LD), mental retardation, and language disorders.

Walking on a treadmill is an activity that adapts the task and environment to work on goals of increased functional mobility (Schindl, Forstner, Kern, & Hesse, 2000). The treadmill adapts the task by providing support for weight bearing and guiding the timing and direction of the steps.

Functional electrical stimulation (FES), also called neuromuscular electrical stimulation (NMES), is an impairment-level intervention that is provided in the context of functional activity. It complements active practice by addressing limitations in production, selective control, and timing of muscle activity. NMES theoretically increases strength and enhances motor reeducation during the performance of gait and other functional activities. In most cases, an electrical current is delivered to the skin with a portable battery-operated device. A particular muscle or group of muscles is stimulated as the child actively performs functional movement (e.g., gait or reaching). The timing of the stimulation provides a sensory cue and assists the

muscle activation patterns that will help to achieve the goal. The efficacy of NMES is supported by a series of case studies by Carmick (1995, 1997) and the work of Commeaux, Patterson, Rubin, and Meiner (1997). Bertoti et al. (1997) reported gains in ambulation and other functional tasks with a variation of NMES, percutaneous intramuscular functional electrical stimulation, in two case studies involving young children with spastic diplegia. Kerr, McDowell, and McDonough (2004) have completed a current review of the evidence on NMES. One precaution with NMES is a history of seizures, because some systemic absorption of the electric current might occur (Reed, 1997).

Biofeedback has also been used to improve muscle activation, selective control, and timing in the context of functional tasks. With biofeedback, the motor output is displayed to reflect muscle activity measured by electromyography or force production. A visual or auditory signal helps to focus attention to the motor response and supplement that with information not naturally available to the learner. Augmented biofeedback can be effective in increasing head and neck posture, reducing hytertonia, improving weight bearing, and reducing drooling. However, carryover without feedback is limited. Furthermore, generalization of muscle control or components of movement to real-life tasks has not been consistent (Bertoti & Gross, 1988; Floodmark, 1986; Seeger, Caudrey, & Scholes, 1981).

Active Impairment-Focused Interventions That Involve Therapeutic Activity

Resistive exercise with free weights or isokinetic devices by children is an example of therapeutic activity focused on impairments in body functions and structures, rather than a functional task or developmental play activity. Resistive exercise addresses force production deficits. In recent years, considerable evidence has been put forth in support of resistive exercise for increasing strength in children with CP. In the past, vigorous strengthening was considered contraindicated in children who demonstrated increased tone because of the fear that resistive work would increase spasticity in children with CP. In fact, over the past few years, there have been many studies that have demonstrated major gains in strength and function without detrimental effects on spasticity (Darrah, 1997, Damiano & Abel, 1998; Damiano, Dodd, & Taylor, 2002). O'Connell and Barnhart (1995) reported gains associated with resistive exercise in subjects with spasticity as well as subjects with MM. It is important that the effects of strengthening programs be investigated in children who demonstrate functional weakness associated with hypotonia, such as children with Down syndrome (Dichter, 1994; Mercer & Lewis, 2001).

Proprioceptive neuromuscular facilitation (PNF) (Eckersley & King, 1993) is an alternative to traditional resistive strengthening with weights that has been applied to children with neurological impairments. This technique integrates neural concepts into strengthening activities. The premise is that muscle actions are more efficient when working in patterns in which movements are diagonal and rotational and when the movement goes from distal to proximal. The active movements in PNF are guided by the physical therapist. Hand placement is carefully planned to provide an appropriate level of resistance, guidance, or sensory feedback. Stretch and traction make use of the elastic properties of the muscle. Verbal prompts serve a motivating function. The efficacy of PNF has not been studied systematically in children with neurological impairments. Eckersley and King (1993) reports her clinical impression of increased strength after using PNF in children with MM.

Passive Impairment-Focused Interventions That Do Not Involve Purposeful Activity

Passive procedures do not involve active participation in purposeful activity on the part of the child. They might be grouped into (1) procedures directed toward the impairment of body function or structures, not administered in the context of a purposeful task or activity, and (2) passive procedures that are preparatory to or administered during a purposeful task or activity. Passive procedures are usually directed toward musculoskeletal limitations associated with abnormal muscle tone findings and are not administered in the context of a purposeful task. Included in this category are interventions directed toward reducing joint limitations or soft tissue contractures. Examples are passive ROM exercises or application of night splints. We intuitively incorporate passive ROM exercises to maintain or increase flexibility. However, there is limited evidence to guide this intervention (Cadenhead, McEwen, & Thompson, 2002; Harris, 1990). Two studies reported only limited advantages of passive ROM exercises (McPherson, Arends, Michaels, & Trettin, 1984; Miedaner & Renander, 1987). Miedaner and Renander (1987) demonstrated an advantage of passive ROM provided twice weekly compared with lower frequency. However, there were limitations to the design of this study, which lacked a control group. Fragala, Goodgold, and Dumas (2003) suggest that the effects of passive ROM exercises vary and may depend on many factors, including child-related factors (growth, underlying motor control, and capability for active movement) and external factors (frequency of passive exercise, positioning, and use of orthoses). They propose that the evidence favors prolonged stretching over brief and intermittent passive stretching. The findings of a study by Tardieu, Lespargot, Tabary, and Bret (1988) demonstrate that to prevent contracture of the soleus muscles for children with CP, prolonged stretch for several hours per day is necessary. In their study, the effects of stretch on contractures were not apparent in those for whom the muscle was elongated 2 hours per day. There was a positive effect on muscles elongated for at least 6 hours per day. Sustained stretch through serial casting or splinting is a method of applying sustained stretch to a muscle. The effects may be enhanced by botulinum toxin A injections, which effect a transient chemical denervation by disturbing the actions of acetylcholine at the neuromuscular junction (Booth, Yates, Edgar & Bandy, 2003).

The findings of Tardieu et al. (1988) support the use of splints and casts (Phillips & Audet, 1990) for prolonged stretch. For children with TBI, splints and serial casting are commonly used to effect a prolonged static stretch (Blaskey & Jennings, 1999; Conine, Sullivan, Mackie, & Goodman, 1990). Limitations in ROM are also addressed by positioning devices such as standing frames (Gudjonsdottir & Stemmons-Mercer, 2002; Stuberg, 1992). Use of a sidelyer or seating devices also provides some passive input to preserve biomechanical integrity (McEwen, 1992).

Manual therapy techniques, including soft tissue mobilization, joint mobilization, massage, and myofascial release, are procedures administered to reduce biomechanical or musculoskeletal impairments. The use of these manual techniques should be guarded, with consideration of developmental factors and risks of injury and fracture (Harris & Lundgren, 1991).

Subthreshold transcutaneous electrical stimulation, another example of a passive procedure, is a variation of electrical stimulation in which the stimulation is delivered during sleeping hours, with intensity below the threshold required to generate a muscular contraction. The objective is to increase blood flow during sleep to promote muscle development (Pape et al., 1993). Pape et al. (1993) concluded in a pilot, single-subject study using electrical stimulation during sleep that there was differential growth of atrophic nonspastic antagonist muscles, thereby reducing the muscle imbalance typical of CP. This intervention addresses the impairment of functional weakness associated with CP. Although there is enthusiastic support for this approach among clinicians and parents of children with CP, there is limited evidence of its efficacy in the literature.

Passive Interventions That Are Preparatory to Purposeful Activity

The second group of passive procedures includes **preparatory procedures** performed by the therapist to create a more optimal readiness for a motor learning experience. Activities that provide tactile, vestibular, or proprioceptive input in a playful manner might be used before functional activity, to regulate sensory reactivity and improve behavioral organization (Miller & Summers, 2001). The effectiveness of these preparatory procedures has not been studied systematically.

Procedures to reduce soft tissue findings associated with symptoms of spasticity are often used by physical therapists. Imbalance of muscle activity often results in increased tension, with shortening in connective tissue, in the relatively active muscles compared with the opposing muscle groups. Preparatory procedures tend to elongate or increase mobility of the affected muscle groups. These theoretically make movement easier and improve the efficiency and quality of movement (Boehme, 1988). Many of these procedures are from the NDT perspective.

According to current models of intervention, the therapist should not create a long-term dependence on these passive procedures. The important question is, Will the child be able to perform the task in the natural environment when the preparatory passive procedures are not available? The need for these procedures should be evaluated on a case-by-case basis. For Katey, the kindergarten student in Figure 7–6, elongation of the ankle plantar flexors is a passive procedure that could prepare her for better active movement of the tibia over the foot during the task of ascending stairs. Figure 7–10A depicts a preparatory activity provided to increase flexibility in the hand before a functional play activity (Figure 7–10B).

Established Approaches to Intervention

Established approaches to intervention, which have traditionally focused on reducing impairments to achieve function, serve as a resource to physical therapists conducting

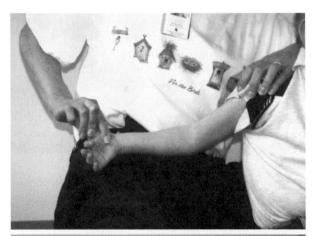

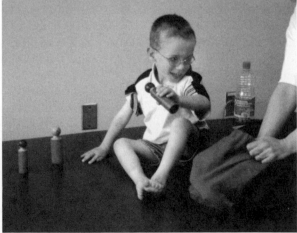

Figure 7-10 (*A*) Preparatory Passive procedure. (*B*) Functional play activity by a boy with cerebral palsy.

therapeutic practice. The established approaches are reviewed in the following section.

Neurodevelopmental Treatment

The **neurodevelopmental treatment** (NDT) approach, also known as the Bobath approach, has had an enormous impact on the intervention of children with neurological impairments. It was introduced in the 1940s and 1950s by Berta and Karl Bobath when approaches to neurological impairments focused primarily on peripheral methods, such as individual muscle strengthening, stretching, and muscle reeducation. Through the years, NDT has been an empirical approach of management techniques and procedures developed by the insights and clinical experience of Berta Bobath and other master clinicians. There have been many advances in the interpretation of the nervous system and the nature of the CP disorder since NDT began, and the theoretical basis for these intervention strategies has evolved. Currently the NDT framework is being refined to include new concepts from movement science (Bly, 1991; Heriza & Sweeney, 1995).

A review of some major concepts from the traditional NDT framework provides a perspective on the issues that have been updated to meet current concepts of neuroscience and motor control. The central concept of traditional NDT theory is the normal postural reflex mechanism. Three components of the normal postural reflex mechanism are considered to be necessary for normal movement: (1) normal postural tone, (2) intact reciprocal innervations (or synergistic interaction of agonist and antagonist for appropriate postural fixation), and (3) normal patterns of coordination, such as automatic postural adjustments necessary to perform functional movement. One of the basic tenets of NDT, derived from the concept of the normal postural reflex mechanism, is the fundamental relationship between muscle tone and movement, and the impact of deviations in muscle tone on functional tasks.

Another central theme of NDT, which persists today, is that motor function can be improved by reducing the impact of spasticity and abnormal movement patterns. Spasticity was thought to be associated with abnormal reflexes in lower levels of control, and the normal movement components, such as righting and equilibrium reactions, were thought to be integrated at higher centers. Traditionally, the major roles of the therapist were to reduce the effects of abnormal tone and encourage the emergence of normal postural components, as a basis for normal movement. The output, or the movement response of the child, was directly related to the input or skillful handling by the therapist, which, if properly executed, would produce immediate positive changes during a treatment session. Although the ultimate goal was function, treatment techniques focused on reducing abnormal reflexes and abnormal tone and developing components of movement. The normal developmental sequence provided a framework for movement (Bobath & Bobath, 1984; Bryce, 1972; Valvano & Long, 1991).

Bly (1991) presented a thoughtful summary of theoretical changes in the NDT approach that are more compatible with the systems model of motor control and the task-oriented model of motor learning. She presents the following:

1. The construct of the normal postural reflex mechanism is no longer viable. The revised concept of postural tone in NDT is consistent with current models of the nervous system. For example, postural control is no longer considered to be reflex dependent, and the proactive as well as reactive aspects of postural control are recognized.

2. The role of sensation in movement is changed. The original feedback perspective on control (in which the motor output was linked directly with a specific sensory input) is replaced with an appreciation of the feedforward and feedback modes of control.

3. Although the skillful handling of the therapist in discouraging abnormal patterns of movement is still emphasized, there is also an emphasis on the active problem-solving processes by the child.

4. NDT still emphasizes components of normal movement, such as weight shift, elongation, and rotation, that translate into functional movements. However, the therapist is encouraged to "treat beyond the components of movement."

5. Atypical quality is no longer a deterrent to challenging children to try new movement experiences, because findings such as stiffness, which were considered problematic in the past, are normal for the early phases of learning new skills.

6. Good handling techniques and skill of the therapist are still essential in NDT.

Bly (1991) suggests that the skillful use of facilitation and inhibition techniques is valuable to "help inhibit abnormal movement components and facilitate normal components in the process of learning new motor programs."

This current model of NDT is compatible with the practice-oriented model presented in this chapter, because it uses procedures to address impairments in body functions and structures in the context of therapeutic practice. An NDT perspective includes adjunct interventions to manage symptoms of spasticity, such as orthoses, splints, and tone-inhibiting casts intended to maintain ROM and prevent deformity. NDT includes many preparatory interventions to reduce the effects of impairments in muscle tone and some soft tissue restrictions, to allow movement components to occur (Boehme, 1988; Nelson, 2001).

Facilitation and inhibition techniques address atypical muscle tone findings in the context of purposeful activity and provide physical guidance during the performance of activity. In facilitation techniques, the therapist places hands on specified parts of the child's body to help align body segments and to initiate and guide or prevent movement. Facilitation techniques may help with differentiation of movement or with the performance of difficult movement patterns. Current guidelines for the application of facilitation techniques are presented in great detail in a book by Bly and Whiteside (1997). They define facilitation as "hands-on" activities that give direction in how to move. This requires skill by the therapist in terms of body position, placement of hands, pressure, timing, and smoothness of the facilitation technique. They propose that facilitation techniques encourage the development of movement components that will generalize into functional activity. However, motor learning theory does not predict this automatic transfer.

Facilitation techniques go hand-in-hand with inhibition techniques. Inhibition techniques suppress abnormal patterns of movement (Boehme, 1988). Facilitation and inhibition techniques theoretically permit the feeling of normal movement. These techniques involve specific sensory inputs associated with the therapist's hand contact as he or she guides the child's movement. By inhibiting dysfunctional movement, abnormal muscle tone, and abnormal patterns, the therapist is thought to provide the opportunity for more efficient movement adaptations (Boehme, 1988). Other sensory inputs used to affect postural tone include deep pressure, joint traction, joint compression, weight bearing, and tapping. The therapist should be cautious of creating a dependence on these assistive therapeutic techniques and should always focus on independent functioning in the natural environment.

Despite the popularity of the NDT approach, and the ubiquitous use of practical handling principles derived from the approach, there is very little formal evidence of its efficacy. Much of the support for NDT is derived from parents' and clinicians' perceptions of efficacy (DeGangi & Royeen, 1994). A review sponsored by the American Academy of Cerebral Palsy and Developmental Medicine examined the evidence for NDT and concluded that the preponderance of results did not confer any advantage to NDT over the alternatives with which it was compared (Butler & Darrah, 2001). I recommend that the reader review this document and the individual studies. The authors recommend additional research, with operationally defined treatment techniques, clearly defined outcome measures, and samples large enough for adequate power.

Research on the efficacy of NDT presents many challenges, including the fact that there are no standard treatments delivered in a standardized manner, the skill levels and aims of therapists vary, and family influences are difficult to standardize (Butler & Darrah, 2001). Furthermore, NDT strategies are commonly combined with other therapy techniques, medical treatments, and motor learning strategies (Bly, 1991). These combined strategies must be evaluated separately from the hands-on therapeutic procedures historically associated with NDT.

Sensorimotor Approach

The sensorimotor approach is another facilitation approach, less well known than NDT. Certain concepts from this framework are still in use, and activities from this framework are often used in combination with NDT (Harris, 1990; Heriza & Sweeney, 1995). The sensorimotor approach was developed by Margaret Rood, who relied very heavily on a neuroanatomical basis for the treatment. She outlined four stages of development of motor control as a basis for normal movement: (1) reciprocal innervation (which involves flexion and extension patterns), (2) co-contraction, (3) stability superimposed on mobility (when there is movement of a segment over a distal stability point, such as the weight-bearing phase in walking and creeping), and (4) mobility superimposed on stability (which involves free distal part moving on a stabilizing proximal part, such as reaching to grasp an object). The final component, in which phasic movement of a segment such as the arm in reach or the leg in stepping is stabilized by tonic contraction of the trunk and limb girdles, represents the high level of control required for advanced movement. These stages of development of motor control occur in key patterns of posture and movement: supine flexion, prone extension (pivot prone), prone on elbows, prone on hands, all fours, semisquat, and walking. Trends in development, such as proximal-to-distal and cephalocaudal, are emphasized in the approach (Stockmeyer, 1972). This approach is obviously based on a hierarchical model of motor control and assumes that lesions in the CNS result in lack of higher-level control over movements. Although the rigid adherence to the developmental progression emphasized in the approach is not consistent with current models of motor control and motor learning, therapists may find the categories of movement, such as mobility superimposed on stability, useful in planning activities for children with impairments in strength or postural control.

Rood also formulated treatment techniques using specific sensory stimuli to elicit desired movement and postural responses on an automatic level. These stimulation techniques include icing and brushing, which are mediated through the tactile system; and stretch, resistance, vibration, pressure, and joint compression, which are mediated through the proprioceptive sense (Eckersley & King, 1993; Harris, 1990). These passive procedures may be useful for children with severe involvement who have limited ability for active movement. On the other hand, the safety of passive stimulation of a compromised nervous system must be monitored carefully. There has been no systematic study of the effectiveness of this intervention approach.

Sensory Integration Approach

Sensory integration (SI) theory and therapy were developed by A. Jean Ayres (1972) in the 1960s to address the sensory processing and the motor and perceptual impairments of children with learning disabilities. According to SI theory, learning is dependent on the ability to take in sensory information derived from the environment and from movement of the body, process and integrate these sensory inputs within the CNS, and use this information to plan and produce organized behavior. Sensory systems, including tactile, proprioceptive, and vestibular systems, contribute to the development of muscle tone, automatic reactions, and emotional well-being (Ayres, 1972, 1979; Spitzer & Roley, 2001). Children who have deficits in processing and integrating sensory inputs are likely to develop deficits in planning and producing motor behaviors. The SI treatment perspective provides guidelines for activity that organizes behavior, elicits adaptive responses, and improves sensory modulation (Bundy, Lane, Murray, & Fisher, 2002; Spitzer & Roley, 2001; Parham & Mailloux, 1996).

SI is most well known as an intervention strategy for children with mild motor involvement as might be seen in children with DCD and LD. However, therapists apply interventions from an SI approach to children with multiple neurological impairments, including mental retardation, CP, premature birth, and fragile X syndrome. There are reports of the effectiveness of a program of SI in children with severe and profound cognitive delays (Lunnen, 1999; Montgomery & Richter, 1980; Norton, 1975). Roley, Blanche, and Schaaf (2001) have addressed the applications of SI to diverse populations.

SI interventions are ultimately directed toward better CNS organization. The interventions facilitate the child's ability to make adaptive responses to specific sensory stimulation (including tactile, vestibular, proprioceptive), while engaging in purposeful motor activity. This purposeful motor activity is essential to the intervention process. SI is directed not toward the mastery of specific tasks or skills but rather toward improving the brain's capacity to perceive, remember, and plan motor activity (Lunnen, 1999). SI therapy frequently uses activities that provide vestibular stimulation to influence balance, muscle tone, ocular-motor responses, movements against gravity, postural adjustments, and arousal or activity level. Suspended equipment, such as hammocks, tier swings, and trapeze bars, is often used to provide controlled vestibular challenges. Linear movement and low-to-ground vestibular activities are sometimes used with children who are hypersensitive to movement. Inputs, such as weight bearing, resistance, movement against gravity, traction, vibration, and weighted objects, are also used to encourage adaptive postural and movement responses.

SI is frequently used as an intervention for children having tactile defensiveness or abnormally increased sensitivity to tactile input. This hypersensitivity is a phenomenon of the tactile system that results in feelings of discomfort from certain types of tactile stimulation. Sensitivity to touch may be environmental (e.g., a child experiencing discomfort with equipment or clothing, such as socks) or people related (e.g., a child avoiding other children). Limited motor activity may render children with significant physical limitations unable to engage in normal sensory activities that tend to normalize sensory responses. Children with neuromuscular dysfunction, such as CP or TBI, may display tactile defensiveness by fisting hands and arching away from the stimulus. In some cases, tactile defensiveness may contribute to toe-walking. SI focuses on techniques, such the use of tactile deep-pressure and graded exposure to tactile stimuli in the context of adaptive play activities, to normalize responses to environmental tactile stimulation (DeGangi, 1990).

Evidence for the efficacy of SI for children with LD and DCD is equivocal. Critics of this approach argue that the use of behavioral or cognitive strategies in the context of actual functional tasks may be associated with better outcomes in terms of functional motor behaviors (David, 2000; Mandich, Polatajko, Missiuna, & Miller, 2001; Polatajko, Mandich, Miller, & Macnab, 2001).

Conductive Education

Another approach to serving children with CP and similar movement dysfunction is conductive education (CE). A Hungarian neurologist, Professor Andras Peto, developed this approach in the 1940s. CE is a holistic approach to development and education of children with neurological impairments. It is not a therapy system but a system of education that aims to teach children to be active and self-reliant participants in the world. Emphasis is on motivation, developing self-esteem, and emotional and cognitive growth along with motor function (Hari & Tillemans, 1984; Kozma & Balogh, 1995; Tatlow, 1993).

CE is an intensive, integrated curriculum that includes cognitive, motor, personal care, and communication learning in real-life contexts. Motor skills are integrated into everyday tasks. The close relationship between language and movement is recognized; therefore rhythmical intention, the use of conscious vocalization with repetitive, dynamic words or rhythmical song, is used before and during movement. Children must learn to prepare mentally for action. They learn to move their bodies, constantly transitioning from one position to the next. Basic wooden equipment, ladder frames, and slatted tables are used almost exclusively (Figure 7–11). Individuals trained in Hungary in this approach are called "conductors". They have been educated to meet a Hungarian personnel shortage for highly skilled special educators, physical therapists, occupational therapists, and speech-language pathologists. There is no evidence to suggest that CE is any more effective than special education and therapy, as practiced in most parts of the developed world, in meeting the developmental needs of children with CP (Bairstow, Cochrane, & Hur, 1993; Bochner, Center, Chapparo, & Donelly, 1999; Reddihough, King, Coleman, & Catanese, 1998; Stiller, Marcoux, & Olson, 2003). CE involved integrated therapeutic programs in the natural environment long before it was standard practice in the United States. In fact, today there is a remarkable similarity among CE and integrative, interdisciplinary, special education, and therapeutic interventions (Effgen, 2001; O'Shea, 2000). If therapists are doing interdisciplinary intervention with a functional focus, in natural environments using extensive repetition

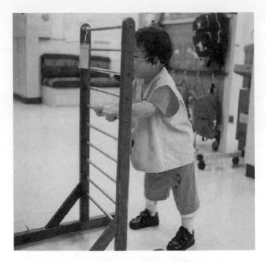

Figure 7-11 Child in Conductive Education Program using ladder frame for walking.

and practice for motor learning, they are doing CE, just perhaps without wooden equipment and singing. Recent research suggests that children with CP develop further under an intensive therapy program than when receiving CE or just special education (Stiller et al., 2003).

This approach focuses on active learning in the context of a functional environment. It emphasizes motor learning strategies such as observational learning from the group; cognitive strategies from rhymes and songs; and practice. The focus is not on impairment level interventions; there is the assumption that they will be ameliorated in the context of functional activity.

Tscharnuter Akademie for Movement Organization Approach

A relatively new approach to improving movement for children with neurological impairments is referred to as the Tscharnuter Akademie for Movement Organization (TAMO) approach (Tscharnuter, 1993, 2002). The approach, developed by Ingrid Tscharnuter, is based on concepts such as self-organization of complex systems from dynamic systems theory. Emphasis is placed on skillful handling by the physical therapist. This approach distinguishes itself from traditional models in that specific movement responses are not elicited through specific sensory input. Rather, the therapist sets up a movement challenge and guides the mover to gather information relevant to the task and initiate a movement response. The practitioner analyzes movement from the perspective of internal forces (neuromuscular forces produced by the child) and external or environmental forces, including gravity, ground reaction forces from the support, and inertia, which complement the internal forces. The child is guided to adapt and use the support surfaces optimally to hold postures and initiate movement.

The contact by the therapist effects a force vector that loads a body segment and encourages the child to activate movement from the support surface contact. These techniques encourage balance between stability and mobility, with a focus on using and integrating neuromuscular forces with forces of gravity and inertia. These techniques encourage adaptations or movement from a stable surface and are performed in the context of a task. Principles from the dynamic systems perspective, such as functional coupling between the child and the environment, and the natural process of picking up task-specific information for movement production, are stressed.

Summary

This chapter offered guiding principles for developing and applying the intervention plan for children with a range of neurological impairments causing limitations in body structures and functions and restrictions in activity and participation. It outlined the theoretical perspectives from which current motor learning principles are derived. An activity-focused model of intervention, based on concepts of change from a dynamic systems perspective, was introduced to structure the intervention of physical therapists. The model stresses practice of functional motor skills by children with neurological diagnoses. The reader is challenged to develop personal guidelines for best practice by reviewing the information presented in this chapter, investigating the evidence, and integrating personal experience and communication with other therapists and families of children with neurological impairments.

DISCUSSION QUESTIONS

1. How do cognitive aspects of motor learning (information processing, memory, and attention) contribute to the learning of functional motor activities by children with neurological impairments?

2. Discuss the role of the pediatric physical therapist as a "change agent" in the process of

promoting functional goals in the intervention plan of care.

3. Discuss three practical ways in which a physical therapist can intervene with task constraints to promote the acquisition and learning of functional motor skills.

4. Discuss three practical ways in which a physical therapist can intervene with environmental constraints to promote the acquisition of functional motor skills. Refer to the physical environment as well as the performance environment.

5. Impairments in multiple body systems affect motor learning. Describe a strategy for addressing impairments of body functions and structures in the context of an intervention plan that focuses on improving functional activity.

RECOMMENDED READINGS

Dynamic Systems Perspective

Heriza, C.B. (1991). Motor development: Traditional and contemporary theories. In Lister, M.J. (Ed.), *Contemporary management of motor control problems: Proceedings of the II STEP Conference* (pp. 99–126). Alexandria, VA: American Physical Therapy Association.

Scholz, J.P. (1990). Dynamic pattern theory—some implications for therapeutics. *Physical Therapy, 70,* 827–843.

Information-Processing Perspective

Light, K.E. (2003). Issues of cognition for motor control. (pp. 245–268). In P.C. Montgomery & B. H.Connolly (Eds.), *Cinical applications for motor control.* Thorofare, NJ: Slack.

Schmidt, R.A., & Wrisberg, C.A. (2000). *Motor performance and learning.* Champaign, IL: Human Kinetics.

Practice Variables

Duff, S., & Quinn, L. (2002). Motor learning and motor control. In D. Cech & S. Martin (Eds.), *Functional movement development across the life span* (2nd ed.) (pp. 86–117). Philadelphia: W.B. Saunders.

Gentile, A.M. (1992). The nature of skill acquisition: Therapeutic implications for children with movement disorders. In H. Forssberg & H. Hirschfeld (Eds.), *Movement disorders in children. Medical Sport Science, 36,* 31–40. Basel, Switzerland: Karger.

Larin, H. (2000). Motor learning: Theories and strategies for the practitioner. In S.K. Campbell, D.W. Vander Linden, & R.J. Palisano (Eds.), *Physical therapy for children* (2nd ed., pp. 170–195). Philadelphia: W.B. Saunders.

Schmidt, R.A., & Wrisberg, C.A. (2000). *Motor performance and learning.* Champaign, IL: Human Kinetics.

REFERENCES

Adams, M., Chandler, L., & Schulman, K. (2000). Gait changes in children with cerebral palsy following a neurodevelopmental treatment course. *Pediatric Physical Therapy, 12,* 114–120.

Adams, R.C., & Snyder, P. (1998). Treatments for cerebral palsy: Making choices of intervention from an expanding menu of options. *Infants and Young Children, 10,* 1–22.

Adolph, K., Eppler, M., & Gibson, E. (1993). Development of perception of affordances. In C. Rovee-Collier & L. Lipsitt (Eds.), *Advances in infancy research,* Vol. 8 (pp. 51–98). Norwood, NJ: Ablex Publishing.

Adolph, K.E., Vereijken, B., & Shrout, P.E. (2003). What changes in infant walking and why. *Child Development, 74,* 475–497.

Alberto, P.A., & Troutman, A.C. (2002). *Applied behavior analysis for teachers* (6th ed.). Englewood Cliffs, NJ: Merrill.

Alley, G.R., & Deshler, D.D. (1979). *Teaching the learning disabled adolescent: Strategies and methods.* Denver: Love Publishing.

American Physical Therapy Association (2001). *Guide to physical therapist practice* (2nd ed.). *Physical Therapy, 81,* 1–768.

Ayers, A.J. (1972). *Sensory integration and learning disorders.* Los Angeles: Western Psychological Services.

Ayers, A.J. (1979). *Sensory integration and the child.* Los Angeles: Western Psychological Services.

Bairstow, P., Cochrane, R., & Hur, J. (1993). *Evaluation of conductive education for children with cerebral palsy. Final report (Parts I and II).* London: Her Majesty's Stationery Office.

Barry, M.J. (1996). Physical therapy interventions for patients with movement disorders due to cerebral palsy. *Journal of Child Neurology, 11*(suppl. 1), S51–S60.

Bernstein, N. (1967). *The co-ordination and regulation of movements.* New York: Pergamon.

Bertoti, D.B. (1988). Effect of therapeutic horseback riding on posture in children with cerebral palsy. *Physical Therapy, 68,* 1505–1512.

Bertoti, D.B., & Gross, A.L. (1988). Evaluation of biofeedback seat insert for improving active sitting posture in children with cerebral palsy. A clinical report. *Physical Therapy, 68,* 1109–1113.

Bertoti, D.G., Stanger, M., Betz, R.R., Akers, J., Maynahon, M.,

& Mulcahey, M. (1997). Percutaneous intramuscular functional electrical stimulation as an intervention choice for children with cerebral palsy. *Pediatric Physical Therapy, 9,* 123–127.

Blaskey, J., & Jennings, M.C. (1999). Traumatic brain injury. In S.K. Campbell (Ed.), *Decision making in pediatric neurologic physical therapy* (pp. 84–140). Philadelphia: Churchill Livingstone.

Bly, L. (1991). A historical and current view of the basis of NDT. *Pediatric Physical Therapy, 3*(3), 131–135.

Bly, L., & Whiteside, A. (1997). *Facilitation techniques based on NDT principles.* San Antonio: Therapy Skill Builders.

Bobath, K., & Bobath, B. (1984). The neuro-developmental treatment. In D. Scrutton (Ed.), *Management of the motor disorders of children with cerebral palsy* (pp. 6–16). Philadelphia: J.B. Lippincott.

Bochner, S., Center, Y., Chapparo, C., & Donelly, M. (1999). How effective are programs based on conductive education? A report of two studies. *Journal of Intellectual and Developmental Disability, 24,* 227–242.

Boehme, R. (1988). *Improving upper body control.* Tucson: Therapy Skill Builders.

Booth, M.Y., Yates, C.C., Edgar, T.S., & Bandy, W.D. (2003). Serial casting vs combined intervention with Botulinum toxin A and serial casting in the treatment of spastic equinus in children. *Pediatric Physical Therapy, 15*(4), 216–220.

Bower, E., McLellan, D.L., Arney, J., & Campbell, J.J. (1996). A randomized controlled trial of different intensities of physiotherapy and different goal-setting procedures in 44 children with cerebral palsy. *Developmental Medicine and Child Neurology, 38,* 226–237.

Bryce, J. (1972). Facilitation of movement: The Bobath approach. *Physiotherapy, 58,* 403.

Bundy, A.C., Lane, S., Murray, E.A., & Fisher, A.G. (2002). *Sensory integration: Theory and practice.* Philadelphia: F.A. Davis.

Butler, C., & Darrah, J. (2001). Effects of neurodevelopmental treatment (NDT) for cerebral palsy: An AACPDM evidence report. *Developmental Medicine and Child Neurology, 43,* 778–790.

Cadenhead, S.L., McEwen, I.R., & Thompson, D.M. (2002). Effects of passive range of motion exercises on lower extremity goniometric measurements of adults with cerebral palsy: A single-subject design. *Physical Therapy, 82,* 858–869.

Campbell, P.H. (1991). Evaluation and assessment in early intervention for infants and toddlers. *Journal of Early Intervention, 15,* 36–45.

Campbell, S.K. (1991). Framework for measurement of neurological impairment or disability. In M.J. Lister (Ed.), *Contemporary management of motor control problems: Proceedings of the II STEP Conference* (pp. 49–64). Alexandria, VA: American Physical therapy Association.

Campbell, S.K. (1999). Models for decision making in pediatric neurologic physical therapy. In S.K. Campbell (Ed.), *Decision making in pediatric neurologic physical therapy.* Philadelphia: Churchill Livingstone.

Carmick, J. (1995). Managing equinus in children with cerebral palsy: Electrical stimulation to the triceps surae muscle. *Developmental Medicine and Child Neurology, 37,* 965–975.

Carmick, J. (1997). Use of neuromuscular electrical stimulation and dorsal wrist splint to improve the hand function of a child with spastic hemiparesis. *Physical Therapy, 77,* 661–671.

Carr, J.H., & Shepherd, R.B. (1987). *A motor learning programme for stroke.* London: Heinemann.

Cesari, P., & Newell, K.M. (2000). Body scaling of grip configurations in children aged 6–12 years. *Developmental Psychobiology, 36*(4), 301–310.

Charles, J., Lavinder, G., & Gordon, A.M. (2001). Effects of constraint-induced therapy on hand function in children with hemiplegic cerebral palsy. *Pediatric Physical Therapy, 13*(2), 68–76.

Clark, J.E. (1995). Dynamic systems perspective on gait. In R.L. Craik & C.A. Oatis (Eds.), *Gait analysis: Theory and application* (pp. 79–86). St. Louis: Mosby.

Commeaux, M.S., Patterson, N., Rubin, M., & Meiner, R. (1997). Effect of neuromuscular electrical stimulation during gait in children with cerebral palsy. *Pediatric Physical Therapy, 9,* 103–109.

Conine, T.A., Sullivan, T., Mackie, T., & Goodman, M. (1990). Effect of serial casting for the prevention of equinus in patients with acute head injury. *Archives of Physical Medicine and Rehabilitation, 71,* 310–312.

Damiano, D.L., & Able, M.F. (1998). Functional outcomes of strength training in spastic cerebral palsy. *Archives of Physical Medicine and Rehabilitation, 79,* 119–125.

Damiano, D.L., Dodd, K., & Taylor, N.F. (2002). Should we be testing and training muscle strength in cerebral palsy? *Developmental Medicine and Child Neurology, 44,* 68–72.

Darrah, J., Fan, J.S., Chen, L., Nunweiler, J., & Watkins, B. (1997). Review of the effects of progressive resistive muscle strengthening in children with cerebral palsy: A clinical consensus. *Pediatric Physical Therapy, 9,* 12–17.

David, K.S. (1985). Motor sequencing strategies in school-aged children. *Physical Therapy, 65,* 883–889.

David, K.S. (1995). Developmental coordination disorders. In S.K. Campbell (Ed.), *Physical therapy for children* (pp. 425–458). Philadelphia: W.B. Saunders.

David, K.S. (2000). Developmental coordination disorders. In S.K. Campbell, D.W. Vander Linden, & R.J. Palisano (Eds.), *Physical therapy for children* (2nd ed., pp. 471–501). Philadelphia: W.B. Saunders.

Dawson, M.M., Hallahan, D.P., Reeve, R.E., & Ball, D.W. (1980). The effect of reinforcement and verbal rehearsal on selective attention in learning disabled children. *Journal of Abnormal Child Psychology, 8,* 133–144.

DeGangi, G. (1990). Perspectives on the integration of neurodevelopmental treatment sensory integrative therapy. *NDTA Newsletter,* March, pp. 1, 6.

DeGangi, G.A., & Royeen, C.B. (1994). Current practice among Neurodevelopmental Treatment Association members. *American Journal of Occupational Therapy, 48,* 803–809.

Dichter, C.G. (1994). Relationship of muscle strength and joint range of motion to gross motor abilities in school-aged children with Down syndrome. Unpublished doctoral dissertation, Hahnemann University, Philadelphia.

Dichter, C.G., DeCicco, J., Flanagan, S., Hyun, J., & Mongrain, C. (2001). Acquiring skill through intervention in adolescents with Down syndrome. [Abstract]. *Pediatric Physical Therapy, 12,* 209.

Duff, S., & Quinn, L. (2002). Motor learning and motor control. In D. Cech & S. Martin (Eds.), *Functional movement development across the life span* (2nd ed., pp. 86–117). Philadelphia: W.B. Saunders.

Dumas, H., & Francesconi, S. (2002). Aquatic therapy in pediatrics: Annotated bibliography. *Physical and Occupational Therapy in Pediatrics, 20*(4), 63–78.

Eckersley, P.M., & King, J. (1993). Principles of treatment. In P.M. Eckersley (Ed.), *Elements of paediatric physiotherapy* (pp. 323–341). New York: Churchill-Livingstone.

Effgen, S.K. (2001). Occurrence of gross motor behaviors in US preschools and conductive education preschools in Hong Kong. [Abstract]. *Physical Therapy, 81,* A78.

Eliasson, A.C., Gordon, A.M., & Forssberg, H. (1992). Impaired anticipatory control of isometric forces during grasping by children with cerebral palsy. *Developmental Medicine and Child Neurology, 34,* 216–225.

Eliasson, A.C., Gordon, A.M., & Forssberg, H. (1995). Tactile control of isometric forces during grasping in children with cerebral palsy. *Developmental Medicine and Child Neurology, 33,* 661–670.

Fetters, L., Harris, S., & Palisano, R. (2002). Developing student competency in evidence-based practice in pediatrics. Paper presented at the APTA Combined Sections Meeting, Boston, MA.

Fetters, L., & Kluzik, J. (1996). The effects of neurodevelopmental treatment vs practice on the reaching of children with spastic cerebral palsy. *Physical Therapy, 76,* 346–358.

Floodmark, A. (1986). Augmented auditory feedback as an aid in gait training of the cerebral palsied child. *Developmental Medicine and Child Neurology, 28,* 147–155.

Fragala, M.A., Goodgold, S., & Dumas, H. (2003). Effects of lower extremity passive stretching: Pilot study of children and youth with severe limitations in self-mobility. *Pediatric Physical Therapy, , 15,* 167–175.

Gallagher, J.D., & Thomas, J.R. (1989). Effect of varying post-KR intervals upon children's motor performance. *Journal of Motor Behavior, 12,* 41–46.

Gentile, A.M. (1987). Skill acquisition: Action, movement, and neuromuscular processes. In J.A. Carr & R.B. Shepherd (Eds.), *Movement science: Foundation for physical therapy in rehabilitation* (pp. 93–154). Rockville, MD: Aspen Publications.

Gentile, A.M. (1992) The nature of skill acquisition: Therapeutic implications for children with movement disorders. In H. Forssberg & H. Hirschfeld (Eds.), *Movement disorders in children. Medical Sports Science, 36,* 31–40, Basel, Switzerland: Karger.

Gibson, J.J. (1979). *The ecological approach to visual perception.* Boston: Houghton-Mifflin.

Giuliani, C.A. (1991). Theories of motor control: New concepts for physical therapy. In M.J. Lister (Ed.), *Contemporary management of motor control problems: Proceedings of the II STEP Conference.* Alexandria, VA: American Physical Therapy Association.

Goodgold-Edwards, S., & Gianutsos, J.G. (1991). Coincidence anticipation performance of children with spastic cerebral palsy and nonhandicapped children. *Physical and Occupational Therapy in Pediatrics, 10,* 49–82.

Gordon, A.M., & Duff, S.V. (1999). Fingertip forces during object manipulation in children with hemiplegic cerebral palsy: Anticipatory scaling. *Developmental Medicine and Child Neurology, 41,* 166–175.

Gudjonsdottir, B., & Stemmons-Mercer, V. (2002). Effects of a dynamic versus static prone stander on bone mineral density and behaviour in 4 children with severe cerebral palsy. *Pediatric Physical Therapy, 14,* 38–46.

Haken, H., Kelso, J.A.S., & Bunz, H. (1985). A theoretical model of phase transitions in human hand movements. *Biological Cybernetics, 51,* 347–356.

Hari, M., & Tillemans, T. (1984). Conductive education. In D. Scrutton (Ed.), Management of the motor disorders of children with cerebral palsy. *Clinics in Developmental Medicine, 90,* 19–35.

Harris, S.R. (1997). The effectiveness of early intervention for children with cerebral palsy and related motor disabilities. In M.J. Guralnick (Ed.), *The effectiveness of early intervention* (pp. 327–348). Baltimore: Paul H. Brookes.

Harris, S.R. (1990). Therapeutic exercise for children with neurodevelopmental disabilities. In Basmajian (Ed.), *Therapeutic exercise* (5th ed., pp. 163–173). Baltimore: Williams & Wilkins.

Harris, S.R., & Lundgren, B.D. (1991). Joint mobilization in children with central nervous system disorders: Indications and precautions. *Physical Therapy, 71,* 890–896.

Heriza, C.B. (1991). Motor development: Traditional and contemporary theories. In M.J. Lister (Ed.), *Contemporary management of motor control problems: Proceedings of the II STEP Conference* (pp. 99–126). Alexandria, VA: American Physical Therapy Association.

Heriza, C.B., & Sweeney, J.K. (1994). Pediatric physical therapy: Part I. Practice, scope, scientific basis, and theoretical foundation. *Infants and Young Children, 7,* 20–32.

Heriza, C.B., & Sweeney, J.K. (1995). Pediatric physical therapy: Part II. Approaches to movement dysfunction. *Infants and Young Children, 8,* 1–14.

Hood, B., & Atkinson, J. (1990). Sensory visual loss and cognitive deficits in selective attentional system of normal infants and neurologically impaired children. *Developmental Medicine and Child Neurology, 32,* 1067–1077.

Horak, F.B. (1991). Assumptions underlying motor control for neurologic rehabilitation. In M.J. Lister (Ed.), *Contemporary Management of Motor Control Problems: Proceedings of the II STEP Conference* (pp. 11–28). Alexandria, VA: American Physical Therapy Association.

Horgan, J. (1985). Mnemonic strategy instruction in coding, processing and recall of movement-related cues in mentally retarded children. *Perceptual and Motor Skills, 57,* 547–557.

Horne, E.M., Warren, S.F., & Jones, H.A. (1995). An experimental analysis of neurobehavioral motor intervention. *Developmental Medicine and Child Neurology, 37,* 697–714.

Huang, H., & Mercer, V. (2001). Dual task methodology: Application in studies of cognitive and motor performance in adults and children. *Pediatric Physical Therapy, 13,* 133–140.

Iarocci, G., & Burack, J.A. (1998). Understanding the development of attention in persons with mental retardation: Challenging the myths. In J. A. Burack, R.M. Hodapp, et al. (Eds.), *Handbook of mental retardation and development* (pp. 349–381). New York: Cambridge University Press.

Jensen, J.L., Ulrich, B.D., Thelen, E., Schneider, K., & Zernicke, R.F. (1994). Adaptive dynamics of leg movement patterns of human infants: 1. The effects of posture on spontaneous kicking. *Journal of Motor Behavior, 26,* 303–312.

Jonsdottir, J., Fetters, L., & Kluzik, J. (1997). Effects of physical therapy on postural control in children with cerebral palsy. *Pediatric Physical Therapy, 9,* 68–75.

Karnish, K., Bruder, M.B., & Rainforth, B. (1995). A comparison of physical therapy in the school-based treatment contexts. *Physical and Occupational Therapy in Pediatrics, 15,* 1–25.

Kelso, J.S. (1984). Phase transitions and critical behavior in human bimanual coordination. *American Journal of Physiology, 15,* R10000–R10004.

Kernodle, M.W., & Carlton, L.G. (1992). Information feedback and the learning of multiple-degree of freedom activities. *Journal of Motor Behavior, 24,* 187–196.

Kerr, C., McDowell, B., & McDonough, S. (2004). Electrical stimulation in cerebral palsy: A review of effects on strength and motor function. *Developmental Medicine and Child Neurology, 46,* 205–213.

Kluzik, J., Fetters, L., & Coryell, J. (1990). Quantification of control: A preliminary study of effects of neurodevelopmental treatment on reaching in children with spastic cerebral palsy. *Physical Therapy, 70,* 65–78.

Knox, V., & Evans, A.L. (2002). Evaluation of the functional effects of a course of Bobath therapy in children with cerebral palsy: A preliminary study. *Developmental Medicine and Child Neurology, 44,* 447–460.

Knutson, L.M., & Clark, J.E. (1991). Orthotic devices for ambulation in children with cerebral palsy and myelomeningocele. *Physical Therapy, 71*(12), 947–960.

Konczak, J. (1990). Toward an ecological theory of motor development: The relevance of the Gibsonian approach to vision for motor development research. In J.E. Clark & J.H. Humphrey (Eds.), *Advances in motor development research,* Vol. 3, (pp. 201–223). New York: AMS Press.

Kozma, I., & Balogh, E. (1995). A brief introduction to conductive education and its application at an early age. *Infants and Young Children, 8,* 68–74.

Larin, H. (2000). Motor learning: Theories and strategies for the practitioner. In S.K. Campbell, D.W. Vander Linden, & R.J. Palisano (Eds.), *Physical therapy for children* (2nd ed.) (pp. 170–195). Philadelphia: W.B. Saunders.

Latash, M.L., & Anson, J.G. (1996). What are "normal movements" in a typical population? *Behavior and Brain Sciences, 19,* 26.

Lee, T.D. (1988). Transfer-appropriate processing: A framework for conceptualizing practice effects in motor learning. In O.G. Meijer & K. Roth (Eds.), *Complex movement behavior: The motor-action controversy* (pp. 201–215). Amsterdam: North-Holland.

Lee, D.N., & Cook, M.L. (1990). Basic perceptuo-motor dysfunctions in cerebral palsy. In M. Jeannerod (Ed.), *Attention and performance XVIII: Motor representation and control* (pp. 583–602). Mahwah, NJ: Lawrence Erlbaum Associates.

Light, K.E. (2003). Issues of cognition for motor control. In P.C. Montgomery & B. H. Connolly (Eds.), *Clinical applications for motor control* (pp. 245–268). Thorofare, NJ: Slack.

Logan, L., Byers-Hinkley, K., & Ciccone, C.D. (1990). Anterior vs posterior walkers: A gait analysis study. *Developmental Medicine and Child Neurology, 32,* 1044–1048.

Lunnen, K.Y. (1999). Children with multiple disabilities. In S.K. Campbell (Ed.), *Clinical decision making in pediatric neurologic physical therapy* (pp. 141–197). New York: Churchill Livingstone.

MacKinnon, J.R., Noh, S., Laliberte, D., Lariviere, J., & Allan, D.E. (1995). Therapeutic horseback riding: A review of the literature. *Physical and Occupational Therapy in Pediatrics, 15*(1), 1–15.

Magill, R.A. (1992). Augmented feedback in skill acquisition. In R.N. Singer & L.K. Tennant (Eds.), *Handbook on research in sport psychology* (pp. 143–189). New York: Macmillan.

Majsak, M. (1996). Application of motor learning principles to the stroke population. *Topics in Stroke Rehabilitation, 3*(2), 27–59.

Mandich, A.D., Polatajko, H.J., Missiuna, C., & Miller, L.T. (2001). Cognitive strategies and motor performance in children with developmental coordination disorder. *Physical and Occupational Therapy in Pediatrics, 20*(2/3), 125–143.

Maruff, P., Wilson, P., Trebilcock, M., & Currie, J. (1998). Abnormalities of imagined motor sequences in children with developmental coordination disorder. *Neuropsychologia, 37,* 1317–1324.

McEwen, I.R. (1992). Assistive positioning as a control parameter of social communicative interactions between students with profound multiple disabilities and classroom staff. *Physical Therapy, 72,* 634–647.

McEwen, I.R. (2000). Children with cognitive impairments. In S.K. Campbell, D.W. Vander Linden, & R.J. Palisano (Eds.), *Physical therapy for children* (2nd ed., pp. 502–531). Philadelphia: W.B. Saunders.

McGibbon, H., Andrade, C., Widener, G., & Cintas, H.L. (1998). Effect of an equine-movement therapy program on gait, energy expenditure, and motor function in children with spastic cerebral palsy: A pilot study. *Developmental Medicine and Child Neurology, 40,* 754–762.

McPherson, J.J., Arends, T.G., Michaels, M.J., & Trettin, K. (1984). The range of motion of long term knee contractures of four spastic cerebral palsied children: A pilot study. *Physical and Occupational Therapy in Pediatrics, 4*(1), 17–34.

Mercer, V.S., & Lewis, C.L. (2001). Hip abductor and knee extensor muscle strength of children with and without Down syndrome. *Pediatric Physical Therapy, 13,* 18–26.

Miedaner, J.A., & Renander, J. (1987). The effectiveness of classroom passive stretching programs for increasing or managing passive range of motion in nonambulatory children: An evaluation of frequency. *Physical and Occupational Therapy in Pediatrics, 7*(3), 35–43.

Miller, L.J., & Summers, C. (2001). Clinical applications in sensory modulation dysfunction: Assessment and intervention considerations. In S.S. Roley, E.I. Blanche, & R. Schaaf (Eds.), *Sensory integration with diverse populations* (pp. 247–274). San Antonio, TX: Therapy Skill Builders.

Missiuna, C., Rivard, L., & Bartlett, D. (2003). Early identification and risk management of children with developmental coordination disorder. *Pediatric Physical Therapy, 15*(1), 32–37.

Montgomery, P.C., & Richter, E. (1980). *Sensorimotor integration for the developmentally disabled child: A handbook.* Los Angeles: Western Psychological Services.

Mossberg, K.A., Linton, K.A., & Friske, K. (1990). Ankle-foot orthoses: Effect on energy expenditure of gait in spastic diplegic children. *Archives of Physical Medicine and Rehabilitation, 71*(7), 490–494.

Nelson, C.A. (2001). Cerebral palsy. In D.A. Umphred (Ed.), *Neurological rehabilitation* (4th ed., pp. 259–286). St. Louis: Mosby.

Newell, K.M. (1986). Constraints on the development of coordination. In M.G. Wade & H.T.A. Whiting (Eds.), *Motor development in children: Aspects of coordination and control.* Boston: Martinus Nijhoff.

Newell, K.M. (1991). Augmented information and the acquisition of skill. In R. Daugs & K. Bliscke (Eds.), *Motor learning and training* (pp. 99–116). Schermdorf, Hoffman.

Newell, K.M. (1996). Change in movement and skill: Learning, retention, and transfer. In M.L. Latash & M.T. Turvey (Eds.), *Dexterity and its development* (pp. 339–376). Mahwah, NJ: Lawrence Erlbaum Associates.

Newell, K.M., & Carlton, L.G. (1980). Developmental trends in motor response recognition. *Developmental Psychology, 16,* 550–554.

Newell, K.M., & Kennedy, J.A. (1978). Knowledge of results and children's motor learning. *Developmental Psychobiology, 14*, 531–536.

Newell, K.M., & McDonald, P.V. (1994). Learning to coordinate the redundant biomechanical degrees of freedom. In S. Swinnen, H. Heuer, J. Massion, & P. Casaer (Eds.), *Inter-limb coordination: Neural, dynamical and cognitive constraints* (pp. 515–536). San Diego: Academic Press.

Newell, K.M., Scully, D.M., McDonald, P.V., & Baillargeon, R. (1989). Task constraints and infant grip configurations. *Developmental Psychobiology, 22*, 817–832.

Newell, K.M., & Valvano, J. (1998). Therapeutic intervention as a constraint in the learning and relearning of movement skills. *Scandinavian Journal of Occupational Therapy, 5*, 51–57.

Norton, Y. (1975). Neurodevelopmental and sensory integration for the profoundly retarded multiple handicapped child. *American Journal of Occupational Therapy, 29*, 93–100.

O'Connell, D.G., & Barnhart, R. (1995). Improvement in wheelchair propulsion in paediatric wheelchair users through resistance training: A pilot study. *Archives of Physical Medicine and Rehabilitation, 76*, 368–372.

Olney, S.J., & Wright, M.J. (2000). Cerebral palsy. In S.K. Campbell, D.W. Vander Linden, & R.J. Palisano (Eds.), *Physical therapy for children* (2nd ed., pp. 533–570). Philadelphia: W.B. Saunders.

O'Shea, R.K. (2000). Conductive education in conjunction with inclusive education: Teaming physical and occupational therapists and conductors. [Abstract]. *Pediatric Physical Therapy, 12*, 221.

Pape, K.E., Kirsch, S.E., Galil, A., Boulton, J.E., White, M.A., & Chipman, M. (1993). Neuromuscular approach to motor deficits in cerebral palsy: A pilot study. *Journal of Pediatric Orthopedics, 13*, 628–633.

Parham, L.D., & Mailloux, Z. (1996). Sensory integration. In J. Case-Smith, A.S. Allen, & P. Nuse Pratt (Eds.),. *Occupational therapy for children* (3rd ed., pp. 307–356). St. Louis: Mosby.

Parks, S., Rose, D.J., & Dunn, J.M. (1989). A comparison of fractionated reaction time between cerebral palsied and nonhandicapped youths. *Adapted Physical Activity Quarterly, 6*, 379–388.

Phillips, W.E., & Audet, M. (1990). Use of serial casting in the management of knee joint contractures in an adolescent with cerebral palsy. *Physical Therapy, 70*, 521–523.

Pigott, R., & Shapiro, D. (1984). Motor schema: The structure of the variability session. *Research Quarterly for Exercise and Sport, 55*, 41–55.

Polatajko, H.J., Mandich, A.D., Miller, L.T., & Macnab, J.J. (2001). Cognitive orientation to daily occupational performance: Part II. The evidence. *Physical and Occupational Therapy in Pediatrics, 20*(2/3), 125–143.

Reddihough, D.S., King, J., Coleman, G., & Catanese, T. (1998). Efficacy of programmes based on conductive education in young children with cerebral palsy. *Developmental Medicine and Child Neurology, 40*(11), 763–770.

Reed, B. (1997). The physiology of neuromuscular electric stimulation. *Pediatric Physical Therapy, 9*, 96–102.

Richards, C.L., Malouin, F., Dumas, F., Marcoux, S., Lepage, C., & Menier, C. (1997). Early and intensive treadmill locomotor training for young children with cerebral palsy: A feasibility study. *Pediatric Physical Therapy, 9*, 158–165.

Roley, S., Blanche, E.I., & Schaaf, R.C. (2001). *Understanding the nature of sensory integration with diverse populations.* San Antonio, TX: Therapy Skill Builders.

Salmoni, A.W., Schmidt, R.A., & Walter, C.B. (1984). Knowledge of results and motor learning: A review and critical reappraisal. *Psychological Bulletin, 95*, 355–386.

Scherzer, A.L., & Tscharnuter, I. (1990). *Early diagnosis and therapy in cerebral palsy: A primer on infant development problems.* New York: Marcel Dekker.

Schindl, M.R., Forstner, C., Kern, H., & Hesse, S. (2000). Treadmill training with partial body weight support in nonambulatory patients with cerebral palsy. *Archives of Physical Medicine and Rehabilitation, 81*, 301–306.

Schmidt, R.A. (1988). *Motor control and learning: A behavioural emphasis* (2nd ed.). Champaign, IL: Human Kinetics.

Schmidt, R.A. (1991). Motor learning principles for physical therapy. In M.J. Lister (Ed.), *Contemporary management of motor control problems: Proceedings of the II STEP Conference* (pp. 49–64). Alexandria, VA: American Physical Therapy Association.

Schmidt, R.A., & Lee, T.D. (1999). *Motor control and learning* (3rd ed., p. 45). Champaign, IL: Human Kinetics.

Schmidt, R.A., & Wrisberg, C.A. (2000). *Motor performance and learning.* Champaign, IL: Human Kinetics.

Scholz, J.P. (1990). Dynamic pattern theory: Some implications for therapeutics. *Physical Therapy, 70*, 827–843.

Scholz, J.P., & Kelso, J.A.S. (1990). Intentional switching between patterns of bimanual coordination depends on the intrinsic dynamics of the patterns. *Journal of Motor Behavior, 22*, 98–124.

Schoner, G., Zanone, P.G., & Kelso, J.A.S. (1992). Learning as change of coordination dynamics: Theory and experiment. *Journal of Motor Behavior, 24*, 29–48.

Section on Pediatrics, American Physical Therapy Association. (2004). *Physical therapy clinical management guideline for children with spastic diplegia* Working document submitted by M. Fragala & M. O'Neil, chairs of task force to develop a clinical management guideline. Alexandria, VA: Author.

Seeger, B.R., Caudrey, D.J., & Scholes, J.R. (1981). Biofeedback therapy to achieve symmetrical gait in hemiplegic cerebral palsied children. *Archives of Physical Medicine and Rehabilitation, 62*, 364–368.

Shea, J.B., & Morgan, R.L. (1979). Contextual interference effects on the acquisition, retention, and transfer of a motor skill. *Journal of Experimental Psychology: Human Learning and Memory, 5*, 179–187.

Shumway-Cook, A., & Woollacott, M.H. (1985). The growth of

stability: Postural control from a developmental perspective. *Journal of Motor Behavior, 17,* 131–147.

Shumway-Cook, A., & Woollacott, M.H. (1995). *Motor control: Theory and applications.* Baltimore: Williams & Wilkins.

Shumway-Cook, A., & Woollacott, M.H. (2001). *Motor control: Theory and practical applications* (2nd ed.). Philadelphia: Lippincott Williams & Wilkins.

Spitzer, S., & Roley, S.S. (2001). Sensory integration revisited: A philosophy of practice. In S. Roley, E.I. Blanche, & R.C. Schaaf (Eds.), *Understanding the nature of sensory integration with diverse populations* (pp. 3–27). San Antonio, TX: Therapy Skill Builders.

Steinbok, P., Reiner, A., & Kestle, J.R. (1997). Therapeutic electrical stimulation following selective posterior rhizotomy in children with spastic diplegic cerebral palsy: A randomized clinical trial. *Developmental Medicine and Child Neurology, 39,* 515–520.

Stiers, P., Vanderkelen, R., Vanneste, G., Colne, S., DeRammelaere, M., & Vandenbussche, E. (2002). Visual-perceptual impairment in a random sample of children with cerebral palsy. *Developmental Medicine and Child Neurology, 44*(6), 370–382.

Stiller, C., Hall, H., Marcoux, B.C., & Olson, R.E. (2001). The effect of conductive education, intensive therapy, and special education services on motor skills in children with cerebral palsy. *Physical and Occupational Therapy in Pediatrics, 23*(3), 31–50.

Stockmeyer, S.A. (1972). An interpretation of the approach of Rood to the treatment of neuromuscular dysfunction. *American Journal of Physical Medicine, 46,* 900–956.

Stuberg, W. (1992). Consideration related to weight bearing programs in children with developmental disability. *Physical Therapy, 72,* 35–40.

Tardieu, C., Lespargot, A., Tabary, C., & Bret, M.D. (1988). For how long must the soleus muscle be stretched each day to prevent contracture? *Developmental Medicine and Child Neurology, 30,* 3–10.

Tatlow, A. (Ed.). (1993). *The Hong Kong conductive education source book.* Hong Kong, China: Working Group on Conductive Education, Joint Council for the Physically and Mentally Disabled.

Taylor, J. (1999). Blocked and random practice of crutch walking skills in young children. Unpublished master's thesis, MCP Hahnemann University, Philadelphia.

Thelan, E. (1986). Development of coordinated movement: Implication for early human development. In H.T.A. Whiting (Ed.), *Motor development in children: Aspects of coordination and control* (pp. 107–120). Boston: Martinus Nijhoff.

Thelan, E., & Fisher, D.M. (1982). Newborn stepping: An explanation for a "disappearing" reflex. *Developmental Psychology, 8,* 760–775.

Thorpe, D.E., Showokis, R.A., Kilby, J.M., Markham, J.R., Roberson, T.M., & Seymour, S.K. (2003). Does KP-driven internal or external focus of attention facilitate the learning of a novel tossing task in typically developing children? [Abstract]. *Journal of Sport and Exercise Psychology, 25,* Supplement, 132.

Thorpe, D.E., & Valvano, J. (2002). The effects of knowledge of results and cognitive strategies on motor skill learning by children with cerebral palsy. *Pediatric Physical Therapy, 14,* 2–15.

Tscharnuter, I. (1993). A new therapy approach to movement organization. *Physical and Occupational Therapy in Pediatrics, 13,* 19–40.

Tscharnuter, I. (2002). Clinical application of dynamic theory concepts according to Tscharnuter Akademie for Movement Organization (TAMO) Therapy. *Pediatric Physical Therapy, 14,* 38–46.

Valvano, J. (2004). Activity-focused motor interventions for children with neurological conditions. *Physical and Occupational Therapy in Pediatrics, 24,* 79–107.

Valvano, J., Heriza, C.B., & Carollo, J. (2002). The effects of physical and verbal guidance on the learning of a gross motor skill by children with cerebral palsy. Unpublished data.

Valvano, J., & Long, T. (1991). Neurodevelopmental treatment: A review of the writings of the Bobaths. *Pediatric Physical Therapy, 3*(3), 125–130.

Valvano, J., & Newell, K.M. (1998). Practice of a precision isometric grip force task by children with spastic cerebral palsy. *Developmental Medicine and Child Neurology, 40,* 464–473.

Van der weel, F.R., van der Meer, A.L.H., & Lee, D.N. (1991). Effect of task on movement control in cerebral palsy: Implications for assessment and therapy. *Developmental Medicine and Child Neurology, 33,* 419–426.

Warren, W.J. (1984). Perceiving affordances: The visual guidance of stair climbing. *Journal of Experimental Psychology: Human Learning and Memory, 10,* 683–704.

Wenderoth, N., Bock, O., & Krohn, R. (2002). Learning a new bimanual coordination pattern is influenced by existing attractors. *Motor Control, 26,* 166–182.

Wilson, P.H., & McKenzie, B.E. (1998). Information processing deficits associated with developmental coordination disorder: A meta-analysis of research findings. *Journal of Child Psychology and Psychiatry, 39,* 829–840.

Wilson Howle, J.M. (1999). Cerebral palsy. In S.K. Campbell (Ed.), *Decision making in pediatric neurologic physical therapy* (pp. 23–83). Philadelphia: Churchill Livingstone.

Winstein, C.J. (1991). Designing practice for motor learning: Clinical implications. In M.J. Lister (Ed.), *Contemporary management of motor problems: Proceedings of the II STEP Conference* (pp. 65–76). Alexandria, VA: American Physical Therapy Association.

Winstein, C.J., Gardner, E.R., McNeal, D.R., Barto, P.S., & Nicholson, D.E. (1989). Standing balance training: Effects on balance and locomotion in hemiparetic adults. *Archives of Physical Medicine and Rehabilitation, 70,* 755–762.

Winstein, C.J., Pohl, P.S., & Lewthwaite, R. (1994). Effects of physical guidance and knowledge of results on motor learning: Support for the guidance hypothesis. *Research Quarterly for Exercise and Sport, 65,* 316–323.

Winstein, C.J., & Schmidt, R.A. (1990). Reduced frequency of knowledge of results enhances motor skill learning. *Journal of Experimental Psychology: Learning, Memory, and Cognition, 16,* 677–691.

Wulf, G. (1991). The effect of type of practice on motor learning in children. *Applied Cognitive Psychology, 5,* 123–134.

Wulf, G., Shea, C.H., & Matschiner, S. (1998). Frequent feedback enhances complex skill learning. *Journal of Motor Behavior, 30,* 180–192.

Wulf, G., Shea, C.H., & Whitacre, C.A. (1998). Physical-guidance benefits in learning a complex motor skill. *Journal of Motor Behavior, 30,* 367–380.

Zanone, P.G., & Kelso, J.A.S. (1994). The coordination dynamics of learning: Theoretical structure and research agenda. In S. Swinnen, H. Heuer, J. Massion, & P. Casaer (Eds.), *Interlimb coordination.* San Diego: Academic Press.

Zanone, P.G., Kelso, J.A.S., & Jeka, J.J. (1993). Concepts and methods for a dynamical approach to behavioral coordination and change. In G.J.P. Savelsbergh (Ed.), *The development of coordination in infancy* (pp. 89–153). San Diego, Elsevier Science Publishers.

Chapter 8

THE CARDIOPULMONARY SYSTEM

— Julie Ann Starr, PT, MS, CCS
— Carole A. Tucker, PT, PhD, PCS

Cardiopulmonary impairments of body structures and functions that occur during infancy and childhood can, in the short term, be life threatening, with medical and physical therapy intervention focused primarily on acute care issues. However, the long-term effects of cardiopulmonary dysfunction can alter the physical, social, and cognitive growth of a child, resulting in multifaceted restrictions in activities and participation. As physical therapists treating children with cardiopulmonary system dysfunction, we must not limit our focus to only cardiopulmonary system-related interventions. Rather, we should broaden our planning and implementation with careful considerations for long-term compliance, prevention of secondary impairments, and the effects of impairments and interventions on the maturing child's changing social, cognitive, and behavioral development and eventual role in society.

The overall objective of this chapter is to provide the entry-level physical therapy practitioner with the necessary knowledge to develop effective evaluation, examination, and procedural interventions for children with cardiopulmonary dysfunction. In this chapter, we provide the reader with a detailed overview of the development and maturation of the cardiopulmonary system's structure and function, as well as an overview of common cardiopulmonary conditions diagnosed in the pediatric population. Clinical guidelines to assist the reader in determining appropriate examination and intervention techniques for children with cardiopulmonary impairment and related dysfunction are presented. Physical fitness and the emerging issues concerning health promotion and wellness programs for all children are addressed. The physical therapist's emerging role in reducing disability related to long-term cardiopulmonary effects of a potentially less active lifestyle for children of all abilities is the final focus of the chapter.

Structure and Function

Overview of Cardiopulmonary Function

The discussion of cardiopulmonary function is organized according to "systems theory." A systems theory approach can provide a more organized understanding of the dynamic functioning of such a complex system. According to systems theory, a system's components are usually subdivided into three categories: individual (or organismic), environment, and task (Figure 8–1). Individual or organismic components of the cardiopulmonary system would include characteristics such as the ability to generate muscle force of inspiration, range of motion (ROM) of the thorax, or airway responsiveness. Environmental system components for cardiopulmonary function include air quality, temperature, humidity, and oxygen content of the available air. Task components of the cardiopulmonary system include ventilation, circulation, and respiration. These tasks act to exchange, deliver, and remove gases and to maintain the pH level of the body in a range that allows

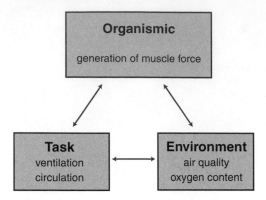

Figure 8-1 Schematic of the systems theory as it applies to the cardiopulmonary system.

for cellular function. The magnitude of gas exchange must be sufficient to provide the body's tissues with enough oxygen and removal of end-product gases to sustain life, and in children to provide enough additional energy for growth and development. At any given time, these cardiopulmonary tasks are performed in concert with the individual and environmental system components.

Constraints on ventilation, circulation, and respiration are often related to the basic forces and laws of physics (e.g., mechanical, fluid, chemical, and electrical laws). Cardiopulmonary system activity is primarily controlled through the nervous system, which is basically constrained by electrical conduction properties, as well as chemical constraints locally.

Ventilation (the flow of gases between the lungs and the external environment) is dependent upon lung compliance, thoracic compliance, airway resistance, and the interplay of forces generated by the respiratory muscles. Ventilation, in particular, is "constrained" or affected by mechanical factors such as the shape and size of the thorax, the rigidity or flexibility of the ribcage, the forces generated by the muscles of respiration, the force-length relationship in muscles, the elastic recoil properties of the thorax, and effective airway diameter.

Circulation (the movement of blood throughout the body) is dependent on pressure gradients, blood flow, blood volume, and the sequence of forces generated by the cardiac muscle. Fluid forces and pressure gradients in the heart and vasculature affect circulation. In addition, muscle force-length properties and electrical activity of the heart muscle are responsible for many of the pressure changes that provide circulation.

In order for **respiration** (gas exchange at the alveolar and tissue level) to be effective, both ventilation and circulation must be accomplished. Respiration is dependent on pressure and chemical gradients, diffusion of chemicals across cell membranes, and capillary interfaces.

The dynamic interplay between ventilation, circulation, and respiration determines the overall level of functioning of the cardiopulmonary system at any given instant. Over a longer time frame, cardiopulmonary system components are altered by growth and maturation, providing a dynamic set of system performance constraints that differ between infancy and adulthood. As a child grows and environmental exploration and societal involvement increase, cardiopulmonary dysfunction will have different levels of impact. In infancy, cardiopulmonary dysfunction can interfere with feeding, growth, and wakefulness, thereby limiting environmental exploration. In a young child, community mobility and socialization with peers through play and school attendance can be affected. During teenage years, socialization, employment, and concerns involving transition into an independent adulthood become increasingly important. In medical management and interventions for cardiopulmonary dysfunction, the broader perspectives need to be considered as the child matures.

Although the structure and function of the cardiopulmonary system reflect the complex interaction between the cardiac and pulmonary systems, the maturation of each system follows a different sequence of events. The heart is one of the first functioning organs within the growing fetus, and it performs the task of circulation in utero. On the other hand, the pulmonary system does not perform its primary task of ventilation until after birth. An understanding of the maturation of the cardiopulmonary system provides an ability to gauge the effect of growth-related interdependence of the two systems and how a small change in one system component can, over time, have an effect on other parts of the system as they mature.

Maturation of the Cardiac System

Development of the heart's structure begins in the first days of embryonic life, with the merging of two epithelial tubes to form the single cardiac tube. Contractions of the heart begin at about 17 days of gestation, although effective blood flow does not occur until the end of the first month. In this early embryonic heart, no intracardiac valves are present; rather, endocardial cushions prevent backflow into the atria with ventricle contraction. At approximately $3^1/_2$ weeks of embryonic life, a process known as *cardiac looping* takes place. The single cardiac tube folds onto itself, effectively forming the right and left sides of the heart, and subsequently the endocardial cushions turn into the cardiac valves. This looping process is critical to ensure correct anatomical formation of the heart, and disruption of this process during the first few weeks of gestation can result in serious cardiac structural defects. Cardiac formation is also dependent on biomechanical forces, such as pressure, flows, and the resultant shearing forces, present in the embryonic heart. Alterations in these forces in early gestation may result in atypical cardiac anatomy. As the embryonic heart continues to grow, coronary circulation is established. Fetal heart sounds can be detected by 8 to 10 weeks of gestation, indicating functioning of the circulatory system.

Despite the relatively early structural development of the heart, fetal circulation remains markedly different from adult circulation. In fetal circulation, only 12% of blood follows the pathway of adult circulation from the right atrium (RA) to the right ventricle (RV), through pulmonary circulation, to left atrium (LA), left ventricle (LV), and finally into the aorta for systemic circulation. Because the fetal blood is oxygenated by the placenta and maternal circulation, passing blood through the fetus's fluid-filled lungs is unnecessary and impractical. Prenatal anatomical differences in the developing cardiac structure allow for two alternative circulation routes that effectively reduce blood flow through the nonfunctioning fetal pulmonary system. The first alternative route uses the **fora**

men ovale, a one-way door in the atrial septum, which allows blood to flow from the RA into the LA (instead of into the pulmonary circulation), then to the LV, and eventually to the systemic circulation via the aorta. The second alternative route uses the **ductus arteriosus**, a vascular link outside the heart between the pulmonary artery and the aorta, allowing blood to exit the pulmonary artery and be delivered directly into the aorta for systemic circulation, effectively bypassing the lungs and the left heart entirely (Figure 8–2). Within the first few hours of life, pressure changes within the cardiac chambers close the foramen ovale. Within a few weeks of life, the ductus arteriosus closes. There remains only one route for blood to flow through the body, that of adult circulation. (For further information, see section on "Initiation of Breathing" in this chapter.)

A child continues to experience altered pressures and forces on the developing chest wall and within the cardiac system as musculoskeletal growth occurs. Transient alterations in pressures and flows within the heart and major vessels can occur. Some of these alterations, such as a transient heart murmur, are considered benign if there is no accompanying symptomatology. Other defects, such as a **coarctation of the aorta** (a stricture in the descending aorta), may become more serious and their effects become more pronounced with growth. Medical professionals routinely assess the cardiac system throughout the child's growth, and any abnormalities noted in a child's cardiac exam deserve documentation and follow-up.

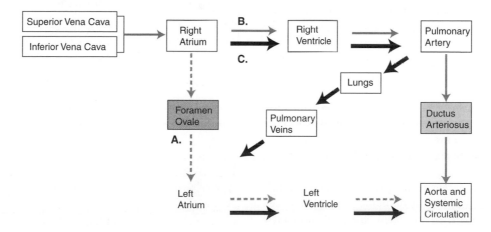

Figure 8-2 Potential routes of blood flow from right atria to aorta in fetal circulation. (*A*) Right atrium through foramen ovale to left atrium to left ventricle to aorta (dashed arrows). (*B*) Right atria to right ventricle to pulmonary artery through ductus arteriosus to aorta (thin arrows). (*C*) Right atria to right ventricle to pulmonary artery to lungs to pulmonary veins to left atria to left ventricle to aorta (thick arrows).

Maturation of the Pulmonary System

The respiratory system begins to develop between 22 and 26 days of gestation, with the formation of a lung bud, a node of endodermal tissue from which the trachea, bronchi, conducting airways, and alveoli arise. The mesodermal tissue surrounding the lung bud develops into the lungs' "support structures," such as pleura, smooth muscle, cartilage, collagen, and blood vessels (Kravitz, 1994). Pathophysiological processes (e.g., maternal and fetal infections) early in gestation can cause widespread systemic or multisystemic effects in both the developing pulmonary and cardiac systems. Between 8 and 16 weeks of gestational age, further branching of the conducting airways occurs down to the terminal bronchioles, and the pulmonary arterial system begins to form. By 17 weeks of gestation, the lung has lobes and the conducting airways have completed branching. In addition, the beginning of the alveolar capillary membranes is formed, providing the first possibility, albeit slight, for the survival of a preterm infant. During 17 to 24 weeks of gestation, the terminal bronchioles form buds and some terminal bronchioles convert to respiratory bronchioles, allowing a potential site for gas exchange. The arterial system continues to grow, and the pulmonary capillary walls that are near to the respiratory bronchioles become thin, narrowing the diffusion distance for improved gas exchange possibilities. During this time, the support tissue becomes more differentiated, with cartilage forming in the bronchi, collagen in the midsize airways, and elastin in the bronchioles. By the 23rd week, the type 2 alveolar cells that produce surfactant appear, and by 28 weeks of gestation some surfactant is present, and the potential for some gas exchange is possible. Surfactant is a lipid-rich substance that allows adequate alveolar expansion by limiting surface tension across the alveolar membrane. Between 28 and 32 weeks gestation, the amount of surfactant increases in quantity, ensuring adequate lung inflation at birth. Infants who are born prematurely often experience respiratory complications secondary to the relative immaturity of the pulmonary system and limited surfactant production.

The pulmonary system is not functional until the first postnatal breath. In utero, the pulmonary system has been immersed in an aquatic environment, and aside from a few hiccups now and then, the respiratory system has not had to perform any function. The first postnatal breath is the initial test of the patency of the pulmonary system. During the first few breaths, the infant has to generate large inspiratory pressures to inflate the lungs and force the fluid within the airways and alveolar units into the lymphatic system. For the first few hours after birth, this diffusing process naturally occurs as the infant breathes. Transient newborn tachypnea, or mild respiratory distress, is not uncommon even in the healthiest of infants.

At birth, the full-term infant has a tracheobronchial tree with approximately 17 branches, yet has a very limited number, only approximately 150 million, of primitive alveoli. During early childhood (until the age of approximately 4 years) the number of branches of the tracheobronchial tree increases to about 23, and the number of alveoli increases to approximately 300 million, similar to the adult lung. Alveolar size and diameter of the airways continue to increase as the child grows.

Important anatomical differences exist between the pulmonary system of an infant and that of an adult, which can predispose an infant to respiratory compromise (Table 8.1). Infants are born with a larynx that is structurally higher, enabling the infant to breathe better while feeding (sucking). It does, however, make the infant an obligatory nose breather, which may become problematic with nasal congestion or nasal obstruction. The diameter of the infant's airway is narrower from the nares all the way to the

Table 8.1 Anatomical Differences in the Cardiopulmonary System of Children Compared With That of Adults

Airway	Higher larynx Smaller diameter of airways Increased resistance to airflow Increased work of breathing Less cartilage within the airway walls for support
Alveolar capillary membrane	Fewer alveoli Less developed collateral ventilation channels Thicker alveolar walls Capillary bed at a greater distance from alveolar wall
Bony thorax	Increased compliance of the rib cage Horizontal alignment of rib cage
Muscles of ventilation	Muscles perform as stabilizers rather than mobilizers Decreased length-tension relationship Diaphragm fibers have fewer fatigue-resistant fibers

terminal bronchioles, making it more susceptible to obstruction (Decesare, Graybill-Tucker, & Gould, 1995). The decreased airway lumen also results in an increased resistance to airflow, increasing the work of breathing. In addition, the smooth muscle within the bronchioles is less developed, providing greater tendency for bronchiolar collapse, until approximately 5 years of age (Doershuk, Fischer, & Matthews, 1975). The alveolar walls of the infants are thicker, and the capillary beds are farther away from the alveolar membrane, impeding respiration by increasing the diffusion distance. Finally, there is less surface area for respiration because there are fewer alveoli.

The compliance, configuration, and muscle action of the chest wall of an infant also differ from those of older children. The healthy newborn's chest wall is primarily cartilaginous, making it extremely compliant (Gaultier, 1995). The cartilaginous ribs allow the distortion necessary for the infant's thorax to travel through the birth canal. However, this increased ribcage compliance results in decreased thoracic stability. The muscles of the infant's chest wall, not the ribs themselves as in adults, are the primary stabilizers of the thorax to counteract the negative pleural pressure of the diaphragm during inspiration. The ribcage of an infant shows a more horizontal alignment of the ribs, rather than the elliptical shape of an older child. This configuration of the infant's ribcage alters the angle of insertion of the costal fibers of the diaphragm, with the orientation being more horizontal than vertical, decreasing the area of apposition (Gaultier, 1995). There is an increased tendency for the diaphragm muscle fibers to pull the lower ribs inward, thereby decreasing efficiency of ventilation and increasing distortion of the chest wall. The chest wall movement of an infant's thorax contributes very little to tidal breathing (Hershenson, Colin, Wohl, & Stark, 1990).

In addition to these differences in ribcage configuration and diaphragm alignment, muscular action associated with ventilation differs in infants. The diaphragm muscle in infants has different fiber-type composition. The diaphragm is the major muscle of respiration in infants as well as adults. However, in the healthy newborn, only 20% of the muscle fibers of the diaphragm are fatigue-resistant fibers, compared with 50% in adults. This difference predisposes infants to earlier diaphragmatic fatigue. Accessory muscles of ventilation are at a mechanical disadvantage in the infant, secondary to the previously mentioned alterations in ribcage alignment and compliance. In addition, the infant uses some accessory muscles, such as the intercostal muscles, to stabilize, not mobilize, the chest wall during inspiration. The upper chest and neck accessory muscles are not well stabilized in young infants.

Until the infant can elongate its cervical spine and stabilize its upper extremities, head, and spine, it is difficult for the accessory muscles to produce the reverse action needed to assist with ventilation. During times of respiratory distress, young infants without head and neck control may exhibit "head bobbing" as they attempt to use accessory muscles of ventilation. Elongation of the cervical spine during musculoskeletal growth will improve the length-tension relationship of some of the accessory muscles of respiration.

As a child grows and is exposed to progressively more upright positions for mobility and activities, muscular and gravitational forces help mold the shape of the thorax and chest wall into a more typical adult configuration. The maturation of thoracic skeletal configuration, in turn, affects muscle mechanics by changing length and alignment of the muscles. The anterior aspects of ribs begin to rotate downward, forming a more elliptical shape. The ribs begin to separate, creating larger intercostal spaces. Ossification of the thorax adds stability and reduces ribcage compliance. As the child gains head and neck control and purposeful upper extremity use, the muscles of the thorax, head, neck, and upper extremities are able to change roles, from stabilizers to mobilizers, and can better be used as accessory muscles of respiration. Greater ribcage motion becomes apparent during tidal breathing. The insertion alignment of the fibers of the diaphragm becomes more vertical with the changing shape of the thorax, resulting in a larger area of apposition. The interaction between trunk and abdominal control also increases the area of apposition, increasing the efficiency of the diaphragm. Overall, the muscular and skeletal maturation has occurred simultaneously, providing a more adultlike thoracic mobility and stability.

Children who do not experience the development of upright antigravity head, neck, and trunk control may not develop the typical ribcage structure and function. Imbalances in muscle forces and support surfaces can lead to asymmetrical chest wall and ribcage formation and may result in eventual impairment in pulmonary function.

Initiation of Breathing

After birth, when the pulmonary system is finally functional, volume and pressure shifts occur in the cardiopulmonary system. Within the first few minutes of ventilation, pulmonary vascular resistance decreases as the alveoli expand. Lower RV heart pressure is required to circulate pulmonary blood flow through the lungs. The umbilical blood flow to the RA stops, lowering the volume and the pressure in the RA. The LA blood volume and pressure increase because of the increased pulmonary venous return. The LV now has more blood to pump from the LA to the systemic arterial system. All of these physiological changes cause a pressure shift within the cardiac chambers. The pressures within the left side of the heart become higher than the pressures within the right side of the heart; aortic pressure becomes higher than the pulmonary artery pressure. These alterations in atrial pressure cause the foramen ovale to close. Over a period of a few hours to a few weeks, the ductus arteriosus also closes because of physiological changes in the neonatal pulmonary and circulatory systems. Atypical persistence of these alternative fetal circulatory routes, that is, through the ductus arteriosus or foramen ovale, is detrimental to normal cardiopulmonary function.

Functional Interaction of Cardiac and Pulmonary Systems

Thus far, we have addressed the maturation of the structure and function of the cardiac and pulmonary systems individually; however, the interaction between the two systems is intimately intertwined, and essentially the two systems function as one. Two short cases illustrate the complex interaction between the cardiac and pulmonary systems.

In the first case, we consider the effect of an isolated cardiac structural abnormality. A **ventricular septal defect (VSD)** is an abnormal opening in the wall (septum) that separates the two ventricles of the heart. With a VSD, when the ventricles contract, there is a tendency for some LV blood to flow through the VSD into the RV, instead of out to the systemic vascular system. This creates a higher-than-expected blood volume, and increased pressure in the RV of the heart as well as in the pulmonary circulation. The pulmonary capillaries respond to this higher blood flow by "leaking" fluid into the pulmonary interstitial spaces, causing pulmonary edema. Lung compliance is reduced, ventilation becomes less efficient, and respiration is impaired. The lungs may respond to this chronic seepage of fluid from its vascular bed by becoming fibrotic over time, resulting in a more permanent pulmonary impairment. All these secondary pulmonary effects are related directly to the primary structural cardiac defect of a VSD.

A second example of the interrelatedness of the cardiac and pulmonary system function is found in the condition of **bronchopulmonary dysplasia (BPD)**. BPD refers to a chronic inflammation and destruction of airways, lung parenchyma, and the alveolar capillary membrane, resulting in a chronic obstructive pulmonary defect. Intrathoracic pressures are altered throughout the respiratory cycle in an obstructive pulmonary disease. These changes in intrathoracic pressures will alter cardiac preload and afterload. The destruction of the alveolar capillary membrane will result in an increased pulmonary vascular resistance. Finally, hypoxia in the pulmonary system causes vasoconstriction, increasing the pulmonary vascular resistance. The RV will have to work harder to push blood through the pulmonary vascular system and, over time, will hypertrophy and may eventually fail (Verklan, 1997). All these secondary cardiac effects are related directly to the primary pulmonary defect of BPD.

Impairments in cardiopulmonary system function can significantly contribute to restrictions in activities within other aspects of a child's development. The social and cognitive developments of children rely on their ability to explore and interact with the environment. Impairments of the cardiopulmonary system in infants can affect endurance and activity tolerance, limiting environmental exploration. The ability to feed orally can be hampered in infants who have high respiratory rates or require mechanical ventilation. Language development and therefore socialization may be delayed in infants who require mechanical ventilation or who cannot adequately control ventilation to allow phonation. Cardiopulmonary impairments can also contribute to slowed physical growth, resulting in less muscle bulk and smaller stature because less oxygen is being delivered to the system and more calories are used to sustain the work of breathing. Therapists serving the needs of children must consider the wide-ranging effects of cardiopulmonary dysfunction, particularly during infancy and early childhood, and provide physical therapy intervention for the whole child.

Diagnosed Conditions

Pediatric cardiopulmonary conditions encompass a variety of diseases less often encountered in the practice of cardiopulmonary physical therapy in adults. Some of these conditions are not seen as frequently in the adult population because (1) the defects may be surgically corrected by adulthood and no longer create dysfunction, (2) children may physically "outgrow" their symptoms, or (3), in unfortunate cases, children die from their disease before reaching adulthood.

Many different pathophysiological processes can cause similar patterns of impairments in body structures and functions and restrictions in activities and participation. Therefore, in this section, as is done in the American

Physical Therapy Association (APTA)'s *Guide to physical therapist practice* (2001), conditions are grouped according to their resultant primary impairments to ventilation, circulation, and respiration. For the most common conditions, the definition, etiology, and pathophysiology for each diagnosis are described, followed by a brief discussion of diagnosis and management. Important but less common conditions are described in Tables 8.2 to 8.7.

Conditions That Impair Ventilation

Ventilation is dependent on airflow through the airways to the respiratory unit of the lung. Factors that affect ventilation include abnormalities of the airway and lung parenchyma, musculoskeletal abnormalities of the thoracic pump, neuromuscular abnormalities of the ventilatory muscles, disorders of central respiratory control, and integumentary conditions that affect the thorax.

Airway and Parenchymal Conditions

Ventilatory impairments are pathophysiological processes that create airway narrowing, cause increased airway secretions effectively reducing the size of the airway, or cause changes in the pulmonary parenchyma. Asthma, cystic fibrosis (CF), infant respiratory distress syndrome (RDS), bronchopulmonary dysplasia (BPD), congenital pulmonary structural abnormalities, and immunological disorders are covered in this section.

Asthma

Asthma is an obstructive pulmonary disease characterized by episodic periods of reversible airway narrowing caused by airway inflammation, increased secretions, and smooth muscle bronchoconstriction. Even during periods of remission, some degree of airway inflammation is present. Asthma is the most common chronic childhood disease affecting 5 million American children. The number of asthma cases increased by more than 160% in children under the age of 5 years, and by 74% in children 5 through 14 years of age, between 1980 and 1994 (Mannino et al., 1998). Asthma accounts for an estimated 11.8 million missed schooldays in the United States and is the third leading cause of preventable hospitalizations in the United States (Lara et al., 2002).

Exercise-induced bronchospasm (EIB), a subset of reversible airways disease, is classically defined by symptoms of shortness of breath, wheezing, cough, or tightness of the chest that occur 8 to 10 minutes into an exercise program with an exercise intensity of 70% to 85% of VO_{2max}. However, symptoms of airway narrowing that occur anytime during exercise, or immediately after exercise, that resolve spontaneously within 20 to 30 minutes, are considered indicative of EIB. A 15% decrease from baseline pulmonary function testing (peak flow or forced expiratory volume in 1 second [FEV_1]) after exercise can confirm the diagnosis. Although some children have EIB without a diagnosis of asthma, many children who have asthma will demonstrate that exercise is one of their triggers for bronchospasm.

Etiology. The exact etiology of asthma is unknown, although genetics, environment (air quality, environmental allergens, cold, dry air), and infection have been implicated as possible causes. For EIB, the most likely etiology is a response to the cooling and drying of the airway that occurs during exercise.

Pathophysiology. Exacerbations of asthma occur in response to an inducer or a trigger, whether an environmental irritant, a virus, cigarette smoke, or another factor. Physiologically, the bronchial mucosa becomes inflamed, decreasing the size of the airway lumen. The bronchial smooth muscle contracts, further decreasing the diameter of the airways. Mucus plugging narrows the airway even further. The result of these changes is an impaired ability to ventilate, or move air through the airway.

During inspiration, the respiratory muscles pull open the chest wall, the attached pleurae, the lung parenchyma, and the airways. Therefore, during inspiration, the airways are as wide as they will be during the respiratory cycle, and inspiratory airflow may not be impaired. However, the lumen of the airways decreases in size throughout exhalation. Given the combined effects of bronchoconstriction, inflammation, and increased airway secretions, the airway lumen abnormally narrows during the exhalation phase of an asthma exacerbation. Clinically, the child with an exacerbation of asthma will present with a prolonged exhalation time. Wheezing at the end of exhalation may be present in a mild exacerbation. As the severity of exacerbation increases, wheezing occurs for a greater portion of the expiratory cycle. In severe airway constriction, the wheezing may occur during both inhalation and exhalation.

Diagnosis. The diagnosis of asthma is clinically based on a history of episodic wheezing, shortness of breath, tightness in the chest, and/or coughing in the absence of any other obvious cause. Symptoms often worsen in the presence of aeroallergens, irritants, or exercise. Symptoms typically occur or worsen at night and/or upon awakening. There may be a family history of asthma, allergy, sinusitis or rhinitis, or allergic skin problems. Physical findings during an exacerbation include cough, hyperexpansion of the thorax, and wheezing during quiet or forced exhalation. Increased nasal secretions (e.g., sinusitis, rhinitis) and/or allergic skin problems (e.g., atopic dermatitis, eczema) may also be present. For older children who are able to participate in pulmonary function testing (PFT), an obstructive pattern will be demonstrated during periods of exacerbation. The FEV_1 will be less than 80% of the predicted value. With the use of a rescue drug (inhaled beta$_2$-agonist), an improvement in FEV_1 of at least 15% should be demonstrated.

Management. Pharmacological management of airway inflammation is the most effective long-term management strategy for the control of the symptoms of asthma (Van Essen-Zandvliet et al., 1992). Inhaled anti-inflammatory drugs are the most commonly used drugs to achieve the control of airway inflammation. These drugs need to be administered on a regular basis, regardless of the child's symptoms, for continued long-term pharmacological management. EIB without asthma does not demonstrate chronic inflammation of the airway; therefore, anti-inflammatory drugs are not used as maintenance drugs. Stabilizing drugs, such as cromolyn sodium, may be useful in children with EIB to manage their airway stability.

A "rescue" drug, usually a beta$_2$-adrenergic inhaled bronchodilator, may be added to the pharmacological management of reactive airway disease for the quick relief of breakthrough symptoms such as cough, chest tightness, wheezing, or shortness of breath. These rescue drugs are used on an "as-needed" basis.

Physical therapy intervention includes secretion removal techniques and proper timing and use of inhaled medications. Breathing exercises with emphasis on exhalation have been used to improve ventilatory patterns of those with an exacerbation of their symptoms. More scientific evidence is needed to support the use of varied breathing exercises for asthma treatment (Holloway & Ram, 2002). Aerobic conditioning should be encouraged in those with reactive airways disease. Special consideration should be given to (1) appropriate premedication with a *beta$_2$-agonist* or cromolyn sodium before exercise, as needed; (2) temperature, humidity, and air quality of the exercise environment; and (3) a longer warm-up period that may decrease breakthrough symptoms. Aerobic exercise has been shown to be beneficial in children with asthma and EIB (Nixon, 1996).

Cystic Fibrosis

Cystic fibrosis (CF) affects the excretory glands of the body. Secretions made by these glands are thicker and more viscous and can obstruct various systems of the body: pulmonary, digestive, hepatic, and male reproductive. The enzymes of the gastrointestinal (GI) tract are often inadequate, causing malnutrition and a picture of "failure to thrive" in the face of adequate caloric intake. The pancreas can be affected, resulting in diabetes. Dysfunction of the pulmonary system is the most common cause of morbidity and mortality in children with CF. Thickened pulmonary secretions narrow or obstruct airways leading to hyperinflation, infection, and tissue destruction.

Etiology. CF is an autosomal recessive, genetically inherited disease. Two gene-carrying parents statistically have a 25% chance of having a child with CF, a 50% chance of having a child who is a carrier of the disease, and a 25% chance of having a child who is genetically free of the disease. Both parents must be carriers of the defective gene to produce a child with the disease. The incidence of CF in the white population is 1:2500 live births. There is a much lower incidence of CF in African American and Asian populations.

Pathophysiology. The prevailing defect in CF is within the chloride ion channels of the body. The chloride channels on the epithelial cells are either absent or fail to open appropriately (Aitken, 1996). There is increased sodium absorption of this membrane, causing a fluid imbalance within the tissues of the body. There is evidence that the altered epithelium in the airways also has a decreased ability to defend itself against bacterial pathogens, making it more susceptible to infection (Smith, Travis, Greenberg, & Welsh, 1996). Thickened and infected pulmonary secretions cause obstructive changes in the airways, hyperinflation of the lung parenchyma, and destruction of alveoli.

Diagnosis. The diagnosis of CF can be made by analyzing the amount of chloride found in the sweat of a child. A positive test for CF is a sweat chloride content over 60 mEq/L. The diagnosis of CF can also be made through genetic testing. Genetic testing is considered positive if mutations in the cystic fibrosis transmembrane conductance regulator (CFTR) gene are noted.

Often a diagnostic workup for CF will begin when a child presents with repeat pulmonary infections, especially if the causative agent is either *Staphylococcus aureus* or

Pseudomonas aeruginosa. A newborn with meconium ileus, a small bowel obstruction indicating dysfunction of the digestive system, should also raise suspicions for the diagnosis of CF. The diagnosis of CF may also be considered in children with GI dysfunction and failure to thrive. If one child in a family is diagnosed with CF, all siblings should be tested for the disease.

Management. Improvements in the management of CF have resulted in a life expectancy of 32.5 years. The management of CF crosses many disciplines, including the physician, nutritionist, nurse, physical therapist, respiratory therapist, and social worker. Recent advances in gene-related therapy are offering better targeted treatment at the cellular level.

The primary intent of pulmonary care in children with CF is to prevent, or at least delay, any decline in lung function. Reducing bacterial load, improving secretion clearance, and treating airway inflammation are the mainstays of pulmonary care. Potent antibiotics, often using two or three different drugs to ensure success, may be necessary to treat the gram-negative pulmonary infections that commonly cause an exacerbation of CF. Resistance to antibiotics in the long term versus freedom from infections in the short term is a constant source of controversy concerning antibiotic coverage. The use of aerosolized antibiotics has been successful in decreasing the number of acute exacerbations and improving lung function in children with CF, but there is an increase in resistant organisms to the antibiotics over time, limiting its widespread use (Mukhopadhyay et al., 1995). Aerosolized recombinant DNA (DNase, Pulmozyme) may be helpful in decreasing the viscoelastic properties of airway secretions, making them easier to clear from the tracheobronchial tree (Shah, Scott, Knight, & Hodson, 1996). Aerosolized saline has also been used to enhance clearance of secretions (Eng et al., 1996). Direct treatment of airway inflammation with corticosteroids and ibuprofen has been studied. Although the use of prednisone, a corticosteroid, was shown to be beneficial by the measurement of FEV_1, there were significant growth retardation side effects in the children studied, limiting its incorporation into CF protocols (Nikolaizik & Schonl, 1996; Van Essen-Zandvliet et al., 1992). Inhaled steroids may have fewer systemic side effects and still help in controlling airway inflammation. Individuals with significant pulmonary involvement may be candidates for lung or heart-lung transplants.

The pulmonary management of CF is critical, but the GI component must also be managed. Malabsorption of nutrients caused by pancreatic insufficiency can lead to malnutrition. Fifteen percent of adults with CF are insulin-dependent diabetics, and 75% have glucose intolerance. Poor nutrition has a negative impact on the pulmonary course of the disease (Borowitz, 1996). In fact, malnutrition has been shown to be an independent predictor of mortality (Corey & Farewell, 1996). Nutritional support, including a high-calorie diet and pancreatic enzyme replacement therapy, is often needed to maximize GI function.

Physical therapy intervention for children with CF includes the performance and teaching of secretion removal techniques, an aerobic exercise program as an adjunct to secretion removal and for overall health and fitness, and education concerning medications, environmental controls, compliance with medical care, and benefits of aerobic conditioning. More information on the intervention for a child with CF can be found in the case study on CF in Chapter 19.

Infant Respiratory Distress Syndrome

Infant respiratory distress syndrome (RDS) is a restrictive pulmonary disease that results from inadequate levels of pulmonary surfactant and lung immaturity.

Etiology. Type 2 alveolar cells begin to produce surfactant at about 20 weeks of gestation. Increasing amounts of surfactant are produced each week as gestational age progresses. Surfactant reaches adequate levels 2 weeks before birth. Therefore the incidence of RDS is related to gestational age. Infants with a gestational age of greater than 36 weeks have a 5% incidence of RDS, whereas infants with a gestational age of 26 to 28 weeks have a 75% incidence of RDS (Fishman, 1988). Race, gender, and maternal health, especially maternal diabetes, are also contributing factors in the development of RDS.

Pathophysiology. RDS is associated with inadequate amounts of surfactant in the lungs of a premature infant. Without adequate amounts of surfactant, there is a decrease in lung compliance, an increase in the work of breathing, collapse of airways and respiratory units, and mismatching of ventilation and perfusion. In premature infants, the alveolar wall is thicker and the pulmonary capillary is farther from the alveoli, making diffusion of gas all the more difficult. The resultant hypoxemia and hypoxia may lead to pulmonary vascular constriction and pulmonary hypertension.

Diagnosis. Respiratory distress caused by alveolar collapse in a premature infant is the presenting sign of RDS. Typical signs of RDS include tachypnea, nasal flaring, intercostal and substernal retractions, and cyanosis within 4 hours of birth. Chest radiographs show a typical "ground-glass" pattern, which indicates interstitial involvement.

Management. Infants with RDS are provided with supplemental oxygen to avoid hypoxemia. Intubation and mechanical ventilation are necessary if oxygen therapy alone is not sufficient. Surfactant replacement therapy has been used to prevent and treat infants with RDS. Although surfactant has had a significant positive impact on survival and quality of life for premature infants, chronic lung disease continues to develop in a significant number of premature infants (McColley, 1998). Often these infants are placed on "stress precautions," which act to reduce environmental stimulation including visual, auditory, and tactile stimulation. Necessary procedures are often grouped to minimize the number of disturbances for the infant. Close coordination between nursing staff and other medical team members is helpful in reducing such stress. Physical therapy intervention includes direct care and consultation with nursing to provide positioning suggestions to optimize ventilation and pulmonary perfusion matching, enhance motor development, and improve secretion removal techniques if appropriate.

Bronchopulmonary Dysplasia

Bronchopulmonary dysplasia (BPD) is an obstructive pulmonary disease that is usually considered a sequela of RDS (Northway, Rosan, & Porter, 1967). The clinical definitions of BPD include (1) the need for ventilatory assistance for at least 3 days and the need for supplemental oxygen at 28 days of life (Bancalari, Abdenour, Feller, & Gannon, 1979); (2) the need for supplemental oxygen at 36 weeks gestational age (Bernstein, Heimler, & Sasidhara, 1998); and (3) radiographic abnormalities and chronic ventilation beyond the initial period of RDS (Korhonen, Tammela, Koivisto, Laippala, & Ikonen, 1999).

Etiology. The exact etiology is not precisely understood, but it is related to exposure of immature lung tissue to high concentrations of oxygen, positive pressure mechanical ventilation, inadequate surfactant production, and infection. Pre-eclampsia, low birth weight, rapid birth weight recovery, packed red cell infusions, the presence of a patent ductus arteriosus, hyperoxia, and long duration of ventilator therapy have been correlated with an increased risk of developing BPD (Korhonen et al., 1999).

Pathophysiology. BPD is characterized by inflammation (Hulsmann & Van den Anker, 1997). Acutely this results in persistent hyaline membranes, necrosis of airway, and alveolar epithelium and inflammation. In the subacute phase, there is hypertrophy of bronchial smooth muscle, and parenchymal fibrosis. In the chronic phase, airway remodeling occurs (Hulsmann & Van den Anker, 1997). Infants with BPD may have chronic hypoxemia, often further exacerbated during feeding, crying, and activity. These children are more likely to have feeding disorders, with a resultant poor growth pattern; and are more likely to require rehospitalization within 2 years of discharge from the hospital compared with preterm infants without BPD. When they reach school age, children who had BPD as infants are more likely to have airway obstruction and airway reactivity than their counterparts without BPD (Gross, Iannuzzi, Kveselis, & Anbar, 1998). However, exercise capacity in long-term survivors of BPD did not differ from matched premature infants without BPD, although the children with BPD did use a greater percentage of their ventilatory reserve (Jacob et al., 1997).

Diagnosis. The diagnosis is based on the infant's clinical course and radiographic evidence.

Management. The medical management of BPD consists of surfactant replacement therapy, nutritional support, oxygen and ventilation support, diuretics, steroids, bronchodilators, and/or antibiotics. Physical therapy intervention may include positioning to optimize cardiopulmonary function, secretion removal techniques, and provision of developmental stimulation activities to promote developmentally appropriate activities.

Congenital Structural Abnormalities

Congenital structural abnormalities of the pulmonary and associated systems are relatively uncommon and yet, when they occur, they can cause significant respiratory compromise. Congenital malformations, including pulmonary sequestration, pulmonary agenesis or hypoplasia, diaphragmatic hernias, and tracheoesophageal fistulas, often have significant effects on pulmonary function. See Table 8.2 for details of congenital structural abnormalities.

Immunological Disorders

Pediatric immunological disorders include (1) allergies, such as asthma, (2) autoimmune disease, such as juvenile rheumatoid arthritis (JRA) and systemic lupus erythematosus (SLE), and (3) immunodeficiency disorders, such as

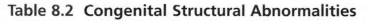

Table 8.2 Congenital Structural Abnormalities

Diagnosis	Definition	Etiology	Impairments of Body Functions and Structures	Potential Activity Limitations and Participation Restrictions	Potential Management
Pulmonary sequestration agenesis hypoplasia	Pulmonary sequestration refers to a portion of the lung that is ventilated but not perfused Pulmonary agenesis or hypoplasia refers to lack of or decreased development of pulmonary tissue	Unknown etiology	• Potential for significant respiratory compromise • Recurrent infection in abnormal lung tissue	• Decreased activity tolerance • Poor growth • Poor feeding • Delay of developmental milestones	• Majority require surgery to either remove abnormal tissue or repair defect in infancy • Physical therapy may include preoperative and postoperative pulmonary care, breathing exercises, positioning for improved ventilation to the affected areas, early intervention to achieve developmental milestones, and parental instruction
Congenital diaphragmatic hernia (CDH)	Incomplete formation and closure of the diaphragm resulting in herniation of abdominal contents into thorax	Unknown etiology Alteration in development between weeks 6–10 of gestation	• Decreased pulmonary formation because thoracic space is occupied by abdominal contents	• Decreased activity tolerance • Poor growth • Poor feeding	• Surgical repair as fetus or neonate
Tracheoesophageal fistula (TEF)	Incomplete separation of the trachea and esophagus	Unknown etiology Alteration in development before 12 weeks gestation	• Impairments in esophageal motility • Impaired tracheal patency • Ventilatory impairments related to aspiration, airway narrowing, and secretions	• Difficulty feeding • Poor growth • Position restrictions (head elevated) to improve esophageal emptying and reduce risk of aspiration. • Tracheomalacia or strictures	• Surgical repair • Positioning to prevent aspiration and to improve gastric absorption • Physical therapy for bronchial hygiene and developmental intervention

HIV/AIDS, and post-transplant immunosuppression. A discussion of asthma is given earlier in this chapter. JRA is a connective tissue disorder more common in the peripheral extremities (ankles, knees, wrists, and elbows), but the shoulder, spine, and thoracic mobility may be affected, which in turn will affect the pulmonary system. SLE is an autoimmune disease that results in inflammation of joints, skin, kidneys, and the pleura, causing pain, poor breathing patterns, and atelectasis. A common cardiopulmonary disorder of the pediatric population with immunocompromise is the presence of opportunistic pulmonary infections, especially *Pneumocystis carinii* pneumonia.

Pathophysiology of Opportunistic Pulmonary Infections. The smaller airway diameter can predispose children to more significant ventilatory impairments during the pulmonary infectious process. Over the short term, acute pulmonary infections can result in increased airway secretions, hypoxemia, and airway inflammation. Chronic infection over the long term can result in destruction of the parenchyma or airway. Infectious and immune disorders can also cause interstitial lung disease, which is covered later in the section on respiration impairments.

Diagnosis of Opportunistic Pulmonary Infections. Signs and symptoms of respiratory distress (e.g., tachypnea, retractions) in combination with clinical signs of respiratory infections and immunocompromise are commonly used for diagnosis. The specific infectious agent can generally be isolated from sputum cultures or throat swabs. Tissue cultures from an open lung biopsy or washings from a bronchoalveolar lavage may need to be obtained to detect the causative agent.

Management. Antimicrobial or antiviral agents, in combination with supportive care as needed (e.g., oxygen, bronchodilators, mechanical ventilation), are the usual courses of treatment during acute infections. Physical therapy interventions may include provision of airway clearance techniques, frequent monitoring of the child's respiratory status, and instructing children in effective coughing and deep breathing exercises, as appropriate for their age. Child and parent education concerning bronchial hygiene programs, environmental controls, and signs and symptoms of infection is important. Any reduction in activity tolerance or delays in development should warrant a physical therapy evaluation.

Musculoskeletal System Impairments

Optimal ventilation relies on a balance between the forces that act on the chest wall and abdomen—the compliance of the musculoskeletal thorax, the strength of the muscles of ventilation, and the compliance of the underlying lung tissue. Arthritis and arthrogryposis of the shoulders or spine can decrease joint ROM and restrict ribcage movement. Primary skeletal processes, such as achondroplasia or osteogenesis imperfecta, that alter the skeletal formation can affect muscle alignment, making the muscles less efficient at generating the necessary forces for ventilation. The following brief description illustrates how musculoskeletal abnormalities can impact cardiopulmonary function.

Thoracic scoliosis, a lateral curvature of the thoracic spine, can alter ribcage movement, resulting in a ventilatory impairment. A thoracic scoliosis results in the rotation of the vertebral bodies. On the side of the concavity, there is decreased costovertebral motion and a decreased intercostal space. On the side of the convexity, the vertebral body rotation causes the ribs to move posteriorly, resulting in the classic posterior rib hump, decreased costovertebral motion, and widening of the intercostal spaces. Thoracic scoliosis, if severe enough, can restrict ventilation and decrease the efficiency of the ventilatory muscles. The lung tissue under a severe concavity is chronically underventilated and may become a source of infection. Changes in skeletal configuration may alter the force-length relationship of the attached muscles, often reducing their effectiveness of force generation.

Interestingly, sternal abnormalities, such as pectus excavatum or pectus carinatum, typically have minimal effects on ventilation (Figure 8–3). Cardiopulmonary physical therapy intervention for these disorders may include thoracic mobility and breathing exercises, positioning to improve ventilation, preoperative and postoperative care, and secretion removal techniques as indicated. More in-depth discussions of musculoskeletal disorders can be found in Chapters 4 and 5.

Neuromuscular System Impairments

Ventilation requires a coordinated interplay between passive forces and active forces generated by muscle contractions. Any alteration in the ability to generate the force of muscle contraction, such as muscular dystrophy, spinal cord injuries, or myelomeningocele, will affect the ability to ventilate. In addition to decreased ventilatory forces, atypical patterns of muscle strength caused by neuromuscular weaknesses can lead to alterations in ribcage and skeletal growth. Pathophysiological processes that result in decreased muscle coordination, such as cerebral palsy (CP) or upper motor neuron lesions, can affect not only extremity and trunk coordination but also respiratory coordination and coughing abilities. A child who has difficulty controlling respiratory muscle force generation and coordinating the timing of respiratory muscle force may present with impaired ventilation, speech, and feeding. Localized and generalized muscle weakness can decrease ventilation in specific lobes or throughout the thorax, depending on the location and degree of weakness. Typically, infants with neuromuscular impairments have healthy pulmonary parenchyma. However, infectious processes, repeated aspiration in individuals with swallowing dysfunction, and atelectasis from hypoventilation can

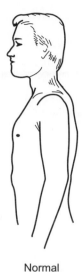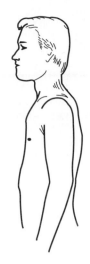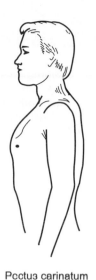

Normal   Pectus excavatum   Pectus carinatum

Figure 8-3 Structural abnormalities of the thoracic cage: Pectus excavatum and pectus carinatum. (Adapted from Swartz, M.H. [1994]. *Textbook of physical diagnoses: History and examination* [2nd ed.]. Philadelphia: W.B. Saunders.)

cause progressive ventilatory impairments. As the child with neuromuscular impairments grows and the disease progresses, movement may become less efficient, the child becomes less physically active, and a decreased exercise and activity tolerance results.

The management of neuromuscular system impairments is discussed in greater depth in Chapters 6 and 7. Cardiopulmonary physical therapy intervention for these disorders may include thoracic mobility and breathing exercises, strengthening of the ventilatory muscles, adaptive seating that optimizes body and thoracic positioning to improve ventilation, providing and teaching assisted coughing techniques, and secretion removal techniques as indicated.

Disorders of Central Respiratory Control

Ventilation requires neural output from brainstem respiratory centers in response to increases in arterial carbon dioxide and decreases in arterial oxygenation. Congenital central hypoventilation syndrome (CHS), and Arnold-Chiari malformation type II are the most commonly encountered disorders of central respiratory control (Pilmer, 1994). Table 8.3 provides details of disorders of central respiratory control.

Integumentary System Impairments

There are relatively few integumentary system impairments that result in significant cardiopulmonary dysfunction in children. Worthy of brief mention is the effect of burns on the cardiopulmonary system. The acute complications from burns are related to infection, dehydration, a decreased ability to thermoregulate the body, decreased aerobic capacity, and issues related to smoke inhalation. Medical management, including skin grafting, skin substitutes, and cultured skin, may be used to close or cover the wounds to improve dehydration and thermoregulation and prevent infection (see Chapter 9). Positioning to improve ventilation-perfusion and splinting to maintain the joint mobility are appropriate. Ventilatory support, with the objective of keeping both airway pressure and oxygen support as low as possible, may be critical to the pulmonary parenchymal outcomes. Aerobic conditioning should begin as soon as the child is able to tolerate activity.

Long-term ventilatory impairments from thoracoabdominal burns may occur secondary to the contraction of scar tissue as well as the outgrowing of the scar tissue during normal growth and development. Physical therapy intervention includes burn care and scar management, as well as thoracic mobility and breathing exercises.

Children with restrictive skin disorders such as juvenile scleroderma can have similar restrictions of their chest wall growth and mobility that may eventually result in ventilatory impairments.

Conditions That Impair Circulation

Circulation is dependent on blood flow, blood volume, vascular resistance, pressure gradients, and the force of

Table 8.3 Disorders of Central Respiratory Control

Diagnosis	Definition	Etiology	Impairments of Body Functions and Structures	Potential Activity Limitations and Participation Restrictions	Potential Management
Congenital central hypoventilation syndrome (CCHS) or "Ondine's curse"	Failure of autonomic control of respiration resulting in decreased output from the brainstem respiratory centers	Unknown, may have a genetic basis	Most likely a defect in CO_2 and O_2 chemoreceptors	• Fatigue • Decreased activity tolerance • Limitations in activity and environmental exploration	• Diaphragmatic pacing • Mechanical ventilation • Physical therapy to promote bronchial hygiene, developmental interventions, or exercise programs for those requiring 24-hour mechanical ventilation. Parental instruction
Arnold-Chiari malformations (type 2)	Cerebellar tonsils descending through the foramen magnum causing brainstem and spinal cord compression	Often associated with myelomeningocele	Apnea, bradycardia, hypoventilation, cyanosis, and breath-holding spells	• Swallowing or feeding difficulties • Irritability	• Surgical decompression of Arnold-Chiari malformation • Mechanical ventilation • Physical therapy may include monitoring respiratory status, and pulmonary hygiene

muscle contraction of the heart. Circulatory defects in children are most often related to congenital cardiovascular structural defects. Congenital heart defects are the most common major birth defects, occurring in approximately 8:1000 live births (Rosenkranz, 1998). The other significant conditions associated with circulatory impairment in children are pediatric myocardial disease, Kawasaki disease, and arrhythmias. Hypertensive disorders and dyslipidemias are less common in children and are not addressed in this chapter.

Cardiovascular Structural Defects

Congenital cardiac defects are structural anomalies that either allow for an alternative route of blood through the cardiopulmonary system or obstruct the usual route of blood flow (Figure 8–4). The new routes for blood flow are called **shunts**. A shunt is termed either a right-to-left shunt or a left-to-right shunt, depending on which way blood is rerouted through the congenital cardiac structural defect. The direction of blood flow through the cardiac structural defect is dictated by the pressure gradient on either side of the defect. A cardiac defect is categorized as a left-to-right shunt when oxygenated blood (left heart blood) does not go out to the periphery but, rather, is returned back to the lungs. A right-to-left shunt occurs when unoxygenated blood (right heart blood) bypasses the lungs and is sent directly out to the systemic circulation. In this section, we will discuss congenital cardiac defects based on three categories: those defects that create a left-to-right shunt, those that create a right-to-left shunt, and those that cause obstruction to the usual route of blood flow.

Etiology. The exact etiology of congenital cardiac defects is unknown. Genetic, environmental, and infectious factors

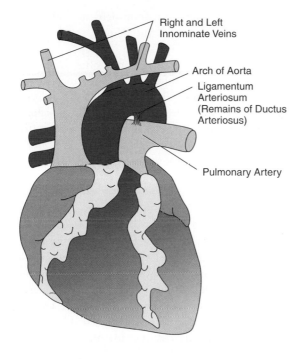

Right and Left
Innominate Veins

Arch of Aorta

Ligamentum
Arteriosum
(Remains of Ductus
Arteriosus)

Pulmonary Artery

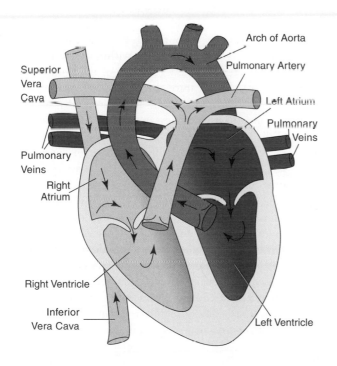

Arch of Aorta

Pulmonary Artery

Superior
Vena
Cava

Left Atrium

Pulmonary
Veins

Pulmonary
Veins

Right
Atrium

Right Ventricle

Inferior
Vena
Cava

Left Ventricle

Figure 8-4 Blood flow through a structurally sound heart. (From Pryor, J., & Prasad, S. [2001]. *Physiotherapy for respiratory and cardiac problems* [3rd ed., p. 445]. Philadelphia: Churchill Livingstone, with permission.)

play various roles in the disruption of the normal cardiac embryological formation. More severe defects are caused by disruption early in the cardiac formation process, whereas less severe defects generally occur later in gestation.

Pathophysiology of Left-to-Right Shunts. Defects that result in left-to-right shunts are sometimes referred to as "acyanotic" defects and include ventricular septal defects, atrial septal defects, and a patent ductus arteriosus.

Ventricular septal defect (VSD) is the term used to describe an opening in the ventricular septum. VSDs account for 20% of congenital cardiac defects and occur in approximately 2.5:1000 live births. A new route for blood to flow, from ventricle to ventricle, is now possible through the opening in the intraventricular septum (Figure 8–5). Given that the pressures in the LV are normally greater than the pressures in the RV, blood flow through a VSD will be from the LV to the RV. This new route of blood will allow already oxygenated blood from the LV to flow back to the RV, back into the pulmonary arteries, and back into the lungs, bypassing the systemic circulation. The amount of blood shunted through a VSD is usually correlated to the severity of symptoms present in the child.

An **atrial septal defect (ASD)** is an opening in the atrial septum, the wall that separates the RA and LA. This defect also results in a left-to-right shunt attributable to the slightly higher pressure within the LA than the RA. The new route for this LA oxygenated blood will be as follows: LA to RA, to the RV, pulmonary artery, and back to the lungs. Typically, ASDs are less symptomatic than VSDs of similar size.

Another common congenital cardiac defect is **patent ductus arteriosus (PDA)**, which occurs in 1:2500 to 5000 live births in full-term infants. Premature infants have an increased incidence of PDA, occurring in approximately 8:1000 live births. The ductus arteriosus is the anatomical communication between the pulmonary artery and the aorta, which is present in fetal circulation. The ductus arteriosus typically closes within the first few days to weeks of a newborn's life, completely separating the aorta from the pulmonary artery. If this channel does not close, that is, the ductus arteriosus remains patent, there is an alternative route for blood flow. The direction of blood flow is dependent on the pressure difference between the ends of the ductus arteriosus. Within the first few minutes after the child's birth, the pressure changes within the heart chambers cause the left heart pressures (LA, LV, and aorta) to be greater than the right heart pressures (RA, RV, and pulmonary artery). Therefore the blood flow through a patent ductus arteriosus after birth will be from the aorta to

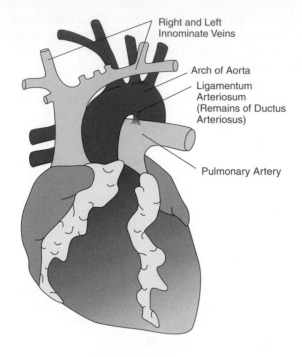

Right and Left
Innominate Veins

Arch of Aorta

Ligamentum
Arteriosum
(Remains of Ductus
Arteriosus)

Pulmonary Artery

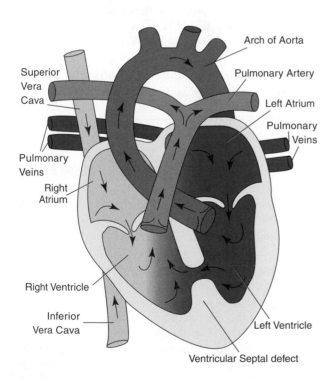

Superior
Vera
Cava

Pulmonary
Veins

Right
Atrium

Right Ventricle

Inferior
Vera Cava

Arch of Aorta

Pulmonary Artery

Left Atrium

Pulmonary
Veins

Left Ventricle

Ventricular Septal defect

Figure 8-5 Ventricular septal defect. (From Pryor, J., & Prasad, S. [2001]. *Physiotherapy for respiratory and cardiac problems* (3rd ed., p. 447). Philadelphia: Churchill Livingstone, with permission.)

the pulmonary artery, or from left to right, causing oxygenated blood to return to the lungs.

Diagnosis. Prenatal ultrasounds can often detect cardiac and great vessel anatomical abnormalities. Postnatal echocardiography and radiological studies can also confirm congenital structural defects. In infancy, suspicion of a cardiac defect may begin with a murmur, either systolic or diastolic, heard on cardiac auscultation. In some cases, when a cardiac murmur is the only sign of a cardiac defect, the physician may choose a "wait and see" approach, as some slight cardiac defects may close with time and with the child's growth. Other cardiac defects are more severe, and the auscultatory findings of a murmur is just one of many signs and symptoms being presented by the child. Infants with severe circulatory impairments are often poor feeders, acting disinterested or requiring prolonged feeding times. These children may also exhibit excessive fatigue, diaphoresis, tachypnea, and dyspnea. The severity of the signs and symptoms is directly related to the severity of the cardiac defect and the amount of blood being shunted.

A child with a left-to-right shunt will have an over-whelmed pulmonary vascular system because a portion of the systemic cardiac output will be returning to the pulmonary capillaries. The pressure within the pulmonary capillaries is increased, causing seepage of fluid out of the pulmonary capillaries into the interstitial space (i.e., congestive heart failure). Signs and symptoms of this increased pulmonary blood flow include crackles on auscultation of the lungs. Arterial oxygen saturation (SaO_2) values may be decreased depending on the extent of congestive heart failure present. Heart rates (HR) may be high. Depending on the extent of respiratory compromise, there may be nasal flaring, intercostal and substernal retractions, and rapid respiratory rate (RR). As a portion of the cardiac output returns to the pulmonary circulation, there is a decreased amount of blood flow systemically. Signs and symptoms of a decreased blood flow to the periphery will be decreased skin temperature; decreased muscle mass, especially in the extremities; decreased energy for crying or playing; decreased endurance for activity including feeding; mottled skin; and delayed motor milestones.

Management. The majority of symptomatic congenital cardiac defects require repair. Repair of cardiac defects is based on the amount of cardiac dysfunction and presenting symptoms. Interventional cardiac catheterization can, in certain instances, repair a PDA by introducing a coil into the ductus arteriosus, thereby closing the vessel. A small ASD or VSD may be sealed by placing a patch (Cardioseal) over the defect via a cardiac catheter. Surgery may be indicated for a more complicated defect repair.

The primary goals in the medical management of children with left-to-right shunts are (1) to reduce the volume of pulmonary circulation that is overloading the system (i.e., reducing congestive heart failure) and (2) to encourage growth.

Physical therapy intervention may include preoperative and postoperative care, positioning to encourage age-appropriate activities with lowered metabolic costs, monitored exercise programs, and aerobic conditioning. Child and family education concerning the prevention of pulmonary infections, use of supplemental oxygen, and exercise guidelines are also areas for intervention.

Pathophysiology: Right-to-Left Shunts

Right-to-left shunts typically result in significant systemic cyanosis as blood flow through the pulmonary system is decreased. Hence, these defects are often referred to as "cyanotic" defects.

Tetralogy of Fallot (TOF) accounts for 50% of all right-to-left shunts. The four cardiac anomalies that make up the tetralogy include (1) a VSD, (2) an impaired pulmonary outlet (a defect such as a stenotic pulmonic valve, a stricture in the pulmonary artery, or a narrowed infundibulum within the RV), (3) a malpositioned aorta (overriding the VSD), and (4) RV hypertrophy (Figure 8–6). As an isolated defect, a VSD is considered a left-to-right cardiac shunt, but in TOF, the pulmonary outflow tract defect is usually severe enough to hinder blood flow out of the RV into the pulmonary circulatory system. The blood volume and therefore pressure within the RV exceed the pressure in the LV. Blood will flow from the RV to the LV through the ventricular septal defect, delivering unoxygenated blood to the periphery. The malpositioned aorta only seems to ease the blood flow from RV blood into the aorta. RV hypertrophy is a result of the increased workload of the RV.

Diagnosis. A child with a right-to-left shunt will have a decreased blood flow through the pulmonary capillaries, resulting in normal pulmonary auscultation findings on physical examination. Although systemic blood flow is adequate in volume, it is inadequate in the amount of oxygen transported. SaO_2 values will be low because some blood has bypassed the lungs, bringing down the overall oxygen content of the blood. Cyanosis may be present. The low oxygen content of the blood may cause decreased muscle mass, especially in the extremities; decreased energy for crying or playing; decreased endurance for activity, including feeding; and delayed motor milestones.

Management. Right-to-left shunts create concerns related to the degree of systemic cyanosis. In infants with severe structural defects, pharmacological management, oxygen therapy, and artificial cardiac assistive devices may be used to support the infant until surgical repair is possible. See Table 8.4 for further details of right-to-left shunt abnormalities.

Pathophysiology of Obstructive Cardiac Defects

Coarctation of the aorta and valvular stenosis are forms of obstructive cardiac defects. Coarctation of the aorta, a stricture or narrowing of the aortic lumen, and valvular stenosis, a narrowing of the cardiac valves, disrupt normal blood flow through the heart or aorta. Pressure build-up behind the narrowing can cause considerable cardiac and vascular compromise. Decreased blood volume beyond the narrowing can result in decreased growth and development. Table 8.5 provides information about obstructive cardiac defects.

Myocardial Disease

Pediatric myocardial disease refers to structural or functional abnormalities of the myocardium that are not secondary to hypertension, pulmonary vascular disease, or valvular or congenital heart disease (Towbin, 1999). This category includes dilated or congestive cardiomyopathies, idiopathic hypertrophic cardiomyopathies, and restrictive cardiomyopathies. The most common cause of acquired heart disease in children is Kawasaki disease, in which vasculitis of the coronary vessels is a predominant feature. Table 8.6 provides details of cardiomyopathy and Kawasaki disease.

Conditions That Impair Respiration

Respiration refers to the diffusion of gases across the alveolar-capillary membrane (Figure 8–7). For respiration to occur, oxygen and carbon dioxide must diffuse across the surfactant layer of the alveoli, the alveolar membrane, the interstitial space, the capillary membrane, the plasma, the red blood cell membrane, and finally into the

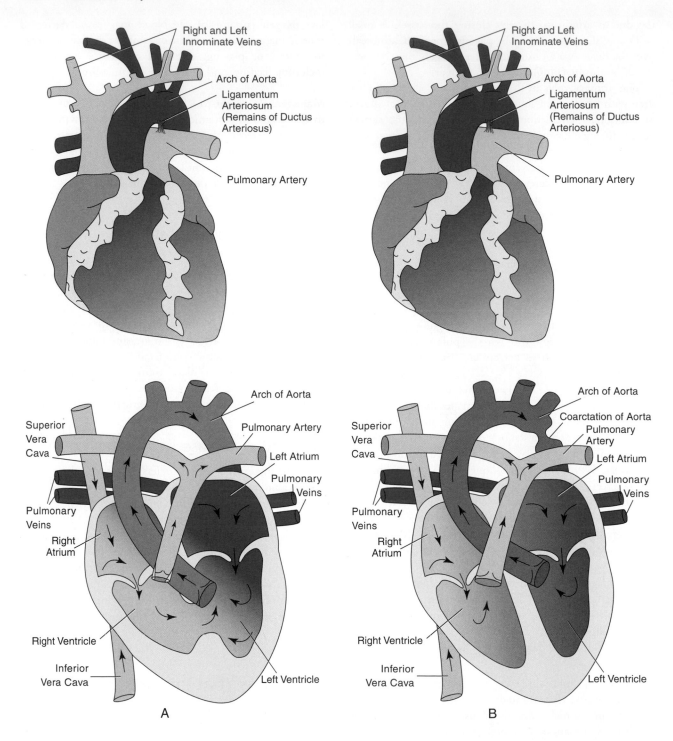

Figure 8-6 (*A*) Tetralogy of Fallot. (*B*) Coarctation of the aorta. (From Pryor, J., & Prasad, S. [2001]. *Physiotherapy for respiratory and cardiac problems* (3rd ed., p. 447). Philadelphia: Churchill Livingstone, with permission.)

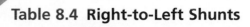

Table 8.4 Right-to-Left Shunts

Diagnosis	Definition	Etiology	Impairments of Body Functions and Structures	Potential Activity Limitations and Participation Restrictions	Potential Management
Tricuspid atresia	Dysfunctional tricuspid valve in the right atrioventricular septum	Unknown etiology	Blood from right atrium cannot flow through tricuspid valve to the right ventricle; therefore must go through the foramen ovale into left atria. Low oxygen saturation	• Poor growth • Poor feeding • Decreased activity tolerance	• Surgical palliation or correction • Physical therapy for pre/postoperative care, early intervention to encourage development, exercise programs, and parental instruction
Truncus arteriosus	A combined pulmonary artery and aorta, commonly with a ventricular septal defect	Unknown etiology	The aorta and pulmonary artery fail to separate, carrying both oxygenated and unoxygenated blood. Hypoxemia	• Poor growth • Poor feeding • Decreased activity tolerance	• Early (younger than 6 months) surgical repair (Grifka, 1999) • Physical therapy for pre/postoperative care, early intervention, and parental instruction
Transposition of great arteries (TGA)	Aorta arises from right ventricle, pulmonary artery from the left ventricle or from the (double outlet) right ventricle	Unknown etiology	Unoxygenated blood is pumped from the right ventricle to systemic circulation. Oxygenated blood returns to the lungs	• Defect is not compatible with life, so surgical palliation as neonate is necessary	• Medical management to pharmacologically maintain a patent ductus arteriosus until surgery is possible • Early surgical correction via arterial switch • Physical therapy for pre/postoperative care, early intervention, and parental instruction
Total anomalous pulmonary venous return (TAPVR)	Pulmonary venous blood returns to the right atrium or systemic veins rather than to left atrium	Unknown etiology	Increased blood return to right atrium with right-sided hypertrophy and increased volume through pulmonary system. An ASD, when present, is the only means for entry to the left atrium. Hypoxemia.	• Poor growth • Poor feeding • Decreased activity tolerance	• Surgical correction in infancy by anastomosis of pulmonary veins to left atrium • Postoperatively may have difficulty with ventilation secondary to stiff, wet lungs from the earlier hyperperfusion caused by defect
Hypoplastic left heart syndrome (HLHS)	Hypoplasia or absence of a left ventricle and hypoplasia of the ascending aorta	Unknown etiology	Initially, PDA may allow adequate systemic blood flow. As PDA closes, systemic flow decreases. Hypoxemia	• Poor growth • Poor feeding • Decreased activity tolerance	• Fatal within first month of life if untreated (Fedderly, 1999). Medical management: supportive care • Multi-stage reconstruction of the heart or cardiac transplantation

Table 8.5 Obstructive Cardiac Diseases

Diagnosis	Definition	Etiology	Impairments of Body Functions and Structures	Potential Activity Limitations and Participation Restrictions	Potential Management
Coarctation of the aorta	Stricture, or narrowing, of the aortic lumen, usually at or near site of the ductus arteriosus Increased pressure proximal to the coarctation and decreased distal pressure	Unknown etiology	Significant differences in pulse intensities and blood pressures are found between upper and lower extremities. Increased proximal pressure impedes left ventricular ejection, leading to congestive heart failure and an increased risk for intracranial hemorrhages.	• The decreased distal pressure results in lower extremity changes • Decreased skin temperature • Delayed growth and development • Decreased exercise tolerance • Increased activity can further increase existing hypertension, necessitating a stress test before participation in an exercise program.	• Surgical repair optimal, between 3 to 10 years of age, reduces the incidence of residual hypertension and associated morbidity and mortality (Fedderly, 1999). • Cardiac stent may be used to enlarge some strictures. • Larger and more complex defects require surgical repair which may be staged over months or years to accommodate growth related changes in the cardiac system. • Early surgical correction allows for more normal growth and development, but an increased risk of recurrent stenosis (Toro-Salazar et al., 2002).
Aortic or pulmonary stenosis	Aortic or pulmonary valvular stenoses cause obstruction of blood flow from the respective ventricle.	Unknown etiology	Involved ventricle will hypertrophy in response to resistance provided by the valve's defect.	• With growth, involved ventricle may fail to meet demands of activity, decreasing activity tolerance.	• Surgical repair or replacement of valve according to severity of symptoms. • Physical therapy for pre/postoperative care, early intervention, and parental instruction.

hemoglobin in the red blood cell. Conditions that increase the diffusion distance by widening any of these layers, or otherwise impair gas exchange, will hinder respiration. The most common pediatric conditions that impair respiration are interstitial lung diseases and congestive heart failure. Sickle cell anemia also affects respiration, as well as circulation, by hindering oxygen bonding to hemoglobin and causing vaso-occlusion. Table 8.7 provides details of interstitial lung disease, congestive heart failure, and sickle cell anemia.

Examination and Evaluation

Tests and measurements of the cardiopulmonary system are outlined in the *Guide* (APTA, 2001). Many of the measurements used with adults who have cardiopulmonary dysfunction can, with some modifications in implementation and interpretation, be used when examining infants and children with cardiopulmonary dysfunction. Specialized equipment is needed to obtain accurate measurement, such as smaller pediatric stethoscopes, SaO_2

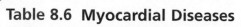

Table 8.6 Myocardial Diseases

Diagnosis	Definition	Etiology	Impairments of Body Functions and Structures	Potential Activity Limitations and Participation Restrictions	Potential Management

Dilated cardiomyopathy	Biventricular dilation with loss of systolic contraction, resulting in congestive heart failure. Atrioventricular valves may be unable to fully close during systole secondary to ventricular dilation.	Unknown etiology	• Typically presents with symptoms of congestive heart failure
			  • Systolic heart murmur
			  • Fatigue
			  • Chest pain
			  • Syncope
			  • Impaired consciousness
			• Limitations associated with circulatory impairments
			  • Tachypnea
			  • Diaphoresis
			  • Poor peripheral circulation
			  • Cyanosis
				• Failure to thrive
				• Poor feeding
				• Decreased activity tolerance
					• Medical management in myocardial disease is to pharmacologically optimize cardiac function, control associated arrhythmias, and minimize risk of thromboembolism. Antibiotic prophylaxis can be important to prevent bacterial endocarditis.
					• Surgery may be indicated in children with left ventricular outflow obstruction to relieve the obstruction.
					• In children for whom medical therapy has failed, heart transplantation may be an option.
					• Physical therapy to reduce secondary complications associated with progressive congestive heart failure and deconditioning. Parental instruction.

Hypertrophic cardiomyopathy	Hypertrophy of the myocardium and intraventricular septum. Chamber size is lessened limiting preload and reducing cardiac output.	Unknown etiology	• Typical complications are:
			  • Arrhythmias
			  • Hypertrophied septum and ventricular wall obstructs blood flow to aorta.
			  • Sudden death		

(Continued)

Table 8.6 Myocardial Diseases (Continued)

Diagnosis	Definition	Etiology	Impairments of Body Functions and Structures	Potential Activity Limitations and Participation Restrictions	Potential Management
Restrictive cardiomyopathy	Restrictive cardiomyopathy results from an abnormal relaxation phase of the ventricle.	Unknown etiology	• Ventricles cannot accept atrial blood volume, resulting in atrial dilation and decreased cardiac output. • Complications related to congestive heart failure and formation of thrombus		
Kawasaki disease	Vasculitis of coronary vessels in children between ages 6 months and 4 years. Resolution within 6 to 8 weeks of onset. May result in aneurysms and coronary artery disease.	Unknown etiology May be response to infectious exposure	• Massive myocardial infarction secondary to coronary thrombosis during weeks 3 to 4 of illness (Rowley & Shulman, 1999) • Myocardial infarction symptoms may include shock, vomiting, and unrest rather than chest pain.	• Activity restriction during acute illness • Decreased activity tolerance with significant cardiac involvement	• Pharmacological support including intravenous gamma globulin and aspirin in children with cardiac manifestations • Precautions for competitive contact athletics or endurance training are followed. • Stress tests may be necessary for those with resultant cardiac manifestations before participation in exercise programs.

sensors, and blood pressure cuffs. Inherent in all pediatric practice is the effect of age on the ability to communicate, follow commands, and remain attentive to physical therapy examination and intervention. In this section, history, systems review, tests and measures, laboratory tests, and exercise testing are described.

History

Interviewing a child should yield information not only from the child but also from parents, guardians, or other caregivers. The information obtained from an interview includes demographics (age, primary language, race/ethnicity, and gender), social history (family culture, resources, social interactions, and support services), growth and development history (gestational age at birth, labor, delivery, and neonatal events), and details of the living environment (e.g., home, school, daycare). A history of present illness, past medical and surgical history, present medications, and pertinent family history can be obtained with help from a parent or guardian as described in Chapter 2. Activity level can be determined by watching the child play during the interview and by asking questions concerning

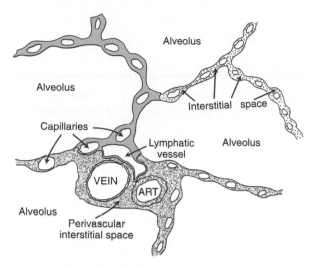

Figure 8-7 Alveolar capillary membrane. (From Guyton, A. [1996]. *Textbook of medical physiology* [9th ed., p. 487]. Philadelphia: W.B. Saunders.)

the child's participation in physical activity, such as feeding, crying, playing, amount of time napping, age at acquisition of motor milestones, and preferred activities. In infants, prolonged feeding times, increased sleeping, or irritability can be symptoms of cardiopulmonary dysfunction. Children with cardiopulmonary compromise may demonstrate age-appropriate fine motor skills but delays in gross motor skills caused by energy constraints. In children with cardiopulmonary impairments, determining the parents' or caregiver's perception of their child's activities of daily life can also provide important information regarding their comfort with the child's participation in physical activities. Parents or caregivers may place limits on their child's activity, partly because of their own apprehension rather than physical restrictions related to the actual cardiopulmonary impairment. The interview process should be performed with the child in view, allowing for an initial observation of the child.

Table 8.7 Conditions That Impair Respiration

Diagnosis	Definition	Etiology	Impairments of Body Functions and Structures	Potential Activity Limitations and Participation Restrictions	Potential Management
Interstitial lung disease	Chronic inflammation of alveolar walls, small airways, arteries, and veins. More peripheral regions of the lungs are generally affected (Bokulic & Hilman, 1994)	Results from infection (e.g., HIV, RSV, CMV), environmental inhalants or toxins (e.g., talcum powder, chlorine, ammonia), treatment induced (e.g., antineoplastic drugs, radiation therapy), neoplastic diseases, metabolic disorders, collagen vascular disease, and neurocutaneous syndromes	• Disruption of alveolar capillary structures leads to pulmonary fibrosis. • Common respiratory symptoms are dyspnea, tachypnea with intercostal and subcostal retractions, nonproductive cough, fatigue, and pleuritic chest pain.	• Decreased growth • Decreased activity tolerance	• Corticosteroids and immunosuppressive agents used to reduce inflammation • Oxygen, nutritional support, and avoidance of environmental exposures • Surgical management is lung transplantation.

(Continued)

Table 8.7 Conditions That Impair Respiration *(Continued)*

Diagnosis	Definition	Etiology	Impairments of Body Functions and Structures	Potential Activity Limitations and Participation Restrictions	Potential Management

Congestive heart failure (CHF)	Inability of the heart to advance blood through cardiac chambers, resulting in congestion of pulmonary and/or systemic circulation	Caused by a
		• Congenital left-to-right cardiac defect
		• Obstruction to left ventricular outflow
		• Cardiomyopathy
		• Chronic restrictive lung disease
			• Clinical signs include:
			  • Tachycardia
			  • Tachypnea
			  • Arrhythmias
			  • Ventricular dilatation
			  • Hepatomegaly
			  • Peripheral and/or pulmonary edema
			  • Poor peripheral perfusion
				In infants
				• Poor feeding
				• Lethargy
				• Respiratory tract infections
				In older children
				• Decreased activity tolerance
				• Abdominal distention or pain
					• Surgical correction of causative cardiac defects
					• Medical treatment includes oxygen and pharmacology to increase myocardial contractility and decrease afterload.
					• Physical therapy may include maintenance of pulmonary hygiene, developmental stimulation, aerobic exercise training, and parental instruction.

Sickle cell anemia	Mutation in hemoglobin that causes a distortion or "sickling" of red blood cell. "Sickled cells" reduce life span of the red blood cell as well as causing vaso-occlusion.	Sickle cell anemia is a genetically inherited disorder seen primarily in individuals of African descent. Diagnosis can be made through neonatal screening or genetic testing.	• Primary presentation is pain • Ischemia • Acute chest syndrome: new pulmonary infiltrate, fever, cough, sputum production, dyspnea, hypoxia, and pain • With repeated acute chest syndrome, restrictive lung disease, pulmonary hypertension, and CHF (Lane, 1996)	• Decreased activity tolerance	• Medical management of acute chest syndrome includes oxygen, pain medication, and intravenous hydration. • Physical therapy directed at improving aeration using airway clearance techniques and breathing exercises during acute episodes

Systems Review

General Observation and Palpation

From observing the general appearance of a child, the examiner can garner important information. Initial observation of posture, breathing patterns, and comfort during play activities can provide insight into cardiopulmonary status.

The child's chosen posture may have cardiopulmonary implications. For example, a child whose preferred positioning is supported sitting may have learned the skill of rationing limited energy. Less energy expended for maintaining the upright position means more energy for other

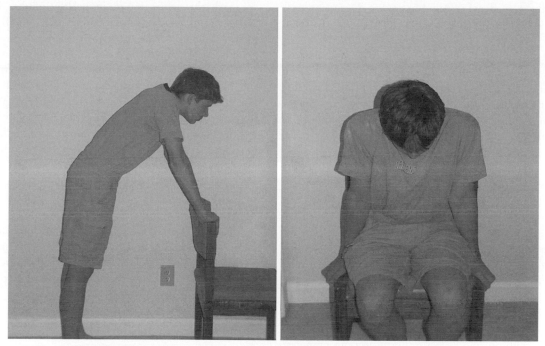

Figure 8-8 Positioning of the upper extremities to assist with ventilation.

tasks. Positions may also be chosen that allow muscles to be used primarily for ventilation rather than posture maintenance. Sitting with upper extremities fixed, supporting the shoulder girdle, allows neck and upper extremity muscles to be used as accessory muscles of ventilation (Figure 8–8). Sleeping in supine position with full shoulder flexion helps elevate the upper chest to assist with breathing. Alterations in speech patterns as a result of breathlessness or changes of position to support speech patterns should be noted.

Skin color can show cyanosis, a sign of acute tissue hypoxia. The bluish-gray skin color of cyanosis is commonly seen about the mouth, eyes, fingertips, and toes. If tissue hypoxia is severe enough, it is also possible to see cyanosis throughout the body. As the oxygenation to the tissues improves, the color change reverses, returning the child to a more normal skin tone. Cyanosis is more difficult to observe in individuals with darker skin tones. Other integumentary changes may include mottling of the skin, common in infants and children with decreased blood flow to the extremities. Children with cyanotic cardiac disease or congestive heart failure may appear diaphoretic, with cool, moist skin. Clubbing of the fingertips may be noted in individuals with chronic peripheral cyanosis (e.g., right-to-left cardiac shunts, CF) (Figure 8–9).

Peripheral edema is often associated with heart or liver

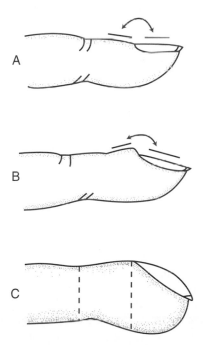

Figure 8–9 Clubbing of the digits. (*A*) Normal. (*B*) Early clubbing with angle present between nail and proximal skin. (*C*) Advanced clubbing. (Reprinted from: Clinical Assessment in Respiratory Care, Wilkins, RL and Drider, SJ (1985), with permission from Elsevier.)

disease. Because edema is found in gravity-dependent areas of the body, edema in an infant may be found on the skull, the back, or posterior aspects of lower extremities.

General muscular development and amount of adipose tissue in the extremities should also be observed. Children may exhibit poor muscle development and lack of adipose tissue for a number of reasons, including prematurity, poor nutrition from a reduced energy to feed, inadequate oxygenation to the extremities, or decreased absorption of calories.

The observed breathing pattern of a young healthy infant is not the coordinated, symmetrical pattern one expects in an older child. The RR of the infant is faster, the tidal volume changes from breath to breath, and there is no rhythmical pattern of breathing or a repeating ratio of inspiratory to expiratory time. Overall, the breathing pattern of an infant is typically uncoordinated and unpredictable. Observation of thoracoabdominal movement and the relative timing of inspiration to expiration should be noted.

During periods of respiratory compromise, nostril flaring, head bobbing, and expiratory grunting can be noted. Significant intercostal, substernal, and subclavicular retractions may also be seen in infants, attributable to the compliant ribcage, lack of accessory muscle fixation, and smaller airways.

Tests and Measurements

Vital Signs

Measurement of vital signs in children includes HR, RR, blood pressure (BP), oxygen saturation of arterial blood (SaO$_2$), and temperature. Body length and weight and extremity pulses can also provide useful information concerning cardiopulmonary function. Higher resting HRs are encountered in healthy children, and a rate that would be considered tachycardic in adults is normal for infants and small children. During periods of high stress, a child's HR can be as high as 180, 190, or even 200 beats per minute. Heart rhythm can be measured through cardiac auscultation, palpation of pulses, or electrocardiography (ECG). Children also have high RR to compensate for the low tidal volumes of the smaller and less compliant thorax. As the pattern of breathing of a child is erratic, RR should be counted for an entire minute to obtain an accurate reporting of breaths per minute. Lower BP in children is partly attributable to the lowered peripheral vascular resistance secondary to shorter blood vessels. As the child grows and develops into adolescence, the vital sign measurements

approach the values found in healthy adults. Table 8.8 compares the expected healthy HR, BP, and RR for an infant, child, and adult.

Serial measurements of length and weight of a child are important. Adequate nutritional intake, nutrient absorption by the GI system, and nutrient delivery to the body by the circulatory system are necessary for healthy growth and weight gain. Lung growth is directly related to overall body length. Children with cardiopulmonary dysfunction should have their height and weight measured periodically and mapped against the normative height and weight charts (see Figure 2–3 in Chapter 2). Any change from the expected will be demonstrated and appropriate follow-up can be suggested.

Palpation of extremity pulses can be helpful in children with cardiac dysfunction. Decreased extremity pulses may indicate decreased blood flow to the extremities. Differences in upper extremity versus lower extremity pulses may indicate obstruction to blood flow, as occurs in coarctation of the aorta, or a change in pulses with stress may indicate cardiac dysfunction.

Auscultation

Because the child's cardiac and pulmonary systems are structurally similar to those of an adult, the same auscultation procedures can be followed. Infants and younger children may have difficulty following commands to breathe in and out for pulmonary auscultation. Asking young children to blow at a tissue or at pretend birthday candles during auscultation may provide deeper breaths and more accurate results. The presence and intensity of pulmonary adventitious sounds (e.g., crackles and wheezes) as well as abnormal cardiac sounds (e.g., murmurs) must be documented. Transmission of abdominal sounds is greater in children because of their smaller size. Warming of the stethoscope's

Table 8.8 Comparison of Vital Signs Between Children and Adults

Vital Signs	Infant	Child	Adult
Heart rate (bpm)	100 to 140	80 to 120	60 to 100
Blood pressure (mm Hg)	80/40	100/60	120/80
Respiratory rate	30 to 40	25 to 30	12 to 18

head and allowing the child to hold or play with the stethoscope before auscultation can decrease apprehension.

Range of Motion

ROM of the upper extremities and chest wall excursion should be measured. Because the infant cannot follow the usual commands to measure thoracic excursion, following the infant's respiratory cycle with the therapist's hands in contact with the child's ribcage can be helpful. Exaggerating the exhalation phase of the child's breath with manual pressure will lead to a greater inhalation on the child's next breath, allowing for a more complete evaluation of thoracic mobility. Thoracic symmetry can be assessed at the same time. Observation of any skeletal chest wall abnormalities should be noted.

Laboratory Studies

Children with cardiopulmonary dysfunction routinely have multiple laboratory tests to assess cardiac and pulmonary status. The physical therapist must be able to integrate the information from multiple laboratory studies into the intervention planning and execution.

Radiology

Radiological laboratory studies are used to define structural and parenchymal abnormalities. Chest radiography, computed tomography (CT) scanning, and magnetic resonance imaging (MRI) can be used to evaluate heart size, amount of pulmonary blood flow, and pulmonary infiltrates or atelectasis. The areas of infiltration identified will direct the physical therapist to the segments of the lung needing intervention. A child's chest radiograph may also demonstrate the alignment of ribs, the amount of ossification of ribs and vertebrae, and the level of the diaphragm.

An echocardiogram uses sound waves to produce a computer-generated picture of the heart. A transthoracic, transesophageal, or even fetal echocardiogram can be performed to look at the structure within the heart. Valvular stenosis or incompetence or congenital defects can be seen and recorded using an echocardiogram.

Right- and left-side heart catheterization can also be used to determine cardiac structural defects in children. A catheter is introduced into the venous system, through which dye is injected to view the right heart. A catheter can be inserted into the arterial system, through which a dye is injected to evaluate the left side of the heart.

Electrocardiography

ECG is performed and interpreted with results normalized for the differences in body size and cardiovascular maturation. Electrocardiographic differences exist between premature infants, newborns, and older children (Park & Guntheroth, 1992). In the full-term newborn, RV mass exceeds LV mass because of the stresses put on these structures during fetal circulation. At birth, as the pulmonary vascular resistance begins to drop and the systemic resistance rises, there is a shift in the relative size of the RV and LV by about 1 month of age. Not surprisingly, there is a reflection of this morphology in the ECG. The full-term newborn's ECG shows an RV dominance that, over a month or so, changes to a more adult LV dominance appearance. The premature infant may not show an RV dominance because the RV did not have the time to increase its mass before birth. With increasing age, the HR decreases and the duration of intervals (PR interval, QRS duration, QT interval) and voltages all increase.

Arterial Blood Gases

Infants have slightly different baseline values for PaO_2, but the interpretation of arterial blood gas values remains the same as in the adult (Table 8.9). Infants with obstructive pulmonary disorders, such as BPD, will demonstrate decreased PaO_2 and increased $PaCO_2$ values. Children with an unrepaired congenital cardiac defect causing a right-to-left shunt will have altered arterial blood gas values, especially a decrease in the PaO_2. It is interesting to note that this lower PaO_2 will not readily respond to supplemental oxygen. Because the blood is bypassing the lungs, more supplemental oxygen to the lungs does not necessarily mean higher PaO_2 values.

Table 8.9 Comparison of Arterial Blood Gas Values of Children and Adults

Value	Infant	Child	Adult
pH	7.35 to 7.45	7.35 to 7.45	7.35 to 7.45
PaO_2	50 to 70	80 to 100	95 to 100
$PaCO_2$	35 to 45	35 to 45	35 to 45
HCO_3^-	22 to 26	22 to 26	22 to 26

Pulmonary Function Tests

Pulmonary function tests are effort-dependent and there-fore require full cooperation of the child. Children who are able to follow commands and control their breathing patterns, often by 6 to 8 years of age, can perform them. Interpretation of the tests must be normalized for body size. Modifications of testing procedures, such as the perform-ance of only certain tests, can make testing possible in younger children. The use of specialized equipment, found predominantly in specialized pediatric pulmonary centers, can make pulmonary function testing possible even in very young children.

Ventilation-Perfusion Scans

Ventilation-perfusion scans are performed to assess the matching of ventilation to perfusion within the lungs, which is helpful in children with cardiac and pulmonary abnormalities. The performance of this test, and interpreta-tion of the results, must take into account the more compli-ant ribcage, and physical maturation, of the child. The results of this test may be helpful in choosing body posi-tions that optimize ventilation and perfusion matching for a child's daily positioning schedule.

Exercise Testing

Exercise testing in children yields information about the cardiopulmonary system (HR, BP, RR, breathing pattern, and oxygen saturation) during different workloads. The results of the exercise test allow a physical therapist to opti-mally prescribe exercise. Exercise and activity tolerance can be assessed at all ages, although different modes of exercise may be used. For infants and children under 3 years of age, "formal" exercise tests are not performed. Activity tolerance in infants and very young children can be assessed during crying, feeding, and play activities. Children older than 3 years of age can perform submaximal treadmill and stair exercise tolerance protocols (Darbee & Cerny, 1995). A more accurate measure of workload can be obtained if the treadmill or stair rails are not used for support, but close supervision is necessary to prevent loss of balance. Children older than 6 years of age can participate in standardized exercise test protocols, with the ergometer workload or treadmill speed adjusted for the motor skill level. Exercise test termination criteria are similar to those used in the adult population. Although the body of literature on pedi-atric exercise testing is growing, children typically serve as their own controls because normative data still need to be developed (Cerny, 1989). The saturation of oxygen in the

arterial blood (SaO_2) should be monitored in any one who has an FEV_1 of less than 50% predicted. If there is evidence of exercise hypoxemia during a graded exercise test, a submaximal steady state test, such as a 6- or 12-minute walk test, should be performed. Sustained submaximal exercise can show a greater change in SaO_2 values than a graded test might provide (Nixon, 2003).

In addition to exercise testing, measures of physical fitness that emphasize health-related fitness components are available. The American Alliance for Health, Physical Education, Recreation and Dance (AAHPERD, 1999), Presidential Physical Fitness Program, and National Child and Youth Fitness Study are common measures of physical fitness in children (Stout & Taber, 1995).

Physical Therapy Intervention

Physical therapy intervention for the child with impair-ments of cardiopulmonary structures and functions, and restrictions in activities and participation, requires a balance between the effects of short-term intervention and long-term outcomes. Children with chronic or progressive cardiopulmonary disorders may require physical therapy intervention for a lifetime. Teaching family and other care-givers how to provide long-term maintenance care should be integrated into the treatment framework from the begin-ning. As the child matures, physical therapy intervention should include methods for more independent physical therapy. The inclusion of mechanical aids and independent exercise programs allows the child with cardiopulmonary impairments to be more independent in and responsible for his or her own care. Physical therapy intervention includes the child's social, family, and medical well-being, in terms of both the immediate needs of a child during an acute illness and activities to promote the long-term development of cardiopulmonary health and functional abilities. In this section, intervention of airway clearance techniques, breathing exercises, and the prescription of aerobic exercise are discussed.

Airway Clearance Techniques

Airway clearance techniques are indicated for the child with retained secretions that obstruct or limit airflow. Improving secretion clearance can take many forms. A daily regimen of the manual secretion removal techniques of postural drainage, percussion, and shaking is the standard management for retained secretions. Other forms of secretion removal techniques—active cycle of breathing, autogenic drainage, positive expiratory pressure, and chest wall oscillation devices—can be instituted if and when the child is ready to become more independent in his or her care. The following is a brief description of each airway clearance technique.

Manual Secretion Removal Techniques

Postural drainage is a term used to identify specific body positions that enlist gravity to drain secretions from a segment of the lung. Manual secretion removal techniques include the use of percussion and shaking in the appropriate postural drainage position to enhance mucociliary clearance of excessive secretions. This combination of techniques requires a caregiver to perform the techniques on the child. It is commonly used with infants, young children, and children who cannot participate in a more independent method of secretion removal.

Optimal body positions used for postural drainage of each lung segment are shown in Figure 8–10. The drainage positions chosen for a treatment session depend on the site of pathology. A child with right middle lobe syndrome will use the position for the right middle lobe only, whereas a child with CF who has involvement of the entire pulmonary system will use all postural drainage positions during the treatment session. The amount of time each body position is maintained is again dependent on the pathology being treated. From 5 to 20 minutes per position is customary, although gravity drainage positions can be incorporated into a child's positioning schedule and therefore maintained for up to 2 hours.

Postural drainage positions can also be useful in improving ventilation. As this technique places a lung segment in a gravity-independent position, improved ventilation to that lung segment is possible. Continual evaluation of the tolerance to positioning is essential. The prone position has been shown to increase oxygenation levels; however, sleeping in the prone position has been associated with an increased risk of sudden infant death syndrome (SIDS). The head of the bed flat and the head down (Trendelenburg) position also requires certain considerations. Children at risk for intraventricular hemorrhage or with acute head injuries may show an increase in their intracranial pressure with the head of the bed flat or in the Trendelenburg position. Acceptable ranges of intracranial pressures should be clear before attempting positioning in this population. Trendelenburg positioning has, in some

instances, been shown to decrease oxygen saturation levels, making it necessary to identify acceptable ranges for SaO_2 before using these positions (Thorensen, Cavan, & Whitelaw, 1988). Gastroesophageal reflux is not necessarily a contraindication for postural drainage in the Trendelenburg position. Rather, physical therapy interventions should be planned around the child's feeding schedule, so that feeding occurs at least 90 minutes before postural drainage. Estimates of the presence of gastroesophageal reflux in premature infants are as high as 80% (Newell, Booth, Morgan, Durbin, & McNeish,1989). Therefore timing postural drainage treatments around feeding schedules is recommended for all premature infants. Special consideration to the child's positioning can be a simple but effective treatment technique.

Percussion is a force applied to the child's thorax by the caregiver's cupped hand to dislodge secretions within the airways, facilitating airway clearance (Figure 8–11). Performance of the technique in the neonate may require tenting of the therapist's fingers, as the therapist's whole hand may be too large. With the child in the appropriate postural drainage position, the percussive force is applied to the area of the thorax related to the lung segment being treated. The customary time frame for percussion is between 2 and 5 minutes, although the time frame should be modified to the child's needs and tolerance. Consideration of the use of percussion as a technique for secretion removal must be weighed against possible untoward outcomes. Children who are experiencing pain, such as during the postoperative period, or after sustaining a trauma may need to be adequately medicated before the intervention. Conditions such as hemoptysis, osteoporosis, coagulation disorders, fractured ribs, stress precautions, and fragile hemodynamics may require modification in or negation of the use of this technique.

A bouncing or vibratory force applied to the thorax during exhalation to enhance the normal mucociliary transport of airway secretions toward the glottis for final removal is called **shaking** (Figure 8–12). The child is asked to take in a deep breath. As the child exhales, the therapist follows the expiratory movement of the thorax with an intermittent manual force, or "bounce." The high RR of an infant and the inability to follow commands can make shaking difficult to perform. Coordination with the infant's respiratory pattern is essential. The increased compliance of the thorax of an infant makes it difficult to determine how much of the external force from shaking is being translated to the underlying lung. The use of five to seven exhalations for shaking is customary. Precautions for use of the shaking technique are similar to those for percussion.

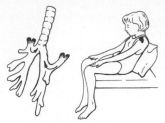

UPPER LOBES Apical Segments

Bed or drainage table flat.

Patient leans back on pillow at 30° angle against therapist.

Therapist claps with markedly cupped hand over area between clavicle and top of scapula on each side.

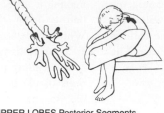

UPPER LOBES Posterior Segments

Bed or drainage table flat.

Patient leans over folded pillow at 30° angle.

Therapist stands behind and claps over upper back on both sides.

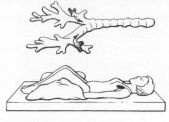

UPPER LOBES Anterior Segments

Bed or drainage table flat.

Patient lies on back with pillow under knees.

Therapist claps between clavicle and nipple on each side.

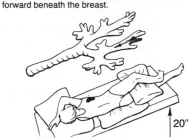

16"

RIGHT MIDDLE LOBE

Foot of table or bed elevated 16 inches.

Patient lies head down on left side and rotates ¼ turn backward. Pillow may be placed behind from shoulder to hip. Knees should be flexed.

Therapist claps over right nipple area. In females with breast development or tenderness, use cupped hand with heel of hand under armpit and fingers extending forward beneath the breast.

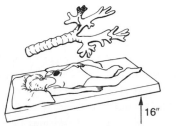

16"

LEFT UPPER LOBE Lingular Segments

Foot of table or bed elevated 16 inches.

Patient lies head down on right side and rotates ¼ turn backward. Pillow may be placed behind from shoulder to hip. Knees should be flexed.

Therapist claps with moderately cupped hand over left nipple area. In females with breast development or tenderness, use cupped hand with heel of hand under armpit and fingers extending forward beneath the breast.

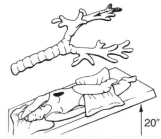

20"

LOWER LOBES Anterior Basal Segments

Foot of table or bed elevated 20 inches.

Patient lies on side, head down, pillow under knees.

Therapist claps with slightly cupped hand over lower ribs. (Position shown is for drainage of <u>left</u> anterior basal segment. To drain the right anterior basal segment, patient should lie on his or her left side in same posture).

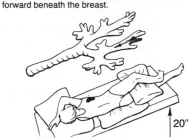

20"

LOWER LOBES Lateral Basal Segments

Foot of table or bed elevated 20 inches.

Patient lies on abdomen, head down, then rotates ¼ turn upward. Upper leg is flexed over a pillow for support.

Therapist claps over uppermost portion of lower ribs. (Position shown is for drainage of right lateral basal segment. To drain the left lateral basal segment, patient should lie on his or her right side in the same posture).

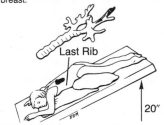

Last Rib

20"

LOWER LOBES Posterior Basal Segments

Foot of table or bed elevated 20 inches.

Patient lies on abdomen, head down, with pillow under hips. Therapist claps over lower ribs close to spine on each side.

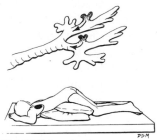

LOWER LOBES Superior Segments

Bed or table flat.

Patient lies on abdomen with two pillows under hips.

Therapist claps over middle of back at tip of scapula on either side of spine.

Figure 8-10 Postural drainage positions for lung segments. (From *The rehabilitation specialist's handbook* (2nd ed., pp. 534–534), by J.M.Rothstein, S.H.Roy, and S.L.Wolf, 1998, Philadelphia: F. A. Davis. Reprinted with permission.)

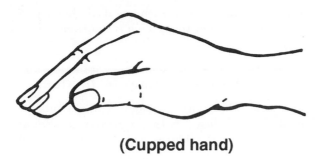

(Cupped hand)

Figure 8-11 Hand position for the technique of percussion. (From National Cystic Fibrosis Foundation, Courtesy of Bettina C. Hilman, MD. From *Cardiopulmonary rehabilitation: Basic therapy and application* (p. 427), by F.J. Brannon, M.W. Foley, J.A. Starr, & L.M. Saul, 1998, Philadelphia: F. A. Davis.)

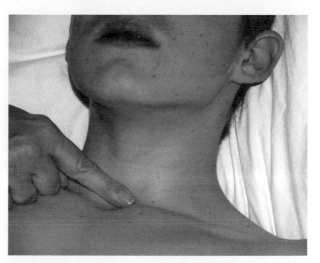

Figure 8-13 Tracheal stimulation for the production of a cough reflex.

After secretions are loosened by the above techniques, clearance of the secretions from the airways is necessary to complete the treatment. Coughing is a natural, often spontaneous, and effective means for clearing secretions from the larger airways. For infants and children who are unable to cough on command because of limitations to cognitive or motor planning abilities, a quick, inward thrust on the trachea, just above the suprasternal notch, will elicit a strong cough reflex (Figure 8–13).

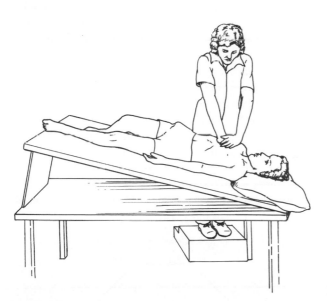

Figure 8–12 Shaking being performed over the involved right middle lobe. (From the National Cystic Fibrosis Foundation, Courtesy of Bettina C. Hilman, MD. From *Cardiopulmonary rehabilitation: Basic therapy and application* (p. 428), by F.J. Brannon, M.W. Foley, J.A. Starr, & L.M. Saul, 1998, Philadelphia: F. A. Davis.)

A child with an obstructive pulmonary disease may have difficulty clearing secretions with coughing because of early closure of the airways. Huffing is a technique that may more effectively clear secretions. The child is told to inhale and then forcefully exhale, producing a breathy "ha ha ha" sound. Modifications of the huff are used in many of the independent secretion removal techniques described in this chapter. This technique may be helpful to clear secretions throughout the day, not just during specified therapy sessions. Children who are able, although somewhat reluctant, to cough on command may become more compliant using coughing or huffing activities. The big bad wolf huffs and puffs, and perhaps can even cough!

For children who are unable to generate the forced expiratory muscle force needed for an effective cough, an assisted cough may improve cough effectiveness. Similar to a coordinated Heimlich maneuver, the therapist's hand is placed just below the xiphoid process (Figure 8–14). As the child attempts a cough, the therapist pushes inward and under the diaphragm, assisting exhalation. The amount of pressure that the therapist uses on the abdomen is dictated by the child's tolerance. A child with muscular dystrophy will have intact sensation, limiting the amount of pressure that can be used to assist the cough. A child with a spinal cord lesion who lacks abdominal sensation can tolerate more pressure. This coughing technique is usually performed in supine position with the child fully supported on a flat surface. It can be used with the child in other positions, such as upright in a wheelchair or sidelying, but the therapist must ensure that the child's position will be

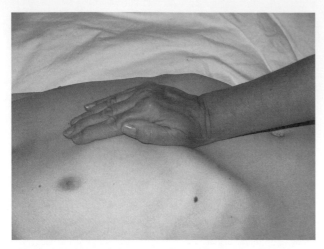

Figure 8-14 Hand placement for an assisted cough.

maintained during the assisted cough. For example, the wheelchair brakes must be locked or pillows placed behind the child to maintain sidelying.

Airway suctioning may be necessary to remove airway secretions in children who are on mechanical ventilation or who are unable to generate an effective cough through any other means. Suctioning techniques for children use a small suction catheter. Neonatal suction catheters are 5 to 6 or 8 French gauge. In older children, a size 10 may be used. When suctioning through an artificial airway, care must be taken not to occlude the airway with the suction catheter. The outside diameter of the suction catheter should be only 50% of the internal diameter of the airway (Pryor & Webber, 1998). Suctioning protocols usually encourage preoxygenation. It is recommended that only a 10% increase above the child's present oxygen settings be used. Even short-term hyperoxemia may lead to retinopathy (Roberton, 1996). The negative pressures used in the suction set-up should be between 75 and 150 mm Hg (Pryor & Webber, 1998). Finally, care must be taken when choosing suctioning as a method of airway clearance because its use is linked with oxygen desaturation, tachycardia, bradycardia, hypertension, hypotension, pneumothorax, and stridor. Nurses, respiratory therapists, physical therapists, and family members may need to perform suctioning, but proper training is essential.

A combination of postural drainage, percussion, and shaking, followed by airway clearance techniques, is used to mobilize secretions in infants and young children. As the child grows and is able to take on some of the responsibility for his or her pulmonary care, more independent methods of secretion mobilization techniques can be introduced.

These often become a primary means of secretion removal when the adolescent or young adult is away from home at college or camp.

Active Cycle-of-Breathing Techniques

Active cycle-of-breathing techniques (ACBT) include a breathing-control phase, thoracic expansion exercises, and the forced expiratory technique to clear secretions from the airways (Figure 8–15). The breathing-control phase is defined as relaxed diaphragmatic tidal volume breathing. This phase is maintained for a few minutes and is used almost as a physiological and psychological warm-up for what is to come. Thoracic expansion exercises are defined as deep breathing, with a 3-second hold, if possible, at the top of inhalation, followed by a passive exhalation. Three or four thoracic expansion exercises are performed during this phase of ACBT. A return to the breathing-control phase (lasting seconds to minutes depending on the child's level of fatigue) follows thoracic expansion exercises as a rest period and an evaluation time. If the child feels that there are secretions ready to be moved upward, the forced expiratory technique completes the cycle. If secretions are not ready to be moved, the child returns to thoracic expansion exercises, followed by another period of breathing control for rest and evaluation of status. The forced expiratory technique, defined as one or two huffs from tidal volume down to low lung volumes, is used to expel secretions from the airways rather than coughing. The forced expiratory technique is followed by a rest period of breathing control.

Using the active cycle of breathing techniques, secretions are milked from smaller to larger airways. Once the secretions have moved into the larger airways, huffs or coughs from mid or high lung volumes remove the secretions. Self-percussion and postural drainage can be added to this technique if warranted. This technique relies on collateral ventilation via the pores of Kohn and channel of Lambert,

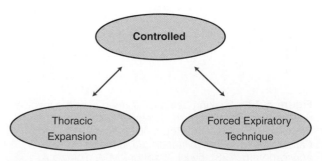

Figure 8-15 Active cycle of breathing technique.

which develop as the child ages, making this an appropriate technique for older children. Children 8 years of age and older are usually able to participate with this type of independent exercise program. The benefits of this technique have, in some instances, been demonstrated to be as effective as postural drainage, percussion, and shaking, with the added benefit of independence from the caregiver (Wilson, Baldwin, & Walshaw, 1995).

Autogenic Drainage

Autogenic drainage uses controlled breathing volumes and velocities in sitting to clear excessive secretions from the airways. There are three phases to autogenic drainage: the unstick phase, the collect phase, and the evacuation phase (Figure 8–16). Phase 1 uses quiet breathing at low lung volumes (essentially breathing in the expiratory reserve volume) to affect the secretions in the most peripheral airways. Phase 2 uses controlled breathing at low-to-mid lung volumes to mobilize secretions within the middle airways. Phase 3 uses breathing at mid-to-high lung volumes (inspiratory reserve volume) to clear secretions from central airways. Coughing is discouraged during the performance of autogenic drainage. This sequence is repeated until secretions are no longer felt within the thorax. Autogenic drainage requires that the child be able to assess his or her own needs, to locate the position of the secretions within the airways, and to target a segment of the treatment to remove the "felt" secretions. The amount of time spent in each phase is determined by the amount and the location of the pulmonary secretions felt by the child. The entire secretion removal session using autogenic drainage usually takes 30 to 45 minutes to perform. Autogenic drainage has been shown in some instances to be as effective in clearing secretions as postural drainage, percussion, and shaking in children with CF (Davidson, Wong, Pirie, & McIlwaine, 1992). In addition, autogenic drainage offers independence from caregivers and was preferred to manual secretion removal techniques in the above study. Learning the techniques of autogenic drainage requires considerable amounts of time, high concentration, and an ability to "read" the body. It is suggested that a child be at least 8 years old before attempting to use this technique.

Oral Airway and Chest Wall Oscillation Devices

The Flutter device uses an external apparatus to oscillate the airflow throughout the airways. The device itself resembles a pipe with a mouthpiece, a stem, and a covered bowl (Figure 8–17). Inside this bowl is a steel ball that rests in a plastic seat. The child inhales a breath somewhat greater than tidal volume, approximately three-quarters of vital capacity. A 2- to 3-second hold of the inhaled breath is followed by an active exhalation through the Flutter device. During exhalation through the mouthpiece, the force of the exhaled air begins to raise the steel ball within the pipe

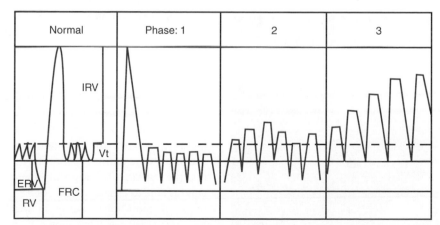

Figure 8-16 Phases of autogenic drainage shown on a spirogram of a normal person. Phase 1: Unstick. Phase 2: Collect. Phase 3: Evacuate. (Vt = tidal volume, IRV = inspiratory reserve volume, ERV = expiratory reserve volume, RV = residual volume, FRC = functional residual capacity.) (From Schoni, M.H. [1989]. Autogenic drainage: A modern approach to physiotherapy in cystic fibrosis. *Journal of the Royal Society of Medicine, 82*(suppl 16), 32–37. Reprinted with permission.)

bowl. The ball reaches its peak height within the device and then drops back into its plastic seat, causing a backward air pressure that jars the airways. The repeated raising and dropping of the ball throughout the exhalation phase provides an intermittent backward pressure, or oscillation, to the airway. The measurement of expiratory pressure varies from 10 to 25 cm H_2O. The usual procedure is to exhale 5 to 10 somewhat greater than tidal volume breaths through the Flutter device, followed by two large exhaled volumes through the Flutter device, and finally a huff or cough to clear mobilized secretions. This routine is repeated until all secretions are cleared from the lungs. The Flutter device has been shown, in some instances, to help in the removal of secretions from airways (Gondor, Nixon, Mutich, Rebovich, & Orenstein, 1999; Konstan, Stern, & Doershuk, 1994). The benefits of a Flutter device are the relatively quick instruction period, ease of use, and independence from a caregiver. Children older than 5 to 6 years can use the Flutter device effectively. The Flutter needs to be performed in a position that provides for maximum oscillations of the airways, usually in a seated position, limiting its use in postural drainage positions. Finally, children need to keep their Flutter devices with them on overnights, or at school. Forgetting the Flutter means that no airway clearance is performed.

Other means of airway oscillations include the Acapella device, which provides positive pressure and vibration to the airway to help mobilize secretions, similar to the Flutter (see Figure 8–17). The benefit of the Acapella is that it can be used in postural drainage positions.

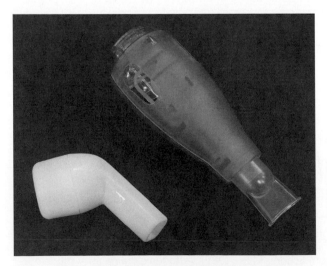

Figure 8-17 Airway oscillation devices: (Left) Flutter device. (Right) Acapella.

High-frequency airway oscillations can also be generated through commercially available ventilators. Research on secretion clearance with high-frequency oscillations versus manual secretion removal techniques has shown similar abilities in clearing secretions (Konstan et al., 1994; Schere, Barandun, Martinez, Wanner, & Rubin, 1998).

High-frequency chest wall oscillation (HFCWO) is another option for achieving the goal of secretion removal. The device is a chest vest that is inflated with an air pulsed generator that delivers an external force to the thorax up to 25 times per second. One benefit of HFCWO is that there is no specific position or breathing pattern required on the part of the child. HFCWO has been shown to be comparable to manual secretion removal techniques in clearing secretions and in improving pulmonary function tests during exacerbations of individuals with CF (Arens et al., 1994). Other studies have also shown similar results in individuals during exacerbation of their CF (Braggion, Cappelletti, Cornacchia, Zanolla, & Mastella, 1995) and in patients with stable CF (Kluft et al., 1996; Schere et al., 1998).

Positive Expiratory Pressure

The **positive expiratory pressure (PEP)** uses a tight-fitting mask or mouthpiece with a one-way valve to regulate expiratory resistance (Figure 8–18). The child is seated, breathing at tidal volumes with the mask or mouthpiece securely in place. Inhalation with the mask or mouthpiece in place is unresisted. Because of the PEP provided, exhalation will be an active phase of breathing. Low-pressure PEP uses a resistance that will measure 10 to 20 cm H_2O during mid-exhalation. After approximately 10 breaths, the mask is removed and the child huffs to clear secretions. After a brief rest period, the routine is repeated until all secretions have been cleared from the airways. For children with unstable airways, high-pressure (50 to 120 cm H_2O) PEP can be used. The child breathes up to 10 breaths with the high-pressure PEP mask in place. Huffing is done from high to low lung volumes with the mask in place, helping to stabilize the airways during the huff. High-pressure PEP requires that the resistance be individually set at the point where the child is able to exhale a larger forced vital capacity with the mask or mouthpiece in place than without. In some instances, PEP has been shown to be equally effective to postural drainage, percussion, and shaking (Hofmeyr, Webber, & Hodson, 1986; Oberwaldner, Evans, & Zach, 1986; Steen, Redmond, O'Neill, & Beattie, 1991; Tyrrell, Hiller, & Martin, 1986; Van Asperen, Jackson, Hennessy,

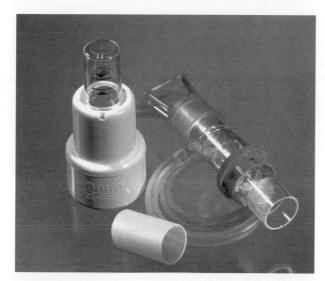

Figure 8-18 Positive expiratory pressure device. (Photo courtesy of DHD Healthcare Corporation, Wampsville, NY 13163.)

& Brown, 1987). High-pressure PEP was shown to improve expiratory flow rates, decrease hyperinflation, and improve airway stability when compared with postural drainage, percussion, and shaking, in individuals with CF (Oberwaldner, Theiss, Rucker, & Zach, 1991).

The Flutter device, PEP, HFCWO, autogenic drainage, and active cycle of breathing have all been compared with manual secretion removal techniques with a range of results. Variations in the performance of each secretion removal technique and differences in measurement make it difficult to conclude efficacy of one treatment over another (Thomas, Cook, & Brooks, 1995). Determination of a treatment plan should consider the availability of care providers, the child's level of responsibility and desire for independence, and the preference of the child (Oermann, Swank, & Sockrider, 2000).

Exercises to Increase Ventilation

Breathing exercises as a means to increase ventilation are the basis for many independent exercise programs for children. In this section, the techniques of diaphragmatic breathing exercises, segmental breathing exercises, ROM exercises, and positioning will be discussed. It is always more enjoyable for the child and the therapist to incorporate a breathing exercise program into age-appropriate play. Blowing bubbles, a toy pinwheel, or tissues can make breathing exercises fun. Blowing a ping-pong ball or a cotton ball across

the table into a goal can add a more competitive aspect to a simple set of breathing exercises. The use of pediatric-sized incentive spirometers can also achieve the goal of improved ventilation. Providing written reminders with checklists at the bedside and age-appropriate motivators, such as sticker charts or video game time, may help to increase compliance with breathing exercises.

Diaphragmatic Breathing Exercises

Diaphragmatic breathing can be used to improve ventilation, decrease the work of breathing, and promote relaxation in children. With the child in a semireclining position, place the child's hand just below the xiphoid process. The therapist's hand is now placed over the child's hand. The child is asked to try to feel the therapist's hand rise up during inspiration and fall down during exhalation. Asking the child to forcefully "sniff in" may help the child feel the difference between movement of the diaphragm and abdominal muscle action. The child is asked to take in a slow deep inhalation, using that same movement of the diaphragm. The therapist's hand can provide pressure inward and under the diaphragm during exhalation, making diaphragmatic motion on inhalation more obvious. When the child begins to perform the technique correctly, the tactile cues are slowly taken away. The child should learn diaphragmatic breathing because it is used in breathing control, relaxation, and many independent secretion removal techniques. Diaphragmatic breathing can be encouraged in infants and children by positioning their trunks in flexion while sidelying; prone; on their knees; or supine with the head, neck, hips, and knees supported in flexion. Upper extremities in a combination of shoulder adduction, extension, and internal rotation will limit upper chest mobility, encouraging diaphragmatic breathing.

Segmental Breathing Exercises

Segmental breathing exercises use a combination of positioning, verbal commands, and tactile cues to enhance ventilation to a particular lung region. Positioning can be used to restrict thoracic motion elsewhere in the chest wall, encouraging the indicated lung segment to expand more fully. For example, a child with right middle lobe collapse can perform segmental breathing exercises while sitting in an armchair. The child places his or her right arm over the back of the chair and leans toward the left armrest. In essence, the left chest has been constrained by the resulting left lateral trunk flexion. The right chest has been opened by the position of the right upper extremity in abduction and by the positioning of the trunk. The child is instructed to inhale slowly and deeply to completely fill his or her chest with air. The therapist's hands can be placed over the right middle lobe. As the child exhales, a firm pressure, or even the shaking technique, can encourage complete exhalation. Pressure is released, although manual contact is maintained, during the next deep inhalation. Once the child is effective in segmental expansion, the therapist's verbal and tactile cues are slowly withdrawn, leaving the child with an independent breathing exercise program.

Positioning for segmental expansion can use positions other than sitting. Using the appropriate postural drainage position described earlier in this chapter will put the affected lung segment in a gravity-independent position that will enhance ventilation to that segment. Tactile cues from the therapist's hands and appropriate verbal cues can be used to improve ventilation.

Range-of-Motion Exercises

The positions of the upper extremity, trunk, and neck have an effect on thoracic mobility. Shoulder flexion, abduction, and external rotation seem to encourage inhalation. Shoulder extension, horizontal adduction, and internal rotation encourage exhalation. Trunk extension encourages inhalation, and trunk flexion encourages exhalation. Neck extension promotes inhalation, and neck flexion seems to be a natural accompaniment to exhalation. A game of "stretch to the ceiling and inhale; now touch your toes while you exhale" can be used to coordinate the inhalation motions of upper extremity, trunk, and neck with deep inhalation and the exhalation motions of the body with exhalation. Proprioceptive neuromuscular facilitation patterns for upper extremity ROM, when coordinated with the breathing cycle, can also be used to enhance ventilation.

Positioning Considerations

Thoughtful positioning can be beneficial to a child's cardiopulmonary system as well as motor development and social interactions. Infant positioning should consider ventilation-perfusion matching, feeding needs, skin integrity, arterial supply and venous return, energy requirements, movement possibilities, and disorder precautions. Eventually, children are meant to assume an upright posture. This posture allows them to locomote, to use their upper extremities freely, and to connect with the world face on. It also allows the ribcage to be affected by gravity and angle downward, thus changing the shape of the thorax and the alignment of the ventilatory muscles. Children must be allowed to come to the upright posture, whether independently or with help from assistive devices such as infant seats, adaptive seating, or adaptive standers. See the section on postural drainage for further clarification of contraindications to certain positioning.

Exercise and Aerobic Fitness

Aerobic exercise is an integral component of prevention and wellness programs for individuals of all ages. Physical fitness programs in children are beneficial to the establishment of life-long physical fitness. The national initiative *Healthy people 2000* (United States Department of Health and Human Services, 1995) has identified aerobic exercise as a key component of health promotion and wellness. In this section, a brief comparison of child and adult exercise physiological parameters is provided. Issues concerning the development of physical fitness programs for children with cardiopulmonary dysfunction, as well as for children of any ability, are also presented.

Exercise Response in Children

The exercise response of children demonstrates several differences in physiological exercise measurements when compared with that of adults. Many of the differences are related to body size. Therefore the absolute measurement of an exercise parameter may show a significant difference between an adult and a child, but the relationship of the relative value, that is, when corrected for body size and/or mass, may not.

The cardiac response to exercise in children includes higher resting HR and higher submaximal and maximal HR compared with those of an adult. There is also a lower absolute resting stroke volume, as well as a lower submaximal and maximal stroke volume attributable to the smaller size of the heart itself. Cardiac output is the product of HR × stroke volume. At rest, there is an absolute decrease in a child's resting cardiac output when compared with that of an adult because the higher HR is not sufficient to counter the lower stroke volume. However, relative resting cardiac output, that is, a cardiac output corrected for size and mass, of a child is actually higher than the resting cardiac output of an adult. Relative cardiac outputs at submaximal and maximal exercise are decreased in children compared with those of adults. Resting BP values in children are also typically lower than adult values. During exercise, the pattern of BP response to workload is similar to that in the adult, with systole increasing and diastole remaining essentially stable. However, the slope of the systolic rise is less dramatic in children.

Pulmonary system differences between children and adults are often related to the differences in body size and mass as well. The maturation of the child's pulmonary system also plays a role in exercise ability because the efficiency of the pulmonary system changes over time. Absolute lung volumes, including vital capacity and tidal volume, are directly related to body size and therefore are decreased in children. Higher resting RRs are noted in children. Minute ventilation is the product of RR × tidal volume. At rest, there is an absolute decrease in resting minute ventilation because the higher RR is not sufficient to overcome the lower tidal volume. Absolute minute ventilation is also lower at submaximal and maximal workloads. However, when corrected for size and mass, relative minute ventilation at submaximal and maximal exercise is increased in children compared with that of adults. The work of breathing during exercise is higher in children than in adults because the efficiency of their pulmonary system is not yet optimal. As with adults, ventilation is rarely the limiting system to exercise in healthy children.

Absolute maximal aerobic capacity, or $\dot{V}O_{2max}$, is smaller in children than adults. Absolute $\dot{V}O_{2max}$ increases from childhood through adolescence, mostly caused by an increase in body size. At puberty, males continue to increase their absolute $\dot{V}O_{2max}$ into adulthood; females tend to plateau (Cerny & Burton, 2001; Krahenbuhl, Skinner, & Kohrt, 1985). The difference between a child's relative $\dot{V}O_{2max}$ and that of an adult, although still decreased, is not as dramatic as the difference in absolute $\dot{V}O_{2max}$ values.

Temperature regulation is also different in children. Although children have a relatively higher skin surface area to body mass ratio, their lower number of sweat glands and lower output from these glands impairs their ability to dissipate heat during exercise at higher environmental temperatures. Children are therefore at a higher risk for heat-related injuries. The same high skin surface area also predisposes children to increased heat loss during exercise in cold environmental conditions, making them more susceptible to cold-related injuries. Excellent in-depth overviews of exercise response in children are available (Darbee & Cerny, 1995; Stout, 2000).

Exercise Prescription for Children

Physical fitness programs typically address cardiorespiratory endurance, flexibility, muscular strength, and body composition. Age-appropriate measures of physical fitness can be used to assess general physical fitness levels (Stout, 2000), and exercise testing can be used to assess more specifically cardiorespiratory endurance. (Refer to section on laboratory studies for more information on exercise testing.) The same exercise prescription parameters of intensity, frequency, duration, and mode that are used to improve cardiopulmonary endurance in adults also pertain to children.

Intensity

The intensity of physical activity should be prescribed at 50% to 85% of the child's maximum capacity, or $\dot{V}O_{2max}$. In children with particularly low initial levels of fitness, 40% to 50% of $\dot{V}O_2$ may be appropriate. Using the Karvonen formula for prescribing exercise intensity accounts for the child's higher resting HR and the higher maximal exercise HR (Table 8.10). By using 50% to 85% of HR reserve or 40% to 50% in a child with a low fitness level, one can calculate exercise target HR ranges to ensure exercise training while maintaining a safe exercise session. Rate of perceived exertion (RPE) can also be used with older children to monitor exercise intensity (Table 8.11).

Duration

The duration of aerobic activity is optimally approximately 30 minutes but it should be adjusted to the child's attention span and kept "fun." Younger children may need a variety

Table 8.10 Karvonen's Formula for the Prescription of Exercise Intensity

(Heart rate max − Heart rate rest) × 85% + Heart rate rest = High end of target heart rate range
(Heart rate max − Heart rate rest) × 50% + Heart rate rest = Low end of target heart rate range
(Heart rate max − Heart rate rest) × 40% + Heart rate rest = Low end of target heart rate range with initial low levels of fitness

Table 8.11 Borg Scale of Perceived Exertion

6	
7	Very, very light
8	
9	Very light
10	
11	Fairly light
12	
13	Somewhat hard
14	
15	Hard
16	
17	Very hard
18	
19	Very, very hard

Source: Adapted from Borg, G.A. (1982). Psychophysical bases of perceived exertion. *Medicine and science in sports and exercise, 14,* 377–387. Copyright by the American College of Sports Medicine.

of different activities to keep them interested and challenged for 30 minutes at a time. Older children are better able to understand complex rule sets and want to engage in longer games with more complex play.

Frequency

Frequency of exercise is dependent on duration. If the duration of exercise can be 30 minutes, a frequency of 3 to 5 times per week is appropriate. If the duration is less than 30 minutes, the frequency should increase. Shorter, more frequent bouts of physical activity can be used to improve fitness.

Mode

Activity modes for children can often be found in age-appropriate forms of play. For infants, encouraging parents and caregivers to place toys slightly out of the infant's reach will require the infant to use larger muscle masses, such as the shoulder, abdominal, and trunk musculature. The additional physical effort required with this activity benefits the cardiopulmonary system. Creeping and crawling in safe, interesting, open spaces encourages cardiopulmonary endurance and promotes motor development. Encouraging the family to take walks together, even if the infant is sitting upright in a stroller, can require greater physical effort than simply sitting or resting at home.

Modes of activities for toddlers and young children are also forms of age-appropriate play. Locomotion in any form—scaling obstacle courses, playing ball, walking, running, chasing soap bubbles, or riding a bike—uses larger muscles and will encourage cardiopulmonary endurance. Young children enjoy music and dancing. Songs of appropriate tempo and duration can help encourage longer periods of physical activity. School-age children continue to enjoy physical activity with daily periods of typical "playground" activities. Gym class, after-school programs, and simple ball games can promote cardiorespiratory endurance.

As organized sports become more competitive in late elementary school, the distinction between the more athletic and the less athletic child becomes more evident. At this same time, a transformation in body composition related to puberty and changes in interests converge, often resulting in a decline of physical activity. Walking programs, aerobic dance programs, fitness courses, hiking, gardening, or other physical activities that are noncompetitive in nature can provide important alternative aerobic activities to organized sports programs.

Concerns about body composition can be a positive factor in promoting participation in physical fitness for some adolescents, but by high school, adolescents find their "free time" reduced by homework, employment, and other after-school activities. Sports are more competitive than ever, with children eliminated from participation based on ability. Less time is allotted to physical education during school, with gym class often held only once or twice a week. If physical fitness habits are not already in place by this age, participation in physical activity will likely be dropped when time is short. Health promotion and wellness programs targeted at the adolescent could be an integral component in promoting physical fitness throughout the life span.

Resistance activities can also be encouraged, provided the proper guidelines and techniques are followed. Strength training that allows for proper breathing, 10 to 15 repetitions with the chosen amount of resistance, and movements that use multiple muscles and span multiple joints can be included into a child's activity program on a twice-weekly basis.

Aerobic Exercise in Children With Impairment of Pulmonary Structures and Function

The potential benefits of aerobic activity in children with chronic cardiopulmonary disease include (1) an improved sense of well-being, (2) an increase in aerobic capacity, (3) an increase in ventilatory muscle strength and endurance, and (4) enhanced secretion clearance. To ensure safety as well as training, an exercise prescription for children with cardiopulmonary system impairments should specify intensity, frequency, duration, and mode. Monitoring and documenting vital signs, including HR, RR, BP, breathing pattern, SaO_2, and RPE during exercise, will help maintain a safe exercise session. Supplemental oxygen should be considered in children with documented hypoxemia during exercise.

The pulmonary system is not usually a limiting factor in aerobic capacity. However, in children with chronic pulmonary disease, exercise tolerance may be limited by pulmonary impairments. To appropriately prescribe exercise intensity for this population, it is helpful to consider pulmonary reserve, the amount of ventilation that is available for exercise, or the difference between resting minute ventilation and maximal minute ventilation. When the pulmonary reserve is very low (i.e., the child has a severe pulmonary limitation), the child will have a higher minute ventilation at rest, will be using a higher percentage of his or her ventilatory ability at lower workloads, and will have a limited ability to perform exercise as a result of pulmonary impairments. In this population, short bursts of high-intensity exercise with interspersed rest periods can be used to produce training. If the pulmonary reserve is larger, a more moderate exercise intensity for a longer duration may be possible. Resumption of a familiar exercise program after a pulmonary exacerbation may require altering the usual exercise intensity until the child can be progressed back to pre-exacerbation levels of exercise. Pediatric physical therapists can encourage children with cardiopulmonary system impairments to participate in exercise programs that, even at low intensities, can provide aerobic training and encourage long-term participation in physical fitness programs.

Frequency and duration of aerobic exercise are related to the intensity of the activity prescribed. If the duration of exercise can be maintained for 30 minutes, the frequency of that activity should be 3 to 5 times per week. On the other hand, if the activity consists of short bouts of high-intensity exercise, then the exercise needs to be performed on a daily basis. Exercise progression is usually focused on increasing exercise duration until 20 to 30 minutes of continuous exercise is achieved. Exercise intensity can then be progressed to continue aerobic training.

The mode of activity should be judged based on the ability to provide safe and effective conditioning. Activities should be aerobic in nature and have the potential for adjustments in workload. Limitation, or at least modification, of collision sports is necessary in many instances.

The typical environment for the activity mode should be evaluated. Winter sports, including figure skating, ice hockey, and skiing, are performed in an environment that is cold and dry, which may not be optimal for a child with reactive airway disease. Different modes of exercise performed in a warm or more humid environment may allow for longer exercise duration and higher exercise intensity. The timing of pharmacological interventions, particularly the use of bronchodilators and sodium cromolyn, before the exercise session should ensure that the child is optimally medicated during the exercise program. Gentle warm-up activities before the actual exercise session may also help to diminish airway reactivity. The limited thermoregulation ability of children should be considered if the typical environment for an activity is either very hot or very cold. Children with CF need to be concerned with salt depletion in warmer environments, making it more important to replenish both fluids and electrolytes during the exercise session.

Children with secretion retention as part of their pulmonary disease, specifically CF, often find that aerobic exercise aids in secretion clearance. Exercise in conjunction with manual secretion removal techniques has been found to enhance secretion clearance in children with CF. Although exercise alone was not found to be as effective, the combination of exercise and secretion removal techniques seems to be complementary (Bilton, Dodd, Abbot, & Webb, 1992; Sahl, Bilton, Dodd, & Webb, 1989). The benefit of long-term aerobic exercise in children with CF is a slower rate of decline in pulmonary function and an improved sense of well-being (Schneiderman-Walker et al., 2000).

Inspiratory muscle training has been a treatment technique for adults with chronic lung disease. Inspiratory muscle training, using an inspiratory threshold loading device, has been shown to improve the inspiratory muscle endurance in children with CF. The ability to translate this improvement into an improvement in exercise capacity, dyspnea, fatigue, or pulmonary function test scores has had mixed results (Asher, Pardy, Coates, Thomas, & Macklem 1982; deJong, van Aalderen, Kraan, Koeter, & van der Schans, 2001; Sawyer & Clanton, 1993). The prescription for exercise using an inspiratory muscle training device varied from study to study, especially in the intensity of exercise prescribed, which may account for the differences in results. Activity training programs targeting the thoracic and shoulder muscles, such as swimming and canoeing, has also been shown to increase ventilatory muscle endurance (Keens et al., 1977). In children with lung disease, functional playful activities of the upper extremities may be more appealing and therefore improve exercise compliance.

Children with chronic pulmonary disease have an increased use of the accessory muscles of ventilation. The addition of static stretching of upper extremity, shoulder, back, and neck musculature to a general stretching program can improve flexibility. The American College of Sports Medicine (1995) guidelines for achieving and maintaining flexibility include (1) frequency of 3 times per week, (2) intensity that stretches a muscle group to the point of mild discomfort, and (3) duration of 10- to 30-second hold for each stretch, with 3 to 5 repetitions of each muscle or muscle group.

Aerobic Exercise for Children With Impairments of Cardiac Structures and Functions

Children with cyanotic heart defects will have a decrease in their aerobic capacity. Severe cyanotic cardiac defects may preclude strenuous participation in exercise. However, addressing flexibility or other less cardiac-demanding physical activity, such as modified yoga, can still plant the physical activity seed. After cardiac repair with good outcomes, there may be little or no residual restrictions to aerobic capacity, and children can participate more fully in recreational physical activities. Children with more serious cardiac defects who have continued altered hemodynamics postoperatively will need to participate in a more modified exercise program that can offer a more precise exercise prescription; closer monitoring of vital signs, including arrhythmias; and the ability to supply supplemental oxygen if needed.

Children with certain types of impairments of cardiac structures and functions may have pacemakers implanted to ensure an adequate HR response at all times. There are many different types of pacemakers available. A pacemaker is described by (1) where the pacemaker senses the underlying cardiac rhythm (A = atrium, V = ventricle, D = dual [both atria and ventricle]); (2) where the pacemaker will deliver an electrical impulse (A, V, or D); and (3) what the pacemaker will do when it senses the underlying cardiac rhythm (I = inhibit, T= deliver, or D, either inhibit or deliver an electrical impulse). Therefore, a VVI pacemaker senses the underlying cardiac rhythm within the ventricle, will deliver the impulse to the ventricle, and will inhibit the pacemaker if a timely beat is already sensed within the ventricle. If a child's heart is paced at a constant rate, such as 90 beats per minute, the needed increase in cardiac output during exercise is provided by stroke volume alone. A rate response pacemaker has the ability to consistently readjust its program in response to the child's level of activity. When an increase in the child's activity is sensed, the pacemaker increases its firing rate to account for the increased activity. This increase in HR, along with an increase in stroke volume, will increase cardiac output, similar to what the heart of a healthy child would do.

Children who are candidates for a heart, lung, or heart-lung transplant often participate in a supervised exercise program before and after transplantation. Children who have undergone a heart or a heart-lung transplant have a modified response HR to exercise. Because there is no direct nervous input to the transplanted heart, the increase in HR is dependent on circulating catecholamines rather than the autonomic nervous system. A longer warm-up is beneficial in order to prime the heart for increased exercise intensity. HR will stay higher longer after exercise has ceased because the catecholamines are still in the system. A longer cool-down period will allow slower HR decline back to resting levels. As HR lags behind exercise intensity, using the RPE scale is helpful in prescribing exercise intensity. Familiarity with, and acceptance of, an established exercise routine will allow children to improve their activity tolerance and to benefit fully from the transplant procedure.

Physical Fitness for Children of All Abilities

The increased incidences of childhood obesity, asthma, and diabetes, coupled with declining physical fitness of our nation's youth, present a serious public-health concern. In the past decade, The United States Department of Health and Human Services (2000) has developed objectives for physical activity and fitness programs. *Healthy people 2010: National health promotion and disease prevention objectives related to mothers, infants, children, adolescents, and youth* identifies the need to increase participation in physical activity, improve dietary practices, and reduce the incidence of obesity. The objectives related to increasing physical activity participation focus on the appropriate mode, frequency, duration, and intensity of physical activity to reduce cardiovascular risks. The *Healthy people 2010* directive should be reviewed by all physical therapists (*www.healthypeople.gov*).

The prevalence of obesity among children and adolescents has been increasing in recent years (Salbe, Weyer, Lindsay, Ravussin, & Tataranni, 2002). Early childhood obesity is the greatest predictor of future obesity, indicating that early childhood intervention is necessary to prevent and reduce obesity in later childhood and adulthood. Children, at both 5 and 10 years of age, who demonstrate a decreased participation in organized sports and an increase in television viewing are more apt to develop obesity. Surprisingly, only after the child has become obese is a decrease in physical activity noted. Youth-focused fitness programs could provide the necessary alternatives to bridge the gap between organized sports and sedentary activities. In order to reduce obesity and modify body composition, a physical fitness program should include activities to increase total energy expenditure (Bar-Or, 2000). Energy expenditure can be increased by selecting activities that involve large muscle groups, such as walking, cycling, rollerblading, skating, swimming, or dancing.

The promotion of physical activity of individuals with physical disabilities is also a public health concern (Heath & Fentem, 1997). Optimal physical fitness should be a goal for children of all abilities. Children with disabilities demonstrate decreased physical work capacity that affects their daily physical activities (Dresen, de Groot, Corstius, Krediet, & Meijer,1982). Several studies have shown that measures of cardiorespiratory endurance are decreased in children with a variety of neuromuscular conditions, including CP (Lundberg, 1978), spina bifida (Agre et al., 1984), spinal cord injuries (Janssen, Van Oers, Van der Woude, & Hollander, 1994), muscular dystrophy (Sockolov, Irwin, Dressendorfer, & Bernauer, 1977), and Down syndrome (Dichter, Darbee, Effgen, & Palisano, 1993). Children with neuromuscular impairments may have difficulty in participating in traditional fitness programs, but maintaining physical fitness is still critical. The ability of children to complete their activities of daily life without undue fatigue can be enhanced by improving their overall fitness. Weight-loading activities in children with CP can also provide increased bone stores and play a role in osteoporosis prevention programs (Chad, Bailey, McKay, Zello, & Snyder, 1999).

Equipment

Medical equipment may be helpful in improving, promoting, and maintaining ventilation and mobility. The physical therapist should understand and give careful thought to the type of equipment that would be useful, when that equipment should be used, and the maintenance of that equipment.

Inhalation Devices

Nebulizers and inhalation devices, such as **metered-dose inhalers (MDIs)**, are commonly used to deliver topical medications to the airways of children with airway disease. The encouragement of proper breathing patterns in an appropriate body position can maximize ventilation and optimize deposition of the medication. Physical therapists can assist young children, or children with neuromuscular impairments, in the coordination of breathing with MDI use or suggest the use of adaptive MDIs. Most MDIs now use a spacer device that allows improved particle distribution within the respiratory system.

Vital Sign and Airflow Monitors

Cardiac, apnea, and oxygen saturation monitors are often found within the hospital setting. Premature infants, those at risk for SIDS, or those with sleep apnea are often placed on these monitors at home. Individuals may intermittently use these monitors during rest or sleep. Handheld spirometers are often used to measure expiratory flow rates in individuals with reactive airway diseases to monitor airway function and optimize medical management.

Mechanical Ventilation and Supplemental Oxygen

Equipment to assist with ventilation may include positive and negative pressure ventilators and devices to provide continuous positive airway pressure (CPAP) or bilevel positive airway pressure (BiPAP). Different modes of ventilation are used, depending on the nature of the cardiopulmonary disease, its severity, and the age and size of the child. Description of these different ventilatory modes is beyond the scope of this text. In children with impaired ventilation, such ventilatory assisting equipment may be used intermittently or all of the time, but most often during sleep or rest times. Children with neuromuscular diseases that cause both progressive limitations in activities and impairments of respiratory structures and functions may be able to remain mobile by adapting their electric wheelchair for a portable ventilation device.

Supplemental oxygen is used in children as it is in adults. Criteria for the need of supplemental oxygen are an SaO_2 less than 88%, a PaO_2 less than 55 mm Hg, or a significant decrease in oxygenation with activity or during sleep. Supplemental oxygen can be delivered via nasal cannula or mask set-up. Various types of home and portable oxygen tanks and concentrators are available from home-care companies that deliver and maintain the equipment.

Adaptive Supports

Abdominal supports can be used to improve ventilation in children with strength impairments of the abdominal wall. These supports act to increase abdominal pressure and improve the diaphragm's resting position. The more domed the diaphragm resting position, the more effective will be the diaphragm contraction as a result of the improved length-tension relationship of that muscle. Children who lack postural control may improve their ability to ventilate with proper thoracic positioning in sitting. Head restraints adapted to a wheelchair, stroller, or car seat that minimize neck flexion and/or rotation can improve ventilation and ensure patent airways in infants and children.

Service Delivery Models

A variety of service delivery models are found for children with impairments in structure and function of the cardiopulmonary system. Direct provision of physical therapy services for individuals with cardiopulmonary diseases is common. In the hospital setting, where children with chronic cardiopulmonary disease may be periodically admitted, a primary physical therapist is often assigned to provide continuity of care over years of possible hospital admissions. Providing direct physical therapy service over time allows for a close relationship to develop between the therapist and child. However, with changes in health-care coverage, direct services are often provided only during periods of exacerbation, or as respite for parents and family providing routine care. The physical therapist who provides intermittent direct care should be sure to review the current plan of care and make updates to the program based on the child's age, abilities, tolerance, progression, or current needs. Questions or concerns of the regular caregiver about the implementation of the plan of care should be discussed. Teaching of any new care providers and a review of treatment techniques for any current care provider are important.

Infants and children with complex cardiopulmonary dysfunction benefit from collaboration among the many caregivers, including nutritionists, physicians, psychologists, social workers, nurses, physical therapists, occupational therapists, and respiratory therapists. Collaboration among family, medical providers, school, and community can ensure a consistent and supportive environment for the child with cardiopulmonary dysfunction. Physical therapists also act as consultants to, or are involved as team members in, a number of areas of pediatric care, including pediatric solid organ transplantation programs, pediatric pulmonary clinics, pediatric neuromuscular clinics, and seating clinics.

Physical therapists should play a major role in health promotion and wellness, including promotion of physical fitness in children. The Individuals with Disabilities Education Act (IDEA) has resulted in greater mainstreaming of children into regular education programs, as well as into physical education programs. Physical therapists have become increasingly involved in after-school recreational programs that address physical fitness. In particular, our expertise can promote physical fitness for children of all abilities and physical skill levels.

Physical therapists are also involved in community organizations as consultants for development of appropriate recreational programs for children of all abilities. The design of accessible parks, recreational systems, and sports and fitness programs for children are important health-promotion and wellness roles for the physical therapist. Physical therapists should also be prepared to contribute to their community's emergency response systems to assist within our expertise. The physical therapist's broad area of expertise provides many avenues to improve the quality of medical care and life for children with cardiopulmonary dysfunction.

8. A child with an atrial conduction abnormality is given a pacemaker. Please explain the term AVD and explain why this device was chosen for this situation.

Summary

Physical therapy practice considers both the short-term enablement of a child and ensuring the best possible outcome across the child's future life span. Physical therapy for the child with cardiopulmonary impairments intervenes at multiple levels of care, from secretion management, thoracic flexibility, breathing exercises, and preoperative and postoperative care to aerobic training for a lifetime. Physical therapists need to be actively concerned with promotion of physical fitness for children of all abilities. We are uniquely prepared for this role and can be instrumental in the development and implementation of physical fitness for our youth.

DISCUSSION QUESTIONS

1. How does the timing of the embryonic development of the heart relate to embryonic and neonatal function? How does the timing relate to structural development of the lungs?

2. Please explain the type of shunt created via the ductus arteriosus in utero and how it changes following the first few postnatal breaths.

3. What are the similarities and differences between asthma and exercise-induced bronchospasm?

4. Children with neuromuscular disease may use a wheelchair for locomotion. What effect does seating have on the pulmonary system?

5. Compare the pros and cons of the following two treatment programs for a child with cystic fibrosis: postural drainage positioning, percussion, shaking, and coughing, compared with use of Flutter in the seated position.

6. Explain how an upper extremity strength and endurance exercise program can be beneficial to the pulmonary system.

7. Design an alternative aerobic activity program for girls aged 12 to 15 years who do not compete in your town's sports program.

SUGGESTED READINGS/RESOURCES

American College of Sports Medicine (1995). *ACSM's guidelines to exercise testing and prescription* (5th ed.). Baltimore: Williams & Wilkins.

Brannon, F.J., Foley, M.W., Starr, J.A., & Saul, L.M. (1998). *Cardiopulmonary rehabilitation: Basic theory and application* (3rd ed.) Philadelphia: F.A. Davis.

Cherny, F., & Burton, H. (2001). *Exercise physiology for health care professionals.* Champaign, IL: Human Kinetics.

Durstine, J.L., & Moore, G.E. (2003). *ACSM's exercise management for persons with chronic diseases and disabilities.* Champaign, IL: Human Kinetics.

Goodman, C.C., Boissonnault, W.G., & Fuller, K.S. (2003). *Pathology: Implications for the physical therapist.* Philadelphia: W.B. Saunders.

Patrick, K., Spear, B., Holt, K., & Sofka, D. (2001). *Bright futures in practice: Physical activity.* Arlington, VA: National Center for Education in Maternal and Child Health.

United States Department of Health and Human Services (2000), *Healthy people 2010.* Washington, DC: Author. Available at: *www.healthypeople.gov.*

REFERENCES

Agre, J.C., Findley, T.W., McNally, C., Habeck, R., Leon, A.S., Stradel, L., Birkebak, R., & Schmalz, R. (1984). Physical activity capacity in children with myelomeningocele. *Archives of Physical Medicine and Rehabilitation, 68,* 372–377.

Aitken, M. (1996). Cystic fibrosis, editorial overview. *Current Opinion in Pulmonary Medicine, 2*(6), 435–438.

American Alliance for Health, Physical Education, Recreation, and Dance (AAHPERD) (1999). *The AAHPERD physical best program.* Reston, VA: Author.

American College of Sports Medicine (1995). *ACSM's guidelines for exercise testing and prescription* (5th ed.) (pp. 170–171). Baltimore: Williams & Wilkins.

American Physical Therapy Association (APTA) (2001). Guide to physical therapist practice (2nd ed). *Physical Therapy, 81,* 6–746.

Arens, R., Gozal, D., Omlin, K.J., Vega, J., Boyd, K.P., Keens, T.G., et al. (1994). Comparison of high frequency chest compression and conventional chest physiotherapy in hospitalized patients with cystic fibrosis. *American Journal of Respiratory Critical Care Medicine, 150*(4), 1154–1157.

Asher, M.I., Pardy, R.L., Coates, A.L., Thomas, E., & Macklem,

P.T. (1982). The effects of inspiratory muscle training in patients with cystic fibrosis. *American Review of Respiratory Diseases, 126*(5): 855–859.

Bancalari, E., Abdenour, G.E., Feller, R., & Gannon, J. (1979). Bronchopulmonary dysplasia: Clinical presentation. *Journal of Pediatrics. 95*, 819–823.

Barron, K.S., Shulman, S.T., Rowley, A., Taubert, K., Myones, B.L., Meissner, H.C., et al. (1999). Report of the National Institutes of Health Workshop on Kawasaki Disease. *Journal of Rheumatology, 26*(1), 170–190.

Bar-Or, O. (2000). Juvenile obesity, physical activity and lifestyle changes. *The Physician and Sportsmedicine, 28*(11), 51–58.

Bernstein, S., Heimler, R., & Sasidhara, P. (1998). Approaching the management of the neonatal intensive care graduate through history and physical exam. *Pediatric Clinics of North America, 45*(1), 79–105.

Bilton, D., Dodd, M.E., Abbot, J.V., & Webb, A.K. (1992). The benefits of exercise combined with physiotherapy in the treatment of adults with cystic fibrosis. *Respiratory Medicine, 86*(6), 507–511.

Bokulic, R.E., & Hilman, B.C. (1994). Interstitial lung disease in children. *Pediatric Clinics of North America: Respiratory Medicine II, 41*(3), 543–567.

Borg, G.A. (1982), Psychophysical bases of perceived exertion. *Medicine and Science in Sports and Exercise, 14, 377–387.*

Borowitz, D. (1996). The interrelationship of nutrition and pulmonary function in patients with cystic fibrosis. *Current Opinions in Pulmonary Medicine, 2*(6), 457–461.

Braggion, C., Cappelletti, L.M., Cornacchia, M., Zanolla, L., & Mastella, G. (1995). Short-term effects of three chest physiotherapy regimens in patients hospitalized for pulmonary exacerbations of cystic fibrosis: A cross-over randomized study. *Pediatric Pulmonology, 19*(1), 16–22.

Brannon, F.J., Foley, M.W., Starr, J.A., & Saul, L.M. (1998). *Cardiopulmonary rehabilitation: Basic application.* Philadelphia: F.A. Davis.

Cerny, F.J. (1989). Relative effects of bronchial drainage and exercise for in-hospital care of patients with cystic fibrosis. *Physical Therapy, 69*(8), 633–639.

Cerny, F., & Burton, H. (2001). *Exercise physiology for health care professionals.* Champaign, IL: Human Kinetics.

Chad, K.E., Bailey, D.A., McKay, H.A., Zello, G.A., & Snyder, R.E. (1999). The effect of a weight-bearing physical activity program on bone mineral content and estimated volumetric density in children with spastic cerebral palsy. *Journal of Pediatrics, 135*(1), 115–117.

Corey, M., & Farewell, V. (1996). Determinants of mortality from cystic fibrosis in Canada. *American Journal of Epidemiology, 143*, 1007–1017.

Darbee, J., & Cerny, F.J. (1995). Exercise testing and exercise conditioning for children with lung dysfunction. In S. Irwin & J.S. Tecklin (Eds.), *Cardiopulmonary physical therapy* (3rd ed., pp. 563–578). St. Louis: Mosby.

Davidson, A.G.F., Wong, L.T.K., Pirie, G.E., & McIlwaine, P.M. (1992). Long-term comparative trial of conventional percussion and drainage physiotherapy versus autogenic drainage in cystic fibrosis. *Pediatric Pulmonology Supplement 8,* 298.

Decesare, J., Graybill-Tucker, C.A., & Gould, A.L. (1995). Physical therapy for the child with respiratory dysfunction. In S. Irwin & J.S. Tecklin (Eds.), *Cardiopulmonary physical therapy* (3rd ed., pp. 516–562). St. Louis: Mosby.

DeJong, W., van Aalderen, W.M., Kraan, J., Koeter, G.H., & van der Schans, C.P. (2001). Inspiratory muscle training in patients with cystic fibrosis. *Respiratory Medicine, 95*(1), 31–66.

Dichter, C.G., Darbee, J.C., Effgen, S.K., & Palisano, R.J. (1993). Assessment of pulmonary function and physical fitness in children with Down syndrome. *Pediatric Physical Therapy, 5,* 3–8.

Doershuk, C.F., Fischer, B.J., & Matthews, L.W. (1975). Pulmonary physiology of the young child. In E.M. Scarpelli (Ed.), *Pulmonary physiology of the fetus, newborn and child.* Philadelphia: Lea & Febiger.

Dresen, M.H.W., de Groot, G., Corstius, J.J., Krediet, G.H., & Meijer, M.A. (1982). Physical work capacity and daily physical activities of handicapped and non-handicapped children. *European Journal of Applied Physiology, 48,* 241–252.

Eng, P.A., Morton, J., Douglass, J.A., Riedler, J., Wilson, J., & Robertson, C.F. (1996). Short-term efficacy of ultrasonically nebulized hypertonic saline in cystic fibrosis. *Pediatric Pulmonology, 21*(2), 77–83.

Fedderly, R.T. (1999). Left ventricular outflow obstruction. *Pediatric Clinics of North America: Pediatric Cardiology, 46*(2), 369–384.

Fishman, A.P. (1988). *Pulmonary diseases and disorders* (2nd ed.). New York: McGraw-Hill.

Frownfelter, D., & Dean, E. (1996). *Principles and practice of cardiopulmonary physical therapy* (3rd ed.). St. Louis: Mosby.

Gaultier, C. (1995). Respiratory muscle function in infants. *European Respiratory Journal, 8*(1), 150–153.

Gondor, M., Nixon, P., Mutich, R., Rebovich, P., & Orenstein, D. (1999). Comparison of flutter device and chest physical therapy in the treatment of cystic fibrosis during pulmonary exacerbation. *Pediatric Pulmonology, 28,* 255–260.

Grifka, R.G. (1999). Cyanotic congenital heart disease with increased pulmonary blood flow. *Pediatric Clinics of North America: Pediatric Cardiology, 46*(2), 405–425.

Gross, S.J., Iannuzzi, D.M., Kveselis, D.A., & Anbar, R.D. (1998). Effect of preterm birth on pulmonary function at school age: A prospective controlled study. *Journal of Pediatrics 133,* 188–192.

Guyton, A. (1996). *Textbook of medical physiology* (9th ed., p. 487). Philadelphia: W.B. Saunders.

Heath, G.W., & Fentem, P.H. (1997). Physical activity among persons with disabilities—A public health perspective. *Exercise and Sport Science Reviews, 25,* 216.

Hershenson, M.B., Colin, A.A., Wohl, M.E., & Stark, A.R. (1990). Changes in the contribution of the rib cage to tidal breathing during infancy. *American Review of Respiratory Disease, 141*(4 Pt 1), 922–925.

Hofmeyr, J.L., Webber, B.A., & Hodson, M.E. (1986).

Evaluation of positive expiratory pressure as an adjunct to chest physiotherapy in the treatment of cystic fibrosis. *Thorax, 41*(12), 951–954.

Holloway, E., & Ram, F.S.F. (2002). Breathing exercises for asthma (Cochrane Review). *The Cochrane Library*, Issue 4. Oxford: Update Software.

Hulsmann, A.R., & Van den Anker, J.N. (1997). Evolution and natural history of chronic lung disease of prematurity. *Monaldi Archives for Chest Disease, 52*, 272–277.

Jacob, S.V., Lands, L.C., Coates, A.L., Davis, G.M., MacNeish, C.F., Hornby, L., Riley, S.P., & Outergridge, E.W. (1997). Exercise ability in survivors of severe bronchopulmonary dysplasia. *American Journal of Respiratory and Critical Care Medicine 155*, 1925–1929.

Janssen, T.W.J., Van Oers, C.A.J.M., Van Der Woude, L.H.V., & Hollander, A.P. (1994). Physical strain in daily life of wheelchair users with spinal cord injuries. *Medicine and Science in Sports and Exercise, 26*, 661–670.

Keens, T.G., Krastins, J.R., Wannamaker, E.M., Levison, H., Crozier, D.N., & Bryan, A.C. (1977). Ventilatory muscle endurance training in normal subjects and patients with cystic fibrosis. *American Review of Respiratory Disease, 116*, 853–860.

Kluft, J., Beker, L., Castagnino, M., Gaiser, J., Chaney, H., & Fink, R.J. (1996). A comparison of bronchial drainage treatments in cystic fibrosis. *Pediatric Pulmonology, 22*, 271–274.

Konstan, M.H., Stern, R.C., & Doershuk, C.F. (1994). Efficacy of the Flutter device for airway mucus clearance in patients with cystic fibrosis. *Journal of Pediatrics, 124*, 689–693.

Korhonen, P., Tammela, O., Koivisto, A.M., Laippala, P., & Ikonen, S. (1999). Frequency and risk factors in bronchopulmonary dysplasia in a cohort of very low birth weight infants. *Early Human Development, 54*, 245–258.

Krahenbuhl, G.S., Skinner, J.S., & Kohrt, W.M. (1985). Developmental aspects of maximal aerobic power in children. *Exercise and Sport Sciences Reviews, 13*, 503–538.

Kravitz, R.M. (1994). Congenital malformations of the lung. *Pediatric Clinics of North America: Respiratory Medicine II, 41*(3), 453–472.

Lane, P.A. (1996). Sickle cell disease. *The Pediatric Clinics of North America: Pediatric Hematology, 43*(3), 639–664.

Lara, M., Rosenbaum, S., Rachelefsky, G., Nicholas, W., Morton, S.C., Emont, S., et al. (2002). Improving childhood asthma outcomes in the United States: A blue print for action. *Pediatrics, 109*, 919–930.

Lundberg, A. (1978). Maximal aerobic capacity of young people with spastic cerebral palsy. *Developmental Medicine and Child Neurology, 20*, 205–210.

Mannino, D.M., Homa, D.M., Oertowski, C.A., Ashizawa, A., Nixon, L.L., Johnson, C.A., et al. (1998). Surveillance for asthma—United States, 1960–1995. *Morbidity and Mortality Weekly Report, 47*, 1–27.

McColley, S. (1998). Bronchopulmonary dysplasia: Impact of surfactant replacement therapy. *Pediatric Clinics of North America 45*, 573–584.

Mukhopadhyay, S., Singh, M., Cater, J., Ogston, S., Franklin, M.,

& Oliver, R. (1995). Nebulised anti-pseudomonal antibiotic therapy in cystic fibrosis: A meta-analysis of benefits and risks. *Thorax, 51*, 364–368.

Newell, S.J., Booth, W., Morgan, M.E., Durbin, G.M., & McNeish, A.S. (1989). Gastroesophageal reflux in preterm infants. *Archives of Disease in Childhood, 64*, 780–786.

Nikolaizik, W., & Schonl, M. (1996). Pilot study to assess the effect of inhaled corticosteroids on lung function in patients with cystic fibrosis. *Journal of Pediatrics, 128*, 271–274.

Nixon, P. (1996). Role of exercise in the evaluation and management of pulmonary disease in children and youth. *Medicine and Science in Sports and Exercise, 28*(4), 414–420.

Nixon, P. (2003). Cystic fibrosis. In J.L. Durstine & G.E. Moore, *ACSM's Exercise management for persons with chronic diseases and disabilities* (pp. 111–116). Champaign, IL: Human Kinetics.

Northway, W., Rosan, R.C., & Porter, D.Y. (1967). Pulmonary disease following respiratory therapy of hyaline membrane disease: Bronchopulmonary dysplasia. *New England Journal of Medicine, 176*, 357–368.

Oberwaldner, B., Theiss, B., Rucker, A., & Zach, M.S. (1991). Chest physiotherapy in hospitalized patients with cystic fibrosis: A study of lung function effects and sputum production. *European Respiratory Journal, 4*, 152–158.

Oberwaldner, B., Evans, J.C., & Zach, M.S. (1986). Forced expirations against a variable resistance: A new chest physiotherapy method in cystic fibrosis. *Pediatric Pulmonology, 2*(6), 358–367.

Oermann, C., Swank, P., & Sockrider, M. (2000). Validation of an instrument measuring patient satisfaction with chest physiotherapy techniques in cystic fibrosis. *Chest, 118*, 92–97.

Park, M.K., & Guntheroth, W.G. (1992). *How to read pediatric ECGs* (3rd ed.). St. Louis: Mosby.

Pilmer, S.L. (1994). Prolonged mechanical ventilation in children. *Pediatric Clinics of North America: Respiratory Medicine II, 41*(3), 473–512.

Pryor, J., & Webber, B. (1998). *Physiotherapy for respiratory and cardiac problems* (p. 338). Philadelphia: Churchill Livingstone.

Roberton, N.R. (1996). Intensive care. In A. Greenough, N.R. Roberton, & A. Milner (Eds.), *Neonatal Respiratory Disorders* (pp. 174–195). London: Arnold.

Rosenkranz, E.R. (1998). Caring for the former pediatric cardiac surgery patient. *Pediatric Clinics of North America, 45*(4), 907–941.

Rothstein, J.M., Roy, S.H., & Wolf, S.L. (1998). *The rehabilitation specialist's handbook* (2nd ed., pp. 534–535). Philadelphia: F.A. Davis.

Rowley, A.H., & Shulman, S.T. (1999). Kawasaki syndrome. *Pediatric Clinics of North America: Pediatric Cardiology, 46*(2), 313–329.

Salbe, A.D., Weyer, C., Lindsay, R.S., Ravussin, E., & Tataranni, P.A. (2002). Assessing risk factors for obesity in childhood and adolescence: I. Birth weight, childhood adiposity, parental obesity, insulin and leptin. *Pediatrics, 110*, 299–306.

Salbe, A.D., Weyer, C., Harper, I., Lindsay, R.S., Ravussin, E., &

Tataranni, P.A. (2002). Assessing risk factors for obesity in childhood and adolescence: II. Energy metabolism and physical activity. *Pediatrics, 110,* 307–314.

Sahl, W., Bilton, D., Dodd, M., & Webb, A.K. (1989). Effect of exercise and physiotherapy in aiding sputum expectoration in adults with cystic fibrosis. *Thorax, 44,* 1006–1008.

Sawyer, E.H., & Clanton, T.L. (1993). Improved pulmonary function and exercise tolerance with inspiratory muscle conditioning in children with cystic fibrosis. *Chest, 104*(5), 1490–1497.

Schere, T.A., Barandun, J., Martinez, E.R., Wanner, A., & Rubin, E.M. (1998). Effect of high frequency oral airway and chest wall oscillation and conventional chest physical therapy on expectoration in patients with stable cystic fibrosis. *Chest, 113*(4), 1019–1027.

Schneiderman-Walker, J., Pollock, S.L., Corey, M., Wilkes, D.D., Canny, G.J., Pedder, L., et al. (2000). A randomized controlled trial of a 3 year home exercise program in cystic fibrosis. *Journal of Pediatrics, 136*(3), 304–310.

Schoni, M.H. (1989). Autogenic drainage: A modern approach to physiotherapy in cystic fibrosis. *Journal of the Royal Society of Medicine, 82*(suppl 16), 32–37.

Shah, P.L., Scott, S.F., Knight, R.A., & Hodson, M.E. (1996). The effects of recombinant human DNase on neutrophil elastase activity and interleukin-8 levels in the sputum of patients with cystic fibrosis. *European Respiratory Journal, 9*(3), 531–534.

Smith, J., Travis, S., Greenberg, E., & Welsh, M. (1996). Cystic fibrosis airway epithelia fail to kill bacteria because of abnormal surface fluid. *Cell, 85,* 229–236.

Sockolov, R., Irwin, B., Dressendorfer, R.H., & Bernauer, E.M. (1977). Exercise performance in 6 to 11 year old boys with muscular dystrophy. *Archives of Physical Medicine and Rehabilitation, 58,* 195–201.

Steen, H.J., Redmond, A.O., O'Neill, D., & Beattie, F. (1991). Evaluation of the PEP mask in cystic fibrosis. *Acta Paediatrica Scandinavica, 80*(1), 51–56.

Stout, J. (2000). Physical fitness during childhood and adolescence. In S.K. Campbell, D.W. Vander Linden, & R.J. Palisano (Eds.), *Physical therapy for children* (2nd ed., pp. 141–169). Philadelphia: W.B. Saunders.

Stout, J., & Taber, L.A. (1995). Biomechanics of growth, remodeling, and morphogenesis. *Applied Mechanics Review, 48*(8), August.

Swartz, M.H. (1994). *Textbook of physical diagnoses: History and examination* (2nd ed.). Philadelphia: W.B. Saunders.

Thomas, J., Cook, D.J., & Brooks, D. (1995). Chest physical therapy management of patients with cystic fibrosis. *American Journal of Respiratory Critical Care Medicine, 151,* 846–850.

Thorensen, M., Cavan, F., & Whitelaw, A. (1988). Effect of tilting on oxygenation in newborn infants. *Archives of Disease in Childhood, 63,* 315–317.

Toro-Salazar, O.H., Steinberger, J., Thomas, W., Rocchini, A.P., Carpenter, B., & Moller, J.H. (2002). Long-term follow-up of patients after coarctation of the aorta repair. *American Journal of Cardiology, 89*(5), 541–547.

Towbin, J.A. (1999). Pediatric myocardial disease. *Pediatric Clinics of North America: Pediatric Cardiology, 46*(2), 289–312.

Tyrrell, J.C., Hiller, E.J., & Martin, J. (1986). Face mask physiotherapy in cystic fibrosis. *Archives of Disease in Childhood, 61*(6), 598–600.

United States Department of Health and Human Services (1995). *Healthy people 2000: Progress report for physical activity and fitness.* Washington, DC: Author.

United States Department of Health and Human Services (2000). *Healthy people 2010.* Washington, DC: Author.

Van Asperen, P.P., Jackson, L., Hennessy, P., & Brown, J. (1987). Comparison of a positive expiratory pressure (PEP) mask with postural drainage in patients with cystic fibrosis. *Australian Paediatric Journal, 23*(5), 283–284.

Van Essen-Zandvliet, E.E., Hughes, M.D., Waalkens, H.J., Duiverman, E.J., Pocock, S.J., & Kerrebijn, K.F. (1992). Effects of 22 months of treatment with inhaled steroids and/or beta2 agonists on lung function, airway responsiveness and symptoms in children with asthma. *American Review of Respiratory Disease, 146,* 547–554.

Verklan, M.T. (1997). Bronchopulmonary dysplasia: Its effects upon the heart and lungs. *Neonatal Network, 16*(8), 5–12.

Wilkins, R.L., & Drider, S.J. (1985). *Clinical assessment in respiratory care.* St. Louis: Mosby.

Wilson, G.E., Baldwin, A.L., & Walshaw, M.J. (1995). A comparison of traditional chest physiotherapy with the active cycle of breathing in patients with chronic suppurative lung disease. *European Respiratory Journal, 8*(suppl 19), 171S.

Chapter 9

Integumentary System

— Suzanne F. Migliore, PT, MS, PCS

The role of the physical therapist in wound care has evolved over the last several decades. For the physical therapist, the groundwork for learning wound and burn management occurs in the entry-level curriculum. Mechanisms of healing and systems reviews that enhance the knowledge base for caring for a child with open wounds or burns are taught. Physical therapists who desire to be active in wound management will need to expand their knowledge through continuing education and, as with any specialty, competency-based training with a mentor. Pediatric clinicians need to be prepared to encounter a wide range of integumentary issues with children. Children are at risk for thermal injuries, pressure ulcers, and traumatic wounds. There are also specific congenital integumentary impairments that will challenge the pediatric clinician's ability to provide timely and age-appropriate interventions. This chapter will serve as an introduction to wound and burn management for the physical therapist as part of an interdisciplinary pediatric wound-management team.

Intervention Settings

Clinicians throughout different care settings need to be prepared to provide wound care for the pediatric population. Acute-care physical therapists play an integral role on the wound-management team. Therapists work closely with physicians and nurses to achieve wound closure through a variety of interventions that are discussed in this chapter. In the rehabilitation setting, management of chronic wounds and burns following the acute healing process or after grafting will present many challenges for the physical therapist. In addition to wound management, achieving independence with functional skills must be addressed. In the outpatient setting, therapists are often called on to maximize function and to decrease activity or participation limitations that may occur with open wounds. Therapists also intervene with scar management techniques after wound closure. School-based therapists need to have background knowledge in the areas of wound and scar management because children with traumatic wounds, pressure ulcers, and burns will eventually return to school after their acute care and rehabilitation. Although school-based therapists may not provide direct wound care, there are often interventions that need to be followed throughout the school day. Examples include the use of static or dynamic splints after a thermal injury, pressure-relieving techniques for a child with a pressure ulcer, and reintegration in school activities after an integumentary injury. Working with teachers and other classmates, the school-based therapist can aid the transition back to school for a child who has had a prolonged hospitalization and may face issues surrounding cosmesis, body image, and peer acceptance.

Skin Structure and Function

The skin is the largest external organ of the human body, covering a surface area of 2 m². To best understand the etiology of integumentary impairments, physical therapists need to know the anatomy and physiology of the skin. Its primary functions are sensation, metabolism, thermoregulation, and protection from trauma (Rassner, 1994). The skin has two primary layers, the epidermis and the dermis. A schematic drawing of the layers of the epidermis and dermis is shown in Figure 9–1 and the corresponding color plate.

Epidermis

The **epidermis**, the outermost layer of the skin, is approximately 0.04 mm thick (Sussman, 1998b). There are four layers in the epidermis: the stratum corneum, stratum granulosum, stratum spinosum, and stratum basale. A fifth layer, the stratum lucidum, is found in the soles of the feet and the palms of the hands (Patterson & Blaylock, 1987). Structures in the epidermis include melanocytes, Langerhans' cells, hair follicles, sebaceous and apocrine glands, and eccrine sweat glands. The hair follicle contains primarily epidermal tissue, which plays a key role in re-epithelialization of wounds (Falkel, 1994). The epidermis is nonvascular and forms a defensive covering for the dermis. The epidermis varies in thickness throughout the body, with the surfaces of the hands and feet having the deepest thickness. It limits water evaporation from the surface of the skin and molds itself onto the papillary layer of the dermis, forming the epidermal-dermal junction (Gray, 1977).

Dermis

The **dermis** is the "true skin," which is tough, flexible, and highly elastic. Its thickness varies throughout the body. The

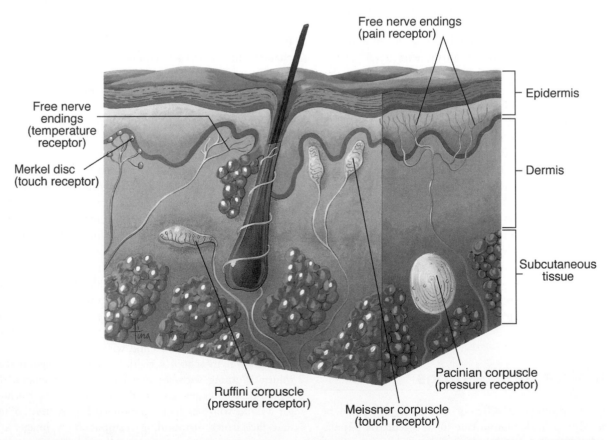

Figure 9-1 Schematic representation of the skin structures. (From Sussman, C., & Bates-Jensen, B. [Eds.]. [1998]. *Wound care: A collaborative practice manual for physical therapists and nurses* [p. 57]. ©Gaithersburg, MD: Aspen Publishing. Reprinted with permission.) See also color plate.

dermal layer is very thick in the palms of the hands and soles of the feet and very thin in the eyelids and genitalia. The thickness of the skin at the location of an open wound or thermal injury plays a role in the severity of injury. For example, pressure at the sacrum has the potential to cause more damage than pressure at the ischial tuberosity because of the thinness of the skin and the lack of depth of subcutaneous tissues. The dermis has two layers: the outermost papillary layer and the deeper reticular layer. The reticular layer contains fibroelastic material, mostly collagen. The dermis is highly vascular and contains structures including lymphatic cells, epithelial cells, connective tissue, muscle, fat, and nerve tissue. The vascular supply of the dermal layer supplies nutrition to the epidermis and aids in regulating body temperature (Gray, 1977).

Phases of Wound Healing

The main phases of wound healing are inflammation, proliferation, and maturation. The phases may overlap in the course of wound healing, but each has unique physiological events. Understanding the phases and being able to identify the phase that a wound is in will guide the clinician in choosing appropriate interventions. The ideal outcome of a wound-management program is to influence healing toward wound closure.

Inflammatory Phase

The hallmark signs of the inflammatory process are changes in color, increased skin temperature, swelling, and the presence of pain. The main goal of the inflammatory phase is to rid the wound of debris and prepare the wound for healing by fighting infection. The first part of the inflammatory phase is the vascular response, with the main goal being to stop the hemorrhage. Catecholamines are then released and produce vasoconstriction; at the same time, collagen and other cells activate platelets and initiate the "clotting cascade" to prevent further bleeding. Increased cell permeability then produces the edema response, which is both immediate and continuous for hours (Greenhalgh & Staley, 1994). This then encompasses the second part of the inflammatory phase, the cellular response.

The cellular response is an elaborate and well-orchestrated array of cells migrating toward the area of injury. Neutrophils tend to migrate toward the wound space within the first 24 hours. Their function is to act as phagocytic cells and fight bacteria. The neutrophil helps to keep the wound clean. Wounds with bacterial counts greater than 10^5 are considered infected (Bates-Jensen, 1998a; Huffines & Logsdon, 1997). Mast cells respond by releasing histamine, which plays a role in cell permeability. During the cellular response, once the body has produced enough platelets for clotting, mast cells change their effect and produce heparin. Heparin then stimulates endothelial cells to migrate toward the wound. Other cells involved in this phase include macrophages, which act to rid the wound of debris. Macrophages have also been linked to the transition to the proliferative phase of wound healing. This is accomplished by the macrophage secreting angiogenesis growth factor (AGF). AGF then stimulates endothelial cells and re-establishes the blood flow to the injured area. Through angiogenesis, nutritional supply is re-established to the wound bed. **Fibroblasts** also appear during the inflammatory phase. Fibroblasts aid in the production of the collagen matrix, which is more clearly defined during the proliferative phase. Late in the inflammatory phase, fibroblasts differentiate into myofibroblasts, which aid in wound contraction. Endothelial and epithelial cells also respond during this phase. From the onset of trauma, the epithelial cells respond from the dermis. These cells begin the resurfacing process known as re-epithelialization. The epithelial cells in the inflammatory phase also aid in ridding the wound of necrotic tissue by releasing lytic enzymes (Sussman, 1998a).

Proliferative Phase

Two key steps toward wound healing occur during the proliferative phase: fibroplasia and wound contraction. These steps provide the wound bed with needed nutrition and oxygen to allow early progression toward wound closure. Ongoing during this phase are angiogenesis and epithelialization.

Fibroplasia

According to Ross (1968), "An optimal inflammatory response appears to be an important, rapid, non-specific stimulus for fibroplasia." **Fibroplasia** is the laying down of the collagen matrix that is known as granulation tissue. The angiogenesis that began in the inflammatory phase supplies nutrition and oxygen to this matrix. Cells that respond to the wound during this phase include fibroblasts, myofibroblasts, and endothelial and epidermal cells. The fibroblast is responsible for producing the collagen matrix, which is called procollagen. The procollagen becomes tropocollagen, which eventually forms a collagen fibril.

These fibrils are laid down in the wound bed in a disorganized manner. Cross-linkage occurs when the collagen matrix comes together; the better the organization of the matrix, the better is the overall improvement in wound tensile strength. When fibroplasia is occurring, the collagen matrix looks like pink or red granules or "buds" piled on top of each other, as seen in Figure 9–2 and the corresponding color plate (Sussman, 1998a). During this stage of the proliferative phase, the granulation buds are fragile and cannot sustain any force from an outside trauma. Such trauma can damage the tissue, causing a regression to the inflammatory phase. This will be important to recall when wound cleansing and dressings are discussed later in this chapter.

Wound Contraction

Myofibroblasts during this phase have the "contractile properties of smooth muscle cells" (Sussman, 1998a). The myofibroblast attaches to the wound edges, pulling the epidermal layer toward the center of the wound. The contracting forces appear to come from the cells that are within the granulation tissue (Ross, 1968). The size and shape of the wound will also have an effect on its ability to contract. A linear wound will contract the fastest; circular wounds, such as pressure ulcers, will contract the slowest (Sussman, 1998a).

Epithelialization

As described earlier under the inflammatory phase, epithelialization begins immediately after trauma. The ongoing

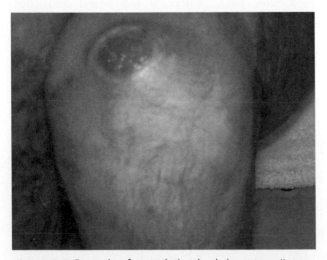

Figure 9-2 Example of granulation buds in a stage II pressure ulcer. See also color plate.

process of **re-epithelialization** or resurfacing of the wound continues during the proliferative phase. The epithelial cells respond to messages from macrophages and neutrophils and advance toward the wound surface in sheets. Epidermal cells in the front of this "sheet" act to rid the wound of debris and allow for resurfacing from the edges of the wound. A moist wound environment is most advantageous for this cell migration. The epidermal cells will have an impossible task of resurfacing a full-thickness (epidermis and dermis destroyed) wound because of the depth. The cells will approach from the wound edges and then appear to roll under the edges, causing epidermal rolling or ridging as seen with a chronic pressure ulcer. Wounds of this depth and chronic nature will not be able to heal by resurfacing (Sussman, 1998a).

Maturation Phase

During the maturation (or remodeling) phase, three processes are seen: collagen lysis, collagen organization, and scar formation. This phase begins a few weeks after trauma and may last for up to 2 to 3 years.

Collagen Lysis/Organization

To regulate fibroplasia during the proliferative phase, the enzyme collagenase is produced. Collagenase has the ability to break the cross-linkages of the tropocollagen; this process is called collagen lysis. During the maturation phase, the balance between collagen synthesis and collagen lysis is a key factor. As a wound matures, collagen lysis takes over and aids in the organization of the collagen bundles. The more organized the bundles, the better is the outcome, as seen with a smooth and elastic scar (Sussman, 1998a).

Scar Formation

While the organization of the collagen is occurring, the fibronectin that is laid down during fibroplasia is eliminated and large bundles of **type I collagen** are present. A decrease in the number of small blood vessels occurs, and the new scar, which usually has a bright red appearance, starts to fade. During the maturation phase, an increase in the cross-linkages of collagen fibers will increase the strength of the scar (Greenhalgh & Staley, 1994).

While the scar is forming, any diversion from the normal processes might lead to abnormal healing. Wounds that take a longer time to heal may develop hypertrophic (thicker/erythematous) scars. This thickening appears to come from prolonged collagen synthesis and angiogenesis. A **hypertrophic scar** will have a raised appearance, as seen in Figure 9–3 and the corresponding color plate. A hypertrophic scar that extends above and beyond the original scar site is considered a keloid. The reason for hypertrophic and keloid type scars is not known. Any event that prolongs the inflammatory phase can lead to excessive scarring. The propensity for raised scars may also be attributed to the location of the wound and to ethnic heritage and age (Greenhalgh & Staley, 1994). Recommended readings for a more comprehensive look at wound healing include *Wound healing: Alternatives in management* (Kloth & McCulloch, 2002) and *Wound care: A collaborative practice manual for physical therapists and nurses* (Sussman & Bates-Jensen, 1998).

Integumentary Impairments

To provide appropriate interventions to children with integumentary impairments, the clinician must possess knowledge of the pathophysiology of each body function. The following is a review of some diagnoses with integumentary impairments.

Pressure Ulcers

Despite the usual correlation of pressure ulcers with the geriatric population, the pediatric population is also at risk. Any child who has decreased sensation, inability to

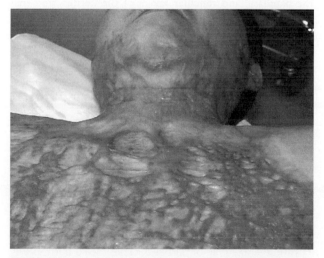

Figure 9-3 Example of hypertrophic scarring after full-thickness burns and skin grafting. See also color plate.

communicate pain and discomfort, prolonged bed rest, poor nutrition, or a known integumentary disorder is at risk for pressure ulcers. Children with spina bifida or spinal cord injury have an increased propensity for skin breakdown caused by impaired sensation. Child and caregiver education for skin care and pressure ulcer prevention is imperative. In order to provide timely interventions, it is important to recognize the stage of the pressure ulcer. Ischemia and hypoxemia occur when pressure occludes blood flow to the local tissues. Four levels of skin breakdown can occur in correlation to the amount of time exposed to pressure. Hyperemia can occur in less than 30 minutes and presents as local redness that dissipates within 1 hour of relief of pressure. Ischemia occurs after 2 to 6 hours of pressure; the erythema that is present takes up to 36 hours to dissipate. Necrosis is the next level of breakdown, and occurs after 6 hours of continuous pressure. Ulceration is the final level of breakdown; it may occur up to 2 weeks after an episode of necrosis. Factors leading to pressure ulcers include immobility, shear, friction, and moisture. **Shear** is a parallel force that causes ischemia by displacing blood vessels. **Friction** occurs when two surfaces move across each other, abrading and damaging the epidermal and upper dermal layers. Friction and shear occur most commonly during position changes in bed and with transfers from bed to other surfaces, including stretchers or wheelchairs. Caution must be taken by all caregivers to avoid friction and shear when moving or transferring children. In children who are incontinent, constant moisture can lead to skin maceration, making the skin more prone to breakdown (Bates-Jensen, 1998c).

Staging of Pressure Ulcers

The Agency for Health Care Policy and Research (AHCPR) has established clinical practice guidelines for treatment of pressure ulcers. They have provided standardized definitions for pressure ulcers and established intervention programs. They define a pressure ulcer as "any lesion caused by unrelieved pressure resulting in damage of underlying tissue" (Bergstrom et al., 1994). Pressure ulcers are described or **"staged"** according to depth and tissue damage. The four stages of pressure ulcers are defined as follows:

- Stage I: Nonblanchable erythema of intact skin, the heralding lesion of skin ulceration. In individuals with darker skin, discoloration of the skin, warmth, edema, induration, or hardness may also be indicators.

- Stage II: Partial-thickness skin loss involving the

epidermis, dermis, or both. The ulcer is superficial and presents as an abrasion, a blister, or a shallow crater.

- Stage III: Full-thickness skin loss involving damage to or necrosis of subcutaneous tissue that may extend down to, but not through, underlying fascia. The ulcer presents as a deep crater with or without undermining of adjacent tissue.
- Stage IV: Full-thickness skin loss with extensive destruction, tissue necrosis, or damage to muscle, bone, or supporting structures (e.g., tendon, joint capsule). Undermining and sinus tracts may also be associated with stage IV pressure ulcers.

Limitations of these definitions require clinical judgments. For example, stage I ulcers are those with intact skin and may not be assessed accurately in children with darker, pigmented skin. If thick, leathery, necrotic, devitalized tissue (**eschar**) is present, the ulcer cannot be correctly staged until it is removed (Bergstrom et al., 1994). Note that as a pressure ulcer heals, it will always be described according to its original stage. Documentation of a "healing stage I, II, III, or IV" ulcer is appropriate; an ulcer should not be downstaged (e.g., from a III to a II) as it heals.

The child's participation in life activities is limited according to the stage, size, and location of the pressure ulcer. Pressure ulcers that are on weight-bearing surfaces will limit mobility, ability to sit, and ambulation. Children may be limited from lying on their backs, sitting up in their wheelchairs, or walking with orthotics. With the most severe pressure ulcers, especially those on the sacrum or ischial tuberosities, the child may be limited to prone positioning while out of bed. For children who are nonambulatory, being restricted from using their wheelchairs will limit their participation in activities in the home and their ability to participate in school or work.

Thermal Injuries

Thermal injuries are the third most common cause of death in children under the age of 1 year, preceded only by nonfirearm homicides and motor vehicle accidents. Between the ages of 1 and 9 years, deaths from thermal injuries are second only to those from motor vehicle accidents. The most common mechanism of burn is scalding, but burns with the highest fatality rate are those from fires, which often include inhalation injuries. The mechanism of thermal injury may also vary by age. Infants have a higher incidence of scald burns from hot beverages or

from being bathed in water that is too hot. Toddlers may pull hot liquids off the stove or sustain electrical injuries from wires or plugs. School-aged children are susceptible to playing with matches and have a higher incidence of flame burns. Adolescents mimic their adult counterparts in the mechanism of injury, including flame, chemical, cooking, smoking materials, or fireworks (Committee on Injury and Poison Prevention, American Academy of Pediatrics, 1997).

Burn Depth Classification

Burns are classified according to the depth of injury and the affected skin structures. The three classifications are superficial, partial thickness, and full thickness.

Superficial Burns

Superficial burns are caused by ultraviolet exposure, sunburn, or a short flash of heat. Only epidermal layers are affected. The skin is erythematous but does not show any signs of blistering. Healing occurs within 3 to 7 days.

Partial-Thickness Burns

Partial-thickness burns are split into two categories, superficial and deep, depending on the involved structures. Superficial partial-thickness burns involve damage to the epidermis and some of the papillary dermis. The skin is blistered or weeping, as seen in Figure 9–4 and the corresponding color plate. These burns usually heal within 7 to 21 days without surgical intervention. Minimal scarring is expected.

Deep partial-thickness burns involve the epidermis and the papillary, and reticular layers of the dermis, and may include fat found in the subcutaneous layer. The skin presents with large blisters or mottled white to cherry-red

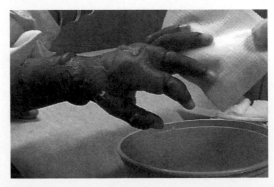

Figure 9-4 Example of partial-thickness scald burn to the hand. Note blistering and weeping of the wound. See also color plate.

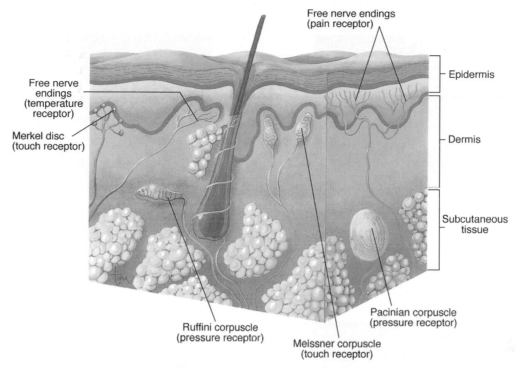

Fig 9-1

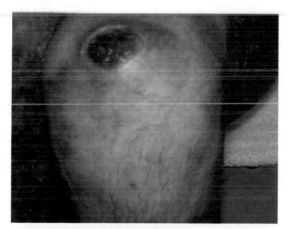

Fig 9-2

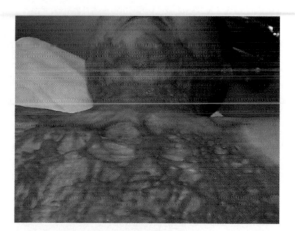

Fig 9-3

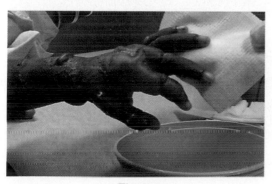

Fig 9-4

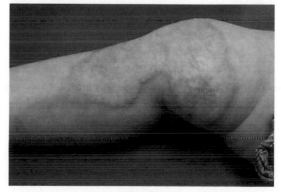

Fig 9-6

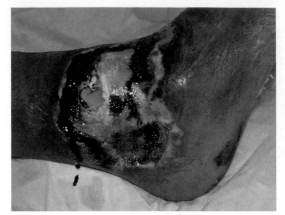

Fig 9-7

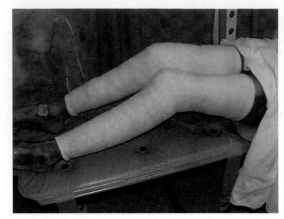

Fig 9-8

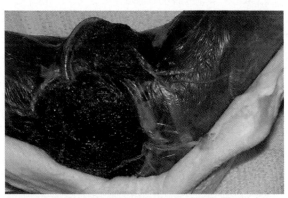

Fig 9-14A

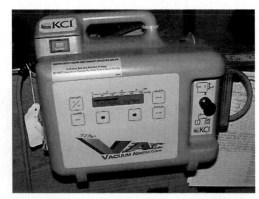

Fig 9-14B

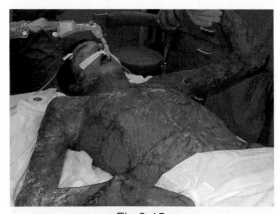

Fig 9-15

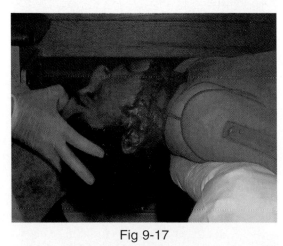

Fig 9-17

coloration. These wounds will heal in 21 to 35 days if not infected. These burns, depending on the burn size, might best be addressed surgically (see section on surgical interventions). Scarring is most likely with a deep partial-thickness burn that is allowed to heal without grafting. With all partial-thickness burns, there is increased pain and sensitivity to temperature.

Full-Thickness Burns

Full-thickness burns involve all of the epidermis, dermis, and subcutaneous tissue, and may include fascia, muscle, tendon, and bone. The skin appears dry or leathery; no blanching is seen with pressure. With the most severe burns, the skin may appear charred. Hair follicles will pull out easily, and there is little or no pain because of the destruction of pain receptors. These burns are best managed surgically by excision and grafting.

One difficulty with using this system of classification is that thermal injuries are not traditionally uniform in their presentation. The most severe portion of the burn is often in the center, with less involved areas surrounding it. Zones of the burn wound classification were established to describe the areas involved. The most central zone is the *zone of coagulation,* with the area of greatest destruction. The center will appear white and leathery, with all viable tissue being destroyed. The *zone of stasis* surrounds the zone of coagulation. It is temporarily without blood supply, but vascular response can be restored and the healing process started. If this zone is allowed to dry out, the vascular supply will not re-establish, killing viable tissue and converting the burn to necrotic tissue. This will be an important premise to remember when topical agents and dressings for burns are reviewed later. The outermost zone is the *zone of hyperemia,* which is equal to a superficial burn with intact vascular supply and blanching on pressure (Johnson, 1994).

Burn Size Estimation

In addition to determining the depth of a burn, it is important to determine the **total body surface area (TBSA)** involved. There are several scales and charts to map out the TBSA; however, they often underestimate the percentage of involved skin in children (Lund & Browder, 1944). For example, the rule of nines, which is often used in adults with burns, is not as useful because of the varying sizes of infants, toddlers, and school-aged children. "The most accurate method of determining surface area burned is by mapping the injured areas on a Lund and Browder–like

body chart and then calculating the burned area from body surface area nomograms" (Herndon, Rutan, Alison, & Cox, 1993). The TBSA is determined by age, as seen in Figure 9–5 and Table 9.1. During the initial burn examination, it is important to use the accompanying body chart to identify where the burns are located. This chart can be updated as additional burned areas are identified.

Burn Severity and Functional Outcomes

The size and location of the burn will determine the child's activity restrictions. Burns over joints will limit range of motion (ROM); loss of muscle mass or prolonged bed rest may affect strength. Severe burns with high TBSA percentages can cause long-standing contractures and permanent body cosmesis changes. Burns on the hands can limit the child's ability to self-feed, and burns on the plantar surface of the feet will limit the ability to ambulate. A child who sustains facial burns may have limitations with swallowing, talking, and adequate nutritional intake. A referral to speech therapy for oral motor skills may be appropriate. The child's ability to participate in activities of daily living (ADLs), school, play, and sports will be affected until acute burn management and rehabilitation have occurred. The child who is burned may face a lifelong battle with episodes of decreased activities caused by scarring, requiring ongoing scar management. If restrictions are severe enough to limit participation in life activities, consideration is given to surgical interventions.

Surgical Interventions for Thermal Injuries

Partial- and full-thickness burns are often examined and re-examined throughout their acute healing course for the need for surgical intervention. Surgery for thermal injuries may be performed in the acute phase by escharotomies, to resume circulation to an area after constriction caused by edema. An **escharotomy** is "a longitudinal incision through the full-thickness burn to the layer of subcutaneous fat of an extremity" (Miller, Staley, & Richard, 1994). This procedure will release the pressure on underlying blood vessels and allow more normal circulation. If the burn is left undressed, ischemia may occur and amputation may be necessary.

After acute management, surgical interventions will focus on the elimination of devitalized tissue. The burn surgeon must remove or excise the devitalized tissue down to healthy bleeding tissue; this is done with an instrument

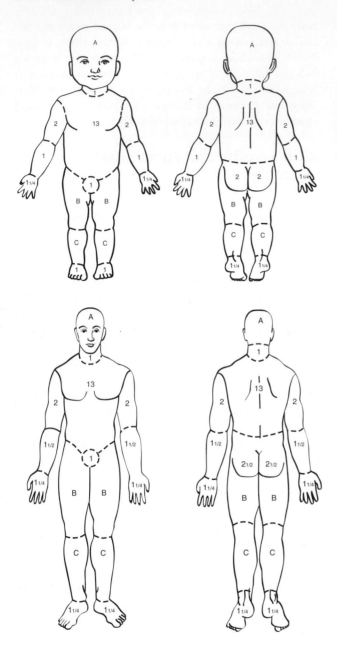

Figure 9-5 Lund & Browder chart for estimation of burn area. (From Lund, C.C., & Browder, N.C. [1944]. The estimation of areas of burns. *Surgery, Gynecology, and Obstetrics, 79,* 352–358. American College of Surgeons. Reprinted with permission.) Caregivers can mark on the figure where partial- or full-thickness burns are with different colors or hatch marks.

Table 9.1 Lund and Browder Chart for Estimation of Burn Area

Area	AGE (YR)				
	0–1	**1–4**	**5–9**	**10–15**	**Adult**
Head	9.5	8.5	8.5	5	3.5
Neck	1	1	1	1	1
Anterior trunk	13	13	13	13	13
Posterior trunk	13	13	13	13	13
Right buttock	2.5	2.5	2.5	2.5	2.5
Left buttock	2.5	2.5	2.5	2.5	2.5
Genitalia	1	1	1	1	1
Right upper arm	2	2	2	2	2
Left upper arm	2	2	2	2	2
Right lower arm	1.5	1.5	1.5	1.5	1.5
Left lower arm	1.5	1.5	1.5	1.5	1.5
Right hand	1.25	1.25	1.25	1.25	1.25
Left hand	1.25	1.25	1.25	1.25	1.25
Right thigh	2.25	3.25	4.25	4.25	4.75
Left thigh	2.25	3.25	4.25	4.25	4.75
Right leg	2.5	2.5	2.75	3	3.5
Left leg	2.5	2.5	2.75	3	3.5
Right foot	1.75	1.75	1.75	1.75	1.75
Left foot	1.75	1.75	1.75	1.75	1.75

Source: Lund, C.C., & Browder, N.C. (1944). The estimation of areas of burns. *Surgery, Gynecology, and Obstetrics, 79,* 352–358. American College of Surgeons. Reprinted with permission.

called a dermatome. Once the eschar has been excised, the surgeon must choose a method to cover the wound. Often this is done with an autograft, or skin graft; skin is taken from another part of the body and used to cover the burn site. If the TBSA percentage is extensive and limited donor skin is available, cultured skin substitutes or biological or synthetic coverings might be used.

Autografts

Split-thickness skin grafts (STSGs) are the most common autografts used in surgical management of children with burns. The skin that is harvested from the donor site includes the epidermis and a portion of the dermis. The donor site will heal in 9 to 14 days and is treated like a superficial or partial-thickness burn. The graft can be applied as a sheet or meshed to cover a greater surface area, as seen in Figure 9–6 and the corresponding color plate. The graft must be secured at the burn site, and after approximately 48 hours, blood vessels in the graft connect with vessels in the wound bed, supplying nutrition to the graft. Grafts should adhere or "take" by the fifth to seventh postoperative day. The surgeon will immobilize the grafted area to ensure that the graft takes.

Full-thickness skin grafts (FTSGs) take the entire thickness of the skin, the epidermis and the dermis, stopping short of the subcutaneous fat. They are often used for coverage on the palms of the hands or pressure points. The donor site of the FTSG will require primary closure or an STSG to heal.

Cultured Skin Substitutes

For children with burns over a large percentage of TBSA, autografts may not be available, or because of frequent reharvesting, the healing process is delayed. With cultured epidermal autografts (CEAs), the child's own epidermal cells are harvested and grown in a laboratory. They are placed on a carrier material that will then be placed on the

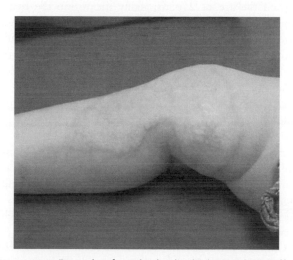

Figure 9-6 Example of meshed split-thickness skin graft. See also color plate.

burn site. These cells take 2 to 3 weeks to grow. Although this is an innovative way to cover burn wounds, these substitutes are often less durable than autografts.

Biological Substitutes

For children without adequate donor sites, an allograft (skin from a cadaver) may be used to cover the wound temporarily. Allografts are harvested and stored in a skin bank for use in burn management. The body will eventually reject the allograft, but it can provide wound coverage for 2 to 3 weeks while previous donor sites heal or until cultured skin is available. Heterografts or xenografts are skin grafts harvested from another species, usually a pig. Heterografts are used as a temporary covering for a wound, protecting it from further external trauma.

Synthetic Substitutes

Synthetic dressings are used to aid in the healing of partial-thickness burns or act as a temporary coverage to deeper burns awaiting autografts. One example is Biobrane, which is "a silastic membrane bonded to a bovine collagen sheet with a nylon backing" (Miller et al., 1994). Another example is Acticoat; this synthetic dressing is placed over a clean wound bed after débridement. The advantage of this dressing is its ability to be left in place for 3 to 5 days, thereby decreasing the amount of painful dressing changes and potential for disrupting healing tissues. Transcyte is another temporary skin substitute. It consists of a polymer membrane and newborn human fibroblast cells that are placed onto a nylon mesh. This provides a temporary protective barrier to partial- and full-thickness burns. Transcyte must be applied in the operating room after débridement, within the first 48 hours after the burn for effective healing. It can be used over wounds that need to be autografted, or those that will heal without further surgical interventions. Advantages of using Transcyte include reduction in painful dressing changes and length of hospital stay.

Traumatic Wounds

Motor vehicle accidents account for one of the highest injury rates in children. Many sequelae occur, including traumatic open wounds. These can be in the form of abrasions or road burns, open fractures, and degloving injuries. **Degloving injuries** are those in which a large portion of the skin is traumatically torn away from the underlying tissue; this often happens in pedestrian-versus-car accidents, in which the pedestrian is pulled underneath the car.

Traumatic wounds often require local care and surgical interventions similar to thermal injuries with skin grafts. If the tissue deficit is large enough, a muscle rotational or free flap might be necessary for wound coverage. Rotational muscle flaps are taken from an adjacent muscle group and rotated over the defect, maintaining their vascular supply. A free flap is one in which muscle is taken from another place in the body (e.g., latissimus dorsi or rectus abdominis) and transferred to the defect site. A free flap will require skin grafting (Miller et al., 1994).

As with skin grafts, muscle flaps must also avoid external trauma during the initial healing phase. The free flaps often appear bulky and do not have a smooth, cosmetic appearance. There also is a risk of failure of the flap resulting from poor circulation or re-establishment of the blood supply and nutrition to the flap.

After a muscle flap and graft, the child will be restricted from normal activities until the graft and flap have taken. Often these wounds are associated with fractures, with the status of the healing bone dictating activity and participation levels. Children with degloving injuries have similar restrictions to those with thermal injuries who require skin grafting.

Toxic Epidermal Necrolysis

The pathophysiology of toxic epidermal necrolysis (TEN) is unknown, but may be linked to a viral illness or drug interaction. TEN is a "severe form of erythema multiforme that results in extensive epidermal sloughing" (Sheridan et al., 1999). It is an acute illness, involving the epithelial layers of the skin and mucous membrane; the conjunctiva is also involved. If the lesions in the conjunctiva are more extensive than those on the skin, the disease is often known as Stevens-Johnson syndrome (SJS). TEN is epidermal sloughing involving 30% or more of the TBSA; sloughing involving less than 30% is called borderline TEN (Schulz, Sheridan, Ryan, MacKool, & Tompkins, 2000). Because of the extensive skin involvement and high mortality rate in children who develop TEN, burn units are the medical centers that are best prepared to deal with their multiple needs. The skin lesions that appear occur at the dermal-epidermal junction. If the disease process affects the oropharyngeal and gastrointestinal systems, there is a high risk of sepsis and death. Children's survival rates improve

with intervention strategies that include local wound care, nutritional support, and early detection of sepsis (Sheridan et al., 1999).

If the mucosal involvement is severe, the child will have limited ability to take in adequate calories by mouth. Nutritional supplementation will need to be considered to allow maximal wound management and increase strength and endurance. Children may encounter the same activity and participation limitations as those with thermal injuries. The severity and TBSA involved will determine the extent of limitations. If medical and wound management is timely and effective, many children will not have long-term sequelae.

Epidermolysis Bullosa

"Epidermolysis bullosa (EB) comprises a heterogeneous group of inherited disorders that produce blister formation in response to minimal skin trauma" (Farmer & Hood, 1990). There are various types of EB, each differing in the way it is inherited, level of separation of the skin, and the clinical manifestations. The major subdivisions of EB are determined by the level of skin involvement. EB simplex is evidenced by the separation in the epidermis. Junctional EB demonstrates separation at the level of the plasma membrane. Dermolytic or dystrophic EB demonstrates separation at the sub-basal reticular zone.

With junctional EB, the most severe type is EB letalis, which appears at birth. The skin and mucous membranes are involved. Infants with EB letalis usually do not survive beyond the age of 2 years; many die within the first 3 months of life. In the milder form of junctional EB (generalized atrophic benign EB), children survive into adulthood. Their appearance at birth is similar to those of the letalis group, but they have less severe skin and mucosal involvement (Farmer & Hood, 1990).

Dystrophic EB (DEB) has a wide range of severity, from mild skin eruptions, in which individuals have a normal life span, to severe, in which individuals have many impairments and limitations in normal activities during a painful and shortened life span. One of the most significant complications of DEB is the propensity to develop squamous cell carcinomas over the bony prominences. This is the major cause of death for persons with severe DEB who survive into adulthood (Atherton, 2000).

Children with EB who survive the neonatal period face a lifetime of skin disruptions, loss of normal joint movement, characteristic loss of fingers and toes, and multiple surgeries and skin grafting procedures. They are often restricted from normal activities because of concern for skin trauma. With the newborn, special attention must be given to positioning and handling to avoid further trauma. These infants will be limited from participating in normal gross motor activities as a result of their skin disruptions. Throughout their lives, children and adolescents will experience different episodes of activity and participation limitations attributable to new blistering, more extensive skin sloughing, or immobilization after surgery.

Prevention

The physical therapist plays a key role in preventing integumentary impairments. Clearly, no one can prevent a congenital skin disorder, but education for families regarding etiology of the disorder and genetic counseling may help parents in family planning. Other injuries, however, are preventable, with child and caregiver education as the key. For children with sensory deficits, teaching them how to do daily skin inspections and proper pressure-relieving techniques can decrease the incidence of pressure ulcers. Prescribing pressure-relieving cushions and wheelchairs that provide pressure-relieving positions will also decrease the incidence. Screening tools such as the Norton Risk Assessment, the Gosnell Scale, the Neonatal Skin Risk Assessment, and the Braden Q Scale were developed to identify children at risk for skin breakdown and allow clinicians to choose appropriate interventions to avoid or reduce skin breakdown (Bates-Jensen, 1998c).

Education is already in place in the school setting for fire safety. Children are taught fire prevention and safety, including the dangers of playing with matches, how to "stop, drop, and roll," and how to practice escape routes in their home and school. For parents, monitoring the temperature of their water heater will decrease the likelihood of scald burns from bath water that is too hot.

Advocating for early referral to physical therapy can aid in preventing skin breakdown in the hospital setting. Even in the intensive care unit, with medically unstable children, positioning programs and devices are appropriate interventions. Often these will prevent secondary limitations from prolonged bed rest after a traumatic accident. The incidence of pressure ulcers should decrease with staff education for use of proper support mattresses, turning and positioning schedules, and routine skin care and inspections.

Examination and Evaluation

Child History

As with any physical therapy examination, taking a detailed history, including information about age, sex, primary language, social history, developmental history, and general health before this episode of care, is important. Knowing the past medical history and related conditions will help the clinician to identify children at risk for skin breakdown or delayed wound healing. For the current integumentary issue, a more detailed history is necessary. The child or caregiver should provide an accurate history of the mechanism of injury, but in some cases you may have to rely on information received in the field from emergency medical personnel. The mechanism of injury is important, especially in the case of traumatic or thermal injuries. For example, with a thermal injury, probing what the child was doing and wearing and what was done immediately after the burn are vital to understanding the resulting injury. The timing of medical care and what procedures or interventions were performed before the physical therapist examined the child are all important pieces of information. In the case of suspected child abuse or neglect, matching the pattern of the burn with the history will be helpful in making the determination of accident versus abuse (Dressler & Hozid, 2001).

Review of the medical chart will provide information regarding prior clinical tests and the medical care of the child. The nutritional history and current nutritional status of the child should be documented. Children who are malnourished are at greater risk of skin breakdown. Laboratory findings, especially albumin levels, will be important. If serum albumin levels are below 3.5 mg/dL, the child is considered malnourished (Bates-Jensen, 1998c). The dietitian should screen all children in the hospital who are at risk for skin breakdown or who have a known integumentary disorder. In the clinic or outpatient setting, a referral to a dietitian might be applicable.

Systems Review

For any child with a potential for integumentary impairments, or with known disorders, it is important to review all of the body systems. If cardiopulmonary comorbidities exist, they may inhibit mobilization, exercise, or wound healing. In the case of a child with a thermal and inhalation injury, the pulmonary sequelae may outweigh the integumentary disruptions. Children with musculoskeletal impairments, such as contractures, might be at greater risk for skin breakdown, as are children with decreased strength or sensation because of neuromuscular disorders. A detailed examination of the integumentary system will be addressed in the Tests and Measures section that follows. It is necessary to examine the child's cognitive level and ability to communicate. If the child is unable to communicate pain or discomfort at a pressure point, he or she is at risk for skin breakdown. Barriers to learning and preferred learning styles must be identified before choosing child and family education materials.

Tests and Measures

There are many tests and measures that might be administered during the initial examination of a child with an integumentary disorder. A more in-depth look into the following categories will be beneficial to the clinician in performing a comprehensive wound examination and evaluation.

Pain

The ability of the child to detect and determine the amount of pain will allow the medical team to address pain management adequately. Therefore, the use of **pain scales** is an important test and measure for any physical therapy examination, but especially for open wounds or burns. Some scales commonly used in the pediatric population include the Attia Behavioral Pain Scale (Attia, Amiel-Tison, Mayer, Schnider, & Barrier, 1987), the CRIES neonatal postoperative pain measurement score (Krechel & Bildner, 1995), the CHEOPS pain scale (McGrath et al., 1985), the Wong-Baker faces pain rating scale (Wong & Baker, 1988), and the 0-to-9-point scale. Each scale is used for specific age ranges or for children who have cognitive or communication disorders that inhibit them from using the appropriate age-related scale. The scales make use of physiological, behavioral, or observational measurements to determine pain (Martin-Herz, Thurber, & Patterson, 2000). Documenting pain scores before, during, and after wound care interventions is vital to identifying the need to change the pain management regimen.

Sensory Integrity

A thorough sensory examination including pain, pinprick, light and deep touch, and temperature will provide valuable information to the clinician regarding body structures and functions that may be intact, impaired, or absent. In the case of a thermal injury, the ability to perceive touch and pain may indicate a less severe burn, rather than the painless presentation of a full-thickness burn. For children with pressure ulcers, identifying areas of decreased sensation will allow the therapist to choose interventions, such as positioning and pressure-relieving surfaces.

Range of Motion

For children who have sustained a thermal injury, initial examination of available ROM is crucial within the first 24 hours. Identifying joints that are at risk or already showing signs of loss of range should lead to immediate interventions (see section on orthotics intervention). Children in the remodeling phase of healing will have scars and scar bands forming. It is a general rule to perform active ROM (AROM) or passive ROM (PROM) for examination purposes within the limits of the scar. "If it's white, it's tight" is a good adage to remember when examining scar tissue. As you are performing PROM, take the scar band/tissue to the point of blanching and then back off by a few degrees; this is the limit of the scar. Pushing the scar past this point may result in skin tears (Humphrey, Richard, & Staley, 1994). Examining the limits of ROM is also important to identify children who are at risk for skin breakdown. A child with significant contractures and decreased ability to move will be more prone to skin breakdown.

Gait, Locomotion, and Balance

Identifying the child's ability to mobilize is an important aspect of the initial examination. For children in an intensive care unit setting, mobility may be restricted because of medical stability and technology. For children who are allowed to move, their effectiveness in repositioning themselves and ambulating will be important. Documentation should include the amount of assistance needed and the ability of the caregiver to provide assistance. If the child is nonambulatory, it is necessary to assess and document wheelchair mobility skills and pressure-relieving techniques.

Orthotic, Protective, and Supportive Devices

If a child has used orthotics before this episode of care, the physical therapist must assess the age, fit, and effectiveness of each device. If a device is older than 1 year or the child has gone through a recent growth spurt or weight gain, the device may be ill fitting and has the potential to cause skin breakdown. Examine wheelchairs and seat cushions to determine their effectiveness in relieving pressure. The therapist should obtain a wearing schedule history; this will aid in the examination and evaluation of the orthotics. If a child is supposed to wear an orthotic for all mobility and is not wearing the device, there may be a greater risk for skin breakdown. An example would be a child with spina bifida who uses hip-knee-ankle-foot orthoses (HKAFOs) for mobility. If the child chooses to crawl around the house and not wear the HKAFOs, he or she runs the risk of creating pressure ulcers or abrasions from friction or shear on the carpet or hard floor on lower extremities that have impaired or absent sensation. On resumption of wearing the HKAFOs, the child and caregiver will need to be diligent in checking the skin and adhering to a wearing schedule. It is important to keep a consistent wearing schedule to avoid problems with poor fit or skin intolerance to the devices.

Integumentary Integrity

Associated Skin

Observation of the skin integrity of the entire body, especially areas prone to skin breakdown (bony prominences, sacrum, occiput, and trochanters), is necessary. Identifying any discrepancy with skin coloration, **turgor** (elasticity/tension), nail growth, hair growth, texture, and temperature, is also part of a comprehensive wound examination.

Thermal Injuries

During the initial examination, determining the TBSA percentage is done by mapping the affected areas on the **Lund and Browder chart** (see Figure 9–5 and Table 9.1). Identifying the structures that have been involved may take several days. Identify the location, joints involved, and depth at each site. For actual burn sites, document the color and texture of the wound, capillary refill, drainage, and odor. Evaluation of these findings will allow the clinician to determine burn depth classifications of superficial, partial-thickness, or full-thickness injuries. Presence or absence of blisters, hair follicles, and pain associated with wound care will also aid in determining burn depth.

For children who are in the remodeling phase of wound healing, identifying the areas of initial thermal injury and those of donor sites will be helpful. Check the scars for texture, smoothness, raised appearance, color, and flexibil-

ity. Newer scar tissue will be bright pink, with more mature scars taking on the coloration of surrounding tissues. Hypertrophic and keloid-type scars will have a raised appearance, with keloids presenting out of the boundaries of the original injury site. Check the scar tissue for hyperpigmentation or hypopigmentation. For children with darker pigmented skin, the scars may often be hypopigmented (Sussman, 1998b).

Pressure Ulcers and Traumatic Wounds

Identification of the location of the wound and its size, depth, and shape are key items in the examination of a pressure ulcer or traumatic wound. Identify any areas of maceration or softening of the skin, which often happens in the periwound area. In intact skin, note the ability to demonstrate capillary refill or blanching. To size the wound, use a tape measure or commercially available plastic measuring tool. Photography, especially with grids, is an excellent adjunct to verbal description of the wound (Figure 9–6). Photographs, whether digital or Polaroid, should be taken on initial examination and subsequent intervals to demonstrate progression of wound healing or failure of the wound to progress through the phases of healing. Cameras that have a specialized focusing system and use grid film allow the clinician to measure the length and width of a wound by the grid lines. For wound depth, use a sterile cotton-tipped applicator. It can be placed into the wound until the base is reached. Mark the depth with a pen or break the applicator at the surface opening of the wound; the applicator length can then be measured for the depth of the wound. Be careful that the applicator tip does not become dislodged in the wound during removal. Other options are to use a plastic or rubber feeding tube or suction catheter. The limitation of using these devices is that they may bend when measuring deep wounds, giving inaccurate dimensions.

With stages II through IV wounds, undermining and tunneling must be examined. **Undermining** occurs when the subcutaneous tissue creates a cave under the wound edges. **Tunneling** occurs when sinus tracts form and travel from the apparent wound, deeper into subcutaneous tissues. Measuring the extent of undermining and tunneling will give insight to the status of the tissues below the surface of the skin. To determine the undermining or tunneling, you can use a moist cotton-tipped applicator under the edges of the wound or into a tunnel. Do not force the applicator once resistance is felt because this can cause further damage. Once the applicator meets resistance, mark the end of the applicator at the wound edge, remove the applicator, and measure it along a centimeter ruler. The location of the undermining or tunneling can be described according to the hands of a clock. Using 12 o'clock as the top of the wound in relationship to the head, the location can be described according to the hands of the clock at 12, 3, 6, and 9 o'clock (Sussman, 1998c).

For pressure ulcers and traumatic wounds, identifying tissue type is the next step. This can be done with a standard three-color description: black for devitalized tissue or eschar, yellow for tissue that is possibly infected and in need of débridement, and red for healthy granulation tissue (Cuzzell, 1988). There will be multiple colors in the wounds during the inflammatory and proliferative phase, with the goal of achieving all red tissue as the wound heals or is ready for surgical intervention, as seen in Figure 9–7 and the corresponding color plate. Progress in wound healing can be documented by percentages of each color, with the goal of 90% red granulation tissue. With grid photography, the boxes that appear on the photo can be counted and a percentage given to each color. The decrease in the percentages for black and yellow tissue and the increase in the percentages for red tissue can indicate progress in wound healing.

Drainage and odor must also be noted. Descriptors for drainage include serous (body fluids), serosanguineous (blood and body fluid), sanguineous (bloody), and purulent (infected and malodorous). Normal wound exudate is clear or yellow. Exudate that is yellow, gray, or green, and malodorous is usually pus. Color and odor, however, are not always an indication of infection. Document the color and amount of drainage seen on removal of the dressings that cover the wounds (Sussman, 1998b).

Identifying any body structure that may be present in an open wound is crucial in your critical decision making for interventions. Having a good anatomy text available during your initial examination or for interventions is essential. Document any muscle, tendon, ligament, bone, or vessel that is seen in the wound. This will also aid in your evaluation of the depth of a partial- or full-thickness wound.

Diagnosis, Prognosis, and Plan of Care

Once your examination findings are evaluated, a diagnosis can be formulated. For thermal injuries and open wounds, this includes staging pressure ulcers and determining the depth of a burn or traumatic wound. The prognosis for each wound will be specific to the child:

- Premorbid status
- Extent of TBSA involved
- Depth of burn
- Stage of pressure ulcer
- System impairments

The plan of care will be specific to the type of wound and other activity or participation restrictions the child encounters. Goals for wound management could include:

- Keeping the wound site free of infection
- Ridding the wound of necrotic tissue
- Preparing the wound bed for surgical intervention
- Aiding in wound closure

Throughout the interventions for wound healing, the concept of maintaining a moist wound environment is key. In a moist wound environment, collagen production is greater than in a wound that is exposed to air and allowed to dry out (Alvarez, Rozint, & Meehan, 1997). In a dry environment, epidermal cells are inhibited from migrating and resurfacing the wound. In contrast, in a moist environment, the epithelialization occurs more rapidly because there is no crust or scab formation.

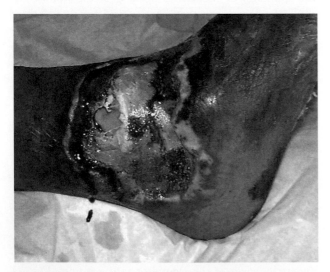

Figure 9-7 Example of red/yellow tissue present in a traumatic wound preoperatively. Black eschar had been surgically removed the day before to reveal underlying tissues. See also color plate.

For wounds in the remodeling phase, scar management is the main wound-care goal. Time frames for goals vary according to the type, size, location, nutritional status, and overall medical stability of the child. For example, a healthy child with no other medical history who sustains a 10% TBSA partial-thickness burn will usually heal in 10 to 21 days. A child with a stage IV pressure ulcer who is insensate and malnourished and has diabetes could take more than 6 months to heal without surgical interventions. Interventions will include those for each identified impairment and for wound care. Frequency of intervention will depend on the phase of healing in which the wound is and what other impairments are found on examination. For a wound in the acute healing phase, for example, a new burn, the physical therapist in a hospital setting should be providing daily interventions. A child in the remodeling phase of healing, without other impairments, may need to be seen only weekly to monthly for child and family education and scar management.

Interventions

According to the American Physical Therapy Association (APTA)'s *Guide to physical therapist practice* (2001), preferred practice patterns for the integumentary system include interventions for primary prevention/risk reduction and interventions for impaired integumentary integrity associated with superficial, partial-thickness, or full-thickness skin loss and scar formation. The following paragraphs describe the interventions.

Coordination, Communication, and Documentation

The complex needs of this population make coordination of care for the child with integumentary disorders crucial. There are often many medical professionals, as well as community and family caregivers, who will be involved in the child's care. Sharing of information regarding the plan of care and appropriate interventions is necessary throughout the continuum of care to ensure proper wound management. Throughout the continuum, one key person should make the decisions surrounding the wound-care needs. This is often the primary-care physician or surgical specialist (plastic or orthopedic surgeon). Documentation surrounding changes to the plan of care or wound interventions must be shared by the physician and disseminated to all caregivers in a timely fashion. Recognizing when referrals to other professionals are necessary is important throughout the episode of care. The collaboration of the hospital-based, school-based, and community therapists is important for integrating one standard of care for the child.

Child-Related Instruction

Child and caregiver instruction is vital to the success of a wound-management program. Often in the care of children, the parent is the primary caregiver in the home and community setting. Identifying any barriers to learning and the learning styles of the child and family is the first step. The family will need specific training for wound-care techniques as well as exercises, positioning, orthotic use, and mobility training. Much of the initial instructions will be done in the acute-care setting, but all members of the care team will need to do ongoing instruction throughout the episode of care. Teaching the child and family about the integumentary disorder and how to prevent further impairments is important. Children and caregivers who are able to incorporate prevention into their daily routines will avoid recurrent hospitalizations and limitations of ADLs. Children with chronic wounds often have multiple medical problems and require increased medical care. Not only is this costly, but it will also put the child at risk for loss of function and social or educational limitations from missing school.

Therapeutic Exercise

ROM and stretching are important interventions for any child with open wounds. For those with pressure ulcers or who are at risk for skin breakdown, maintaining flexibility and avoiding joint contractures is crucial for enhanced quality of life and function for ADLs. For children with thermal injuries, specific attention must be given to ROM. Contraindications to PROM exercises for the child with burns include exposed joints, tendon exposure over the posterior interphalangeal joint, deep vein thrombosis, compartment syndrome, and a new skin graft.

Passive Range of Motion

PROM may be necessary for children who are in the intensive care unit and unable to participate in active exercises. Scar tissue responds well to a slow, prolonged stretch.

Caution must be applied when performing PROM for the extensor tendons of the hand because there is risk of rupturing. Children will often be too afraid to allow PROM; therefore, performing PROM while the child is under anesthesia for surgery may be beneficial to examine fully the available range. Precautions must be taken to avoid tearing the skin or causing joint dislocations while the child is under anesthesia. Identifying the true available ROM will aid the therapist in daily interventions when the child is awake (Humphrey et al., 1994). For a prolonged stretch, serial casting may be used, as seen in Figure 9–8 and the corresponding color plate. This can be done over closed areas or during wound healing with the surgeon's approval.

Active-Assistive Range-of-Motion Exercises

Active-assistive range of motion (AAROM) exercises are used when children are unable to achieve full ROM independently. AAROM can be used for scar contractures, over escharotomy sites, and in children who have increased physiological demands after an extensive TBSA percentage burn. As discussed, be aware of the tissue response to stretch during AAROM and PROM. Ideally, ROM should be performed while dressings are off, allowing close monitoring of skin tension and scar blanching and avoid-

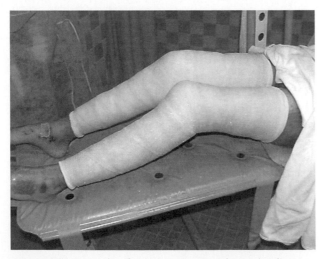

Figure 9-8 Example of serial casting used over healing grafted sites in a child with extensive lower extremity burns. Casts were used for prolonged stretch as well as for wound healing to decrease external trauma to the fragile, healing skin. See also color plate.

ing skin tears (Humphrey et al., 1994). This will allow all caregivers to know the available ROM for all activities on that specific day and not to exceed safe ranges for activity.

Active Range-of-Motion Exercises

AROM exercises are the exercises of choice for children with thermal injuries. The child can be in control during these exercises. The muscle-pumping activity that occurs will aid in edema reduction and increase circulation; it will also prevent muscle atrophy. It is also the exercise format chosen immediately after skin grafting to avoid trauma to the newly grafted site. AROM exercises should not only incorporate the joint involved but also combine movements because this will stretch the scar to the most desired length. For example, for a scar on the anterior shoulder, shoulder flexion and shoulder flexion with elbow extension should be performed to elongate the tissues. Activities such as reaching for a target, shooting baskets, or playing baseball are often fun activities that also achieve AROM in various planes of movement. Choosing age-appropriate play activities will help motivate the child to participate in activities that will gain ROM.

Assistive, Adaptive, Orthotic, Protective, and Prosthetic Devices

Before choosing a device for the child, identify limitations in ROM, strength, and mobility. A positioning program may be used in conjunction with devices such as airplane splints, resting hand splints, or ankle contracture boots. For the child with thermal injuries, there are predictable "at-risk" positions that should be avoided (Figure 9–9). Listed in Table 9.2 are sites of burns and the preferred position for elongation. These positions are used for positioning programs or for splinting.

For the child at risk for a pressure ulcer or with a known skin disorder, a positioning program is also vital. Children should be repositioned at least every 2 hours to avoid unnecessary pressure. Use the times on a clock as a reminder for which position to choose. For example, at 12 o'clock the child lies supine; at 2 o'clock, right sidelying; at 4 o'clock, left sidelying; and at 6 o'clock, prone. Prone positioning is often overlooked, but it is an effective position for complete pressure relief for the posterior aspect of the body and pulmonary function. Take pictures of the

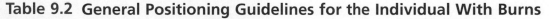

Table 9.2 General Positioning Guidelines for the Individual With Burns

Body Area	Contracture Predisposition	Preventive Positioning
Neck	Flexion	Extension Hyperextension
Anterior axilla	Shoulder adduction	Shoulder abduction
Posterior axilla	Shoulder extension	Shoulder flexion
Antecubital space	Elbow flexion	Elbow extension
Forearm	Pronation	Supination
Wrist	Flexion	Extension
Dorsal hand/finger	MCP hyperextension IP flexion Thumb adduction	Metacarpophalangeal flexion Interphalangeal extension Thumb palmar abduction or opposition
Palmar hand/finger	Finger flexion Thumb opposition	Finger extension Thumb radial abduction
Hip	Flexion Adduction External rotation	Extension Abduction Neutral rotation
Knee	Flexion	Extension
Ankle	Plantarflexion	Dorsiflexion
Dorsal toes	Hyperextension	Flexion
Plantar toes	Flexion	Extension

Source: Apfel, L., et al. (1994). Approaches to positioning the burn patient. In R.L. Richard & M.J. Staley (Eds.), *Burn care and rehabilitation* (p. 223). Copyright F.A. Davis Company. Reprinted with permission.

child in these positions and post the program bedside for all caregivers to follow.

Adaptive Devices

In the acute-care setting, the choice of hospital bed/mattress is the first line of defense for maintaining skin integrity. Each institution may have a policy for when a specialty bed is appropriate for a child with integumentary impairment. For example, a specific score on the Braden Q Scale or Norton Scale may qualify the child for a specialty bed. These devices can be as simple as an air mattress overlay, a low air-loss system, gel mattresses, or air-fluidized therapy. In the home-care setting, more generic, commercially available devices may be an air mattress or foam mattress. When positioning a child in bed, maintain the head of the bed at the lowest degree possible and limit the time that the head of the bed is elevated because, with this elevation, shearing forces occur at the sacrum and buttocks and can impair blood vessel function (Bergstrom et al., 1994). Once the child is medically stable enough to be out of bed, an appropriate seating system must be developed. In the hospital setting this may be done with a wheelchair or other type of chair. Any seating system that is used should demonstrate appropriate fit, support the child, and provide pressure relief at the ischium/buttocks. Using a pressure-relieving cushion, rather than a standard pillow, will decrease the risk of developing pressure ulcers. Positioning the child as upright as possible will avoid friction and shear at the sacrum.

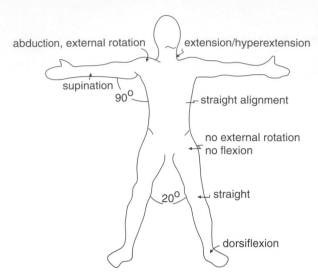

Figure 9-9 General positioning guidelines for the individual with burns. (From Apfel, L., et al. [1994]. Approaches to positioning the burn patient. In R.L. Richard & M.J. Staley [Eds.], *Burn care and rehabilitation* [p. 223]. Copyright F.A. Davis Company. Reprinted with permission.)

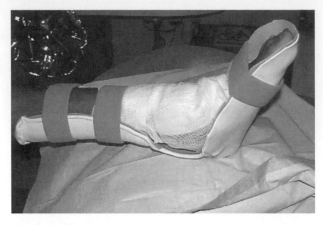

Figure 9–10 Example of orthoplast resting ankle splint fabricated to protect free flap at medial malleolus and maintain ankle range of motion.

Assistive Devices

After a thermal injury or during interventions for a pressure ulcer or traumatic wound, the child may require the use of an assistive device for mobilization. For example, a child with a sacral pressure ulcer may be restricted from sitting in a wheelchair and is nonambulatory. Using a prone cart will enable the child to get out of bed, avoiding all pressure on the ulcer, and provide a means of independent mobility.

Orthotic Devices

While the child is on prolonged bed rest or medically unstable, use of static splints may be necessary to prevent contractures or improve ROM. An example of an orthotic device would be a posterior ankle resting or foot drop splint. These are commercially available in prefabricated sizes and provide neutral ankle positioning and suspend the heel from the support surface. Often, for the pediatric population, these prefabricated orthotics may not fit well, and fabrication of an orthoplast-type splint may be required. Prefabricated splints are time saving but often do not fit over bulky dressings. Use of orthoplast-type materials and fabricating custom splints to accommodate

dressings and protect grafts or flaps might be necessary (Figure 9–10).

For children with thermal injuries, early splinting is the key to preventing further deformities; Table 9.2 lists preventive positions. To maintain or improve ROM, splinting may be necessary, either continuously or during the night to provide a prolonged stretch. Splints may also be used to protect grafted areas after surgery. Splints will decrease external trauma or shear to ensure graft adherence (Figure 9–11). Custom-made orthotics may be prescribed after scar revision surgery to protect the grafted area and to improve ROM (Figure 9–12).

Protective Devices

The use of pressure-relieving cushions is effective in protecting the skin from breakdown. For children at risk or after closure of a pressure ulcer, an appropriate device must be prescribed. There are many types of pressure-relieving cushions, from high-density foam to gel and Roho cushions. Sitting on a standard pillow should be discouraged because this does not relieve pressure. Instructing the child to perform pressure-relieving techniques, such as pushups or shifting weight, every 15 to 30 minutes will also be vital to prevent pressure ulcers.

For children with anterior neck burns, pillows should not be used behind the head. This forces the neck into flexion and places the child at risk for neck flexion contractures. A pillow may be used behind the shoulders to extend the neck slightly while the child sleeps.

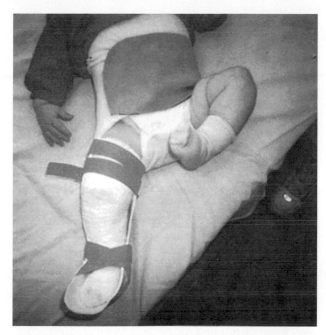

Figure 9-11 Example of orthoplast splint fabricated to restrict right hip and knee flexion to protect skin graft site at the knee.

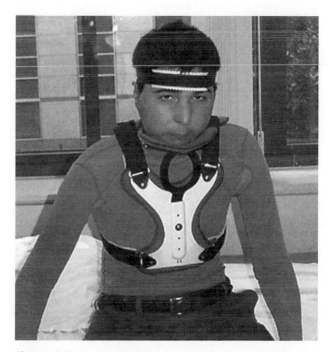

Figure 9-12 Example of a custom head/neck orthosis to protect anterior neck graft site and improve cervical range of motion.

Donut-type or ring-style cushions should be avoided. They may cause circumferential pressure and act as a tourniquet, thus decreasing the blood supply to the area you are trying to protect. Ring-style cushions are known to cause venous congestion and are more likely to cause pressure ulcers than to prevent them. Positioning a child in the sidelying position with direct pressure over the trochanters should be avoided. Use of pillows and blanket rolls will help the child to maintain a quarter-turn toward supine and relieve the pressure over the bony prominences. Elevating the affected area (e.g., heels) off the bed is also effective for relieving pressure and healing (Bergstrom et al., 1994). Alternatives for areas such as the occiput or bony prominences of the ankle or elbow are gel pillows.

Supportive Devices

After thermal or traumatic injuries, a child may have required a skin graft to close the wound. Use of compression devices will aid in vascular support to grafts. Once a graft or flap has reached the remodeling phase, scar tissue is forming and can continue to form for up to 2 years. Compression has been shown to aid in the collagen alignment, thus aiding in scar formation. The one main effect of the use of compression is to balance collagen synthesis and lysis (see Maturation Phase, pages 332–333). Collagen fibers align parallel to the epidermal surface and have a decreased risk of hypertrophy. Use of compression garments will aid in keeping the scars or grafts smoother and less raised and ultimately promote increased cosmesis. During the remodeling phase, hypertrophic scars begin forming early, so the earlier the pressure or compression is applied, the better are the results. Pressure can be applied as early as 2 weeks after wound closure or graft healing. Pressure can initially be in the form see p 332 of elastic bandages, cohesive bandages, elastic tubular support bandages, or custom-made **pressure garments** (Figure 9–13). These garments should be worn for 23 hours per day, with time out of the garment for hygiene and scar management. Inserts may be needed to obtain even pressure over misshapen or bony prominences. Inserts can be foam, silicone elastomer, gel sheets, or silicone gel pads (Staley & Richard, 1994). Compression for facial burns can be accomplished with compression garments or plastic face masks. Groce, Meyers-Paal, Herndon, and McCauley (1999) studied the effectiveness of the garment versus the plastic face mask. They found that the compression garment had lower pressure over the forehead, left cheek, right cheek, and chin in

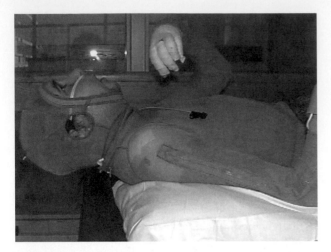

Figure 9-13 Example of custom compression garment for the face, chest, and upper extremities.

comparison to the face mask. They also noted that the full compression garment mask makes the individual appear "sinister" and may cause him or her to withdraw socially. The transparent face mask may give the child a better appearance and improve peer acceptance (Groce et al., 1999).

Integumentary Repair and Protection Techniques

Preprocedure Considerations

The role of the parent or caregiver in wound-care techniques has evolved over the past decade. Where once they may have been banned during painful procedures, parents and caregivers are now being encouraged to assist with the child's coping. Doctor's study in 1994 found that parent participation was "mutually beneficial" for the parent and the child. Parental involvement with wound-care procedures took longer, but the parent was able to provide emotional support to the child and also learned how to provide skin care at home (Doctor, 1994). A child-life specialist or music therapist with expertise in preparation and distraction techniques can help the child cope with the pain and fear of wound-care procedures. Activities should be targeted for each age population. For example, an infant can be bundled or held by a parent for comfort. Singing or blowing bubbles can distract a toddler. A school-aged child may want to sing a song or read a book. An adolescent may find relaxation or distraction in using headphones to listen to music or playing a video game.

Before any painful procedure, whether it is wound care or other interventions, care should be taken to ensure proper premedication for the child. Working with a pain management team in a hospital setting or having the parents administer prescribed pain medicine before an outpatient visit will aid in pain relief for the child. Other techniques that may be beneficial during a therapy session are distraction, relaxation or breathing techniques, and guided imagery. The use of a positive reinforcement program may also be beneficial. These can include progress or reward charts using stickers or other rewards when activities or procedures are completed (Martin-Herz et al., 2000).

Débridement

Débridement is "the removal of necrotic and/or infected tissues that interfere with wound healing" (Loehne, 2002). There are two types of débridement: nonselective and selective. When there is necrotic tissue in a wound, débridement must be done for the wound to progress through the healing phases.

Selective

Selective débridement can be achieved through enzymatic or autolytic débridement, or by surgical excision. Surgical débridement is the most efficient way to selectively débride necrotic tissue. This sharp débridement can be done in the operating room or may occur in a therapy setting. It should be performed when there is gross necrotic tissue. If an ischemic wound is present, sharp débridement is not indicated unless collateral circulation has been evaluated. Sharp débridement should be done by a trained, skilled clinician and under a doctor's order. Other forms of débridement can include the use of scissors and forceps (in the case of removing blisters from a partial-thickness burn) or gauze to remove sloughing blisters. Individual states' practice acts provide guidelines for the physical therapist regarding débridement. A specially educated and experienced clinician must be able to identify body structures that may be present in the wound bed. This is an advanced skill and should ideally be performed by a clinician who has completed a competency-based training program with a mentor (Bates-Jensen, 1998b).

The use of topical enzymatic agents is also selective débridement because enzymes digest only necrotic tissue. Proteolytic enzymes are able to débride heavy eschar and denatured proteins. Some wounds contain eschar with undenatured collagen, which can be débrided with the enzyme collagenase. If a thick crust of eschar is present, the eschar may be scored or cross-hatched with a scalpel to allow permeation of the enzymes (Loehne, 2002).

Autolytic débridement is achieved when the body's white blood cells break down necrotic tissue. This is accomplished with a moisture-retentive dressing. The moist wound environment promotes rehydration of dry, dead tissue, and the fluid that accumulates has white blood cells in it to break down the necrotic tissue. Dressings that can be used include films, hydrocolloids, and hydrogels (see Dressings and Topical Agents).

Nonselective Débridement

Nonselective débridement removes necrotic and viable tissue from the wound. It can be achieved via wet-to-dry dressings, vigorous agitation in a whirlpool, or pulsed irrigation. This form of débridement is used in wounds that have extensive amounts of necrotic tissue. Caution must be used when using wet-to-dry dressings for nonselective débridement. When the dressing is adherent and then removed, there is a risk of damaging healthy epithelial and granulation tissue along with the necrotic tissue (Loehne, 2002).

Physical Agents and Mechanical Modalities

Hydrotherapy

Whirlpool

Whirlpool therapy has historically been used in the care of thermal injuries and pressure ulcers. Care must be taken when determining the efficacy of whirlpool intervention. According to the AHCPR, whirlpool therapy may enhance the removal of necrotic debris from pressure ulcers. Whirlpool therapy should be discontinued, however, when the wound is clean, because of the risk of trauma to healthy granulation tissue (Bergstrom et al., 1994).

In the management of thermal injuries, the whirlpool has often been used to cleanse the wounds and remove old topical agents. Gentle ROM exercises can also be done while the child is in the whirlpool with the dressings removed. Full submersion to partial submersion in a Hubbard tank may be used for children who are unable to participate in wound care. Children who can mobilize may use smaller tanks or showers to cleanse their wounds (Saffle & Schnebly, 1994).

A concern in whirlpool therapy is the risk of cross-contamination from others and the risk of contracting *Pseudomonas aeruginosa*. Despite adequate cleansing between whirlpool users, it is impossible to completely eradicate the risk for contamination of wounds. Use of antiseptic agents should be discouraged in the whirlpool because of the cytotoxic effects of most additives. All commonly used antiseptic agents, such as iodine, sodium hypochlorite, and hydrogen peroxide, have cytotoxic effects, even when diluted. Only tap water should be used in the whirlpool setting (Bergstrom et al., 1994).

Pulsed Lavage

Pulsed lavage or irrigation has emerged as an effective method of wound cleansing and nonselective débridement. According to the AHCPR, irrigation pressures should be between 4 psi and 15 psi. At lower ranges, the wound may not be cleansed appropriately; above 15 psi, tissue damage may occur (Bergstrom et al., 1994). Pulsed-lavage systems incorporate an irrigation solution (most commonly saline) and an electrically powered device to deliver the agent, in conjunction with wall suction. Because this is a portable intervention, it can be done at the bedside and localized to the wound site, in contrast to whirlpool therapy, which would partially or fully submerge a body part. It also has demonstrated an increased rate of granulation tissue formation in comparison to whirlpool treatments (Luedtke-Hoffman & Schafer, 2000).

The suction component of pulsed lavage removes debris, bacteria, and the irrigation solution used, and also provides negative pressure, which has been shown to promote granulation tissue formation (Loehne, 2002). Pressure parameters are usually between 60 and 90 mm Hg of continuous suction. The level of suction should be decreased if bleeding occurs or the child complains of pain (Loehne, 2002). Caution must be taken, as with any nonselective débridement device, with body structures that may be present in the wound bed, including tendon, fascia, joint capsule, and blood vessels.

Dressings and Topical Agents

Dressings are specific to the type of integumentary disorder and vary in their properties. Ideal dressings should be user friendly, protect the surrounding skin from maceration, remove necrotic tissue, maintain a moist wound environment, promote granulation tissue or re-epithelialization, relieve pain, stay in place, and be cost effective (Saffle & Schnebly, 1994).

Thermal Injuries

Burn wounds should be cleansed once to twice a day. Necrotic tissue should be loosened during this cleansing, as well as old topical agents that have lost their antimicrobial effects after application. Warm water or saline should be used to clean the wound. Topical antibiotics are used to reduce the incidence of infection. Topical agents used in burn care include silver nitrate, mafenide acetate (Sulfamylon), nitrofurazone (Furacin), silver sulfadiazine (Silvadene), and bacitracin (Saffle & Schnebly, 1994). Silver sulfadiazine is the most widely used topical agent. It has broad-spectrum antimicrobial coverage, softens eschar and aids in its separation, and maintains a moist wound environment. Topical agents are applied to a contact layer dressing instead of directly to the wound to decrease pain. The contact layer of dressing can be gauze or a nonadherent gauze sheet to avoid adherence of the dressing to the wound. These can be secured via a gauze roll, elastic netting, or elastic bandages. Silvadene can cause allergic reactions and transient leukopenia.

The topical agent for certain body areas requires special attention. The face is usually dressed with a thin cover of transparent ointment instead of Silvadene, which can harden and is difficult to remove. Burns on the ear are best treated with Sulfamylon cream because it penetrates more effectively into the tissues and protects ear cartilage from infection. Burns in the perineum are treated with transparent ointments because of the thinness of the dermis and increased absorptive capacities (Saffle & Schnebly, 1994).

Gauze dressings that are applied to burn sites must be placed so that the child may maintain or increase function. For example, fingers and toes should be wrapped individually to avoid sticking together, and gauze should be placed between the fingers to preserve the web space. Dressings should be applied from distal to proximal to reduce edema. As dressings are applied, the therapist should incorporate proper positioning to avoid losing ROM. Using dressings with uniform thickness is important to allow orthotic use over burned areas. Orthotics are fabricated over a dressing; thus uniform dressing thickness and technique will aid in the appropriate fit of the splint. Burn dressings for an infant or a toddler may need to be more extensively reinforced to prevent the child from pulling or biting on the dressing and disrupting the underlying wound-healing environment. It is often recommended that fingernails be trimmed short to decrease the risk of causing bleeding from scratching.

Once a thermal wound has closed, either by re-epithelialization or by skin grafting, skin care must continue. Use of a moisturizing lotion is important because of the grafted wound's inability to produce normal body oils. An ideal moisturizer is one that is gentle, hypoallergenic, and without alcohol because alcohol has been shown to dry out the skin and may lead to cracking (Saffle & Schnebly, 1994).

In addition to moisturizing the skin, application of lotion can be effective in scar massage. By massaging the skin with lubricating lotion, the scar becomes desensitized via tactile stimulation. The scars should be massaged with hard enough pressure to make them blanch, 3 to 6 times per day. Scar massage may make the skin more mobile; however, no permanent decrease in thickness is usually seen (Staley & Richard, 1994).

Pressure Ulcers and Traumatic Wounds

As with thermal injuries, pressure ulcers and traumatic wounds require cleansing and application of appropriate dressings. Antiseptic agents are cytotoxic to normal tissue and should be avoided. Examples of these are povidone-iodine, iodophor, sodium hypochlorite (Dakin's solution), hydrogen peroxide, and acetic acid. They have been found to be toxic to fibroblasts, which play a key role in the inflammatory and proliferative phases of healing. Normal saline is the preferred topical agent for cleansing wounds because it is physiological and will not harm tissues (Bergstrom et al., 1994).

Film Dressings. Film dressings are moisture and oxygen permeable. They are impermeable to microorganisms and allow easy monitoring of the wound because they are transparent. They provide a moist wound environment. Film dressings can be used for minor abrasions and lacerations and for stage I ulcers. They can also be used as a secondary dressing to hold a primary dressing over a wound. Film dressings should not be used in a wound with excessive exudates. Examples of film dressings include Opsite, Bioclusive, and Tegaderm.

Foam Dressings. Foam dressings are produced from polyurethane. They are able to absorb exudates from the wound and maintain a moist environment. Foam dressings can be used for superficial and deep wounds and can be used over skin grafts and minor burns. They can be a secondary dressing to cover an amorphous hydrogel. They can also be used around a tracheostomy tube or gastrointestinal tube. Foam dressings are not effective for use in a dry wound but do not have any true contraindications to use. Examples of foam dressings are Allevyn, Hydrasorb, and Lyofoam.

Hydrogels. Hydrogels contain organic polymers with a high water content. There are two types: amorphous and fixed. Amorphous hydrogels are able to absorb water; they are free flowing and easily fit into a cavity space. Fixed hydrogels come in a thin, flexible sheet and swell in size until saturated. They can provide moisture to a dry wound but can also absorb fluid from an exuding wound. Hydrogels can also easily conform to wound or body shape. They are chosen for wounds that are dry to rehydrate eschar and allow autolytic débridement. They should not be used in a wound with a large amount of exudates. Amorphous hydrogels are held in place by a secondary dressing (foam or film) and can stay in place for up to 3 days. Sheet hydrogels are fixed to the skin with tape or cohesive bandage and can also stay in place for 3 to 4 days. Examples of hydrogels are Carrasyn gel, DuoDerm gel, and Intrasite gel.

Hydrocolloids. Hydrocolloids contain gel-forming polymers with adhesives, found on a film or foam. Hydrocolloids can also be in the form of granules, powders, or pastes. The dressing will absorb wound exudates, provide a moist wound environment, and conform to body shape. They can be used for superficial wounds, donor sites, and pressure ulcers. Concern for using this type of dressing in a child with fragile skin is high because of the risk for further skin trauma when removing the dressing. The dressing does not need to be changed for up to 3 to 4 days. Hydrocolloids should not be used in a clinically infected wound or a deep cavity. They will aid in autolytic débridement. Examples of hydrocolloids are Comfeel, Duoderm, and Tegasorb.

Alginate Dressings. Alginate dressings contain calcium, or calcium and sodium salts. When they are applied to a wound, the sodium ions in the wound are exchanged for calcium ions in the dressing, thus acting as a hemostatic agent. They provide a moist wound environment, provide a high absorptive capacity, conform to body shape, and are nonadherent. Alginates are used in exudative wounds, pressure ulcers, and postsurgically at bleeding sites. They come in forms such as sheets, rope, or packing alginates. These dressings can stay in place for up to 1 week in clean wounds or changed daily in an infected wound. Examples of alginate dressings are Curosorb, Kaltostat, and Sorbsan (Sussman, G., 1998).

Vacuum-Assisted Closure System. The vacuum-assisted closure (V.A.C.) system was developed for interventions with traumatic wounds with soft tissue defects and pressure ulcers. The technique associated with the V.A.C. was devised to aid in wound treatment and decrease pain and length of hospitalization. The device itself is a subatmospheric pressure system with a polyurethane foam dressing. Before use of this device, all nonviable tissue must be removed via surgical débridement (Argenta & Marykwas, 1997). Mooney, Argenta, Marks, Marykwas, and DeFranzo (2000) conducted a study of the V.A.C. system with children with complex wounds. The children underwent surgical débridement of all nonviable tissue and then application of the system. The V.A.C. system sponge and outflow tube were cut and fit to the appropriate size of the wound and then covered with a transparent film/drape, as seen in Figure 9–14 and the corresponding color plate. Continuous negative pressure was used at 125 mm Hg, as close to 24

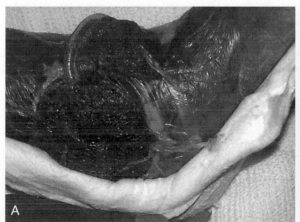
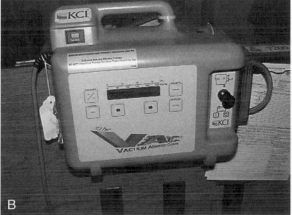

Figure 9-14 (*A*) Vacuum-assisted closure (V.A.C.) system placed on open wound (as seen in Figure 9–7). Black, polyurethane foam dressing in place. (*B*) V.A.C. unit. See also color plate.

hours per day as possible. The dressing was changed 3 times a week. Once a granulating wound bed was achieved, wound coverage was performed through either skin grafting or free flaps. The children required fewer painful dressing changes and less extensive coverage surgeries. The primary goals of the system, stimulating granulation tissue and removing interstitial fluid from the wound, were met. The continuous suction also acted to slowly draw the wound edges together. Mooney et al. (2000) also found that the system was well tolerated by the children and decreased the need for frequent dressing changes that occurs in a more traditional wound management program.

Electrotherapeutic Modalities

Management of wound healing with electrotherapeutic agents has been shown to be safe and effective. These agents include transcutaneous electrical nerve stimulation (TENS) and high-voltage pulsed current (HVPC). These devices can produce physiological responses at the cellular level. TENS causes vasodilation of small blood vessels and increases blood flow to the extremities. HVPC increases tensile strength of the scar, increases collagen synthesis and epithelialization, and increases fibroblast production. With HVPC, on days 1 to 5 use 50 pps, 150 V, and negative polarity for 30 to 60 minutes daily. From day 6 until healing, use 80 pps, 90 V, and positive polarity for 30 to 60 minutes daily. If the wound appears to have plateaued, alternate the polarity daily (Unger, 1992).

Electrical Stimulation

"Several in vitro and in vivo studies have reported that ES [electrical stimulation] has either an inhibitory (bacteriostatic) effect or a killing (bactericidal) effect on microorganisms that commonly colonize or infect wounds" (Kloth, 2002a). Other effects reported for ES include increases in the rates of collagen synthesis and epithelialization and improved revascularization and oxygen levels. Kloth (2002a) also reports effects such as acute wound-related pain reduction, augmentation of autolysis, and accelerated wound healing with the use of ES. Precautions for ES include sensation of a light tingling under the electrodes and potential for skin irritation. Contraindications for ES include basal or squamous cell carcinoma in the wound or periwound tissues or melanoma, untreated osteomyelitis, application to the neck or thorax that may send a current through the pericardial area, or when a pacemaker is implanted. For a more in-depth look at ES, see Kloth and

McCulloch's (2002) chapter on electrical stimulation for wound healing in *Wound healing: Alternatives in management*.

Hyperbaric Oxygen Therapy

Hyperbaric oxygen therapy (HBO) is delivered to an individual by 90% oxygen breathed in a sealed chamber with an atmospheric pressure between 2.0 and 2.5 atmospheres absolute. The use of HBO has been documented for smoke inhalation, enhancement of healing in selected problem wounds, compromised skin grafts and flaps, necrotizing soft tissue infections, and thermal burns (Kloth, 2002b). The improved oxygen delivery will have a great effect at the cellular level. Neutrophils, fibroblasts, and macrophages are all dependent on an oxygen-rich environment. Improved oxygenation has also been correlated with decreasing infection and accelerating wound healing. Precautions for using HBO for wound healing include upper respiratory infections, seizures, high fevers, history of spontaneous pneumothorax, history of thoracic surgery, viral infections, and optic neuritis. Contraindications for HBO include antineoplastic medications and untreated pneumothorax.

Outcomes

Because of the wide range of integumentary impairments that have been reviewed, it is not possible to provide one set of guidelines for outcomes. Outcomes for thermal injuries and open wounds include progression of the wound through the stages of wound healing, absence of infection, and an acceptable scar that does not impede functional mobility, ADLs, or community activities and participation. Good wound management is of paramount importance for the child to return to normal activities and participation in ADLs, school, play, and extracurricular activities. Early detection of skin disorders and timely wound care will aid in the child's return to these activities. Care for children with skin disorders should be done at burn centers or trauma centers capable of handling their complex care. Neonatal intensive care units familiar with congenital skin disorders such as EB will also aid in the timely care of newborns with skin disruptions. Children with large TBSA thermal injuries or TEN will have the highest probability for long-term sequelae. Some integumentary disorders and their subsequent impairments will limit the child's quality of life and ability to participate in age-appropriate activities.

CASE EXAMPLE 9–1 . . . . . .

Child History

Ethan is a 14-year-old boy with autism who, at age 13 years, was in his usual state of good health until December 2000, when he was found lying on a burning mattress in his group home. He was transported to a burn center and underwent acute care for approximately 63% TBSA partial- and full-thickness burns to his face, neck, chest, abdomen, back, and extremities. His eyes, forehead, and scalp were spared, along with his perineum and portions of his back, legs, and feet. He required amputations of digits 2, 4, and 5 on his right hand because of the severity of his injuries. He underwent numerous skin grafting procedures and the use of CEA to cover areas when he had no donor sites available. In March 2001, he was transferred to a rehabilitation hospital, where he underwent intensive therapy and ongoing wound management. He was discharged to his home in June 2001 and readmitted to the acute-care setting in July 2001 for neck scar revisions. He had a brief rehabilitation stay and was discharged back home in his parents' care. Barriers to learning for Ethan include expressive language and cognitive deficits, as well as behavioral problems associated with his autism. Barriers to intervention included Ethan's inability to understand why procedures were being done and overall anxiety with any new caregiver.

Impairments in Body Structures and Functions

Ethan has comorbidities of an extensive TBSA thermal injury and autism. Autism is a syndrome noted in early childhood that can be characterized by abnormal social relationships, language disorders, the presence of rituals, and a compulsive component. In many cases, impaired intellectual development is present (Allison & Smith, 1998).

Integumentary

On arrival at rehabilitation, Ethan had many open wounds and unhealed grafted areas. He was also having intermittent breakdown at the sites that were covered with CEA.

He had begun to develop hypertrophic scarring throughout the burned sites.

Goal: To have complete wound closure and to decrease the risk of further skin breakdown as a result of trauma.

Interventions:

1. Daily wound care in a shower room separate from his room

2. Use of a standard procedure for wound care and a scheduled time for the procedure for all caregivers to follow. Established a routine for his daily care

3. Premedication before interventions for both pain and anxiety

4. Use of a specialty mattress to decrease risk for secondary limitations or pressure sores and to decrease shearing forces on healing tissues

5. Nutrition consultation for adequate intake by mouth with supplemental nasogastric tube feedings at night

6. Use of distraction techniques including favorite DVD movies during dressing changes

7. Use of serial casting not only for prolonged stretching but also to decrease the trauma he would cause to his healing wounds by shearing or scratching

8. Early compression as soon as wounds had healed; initial compression with elastic bandages, then elastic tubular bandages, and eventually custom compression garments

Range of Motion

Ethan had deficits in joint ROM at his neck, upper extremities, lower extremities, and trunk caused by scar tissue and tissue shortening that occurred despite therapy in the acute-care setting.

Goal: Ethan will achieve functional use of his neck and extremities for ADLs.

Interventions:

1. PROM/AROM/AAROM exercises geared to his tolerance.

2. Positioning program posted at bedside.

3. Examination of ROM in the operating room while Ethan was under general anesthesia because of his inability to tolerate PROM to the point of scar blanching. True ROM measurements and restrictions were noted and used for ADLs (Figure 9–15 and the corresponding color plate).

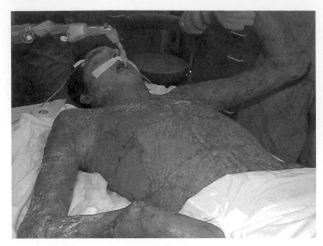

Figure 9-15 Range of motion performed on child while under general anesthesia in the operating room. See also color plate.

4. Orthotic devices such as ankle resting splints, elbow and hand resting splints, knee extension splints, and Watusi rings.

5. Serial casting for elbows, hands, and knees to achieve a prolonged stretch and decrease risk of trauma to healing tissues from shearing and scratching by Ethan.

6. Use of functional equipment, such as stationary bike or adult-sized tricycle that Ethan appeared to enjoy (Figure 9–16).

7. Use of distraction techniques including counting and singing a familiar song during PROM.

Ethan was referred to the plastic surgery department in July for revision of his neck scar because of significant loss of ROM and cosmesis. Preoperatively, he was unable to extend his head to neutral and had minimal to no rotation to either side. He underwent surgical excision of the scar and skin grafting. He spent 9 days in intensive care, 7 of which were under heavy sedation and on the ventilator to allow proper positioning and ensure that the graft would take postoperatively.

Goal: Ethan will increase neck ROM to at least 50% of normal to aid in ADLs.

Interventions:

1. Postoperative positioning while sedated in neck hyperextension

2. Use of a head/neck orthosis to maintain neck in

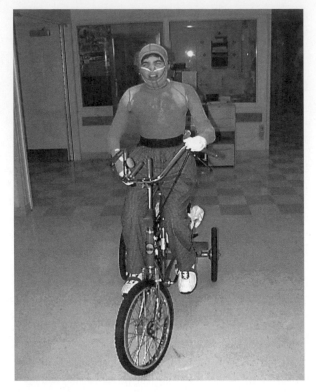

Figure 9-16 Functional and fun activities to gain range of motion and endurance.

neutral to slightly extended position while sitting and mobilizing

3. PROM exercises for neck rotation, side flexion and extension, using singing/counting techniques for distraction and tolerance of intervention (Figure 9–17 and the corresponding color plate)

4. AROM exercises

Mobility

Ethan was limited in his ability to ambulate on level surfaces. He required assistance for bed mobility, transfers, and gait.

Goal: Ethan will be independent with all aspects of household and community mobility.

Interventions:

1. Mobilization out of bed to wheelchair

2. Parent education for transfer and guarding techniques

3. Assisted ambulation with hand-held assistance because of inability of arms to use assistive device

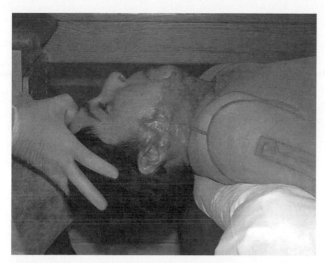

Figure 9-17 Passive range of motion interventions for cervical extension after scar revision. See also color plate.

Endurance

Ethan was limited in participating in long therapy sessions, not only because of his attention span but also because of his low endurance and inability to regulate his body temperature as a result of the extensive thermal injury.

Goal: Ethan will be able to participate in ADLs and household mobility without needing frequent rest breaks.

Interventions:

1. Daily routine and schedule adhered to by all staff members

2. Shortened therapy sessions, looking for signs of fatigue that included sitting down, pointing to his wheelchair, or agitation

3. Encouraged Ethan to drink during therapy session, with water bottle always on hand

4. Cool towel applied to his face and neck during rest period of therapy session

5. Participation of his parents in therapy sessions to encourage and reassure him

Activity and Participation Restrictions

Ethan was limited from participating in normal ADLs, other community activities, and interactions with his peers because of his prolonged hospitalizations. His parents chose

to care for him at home and restrict his participation in school and group home activities because of the nature of the accident.

Outcomes

Ethan continues to have ongoing issues with skin breakdown at sporadic sites throughout his body, now 9 months after the initial injuries. He wears compression garments for his arms, legs, trunk, and face. His skin is slowly starting to appear smoother, with less apparent hypertrophic scarring present. He continues to have decreased use of his right hand caused by amputations and contractures and has some functional use of his left hand. His neck ROM improved after surgery, but he has already lost range because of scarring. Because of poor tolerance, he uses his neck orthosis only intermittently. Since returning home after surgery, he receives therapy several days a week, and his parents are extremely invested in his care. He is independent ambulating in his house, including up and down stairs. He is able to walk 4 miles daily in a rough terrain setting with supervision. He will require ongoing therapy for an extended period because of his risk for contractures caused by the remodeling process. He will likely need numerous scar revision surgeries and faces a lifetime of episodes of care for wound and scar management, ROM, compression garments, and mobility.

Summary

The physical therapist plays an important role in managing children with open wounds and burns. Knowledge of the structure and function of the integumentary system and related impairments that may occur are essential for delivering quality care. Advanced training that can best be accomplished in the clinical setting will enhance the intervention skills needed to best serve this population. Competency-based training programs are essential to ensure clinical competence for interventions, especially for débridement and wound-healing techniques.

The physical therapist must also serve as educator for other health-care professionals. Therapists are often the most extensively trained health-care professionals in the area of wound, burn, and scar management. We must advocate for a wound-management program that enhances moist wound healing and decreases the trauma to the viable tissue. It is vital to keep in mind what phase of healing the wound is in and how best to progress it through all the stages to achieve wound closure, an acceptable-appearing scar, and ultimate function and independence for the child. Continuing education programs that include both didactic and laboratory portions for learning new techniques are highly recommended for clinicians of all levels of experience.

DISCUSSION QUESTIONS

1. Describe the key processes in each of the phases of wound healing.

2. How do hypertrophic scars form, and what interventions can be taken to prevent and control them?

3. How can you differentiate the four stages of pressure ulcers?

4. What objective findings would you include in your open wound/thermal injury examination?

5. Discuss the role of proper positioning and ROM for the child with thermal injuries.

6. Describe one modality, other than traditional gauze dressing changes, for achieving wound cleansing and healing.

RECOMMENDED READINGS

American Burn Association. Retrieved April 1, 2004, from *http://www.Ameriburn.org*

Carrougher, G.J. (Ed.) (1998). *Burn care and therapy*. St. Louis: Mosby.

Dermolytic Epidermolysis Bullosa Research Association. Retrieved April 1, 2004, from *http://www. DEBRA.org*

Kloth, L.C., & McCulloch, J.M. (Eds.) (2002). *Wound healing: Alternatives in management* (3rd ed.). Philadelphia: F.A. Davis.

Sussman, C., & Bates-Jensen, B. (Eds.) (1998). *Wound care: A collaborative practice manual for physical therapists and nurses.* Gaithersburg, MD: Aspen Publishing.

Pain Scale Resources

Attia, J., Amiel-Tison, C., Mayer, M.N., Schnider, S.M., & Barrier, G. (1987). Measurement of postoperative pain and narcotic administration in infants using a new clinical scoring system. *Anesthesiology, 67*, A532.

Krechel, S.W., & Bildner, J. (1995). CRIES: A new neonatal postoperative pain measurement score. Initial testing of validity and reliability. *Paediatric Anaesthesia, 5*(1), 53–61.

McGrath, P.G., Johnson, G., Goodman, J., Schillinger, J., Dunn J., & Chapman, J. (1985). CHEOPS: A behavioral scale for rating postoperative pain in children. *Advances in Pain Research Theory, 9*, 395–402.

Wong, D., & Baker, C. (1988). Pain in children: Comparison of assessment scales. *Pediatric Nursing, 14*(1), 9–17.

REFERENCES

Allison, K.P., & Smith, G. (1998). Burn management in a child with autism. *Burns, 24*, 484–486.

Alvarez, O., Rozuint, J., & Meehan, M. (1997). Principles of moist wound healing: Indications for chronic wounds. In D. Krasner (Ed.), *Chronic wound care: A clinical source book for healthcare professionals* (pp. 49–56). King of Prussia, PA: Health Management Publishers Inc.

American Physical Therapy Association (2001). Guide to physical therapist practice (2nd ed.). *Physical Therapy, 81*, 6–746.

Apfel, L., et al. (1994). Approaches to positioning the burn patient. In R.L. Richard & M.J. Staley (Eds.), *Burn care and rehabilitation*. Philadelphia: F.A. Davis Company.

Argenta, L.C., & Marykwas, M.J. (1997). Vacuum-assisted closure: A new method for wound control and treatment: Clinical experience. *Annals of Plastic Surgery, 38*, 563–576.

Atherton, D.J. (2000). Epidermolysis bullosa. In J. Harper, A. Oranje, & N. Prose (Eds.), *Textbook of pediatric dermatology,* Vol. 2 (pp. 1075–1095). Malden, MA: Blackwell Science.

Attia, J., Amiel-Tison, C., Mayer, M.N., Schnider, S.M., & Barrier, G. (1987). Measurement of postoperative pain and narcotic administration in infants using a new clinical scoring system. *Anesthesiology, 67*, A532.

Bates-Jensen, B. (1998a). Management of exudate and infection. In C. Sussman & B. Bates-Jensen (Eds.), *Wound care: A collaborative practice manual for physical therapists and nurses* (pp. 159–176). Gaithersburg, MD: Aspen Publishing.

Bates-Jensen, B. (1998b). Management of necrotic tissue. In C. Sussman & B. Bates-Jensen (Eds.), *Wound care: A collaborative practice manual for physical therapists and nurses* (pp. 139–150). Gaithersburg, MD: Aspen Publishing.

Bates-Jensen, B. (1998c). Pressure ulcers: Pathophysiology and prevention. In C. Sussman & B. Bates-Jensen (Eds.), *Wound care: A collaborative practice manual for physical therapists and nurses* (pp. 235–270). Gaithersburg, MD: Aspen Publishing.

Bergstrom, N., Allman, R.M., Alvarez, O.M., Bennett, M.A., Carlson, C.E., Frantz, R.A., et al. (1994). *Treatment of pressure ulcers*. Clinical Practice Guideline, No. 15. Rockville, MD:

U.S. Department of Health and Human Services. Public Health Service, Agency for Health Care Policy and Research. AHCPR Publication No. 95–0652.

Committee on Injury and Poison Prevention, American Academy of Pediatrics. Widome, M.D. (Ed.) (1997). *Injury prevention and control for children and youth* (pp. 233–267). Elk Grove Village, IL: Author.

Cuzzell, L.J. (1988). The new RYB color code. *American Journal of Nursing, 88,* 1342–1346.

Doctor, M.E. (1994). Parent participation during painful wound care procedures. *Journal of Burn Care and Rehabilitation, 15,* 288–292.

Dressler, D.P., & Hozid, J.L. (2001). Thermal injury and child abuse: The medical evidence dilemma. *Journal of Burn Care and Rehabilitation, 22,* 180–185.

Falkel, J. (1994). Anatomy and physiology of the skin. In R.L. Richard & M.J. Staley (Eds.), *Burn care and rehabilitation: Principles and practice* (pp. 10–28). Philadelphia: F.A. Davis.

Farmer, E.R., & Hood, A.F. (Eds.) (1990). *Pathology of the skin* (pp. 762–771). New York: McGraw-Hill.

Gray, H. (1977). General anatomy or histology. In T. Pick & R. Howden (Eds.), *Gray's anatomy* (pp. 1135–1143). New York, NY: Bounty Books.

Greenhalgh, D.G., & Staley, M.J. (1994). Burn wound healing. In R.L. Richard & M.J. Staley (Eds.), *Burn care and rehabilitation: Principles and practice* (pp. 70–102). Philadelphia: F.A. Davis.

Groce, A., Meyers Paal, R., Herndon, D.N., & McCauley, R.L. (1999). Are your thoughts of facial pressure transparent? *Journal of Burn Care and Rehabilitation, 20,* 478–481.

Herndon, D.N., Rutan, R.L., Alison, W.E., Jr., & Cox, C.S., Jr. (1993). Management of burn injuries. In M.R. Eichelberger (Ed.), *Pediatric trauma* (pp. 568–605). St. Louis, MO: Mosby-Year Book.

Huffines, B. & Logsdon, M.C. (1997). The Neonatal Skin Risk Assessment Scale for predicting skin breakdown in neonates. *Issues in Comprehensive Pediatric Nursing, 20*(2), *103–114.*

Humphrey, C.N., Richard, R.L., & Staley, M.J. (1994). Soft tissue management and exercise. In R.L. Richard & M.J. Staley (Eds.), *Burn care and rehabilitation: Principles and practice* (pp. 324–360). Philadelphia: F.A. Davis.

Johnson, C. (1994). Pathologic manifestations of burn injury. In R.L. Richard & M.J. Staley (Eds.), *Burn care and rehabilitation: Principles and practice* (pp. 29–48). Philadelphia: F.A. Davis.

Kloth, L.C. (2002a). Electrical stimulation for wound healing. In L.C. Kloth & J.M. McCulloch (Eds.), *Wound healing: Alternatives in management* (3rd ed., pp. 271–315). Philadelphia: F.A. Davis.

Kloth, L.C. (2002b). Adjunctive interventions for wound healing. In L.C. Kloth & J.M. McCulloch (Eds.), *Wound healing: Alternatives in management* (3rd ed., pp. 316–381). Philadelphia: F.A. Davis.

Krechel, S.W., & Bildner, J. (1995). CRIES: A new neonatal post-operative pain measurement score. Initial testing of validity and reliability. *Paediatric Anaesthesia, 5*(1), 53–61.

Loehne, H.B. (2002). Wound débridement and irrigation. In L.C. Kloth & J.M. McCulloch (Eds.), *Wound healing: Alternatives in management* (3rd ed., pp. 203–231). Philadelphia: F.A. Davis.

Luedtke-Hoffman, K.A., & Schafer, D.S. (2000). Pulsed lavage in wound cleansing. *Physical Therapy, 80,* 292–300.

Lund, C.C., & Browder, N.C. (1944). The estimation of areas of burns. *Surgery, Gynecology, and Obstetrics, 79,* 352–358.

Martin-Herz, S.P., Thurber, C.A., & Patterson, D.R. (2000). Psychological principles of burn wound pain in children. II: Treatment applications. *Journal of Burn Care and Rehabilitation, 21,* 458–472.

McGrath, P.G., Johnson, G., Goodman, J., Schillinger, J., Dunn J., & Chapman, J. (1985). CHEOPS: A behavioral scale for rating postoperative pain in children. *Advances in Pain Research Theory, 9,* 395–402.

Miller, S.F., Staley, M.J., & Richard, R.L. (1994). Surgical management of the burned child. In R.L. Richard & M.J. Staley (Eds.), *Burn care and rehabilitation: Principles and practice* (pp. 177–197). Philadelphia: F.A. Davis.

Mooney, J.F., III, Argenta, L.C., Marks, M.W., Marykwas, M.J., & DeFranzo, A.J. (2000). Treatment of soft tissue defects in pediatric patients using the V.A.C. System. *Clinical Orthopedics and Related Research, 376,* 26–31.

Patterson, J.W., & Blaylock, W.K. (1987). *Dermatology* (pp. 1–15). New York: Medical Examination Publishing.

Rassner, G. (1994). *Atlas of dermatology* (pp. 7–8). (Walter Burgdorf, trans.). Philadelphia: Lea & Febiger.

Ross, R. (1968). The fibroblast and wound repair. *Biological Review, 43,* 51–91.

Saffle, J.R., & Schnebly, W.A. (1994). Burn wound care. In R.L. Richard & M.J. Staley (Eds.), *Burn care and rehabilitation: Principles and practice* (pp. 119–176). Philadelphia: F.A. Davis.

Schulz, J.T., Sheridan, R.L., Ryan, C.M., MacKool, B., & Tompkins, R.G. (2000). A 10-year experience with toxic epidermal necrolysis. *Journal of Burn Care and Rehabilitation, 21,* 199–204.

Sheridan, R.L., Weber, J.M., Schulz, J.M. Ryan, C.M., Low, H.M., & Tompkins, R.G. (1999). Management of severe toxic epidermal necrolysis in children. *Journal of Burn Care and Rehabilitation, 20,* 497–500.

Staley, M.J., & Richard, R.L. (1994). Scar management. In R.L. Richard & M.J. Staley (Eds.), *Burn care and rehabilitation: Principles and practice* (pp. 380–418). Philadelphia: F.A. Davis.

Sussman, C. (1998a). Wound healing biology and chronic wound healing. In C. Sussman & B. Bates-Jensen (Eds.), *Wound care: A collaborative practice manual for physical therapists and nurses* (pp. 31–47). Gaithersburg, MD: Aspen Publishing.

Sussman, C. (1998b). Assessment of the skin and wound. In C. Sussman & B. Bates-Jensen (Eds.), *Wound care: A collaborative practice manual for physical therapists and nurses* (pp. 49–82). Gaithersburg, MD: Aspen Publishing.

Sussman, C. (1998c). Wound measurements. In C. Sussman & B. Bates-Jensen (Eds.), *Wound care: A collaborative practice manual for physical therapists and nurses* (pp. 83–102). Gaithersburg, MD: Aspen Publishing.

Sussman, G. (1998). Management of the wound environment. In C. Sussman & B. Bates-Jensen (Eds.), *Wound care: A collaborative practice manual for physical therapists and nurses* (pp. 201–213). Gaithersburg, MD: Aspen Publishing.

Unger, P.G. (1992). Electrical enhancement of wound repair. *Physical Therapy Practice, 80*, 41–49.

Wong, D., & Baker, C. (1988). Pain in children: Comparison of assessment scales. *Pediatric Nursing, 14*(1), 9–17.

Service Delivery Settings

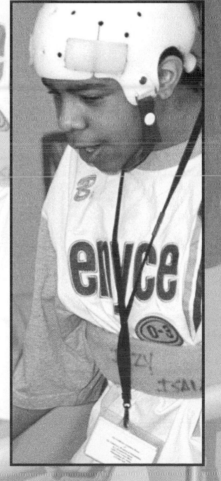

Chapter *10*

Early Intervention

— Jane O'Regan Kleinert, MSPA, CCC
— Susan K. Effgen, PT, PhD

This chapter will discuss early identification, examination, evaluation, and intervention services for very young children from birth to 3 years of age. We will discuss the federal legislation that guides services to this population of children, and current "best practice" procedures for examination and intervention. Guiding principles for this chapter will include family-centered services, interdisciplinary and transdisciplinary team models, providing services in natural environments, and using activity-based instruction whenever possible.

What Do We Mean by "Early Intervention"?

The term *early intervention* (EI) is used in a variety of ways in a variety of disciplines. Conventional wisdom tells us it is best to intervene quickly when problems are suspected, before major problems occur. In medicine, competent physicians practice EI when they strive to provide intervention for illness as soon as symptoms are detected. The kindergarten teacher practices EI when he or she screens the class at the beginning of the school year to determine which children may need extra help in learning to read. Even the wary homeowner who watches for signs of a leaky roof or basement is practicing early identification and intervention in an effort to ward off major and expensive

household repairs. In other words, EI involves early detection and intervention of problems in order to minimize negative effects and reduce future potential problems as cost-effectively as possible.

When we engage in EI with infants and young children with delays, disabilities, or potential disabilities, we are doing essentially the same things as the individuals previously described. Pediatric therapists work with families, physicians, and others interested in the well-being of young children to *identify* potential or emerging problems or established developmental physical and cognitive problems as early as possible and *intervene* quickly and efficiently to *correct* or *minimize* the problem/delay and *maximize* the child's developmental potential, whatever that may be.

Definitions of Early Intervention

Federal legislation (PL 99–457), adopted in 1986, provided federal funding to the states for provision of early identification and intervention services to infants and young children aged 0 to 36 months who have, or are at risk of having, disabilities, and their families. This legislation was part of the Individuals with Disabilities Education Act (IDEA) and is discussed in this and the following chapter. This act and its reauthorization in 1997 define an EI program as "the total effort in a State that is directed at meeting the needs of children eligible under this part (Part C) and their families" (IDEA Practices, 2003).

Although this legislation provides the "legal" definition of EI programs, experts in the field provide additional information regarding EI services and programs. Rune Simeonsson, a renowned educator and researcher in the area of EI, notes that the overall goal of EI "is to prevent disabilities in infants and young children by reducing or removing physical and social barriers and by promoting their growth, development, and well-being through stimulation and provision of support" (Simeonsson, 2000, p. 6). Simeonsson believes that EI must see each child as an individual, be comprehensive, address the child *and his or her family* as a unit, and take the individual family's social and cultural context into account. Guralnick (2000) sees the provision of *early, comprehensive assessment from many disciplines all working in harmony with the family* as a vital element of EI. Bailey (1997) has stressed the importance of addressing the *"at-risk" child* when we speak of EI, and the EI pioneer Carl Dunst (Dunst, Trivette, & Jodry, 1997) reminds us that a *child's and family's social support systems* influence EI programs. Authorities in EI come from many fields of research and study. Those of us learning about EI will benefit from their rich variety in focus. This variety in focus gives a broad, encompassing nature to the definitions of EI programs.

Who Receives Early Intervention Services?

States are allowed to develop their own specific eligibility guidelines, but the federal legislation on EI includes the following description of children who may receive EI services. Children who may receive such services are "infants and toddlers with disabilities...from birth through age two who need EI services because they are experiencing developmental delays, as measured by appropriate diagnostic instruments and procedures, in one or more of the following areas...cognitive development; physical development, including vision and hearing; communication development; social or emotional development; adaptive development" (IDEA Practices, 2003) or the child who has a physical or mental condition that will probably result in a developmental delay, often referred to as an "established risk." Some states also include children who are at risk for having a developmental delay if EI is not provided. Children may receive EI services until the age of 36 months, or their third birthday.

What Services May Be Available to Children in Early Intervention?

Again, IDEA helps answer this question. Services include assessment and intervention in a large variety of areas and disciplines, including primary service coordination; audiology (hearing) and vision services; some health, medical, and nursing services; nutrition; occupational therapy; physical therapy; psychological services; social work services; speech/language pathology services; and some transportation services. Specialized instruction provided by specially trained educators, assistive technology services, and family support and respite services are also included in EI programs. One other very important part of the team is the **primary service coordinator** (**PSC**), who is often an initial contact for the family as they enter the EI system. The PSC is involved with the family from their initial referral and will be available to the family to *help facilitate all areas of the EI process.* The PSC coordinates other team members, evaluations, Individualized Family Service Plan (IFSP) development, interventions, and finally, the smooth transition from EI to public school programs when the child reaches 3 years of age.

Physical therapy examination, evaluation, and intervention are important services needed by many children who participate in EI. It is important to note that physical therapy is considered a *primary* service in EI rather than a related service. This means that, unlike services to public school children in which the physical therapy program must relate to an educational objective, in EI, physical therapy services, when needed, stand alone regardless of a child's educational/cognitive needs. Therefore, an infant with cystic fibrosis or a toddler with juvenile rheumatoid arthritis might receive physical therapy services even though there may not be an educational need for services.

What Are the Components of Early Intervention?

The components of EI are determined by two guiding principles. These are the federal regulations of Part C of IDEA and the concept of "best practice." Best practices are those goals, strategies, interventions, and principles that have been agreed on as reflecting the highest level of quality by certain professions, disciplines, and practitioners in those various fields. Best practices are now slowly being supported by research, as required for evidence-based practice. As noted, the field of EI involves many disciplines. Authorities from these disciplines participated in the development of IDEA, and so for the most part, the federal guidelines and best practice for EI are often the same. These best practices and IDEA guidelines form the major components of quality EI and will compose the rest of this chapter. The following topics will be discussed: individualized planning for *each child and family*; family-centered services; implementation of EI services within natural environments; activity-based, functional intervention; and team-based assessment/evaluation and intervention. In the following sections, the term *assessment* is used frequently because it is the word for the examination and evaluation of the child within the IFSP framework. In addition, many of our colleagues in early childhood, special education, and speech-language pathology use the term "assessment" to refer to the initial and, especially, the ongoing examination and evaluation of a child's status. This is not meant to conflict with the physical therapist's use of the words "examination" and "evaluation," which have specific meaning within physical therapy. Rather, the term "assessment" is used to familiarize you with the terms most commonly used in the overall field of EI, and within IDEA.

Individualized Planning for Each Child and Family

The federal regulations of Part C in IDEA define for us the what, who, where, when, how, and why of EI; however, states have latitude in how these regulations are implemented. Each child and family must have an individualized family service plan (IFSP), mentioned previously. The IFSP has several main components. Each state has an IFSP form to describe the proposed EI program for a specific child and family. Although forms may vary in appearance, the components are standard across states. The following are the major components of an IFSP.

Demographics

These are simply the basic identifying information for the child, family, service providers, and agencies to be involved in the plan.

History

Included in this section might be the child's past medical, prenatal, birth, and developmental histories, family history, and any past intervention the child may have received. See Table 1.12 for content areas important to physical therapists.

Child's Current Level of Functioning

This section includes a summary of the child's current strengths and deficits. This information comes from recent assessments by a team of interventionists and the family and includes the child's abilities in the major developmental areas of cognition, communication, physical, social/emotional, and adaptive skills. It is vitally important that all members of the EI team focus on the child's strengths as well as his or her needs. For too long, parents have had to endure long recitals of their child's deficits when they attended the planning meetings, with no attention being given to the positive, typical aspects of their child. Parents who have had such past experiences often tell us after attending an IFSP meeting in which their child's strengths are recognized, "This is the first time anyone has had positive things to say about my child." This is a chilling commentary on the medical, educational, and therapeutic fields, and an occurrence we can no longer allow.

Family's Concerns, Priorities, and Resources

This is the section of the IFSP in which the family members identify their primary concerns regarding their child, and their own needs in fostering their child's optimal development. They then list the priority *outcomes* they envision from the EI program. We may be more familiar with seeing the word "goals" used rather than "outcomes." Using the word *outcomes*, however, implies a more active program that focuses on the whole team working toward the same result. Finally, the family reflects on the resources that are available to them to assist in achieving the outcomes they have selected. These resources include not only the agencies and providers at the IFSP meeting but also any community resource, family, or friends who may help support the family's and child's optimal development.

Early Intervention Services

Next, the team, including the family as a full participating member, designs the intervention program that is to help achieve the selected outcomes. This section includes the intervention strategies each provider will use and where, when, how often, and for how long the intervention services will be implemented. We discuss this element of the IFSP and the philosophical guidelines that are followed in detail later in this chapter, in the sections on assessment and intervention.

Primary Service Coordinator

Each family is provided with a PSC, who serves as a case manager for the family and child's EI program. The PSC has regular contact with the family and the full team and aids the family, when needed, in coordinating their resources to maximize the child's development. The PSC also helps facilitate the child's transition to any other programs, especially as the child approaches his or her third birthday.

Transition Plan

EI programs seek to provide "seamless" transition of services from EI to the early childhood program offered by the local public school system for the child. Long before the child approaches age 3 years, when he or she must transition out of EI, the local school system should have been advised of the child's needs and become a member of the IFSP team. In this way, the child and family are not left alone when EI services stop at age 3 years. (See Chapter 11 on preschool and school-age services.)

Family-Centered Services and Intervention

The components of family-centered services and intervention are covered in Chapter 3. However, we cannot have a discussion of EI without including this overriding concept. **Family-centered services** and intervention imply the full involvement of the family in *all* aspects of the EI program. This includes active participation of the family in assessment, planning, and intervention. It is easy to see that, as professionals, we cannot address the needs of an infant or toddler without the full participation of the most vital individuals in that child's life. What possible impact can we have on a child by visiting him or her 1 or 2 hours per week? What of the remaining 166 hours of the week? Unless the family has selected the outcomes that are important to them and their child, agrees with the intervention program, and has helped develop and implement that program within their individual abilities, how can we expect to really affect a child's development? Family-centered services and intervention also imply that the family serves as advocate for the child. In this position, they may not always agree with what the professional believes is the "best" for the child. The therapist must be ready to listen and work with the family until the EI program is acceptable to all concerned, if possible.

Remember, as in all aspects of the EI program, communication with the family must be in their primary language, and interpreters should be available when needed. This includes not only those who speak a language other than English but also those individuals who are deaf or hard of hearing. In addition, we must be sensitive to the cognitive abilities of some parents and be sure that they fully understand what is being developed and decided in any EI program.

Implementation of Early Intervention Within Natural Environments

IDEA defines **natural environments** as "settings that are natural or normal for the child's (same) age peers who do not have disabilities" (IDEA Practices, 2003). Research in a variety of disciplines has shown that a child acts and reacts differently in familiar, secure locations, such as his or her home, than he or she may in an unfamiliar setting. We are more likely to achieve the most reliable examination information and the most typical behaviors in intervention if we work with the child and his or her family within their natural environment. In addition, it is frequently much easier for the family if the interventionist can come to their home or the child's daycare setting. This causes less disruption of the family's daily life. Seeing a child for intervention in a hospital or office is using an artificial environment. What if the family does not have the equipment we use in our office? What if we work on activities that never occur in the family's daily life or in the daycare setting? How is the family going to implement intervention strategies the other 166 hours per week, if the intervention strategies and materials are not readily part of their lives? For these reasons, IDEA directs that assessment and intervention occur in the family's natural environments, not that of the therapist or interventionists. Natural environments can include the child's home, daycare setting, local playground, or perhaps a play group site. Natural environments encourage and stimulate the easy carryover of intervention objectives into the family's everyday life. The family can see how everyday materials found in their home can be used to aid in their child's development. Seeing the child in his or her daycare setting helps caregivers to become active in his or her EI program and to use their time with the child to help optimize his or her development. This requires that the therapist become flexible in finding and adapting therapeutic strategies to the equipment, toys, and activities available to the child on a daily basis. In addition, the therapist must be a model and teacher to the child's caretakers so that they can carry out therapeutic activities with the child when the therapist is not present. We will discuss specific strategies for this later in this chapter when we discuss intervention.

Activity-Based Instruction

Conducting EI activities in the child and family's natural environment leads us directly to the concept of **activity-based instruction**. Activity-based instruction is a concept that was developed in the field of special education in which teachers and interventionists strive to make intervention strategies as functional and integrated into the child's daily routine as possible. Working in the natural environment facilitates our ability to develop functional objectives and strategies that fit the family's lifestyle and the desired outcomes they have for their child. In years past, when therapists developed goals and interventions without the family's input, we often selected strategies or goals that could be implemented only by a therapist. Or we showed the family intervention strategies that required them to set aside specific, lengthy time periods of the day in which they did "therapy" with their child. Unfortunately, families have more to do than carry out "homework" assignments that the therapist assigns to them, with no regard to the time, or energy, that must be available to the family for them to complete the assignment each week. In the authors' experience, all too often, a parent would quickly fill in the "homework" data sheets that she or he had been given to complete throughout the week while sitting in the waiting room before the child's therapy session! Therapists need to learn that unless the suggestions we give families for daily activities with their child fit easily into the family's routines, are functional, and are easy to complete while the parent cares for the other children, goes to work, cleans the house, and cares for grandmother, those "home programs" may as well be pitched in the trash. The use of activity-based instruction will be discussed in more detail in the intervention section of this chapter.

Teaming

Teaming is a vital part of the EI process. In Chapter 1, you learned about the various models of teaming and how the members interact; therefore, we will only briefly review these models as they relate to EI. Part C of IDEA requires team input during examination, evaluation, and intervention with the young child and family. Regular interaction and planning among the professional team with the family, and with each other, are necessary in EI. Team collabora-

tion does not stop after the evaluation, but continues as long as the IFSP is in place.

There are several types of teams seen in EI. As you read in Chapter 1, the **multidisciplinary team** is the oldest form of teaming and has the least active interaction among team members. There are no set channels of interaction and consultation among the team members. Indeed, a multidisciplinary team could individually assess and report their findings without ever seeing each other in the same room. This type of team is clearly not sufficient to meet the requirements of Part C, which *requires* that each assessment conducted in EI include *multiple sources* of input and involve *interaction of the family and other evaluators*. The **interdisciplinary team** offers more interaction among the team members than the multidisciplinary team. In this type of teaming, there are typically formal channels of communication established among the professionals, and there is a case manager who coordinates the activities and reporting of the team's information. Often, the team may submit one combined assessment report that includes information from all the professionals involved. Although this is an improved model of teaming, it still does not guarantee well-integrated development of intervention programming. The **transdisciplinary team** is a current model of team assessment and program development in EI. In this model, the team members are encouraged to share information, skills, and programming *across* disciplines and with the family. Some of this sharing involves *role release* and will be discussed in detail under intervention. Team members may assess the child together, and even treat together at times, to ensure themselves and the family that *all team members are sharing goals and strategies for the child's optimal development*. When assessment and programming are developed with all the team members and the family together and strategies are shared across disciplines, the child receives constant reinforcement of all the important outcomes strategies, rather than receiving input only when the physical therapist, speech-language pathologist, or occupational therapist happens to be in the home or with the child.

Keeping best practice and Part C regulations in mind, physical therapists should no longer examine a child and independently develop and implement an intervention program. We must serve as part of a larger team, including a variety of disciplines and the child's family. Somewhat counter to this important concept of team assessment, program planning, and intervention is an unfortunate trend in some locations to have one group of professionals perform the assessment and another group provide the intervention. This is done under the misguided assumption that too many children are being recommended for services by assessment teams that will provide the services. Perhaps this has occurred; however, the use of two teams creates additional work, expense, and duplication of assessment services. In this model, once the assessment team determines that intervention is required, the child is referred for services, and another team provides the intervention. Under most circumstances, though, the second team *reassesses* the child before intervention can be provided.

The composition of the individual child's IFSP team should be individualized, with different team members constituting teams for different children. The primary IFSP team may include smaller teams. For example, the child with orthopedic problems may be seen by a *team* of medical specialists that includes an orthopedist, a physiatrist, a nurse, an occupational therapist, a physical therapist, and an orthotist. These professionals may see the child only a few times each year. We hope that this team will make every effort to include the child's primary physical therapist in any decisions they make about the child's care.

The child may also see teams at a particular center that specializes in a specific disability. Often children who have been diagnosed with autism travel to a center that specializes in that disability for assessment and consultation. There the child may see another set of occupational therapists, physical therapists, speech-language pathologists, psychologists, social workers, physicians, and so on. Again, this specialized team must be careful to include the input of the EI team that sees the child on a regular basis. Unfortunately, this is not always the case, and we, as early interventionists, whether part of the home-based team or the specialized consultation team, must work diligently to be sure that interaction between the two teams occurs so that the child and family are not given conflicting information or confusing input.

How Are These "Best Practice" Components of Early Intervention Integrated Into Assessment/Evaluation and Intervention Strategies?

We have just discussed the primary components of a quality EI program. These components included the IFSP, family-centered services and intervention, assessment/intervention within the child's natural environment, activity-based instruction, and teaming. Now we will see how these components play out in the two major parts of the EI process: assessment/evaluation and intervention.

Assessment/Evaluation

Individualized Family Service Plan and Family-Centered Services

IDEA provides specific timelines regarding how many days may pass between the referral of a child to the EI system and when the first contact with the family must occur. In addition, each state has specific guidelines regarding how many days may pass before an assessment is completed after the child is referred to a provider and how soon the assessment report must be completed. Often a state requires that the results of the assessment must be given to and discussed with the family *before* the IFSP meeting. Therapists must be aware of the guidelines of the state in which they practice and adhere closely to those guidelines at all times.

In addition, each state might have a specific format for reporting assessment/evaluation results. The state may also delineate what particular instrument early interventionists must use to determine "eligibility" for their EI program. This instrument may be (but is not necessarily) a standardized instrument that establishes functioning levels in the five developmental areas outlined by Part C of IDEA. Although this instrument may be sufficient to determine that a child is eligible for the state's EI program, it may not be sufficient to program for a child's individual needs in any particular area. After a child qualifies for EI and the developmental areas of need are determined, a more complete assessment/evaluation is usually conducted by professionals in each appropriate discipline that address the child's specific areas of need. The family's concerns must also be a driving force in determining which assessments are to be completed.

Part C also requires that assessments include *multiple sources of information*. This means not only that *more than one evaluator* gives input *as well as the family*, but that this *input has come from more than one type of measure*. Simply giving the child a commercially available instrument is not sufficient for assessment under Part C. The child should be observed in natural activities and natural environments that allow numerous opportunities for the child to display true functioning levels and strengths.

Part C makes some very clear requirements for the conducting and reporting of the EI assessments. Under Part C, the assessment should include the family's input. Before any interaction with the child, the therapist contacts the family to determine their primary concerns regarding the child's development, a top-down approach to assessment. The family must give written consent for assessment. The family should be present throughout the assessment, whether it is conducted only by the physical therapist or in a team setting involving other disciplines. We have found it to be especially helpful to give the family some form of a family-friendly check list or home assessment to record their own impression of their child's developmental levels. This information is then integrated into the written report as the parental input, information that is required under Part C. Such an activity also allows *parents to give their own assessment input*, if they desire, during the IFSP meeting. The assessment must be in the family's primary language and should be culturally sensitive. If the therapist does not speak the family's primary language, an interpreter should be present, and an interpreter for the deaf or hearing impaired if needed. If any standardized instruments are used in the evaluation, every effort should be made to use only instruments that have been standardized on a population similar to the family's cultural and socioeconomic background. Because this may not always be possible, care *must* be taken in *interpreting and reporting* the results of instruments that do not fit these requirements.

Natural Environments

Assessments should be conducted within the child's natural environment. As stated earlier in this chapter, that setting may be the child's home, daycare setting, the playground, a family friend's home, or any other setting where typically developing children are found. The therapist's office, a hospital, or a developmental center designed specifically for children with special needs usually does not qualify as a "natural environment." The use of the natural environment allows naturalistic observation of play and other daily routines that are required under Part C. The natural environment helps to ensure that we are being culturally sensitive and family centered and provides a much more realistic picture of the child's real, functional abilities. Although a child may be hesitant to climb stairs in our office building, he or she may be quite adept at this skill at home or on the playground.

Activity-Based Assessment

In the field of EI, authorities have long been concerned that standardized assessment/evaluation instruments are not functional or realistic, do not give a "real-life" picture of a child and his or her daily routines, and frequently are not sensitive to the family's culture. Rich information about the child and his or her skills can be drawn from observation and interactions with the child in everyday play and activities. Activity-based assessment can be conducted by using a commercially available, criterion-referenced instrument, or from our own trained observations. Some of the more popular commercial instruments are listed in Appendix 2.B of Chapter 2. These instruments are usually conducted in the child's home or daycare setting and involve a team of early interventionists, as well as the family. The child is observed with his or her siblings or peers during a variety of activities. Professionals record information that applies to their discipline and expertise, and the team discusses and scores the assessment as a group. A commercial instrument is not necessary to complete an activity-based assessment. The physical therapist may choose to observe and "play" with the child in his or her natural environment and allow the child to select favorite, natural, functional activities through which he or she demonstrates strengths and areas of need. This allows the child to demonstrate his or her true functional abilities while enjoying natural activities. Using specific instruments, which allow only certain materials and activities, may severely limit the functionality of the assessment as well as its accuracy. We often try to come to the home at a time when the child is usually going to be involved in activities that will demonstrate his or her skills in a certain area. If a therapist needs to observe a child's self-feeding skills, it makes sense to try to come during the child's typical mealtime. This reduces the disruption of the family's schedule, and increases the likelihood of seeing the child's real skill level.

Teaming

We have already discussed the types of teams that are seen in EI. The type of team you participate in may well influence how your assessments are conducted. The assessment should be at least of an *interdisciplinary* nature. This means that the individuals involved with the assessment of a particular child have (1) discussed concerns with the family; (2) discussed what areas of assessment and what tools are to be used with the other team members; (3) determined, with the family, what are the best times and locations for the assessment, and have coordinated this with other team members so that the family's schedule is not unduly disrupted; (4) discussed the results of assessments with the family and with other team members before the IFSP meeting; and (5) worked to coordinate and integrate assessment information in the reporting process. Each individual interdisciplinary team member then conducts the actual assessment of the child on a one-to-one basis.

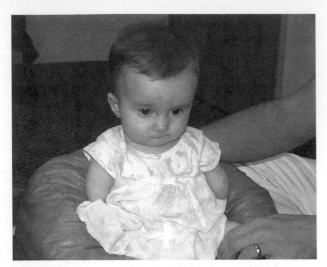

Figure 10-1 Infant with limb deficiencies participating in an arena assessment.

Best practice indicates that *transdisciplinary assessments* may be an especially efficient and effective form of assessment in a child's EI years. We have already discussed how a transdisciplinary team might be constructed and, in general, how such a team operates. Let's look at how that type of team might conduct an assessment.

The initial aspects of the assessment process might be similar to the interdisciplinary approach. Each team member talks to the family before the assessment to secure the family's concerns about their child. The team also decides together which instruments are to be used and, with the family, when and where the assessment will be conducted. How the actual assessment is conducted, however, can be quite different from the way it is conducted in the interdisciplinary team approach.

Transdisciplinary teams frequently use **arena assessment** as discussed in Chapter 1. In this style of assessment, team members are all together for the assessment along with the family and child (Figure 10–1). Which team members will be included in the assessment process for a particular child will be determined by the family's areas of concern for their child's development. A team might include a physical therapist; a speech-language pathologist; an occupational therapist; an early childhood educator (developmental interventionist); possibly a social worker or psychologist and, of course, the PSC as well as the family. In an arena assessment, the team selects one or more assessment instruments that include sections for each of the five developmental areas (cognition, communication, physical, adaptive, and social/emotional skills) typically addressed in

EI. Some commonly used assessments in EI include the Bayley Scales of Infant Development II, Hawaii Early Learning Profile, Carolina Curriculum, and Birth to Three Assessment and Intervention System.

In an arena assessment, all members are present for the assessment, but only one or two may actually interact directly with the child. This reduces the number of adults to whom the child must become accustomed. The team usually selects the members who will be working directly with the child, based on the family's primary concern about the child's development. For instance, if the parent is very concerned about the child's ability to move and walk, the physical therapist may be the primary evaluator. If the child is not yet talking and has a feeding disorder, the speech-language pathologist and occupational therapist may lead the assessment. The other team members observe and prompt the primary evaluator(s) to complete various tasks with the child that they need to observe.

In the arena assessment, the parent will answer developmental and history questions with all team members present. This decreases the repetitious nature of multiple individual assessments. Often, one or more team members can talk with the family quietly during the assessment and secure their opinion of their child's performance *during the assessment*, when adjustments and adaptations can readily be made to enhance the child's performance. One of the team members can quietly suggest to the primary evaluator(s) that they try some alternative activity or input to facilitate the child's participation or interaction that the parent has suggested. Parents are often frustrated when they know that their child could perform a task if the evaluator merely stated a direction differently or allowed the child to use the assessment material in a different manner. Remember, unless we are administering a standardized instrument, our goal is to see if there is any way a child can complete a task by accessing his or her *strengths*, rather than simply noting the weaknesses and what cannot be done. This approach to assessment allows the parent to have a more active role and reinforces to the family how much we value their input. When the primary instrument has been completed, various members of the team may need to complete more specific examinations with the child while the rest of the team observes or interacts with the family. The physical therapist might need to examine body structures and functions that might impair the young child's performance of activities.

Materials and activities should be familiar to the child and be appropriate for his or her age and cultural background. As noted above, the team should make the assessment as functional and activity based as possible. Remember, we want the assessment to be as reflective of the child's actual functional abilities as possible and to be as enjoyable as possible for the child and family.

Assessment Report

When the *written report* is developed, each team member contributes within his or her area of expertise, and *a single, well-integrated report and recommendations* are developed from the assessment. This is easily done if an arena assessment was performed. *Early intervention assessment reports*, as in all EI reports, must use *family-friendly language.* The assessment report should be easily understandable to the child's parents or caregiver. Families vary in their education, cognitive levels, cultural background, and reading skills. If a technical term or professional jargon is necessary in a report, a simple explanation should accompany that term immediately after it is used. For example, if the physical therapy notes that a child appears to be "hypertonic," the therapist might report this as follows: "Muscle tone examination revealed hypertonicity in the legs. This means that Billy's legs are stiff and difficult to bend." The report must be understandable to family members regardless of their educational or language background.

Intervention

Individualized Family Service Plan

The IFSP includes the outcomes decided on by the family and team, and it guides the child's intervention program. These outcomes are written in the family's words. The team then develops strategies that are aimed at accomplishing the outcomes the family desires for their child. These outcomes are similar to intervention goals but they are recorded in the family's words. For example, an outcome may read: "Bob and Nancy want Billy to walk." The therapist then works with the family toward designing programming to fulfill this outcome. The child might need to begin working toward the outcome of "walking" at a much earlier developmental level. The therapist does not try to dash the family's dream of their child walking, even if he or she is not ready for this stage. The IFSP is developed around the family's outcome statements and is being written before the child is even 3 years of age. Remember that few of us can predict what any particular child may achieve at so early an age. On the other hand, we must be honest with families

about the child's current developmental levels. We may discuss with the family the stages a baby passes through on the way to walking and decide with them where to begin therapy. Perhaps you will begin with the child bearing weight and rocking on all fours. Your plan for the child's treatment for the next 6 months becomes the strategies you will use for the "walking" outcome the family has selected. This plan, along with the *functional, activity-based techniques* you will use when working with the child and family, fits well under the "strategies" section of the IFSP. Just remember that the important elements of your strategies must include how you will embed the intervention plan into the family's daily routines, natural environment, and activities.

Family-Centered Intervention

As in all stages of the EI program, intervention must fully include the family, be designed around the family's routines and activities, and be easily completed within the family's busy schedule. Strategies for these requirements will be discussed toward the end of this chapter. In addition, intervention is scheduled as closely as possible to the family's requests in order to not disrupt their daily routine. The therapist works with the family and PSC to find times for home visits that are optimal for the child's performance and the family's full participation.

The family is a full member of the intervention team. We do not enter a child's home, provide therapy alone with the child, make a few written suggestions, and leave. It is very important that the family or caregiver be present throughout the intervention visit and has active participation in the session. Materials, toys, and equipment used should be those found in the home, if possible, so that the family can easily follow through on the activities and strategies. Any interventions that can be taught to the family should be practiced while the therapist is present. When family members cannot be present for a session, consider videotaping the session and leaving it for the family to watch later. This allows them to actively involve themselves in the intervention and learn what activities may be helpful for their child.

Natural Environments

Intervention should be conducted in natural environments (Bruder, 2001). Natural environments are where typical children would be found and include the home, daycare setting, playground, a play group with typical peers, or even at grandma's house. Children are much more interactive and perform better in familiar environments. We have also found that including the siblings in the intervention session gives the child wonderful models. The child is often much more likely to imitate his or her brother or sister than the less-than-appealing adult therapist! By working in the child's natural environment, we increase the likelihood that the primary caregiver can be available to participate in the sessions. This is especially true when we visit the daycare setting. These caregivers are often eager to carry over a child's EI goals if they are included in the sessions and taught what they can do to contribute to the child's EI program.

Activity-Based Instruction

As already described, the concept of activity-based instruction originated in the area of special education and has been contributed to by many individuals (Bricker, Pretti-Frontczak, & McComas, 1998; Pretti-Frontczak, Barr, Macy, & Carter, 2003). In the past, educators found that children with disabilities were often being taught, and received therapy services, in rigid, nonfunctional ways. There was no intrinsic reinforcement for the child in the activity in which he or she was participating. The goals were selected from developmental profiles, without regard to a particular child's interest or functional needs.

Activity-based instruction, on the other hand, looks at what the child enjoys doing, how target skills can be embedded into interesting activities or daily routines, and a the functionality of an activity and goal. Why must a child stack blocks if there is no interest in block stacking? We should analyze the skills block stacking involves (e.g., grasping, alternating use of hands, visual perception, and coordination) and then find ways to stimulate these skills in activities that are interesting to the child. Maybe the child prefers to construct a fort with blocks or to stack cookies. Why not stimulate the same motor skills and make use of the intrinsic reinforcement that fun activities offer the child? Children who have been mistakenly labeled "uncooperative" may merely be telling us that they do not like the activity we have selected for them. Remember, EI is largely child directed, not adult directed. It requires creativity and perseverance at times to fit the goals into the child's daily activities or favorite games, but it can be done, and the payoff is a happily engaged child and a positive caregiver or parent.

Activity-based instruction also means that we fit our therapeutic strategies into the child's and family's daily routine. It certainly makes more sense to schedule a session on sensory or tactile input during bath time than to come at some other time of day that will disrupt the busy schedule of the family. This also allows the parent or caregiver to be fully involved with the session, because they would be bathing the child at the time anyway. Helpful strategies for implementing activity-based instruction will be discussed toward the end of the chapter.

Teaming in Intervention

You are already familiar with the variety of team models available in EI. The most commonly used models are the interdisciplinary model and the transdisciplinary model. As discussed before in the **interdisciplinary model,** the intervention team and the family may talk regularly and meet periodically in IFSP meetings (at least every 6 months) to develop outcomes together. The actual implementation of those outcomes and the strategies that support them, however, are typically completed separately, with each team member visiting the family and child on an individual basis. Hopefully, the team members talk or correspond on a regular basis, sharing their strategies and concerns. Often, written copies of each therapist's programs and suggestions are circulated among the team. The parents or caregivers are present, if possible, at all therapy sessions and are given demonstrations and written suggestions for home carryover of therapeutic goals. Intervention in any team model should incorporate the principles of activity-based, functional instructions and curriculum, and occur in the child's and family's natural environment.

The preferred mode of EI team intervention is that of the interdisciplinary or transdisciplinary team (Mellin & Winton, 2003). As already noted, the **transdisciplinary** team has extensive interaction among the intervention team members and with the family. In this model there is constant communication among team members, and often this is face to face. Team members and the family work together to consolidate programming so that each session, regardless of what discipline is involved, reinforces all outcomes and strategies that have been developed for a child's intervention program. Another version of this approach is termed "coaching," which utilizes conversation and self-observation to support families and other team members in gaining skills to facilitate the child's development in natural situations and then to self-evaluate the result (Rush, Sheldon, & Hanft, 2003). The IFSP may have only three or four outcomes depending on what the parents have prioritized as their main concerns. If the parents have said, perhaps, that they want their child to sit up, eat from a spoon and drink from a cup, and talk, those are the three desired outcomes **all** the therapists work toward. The physical therapist should have very specific strategies to facilitate the child's ability to sit. The physical therapist must provide the other team members with training and demonstrations to allow them to reinforce the sitting outcome, and to be able to have the child sit with stability when working on feeding skills. At the same time, the physical therapist has much to offer the speech-language pathologist in terms of working with the child's respiration to facilitate oral/vocal output that leads to oral speech. And in the middle of all this is the family, who will be with the child all week when no professional is present. The family will want to encourage the child's progress as much as, or more than, any of the therapists.

How does one fulfill all these responsibilities in, perhaps, only an hour per week? Are we not just there to see that the child learns to sit and later walk if possible? How can we also be responsible for reinforcing the goals of other professionals? How can we "allow" others (family and colleagues) to carry out activities with the child for which the physical therapist has trained for years?

There are three very important elements of the transdisciplinary intervention approach that help answer these weighty questions: *integrated programming, cotreatment,* and *role release.*

Integrated programming specifically involves the development of strategies for the parent-selected outcomes that are developed *as a team.* When the team develops the strategies for "talking," the speech-language pathologist and family will, of course, take the lead. However, the speech-language pathologist will ask the physical therapist to include specific strategies that the full team can be taught, which will improve the child's respiration so that vocalization is more likely. If the child is not yet an oral speaker, the speech-language pathologist will develop an augmentative communication system. This could include the use of manual signs, a simple picture board, or an electronic device. In this situation, the speech-language pathologist teaches the other team members to use this system of communication and it becomes as much the responsibility of the physical therapist, occupational therapist, and special educator to utilize this system when communicating with the child, as it is for the speech-language pathologist and family. The strategies section of the IFSP is then developed as a *unit* by the team and family, with all disciplines offering input to *each outcome,* not only the one or two that

seem to fall solely within one's own discipline. An individual therapist might then develop a plan of care to meet those outcomes addressing activities and participation and might also include interventions for impairments in body structures and functions that impede achievement of the activity outcomes.

Cotreatment is a situation in which two or more of the professionals are involved in the child's intervention in a single session. There are situations in which this is a necessity. If a child has severe cerebral palsy and has great difficulty sitting or moving, or even achieving a stable position for oral feeding, it may be almost impossible for a speech-language pathologist to set up a feeding program with the family without the hands-on input and *demonstration and instruction* from the physical therapist, with both the speech-language pathologist and family present and actively involved. Likewise, the physical therapist may be at a loss in communicating with a child with a severe communication disorder. This may occur if a child is nonverbal, has a severe physical handicap, or perhaps has been diagnosed with autism. In this situation, the physical therapist will want the speech-language pathologist to be present to *demonstrate and instruct* during a physical therapy session in order to help the physical therapist learn to interact with the child. If communication is poor, the physical therapist may mistake a child's frustration at not understanding or being understood as a behavioral problem. When such a problem is left unchecked, therapy sessions may become unfruitful. Parents become frustrated with the therapist as well, thinking that the child "does not like the physical therapy sessions," when, in fact, there is only a communication problem. Cotreatment in which the speech-language pathologist helps analyze the problem and offers training and demonstration for improved means of communication, may markedly improve the sessions.

Cotreatment does not have to be on a weekly basis. In fact, some payors mistakenly think that a cotreatment session is not a full session of treatment by each of the professionals present. We know that this is not true. In the cotreatment session, both therapists are actively involved at all times, and the sessions may well be much more productive than a 1-hour, individual session by individual therapists. Nevertheless, the reality is that some payors do not support this mode of intervention, and in truth, it may be difficult to schedule with the family's and therapists' busy schedules. Intermittent, regularly scheduled cotreatment sessions, or cotreatment sessions on an "as-needed" basis, are still highly beneficial to the child, family, and therapists and are usually possible in most situations.

The last strategy, that of **role release,** grows directly out of our cotreatment sessions and integrated planning strategies. In role release, the primary therapist for a specific outcome, say the physical therapist for our independent sitting outcome, decides what are the most important strategies that must be completed with the child on a regular basis in order to learn the task of sitting. Such strategies or therapeutic techniques might include encouraging head control, sitting with support, and then reducing the degree of support and reduction of the limitations of body structure and function, such as increasing range of motion (ROM) and trunk strength. Although the physical therapist will be highly adept at these strategies, we have already said that intervention occurring once a week for 1 hour will not accomplish much progress with the child's development unless some strategies or techniques can be repeated regularly throughout the week. Many of these strategies can be safely demonstrated, practiced, and then carried out by the family and other interventionists. Videotaped demonstrations, photographs, written instructions, hands-on instructions, and regular monitoring by the physical therapist will allow the child to benefit from "intervention" all week long. The "coaching" model would also fit nicely into this paradigm. All professionals will have certain strategies that they can safely share with their colleagues and the child's family. They will also, of course, have strategies that only they are trained or licensed to complete. These are obviously not part of role release. However, unless we make an effort to share some of our expertise, when feasible and safe, with the team, the child will not get the consistent input needed to make rapid and consistent progress. Some therapists like to keep a written log of the strategies they have taught to the family and to the other therapists, and then periodically monitor the use of these strategies.

All of the strategies we have discussed are considered "best practice" in the area of EI. How can therapists implement these excellent ideas when they are bound by a heavy caseload and busy schedule? In addition, how can we ask parents to add more responsibilities to their already full days? The next section of this chapter will try to answer some of these concerns.

Strategies to Encourage Intervention: Cataloging and Matrix Development

Families who have children with disabilities are especially busy and may have difficulty fitting in everything we wish they would do with their child each day. We may make

suggestions about home carryover of the therapy activities that we share with families, but they may not have the time, person power, or energy to follow all our suggestions. When this occurs, many parents or caregivers begin to feel guilty. If we are not sensitive to the many stressors and demands each family has, we may inadvertently contribute to their feelings of "not doing enough" for their child with a disability.

There are some excellent strategies we can use when making suggestions to families for carryover or home implementation of therapy goals and techniques. Let's discuss two of the most effective of these strategies.

Suppose you are working with a family that has three children. They have a set of 3-year-old twins and an 8-month-old infant who has just been diagnosed with cerebral palsy (CP). The father works for a trucking firm and drives several days at a time. This leaves his wife to care for their three children alone, several days per week. There are no grandparents or close relatives nearby. You are the physical therapist seeing the baby who has CP. The baby has poor head control, is not sitting yet, and has difficulty grasping her toys. She "stiffens" when her diaper is changed or when placed on her tummy. You believe that she needs a variety of developmental activities completed throughout the day, and you suggest these to the mother. The mother calmly but clearly tells you that there is no way she can possibly add anything else to her busy schedule. She is distressed that she cannot complete all the activities the therapists are recommending for her child.

What will you do? Two excellent strategies have been developed in the disciplines of special education and early childhood special education that are well suited for this situation. They are called **cataloging** and **matrix development** (Browder & Martin, 1986; Wilcox & Belamy, 1987) and have been used in the areas of education and EI for some time. The following paragraphs illustrate how they can be applied to this situation.

Cataloging

Cataloging involves making a simple log of all of the baby's daily activities from morning to night. The therapist, team, or even the PSC meets with the parents at a convenient time and asks them to outline the baby's day. Activities usually include a sequence such as getting up, changing diapers, eating breakfast (or nursing), taking a bath, and swinging in the baby seat while mother gets the other children up, fed, and dressed. The baby may then ride in the car while her siblings are taken to preschool, go with mom to the grocery, then pick up the siblings, come home, eat, and take a nap. All this is probably done before noon! You can see right away how useful cataloging is for the therapist. We often have no idea what a family deals with daily. Some training programs have their students spend one or more days with "mentor families" who have children with disabilities, just to learn what families experience daily.

When the catalog is completed, we assure the family that we do not want to add any more stress to their daily lives. Rather, we want to see if our therapeutic activities can be embedded into the family's existing schedule. For example, the baby may have her diaper changed up to eight times per day. That is an activity that occurs regularly and cannot be omitted. Why couldn't we just show the parents how they can perform some gentle trunk rotation activities each time the baby's diaper is changed? Mom will place the baby on the changing table, and before taking off the diaper and raising the baby's legs to clean her and place the new diaper on, she bends the hips and knees, gently rocking the legs and trunk from side to side. Remember, we said that the baby stiffens every time her diaper is changed, and this makes diapering unpleasant for her and Mom. By embedding some rotation and muscle tone reduction activities into the diapering routine, we help make diapering more enjoyable for everyone. Later we might add leg abduction activities to also increase ROM. Most of our objectives can be accomplished by embedding them into the baby's daily routine.

Table 10.1 Form for Entering the Activity Catalog on a Matrix

Catalog Information	Communication Outcomes	Physical Outcomes	Cognitive Outcomes	Adaptive Outcomes	Social/Emotional Outcomes
Wake up 7 AM					
Diaper change					
Nurse/eat					
Bath					
Dress					
8 AM Twins get up, eat, dress					
9 AM Take twins to preschool					
Go to grocery					
Run errands					
11:30 AM pick up twins					
Change diaper					
Mom fixes lunch					
Eat					
Change diaper					
1 PM Take nap					

Table 10.2 Completed Matrix With Several Embedded Strategies

Information	Communication Outcomes	Physical Outcomes	Cognitive Outcomes	Adaptive Outcomes	Social/Emotional Outcomes
Wake up 7 AM	Call baby's name				
Diaper change		Do rotation and sensory activity			
Nurse/eat				Assist with lip closure	
Bath		Sensory input			
Dress			Show each item of clothes and name it		
8 AM Twins get up, eat, dress					Twins talk to baby, baby responds with smile
9 AM Take twins to preschool	Sing in the car				
Go to grocery			Have baby look at each item as it goes into the cart		
Run errands					
11:30 AM pick up twins	Twins call baby's name as they get in the car, baby looks				
Change diaper		Rotation and sensory input			
Mom fixes lunch					
Eat				Lip closure	
Change diaper		Rotation and sensory input			
1 PM Take nap		Position for sleeping			

Matrix Development

Once the catalog of the baby's day is completed and we have shown the parents how they can embed specific activities into their daily routine, we place the baby's catalog entries on the first column of a "matrix" (Table 10.1). The matrix is a chart that lists the baby's daily activities down the first column, and lists the main outcome areas or specific outcomes across the top row. In the boxes by each of the baby's main activities, we embed a therapeutic activity that is easily completed within the daily routine. In the transdisciplinary model, all the therapists contribute to one matrix, so as not to overload the family. If the baby has feeding goals, they can be easily inserted into snack times or mealtimes. Occupational therapy sensory programs can fit nicely into bath time. The speech-language pathologist might suggest that the parents call the baby's name each time they intend to pick her up to help her learn to recognize and respond to voice and then words. Do not overload the family. Begin with only one outcome for each therapy at first. When the family becomes familiar with the matrix concept and the activities, they will decide for themselves what to do throughout the day. A completed matrix is presented in Table 10.2. Using the strategies of cataloging and matrix development assists the early interventionist in making maximum use of the child's natural environments, and will utilize activity-based instruction within the family's daily routines.

Occasionally the team will determine that the child requires more intervention than can be provided by the EI team. The intensity and frequency of services generally vary across, and even within, states. This variability is often not based on the child's needs but on the resources available in each individual state. The therapist must discuss with the entire team the extent of required additional services. In some states, the team can request and receive permission to provide additional services. If these needed services are not available through the EI system, the therapist has the ethical obligation to work with the team to seek appropriate services in the community. Children who might require more extensive physical therapy services than the EI system can provide include those with complex medical needs, those who are at critical transition periods, and those whose parents or care providers are clearly unable to carry out any of the recommended activities. Children should not be punished because of the limitations of the EI system or their caregivers, and efforts should be made to obtain necessary services.

What Do Other Disciplines Expect of the Physical Therapist in the Team Setting?

If you are lucky enough to have the opportunity to work in a strong interdisciplinary or transdisciplinary setting, your colleagues in occupational therapy, speech-language pathology, special education, and so on, will expect to be able to ask you for consultation, inservicing, demonstrations, cotreatment, team assessment, and planning. They will also expect that you will come to them for the same type of input. Each member of the team is responsible for these

activities within their area of expertise. Only in this way can a strong team be built. Some of the most common areas of consultation and demonstration that the physical therapist offers to colleagues in EI include positioning and seating for daily activities, feeding, play, and transportation; providing information on age-appropriate movement activities; assisting in improving respiratory development, which will facilitate louder and easier speech sounds and babbling; helping to determine which body part should be used to activate an augmentative communication device or adapted toy play; and identifying proper body mechanics.

The physical therapist will also be expected to carry over and reinforce the therapeutic strategies of other disciplines. The speech-language pathologist may give input regarding how to help the child learn and understand language, and how to use the child's augmentative communication system. The speech-language pathologist may also ask the physical therapist to model certain vocalizations when the baby is in movement activities that often elicit vocalizations. The special educator will have suggestions about what toys are best for play during therapy or what directions the baby needs to learn to follow. The behavioral specialist may ask that all members of the team respond to the child's disruptive behavior in a certain manner because consistency of responses is of critical importance. The occupational therapist may provide suggestions for each team member to follow as he or she introduces activities that include sensory stimulation and functional hand use.

Clearly, the physical therapist has much to offer the EI team and will have many opportunities to learn from colleagues. Inexperienced physical therapists will learn a great deal from all members of the team; however, they should also seek an experienced physical therapist as a mentor so that they can develop skills and knowledge within their own discipline.

Summary

EI is an exciting and challenging area of practice. It provides the opportunity to work closely with numerous different professionals focused on a single goal of meeting the needs of the young child and family. The transition to service delivery in natural environments has been a challenge for some professionals, but as the benefits unfold, the obstacles have been overcome. EI can offer the physical therapist constant learning opportunities and many rewards.

DISCUSSION QUESTIONS

1. What are the benefits of observation and evaluation in the natural environment?

2. Are there any problems with intervention in the natural environment, and if so, how might they be overcome?

3. What is the role of the physical therapist in activity-based instruction?

4. In family-centered care, it is important to understand the family's daily routine. How does cataloging assist the therapist and family?

RECOMMENDED READINGS

Journals Specifically for Early Intervention

Infant-Toddler Intervention: The Transdisciplinary Journal.
Infants and Young Children: An Interdisciplinary Journal of Special Care Practices.
Journal of Early Intervention.

Texts

Bailey, D., & Wolery, M. (1999). *Teaching infants and preschoolers with disabilities* (2nd ed.). New York: Merrill.

Bricker, D., Pretti-Frontczak, K., & McComas, N. (1998). *An activity-based approach to early intervention* (2nd ed.) Baltimore: Paul H. Brookes.<AU3:

Guralnick, M. (1997). *The effectiveness of early intervention.* Baltimore: Paul H. Brookes.

Guralnick, M. (2000). *Interdisciplinary clinical assessment of young children with developmental disabilities.* Baltimore: Paul H. Brookes.

Guralnick, M. (2001). *Early childhood inclusion: Focus on change.* Baltimore: Paul H. Brookes.

Hanft, B.E., Rush, D.D., & Sheldon, M.L. (2004). *Coaching families and colleagues in early childhood.* Baltimore: Paul H. Brookes.

Linder, T. (1996). *Transdisciplinary play-based intervention: Guidelines for developing a meaningful curriculum for young children.* Baltimore: Paul H. Brookes.

McEwen, I. (Ed.) (2000). *Providing physical therapy services under Parts B & C of the Individuals with Disabilities Education Act (IDEA).* Alexandria, VA: Section on Pediatrics, American Physical Therapy Association.

McLean, M.E., Wolery, M., & Bailey, D. (2004). *Assessing infants and preschoolers with special needs* (3rd ed.) Old Tappan, NY: Merrill.

REFERENCES

Bailey, D. (1997). Evaluating the effectiveness of curriculum alternatives for infants and preschoolers at high risk. In M. Guralnick (Ed.), *The effectiveness of early intervention.* Baltimore: Paul H. Brookes.

Bricker, D., Pretti-Frontczak, K., & McComas, N. (1998). *An activity-based approach to early intervention* (2nd ed.). Baltimore: Paul H. Brookes.

Browder, D., & Martin, D.K. (1986). A new curriculum for Tommy. *Teaching Exceptional Children. 18*(4), 261–265.

Bruder, M.B. (2001). Infants and toddlers: Outcomes and ecology. In M. Guralnick (Ed.), *Early childhood inclusion: Focus on change.* Baltimore: Paul H. Brookes.

Dunst, C., Trivette, C.M., & Jodry, W. (1997). Influences of social support on children with disabilities and their families. In M. Guralnick (Ed.), *The effectiveness of early intervention.* Baltimore: Paul H. Brookes.

Guralnick, M. (2000). *Interdisciplinary clinical assessment of young children with developmental disabilities.* Baltimore: Paul H. Brookes.

IDEA Practices (2003). *IDEA regs subpart A–C.* Retrieved March 21, 2003, from *www.ideapractices.org/law/regulations/regs/SubpartA2CpartC.php*

Mellin, A.E., & Winton, P. (2003). Interdisciplinary collaboration among intervention faculty members. *Journal of Early Intervention, 25,* 173–188.

Pretti-Frontczak, K.L., Barr, D.M., Macy, M., & Carter, A. (2003). Research and resources related to activity-based intervention, embedded learning opportunities, and routines-based instruction. *Topics in Early Childhood Special Education, 23,* 29–39.

Rush, D., Sheldon, M., & Hanft, B. (2003). Coaching families and colleagues: A process for collaboration in natural settings. *Infants and Young Children, 16* (1), 33–47.

Simeonsson, R. (2000). Early childhood intervention: Toward a universal manifesto. *Infants and Young Children: An Interdisciplinary Journal of Special Care Practices, 12*(3), 4–9.

Wilcox, J., & Belamy, T. (1987). *A comprehensive guide to the activities catalog: An alternate curriculum for youth and adults with severe disabilities.* Baltimore: Paul H. Brookes.

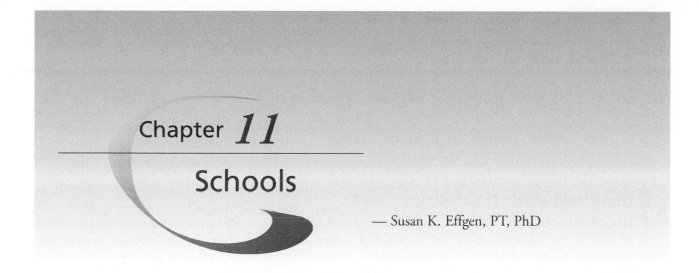

Chapter *11*

Schools

— Susan K. Effgen, PT, PhD

Physical therapists have worked in school settings from almost the beginning of the profession. These school settings require collaboration with teams of individuals, including numerous professionals, paraprofessionals, and, of course, the child's parents. School systems are major employers of pediatric physical therapists and are interesting, fun places to work. In this chapter, the unique aspects of school-based physical therapy will be discussed. Local, state, and federal laws regulate all school services and are discussed in some detail. The most significant law is the Individuals with Disabilities Education Act (IDEA). You have probably gone to school with children with disabilities because of this important United States federal law, first enacted in 1975. This law has a major impact on the education and delivery of related services for preschoolers and school-aged children with disabilities, and is the focus of this chapter.

History of Physical Therapy in Schools

Physical therapists have a long, rich history of serving children with special needs, in special schools set aside for those with physical disabilities. Those schools, many of which were residential, were started in the late 1800s and became common in the early 20th century. Most major cities had special schools for "crippled children" where physical therapists worked. In fact, in the 1930s, a master's

thesis was written on physical therapy in the Chicago city schools (Vacha, 1933). Since that time, services to children with disabilities have expanded from just serving those with physical disabilities to including children having a wide range of disabilities, including those with mental retardation and mental illness, children who were not adequately served until the mid to late 20th century. The role of physical therapists in schools continued to expand slowly, until the exponential increase in responsibility and need resulting from major federal legislation in 1975. In 1975, the United States Congress passed **PL 94–142, the Education of All Handicapped Children Act**. This landmark legislation provided that all children aged 6 to 21 years were entitled to a free appropriate public education that included "related services" such as physical therapy, occupational therapy, speech-language pathology, and transportation. Until that time, each local school system had the privilege of determining which children would receive an education. Some systems, especially in large cities, provided extensive services to many children with special needs. Other systems had requirements, such as that the child must to able to walk, independently use the bathroom, or not have mental retardation, to be eligible to receive an education. This national inequity in the availability of a public education, which forced families to move to areas that would serve their children with special needs, ended with PL 94–42.

Since 1975, the Education of All Handicapped Children Act has been amended six times. In 1986, the reauthorization included the provision of early intervention (EI) services for infants and toddlers with disabilities, as discussed in Chapter 10. In 1990, the act's name was changed to the Individuals with Disabilities Education Act, mentioned in the first paragraph. IDEA and Section 504 of the Rehabilitation Act of 1973 guide physical therapy services in school settings, and a thorough knowledge of these federal laws is critical for the provision of school-based services for children and young adults aged 3 to 21 years.

Individuals With Disabilities Education Act

IDEA 97 (*Federal Register* 34 CFR 111 §300 and §301, 7-1-02 Edition) notes, "Improving educational results for children with disabilities is an essential element of our national policy of ensuring equality of opportunity, full participation, independent living, and economic self-sufficiency for individuals with disabilities." The purpose of IDEA was "to ensure that all children with disabilities have available to them a free appropriate public education that emphasizes special education and related services designed to meet their unique needs and prepare them for employment and independent living" [*Federal Register* 34 CFR §300.1(a)]. The phrase "prepare them for employment and independent living" was new in IDEA 97 and is a critical addition for helping to meet the needs of children with more severe disabilities. It was probably added to expand the very strict interpretation of education as meaning only traditional academic areas, used by some systems. Many school systems have had a difficult time understanding the importance of a life skills curriculum in which children with significant disabilities learn to function in society even though they may never be able to read or write. Congress and advocacy groups believed that being prepared for independent living and, perhaps, employment, was for some children more important and functional than learning to read.

The original Education of All Handicapped Children Act, enacted in 1975, included seven major provisions that were very new, if not radical, regarding the education of children with special needs at that time. These included *Zero Reject, Least Restrictive Environment, Right to Due Process, Nondiscriminatory Evaluation, Parent Participation, Individualized Education Plan,* and *Related Services.* "All children" meant all children. There was to be **Zero Reject** of children in schools, even children with the most severe physical and mental disabilities were to be provided with an education. Children were also to receive their education in what was termed the **Least Restrictive Environment (LRE)**. "To the maximum extent appropriate, children with disabilities … are educated with children who are not disabled" [PL105–17, 111 Stat.61, Part B, Sec. 612, (a)(5)(A)]. Thus, the concept of mainstreaming and, later, integration, natural environments, and inclusion began to influence provision of all educational and related services as discussed later in this chapter.

Parents were now to become active partners in their child's education. They had the **Right to Due Process,** which included impartial hearings, the right to be represented by counsel, and the right to a transcript of meetings. Later legislation provided for reimbursement of legal fees to parents if they prevailed in a court case. Interpreters were to be provided as necessary at meetings. **Parent Participation** was now welcomed, and parents were to be major decision makers in determining their child's educational program.

Nondiscriminatory evaluation was required, and every child receiving special education was to have an **Individualized Education Plan (IEP)**. The IEP is the foundation of service delivery and will be discussed in detail. The IEP team meeting might determine that the child needs **Related Services** "as required to assist a child with a disability to benefit from special education" [*Federal Register* 34 CRF Part §300.24 (A)]. Related services assist children in meeting their educational needs in a variety of ways and include physical therapy, occupational therapy, speech-language pathology, transportation, audiology, psychological services, recreation, rehabilitation counseling, orientation and mobility services, and medical services for diagnostic or evaluation purposes only.

Since the passage of PL 94–142 in 1975, many of the original provisions of the law that were once thought unusual or controversial are well-accepted, routine practice. The components of IDEA that still require some refinement, as now suggested by IDEA Practices (2003), include the *IEP, LRE, School Climate and Discipline,* and *State and District-Wide Assessment.* The management of discipline is a major issue in schools. Advocates fear that, all too often, children with behavior disorders are not being provided with appropriate services and are being expelled from school so that the local education agency (LEA) can avoid dealing with the problem. In IDEA 97, requirements were made that appropriate positive behavioral interventions and strategies be determined for each child. State and district-wide assessment is related to the push for outcomes data that are so critical in *No Child Left Behind.* How to test children with disabilities and whether to include them in state or district-wide assessment are ongoing areas of concern and debate. These two issues, although very important, are not within the province of physical therapy. The IEP and LRE are important to physical therapists and require discussion.

Individualized Education Plan

The IEP is developed after a multidisciplinary team has evaluated the child. The term *multidisciplinary* is used in educational circles to really reflect interdisciplinary services. *Multidisciplinary* is defined by IDEA as "involvement of two or more disciplines or professions in the provision of integrated and coordinated services" (*Federal Register*, 1989). As you can see, that definition of practice is more in keeping with the definition of interdisciplinary. The evaluation process varies from LEA to LEA and state to state. The multidisciplinary team might first screen the child to determine what professionals would be most appropriate to participate in the evaluation. If the child has serious reading problems but no other noticeable problem, the physical therapist would not be involved in the evaluation. On the other hand, if after the evaluation by an educator and psychologist subtle gross motor and coordination problems are noted, a physical therapist might be asked to perform a more in-depth examination of coordination, perceptual motor development, and gross motor skills to determine if these problems affect educational performance.

Examination and Evaluation

In the educational environment, "Evaluation means the procedures used...to determine whether a child has a disability and the nature and extent of the special education and related services that the child needs" [*Federal Register*, 34CRF §300.500(B)(2)]. The evaluation procedures should include tests and materials that are nondiscriminatory regarding race and culture, are administered in the child's native language, and include a range of tools and strategies to gather functional and developmental information about the child [*Federal Register*, 34CFR §300.532(a), (b)]. A child should be evaluated in all areas of suspected disability including motor abilities [*Federal Register*, 34 CRF §300.532(2)(g)]. The initial evaluation of the child will assist in determining eligibility for special education and then whether the child requires related services. The evaluation should also assist in the program planning. Note that in Part C of IDEA, the term *evaluation* is used to

determine eligibility and the term *assessment* is used for program planning and ongoing procedures to determine the child's strengths and needs. Physical therapists working in school settings need to use the terminology dictated in that setting.

Based on the evaluation, the child's eligibility for special education and related services is determined by the multidisciplinary team. The child must fit into one of the diagnostic categories for special education listed in Box 11.1. If the child qualifies for special education, within 30 calendar days, the IEP team, sometimes called the Admissions and Release Committee (ARC), must meet to develop a written IEP. Only after it is decided that the child qualifies for special education, is the extent of need for various related services that will assist the child to benefit from special education determined by the team.

The purpose of therapy in a school setting is to meet the educational needs of the child. To determine how to best meet those needs, a comprehensive physical therapy examination is required to determine the most appropriate

---

BOX 11.1 IDEA 97 Definitions of Child With a Disability

Autism: "A developmental disability significantly affecting verbal and nonverbal communication and social interaction, generally evident before age 3, that adversely affects a child's educational performance. Other characteristics often associated with autism are engagement in repetitive activities and stereotyped movements, resistance to environmental change, change in daily routines, and unusual responses to sensory experiences. The term does not apply if a child's educational performance is adversely affected primarily because the child has an emotional disturbance."

Deaf-blindness: "Concomitant hearing and visual impairments, the combination of which causes such severe communication and other developmental and educational needs that they cannot be accommodated in special education programs solely for children with deafness or children with blindness."

Deafness: "A hearing impairment that is so severe that the child is impaired in processing linguistic information through hearing, with or without amplification, that adversely affects a child's educational performance." *(Continued)*

BOX 11.1 IDEA 97 Definitions of Child With a Disability *(Continued)*

Developmental delay: "The term *child with a disability* for children aged 3 through 9 may, at the discretion of the State and LEA … include a child who is experiencing developmental delays, as defined by the State and as measured by appropriate diagnostic instruments and procedures, in one or more of the following areas: physical development, cognitive development, communication development, social or emotional development, or adaptive development, and who, by reason there of, needs special education and related services."

Emotional disturbance: "A condition exhibiting one or more of the following characteristics over a long period of time and to a marked degree that adversely affects a child's educational performance: (A) An inability to learn that cannot be explained by intellectual, sensory, or health factors. (B) An inability to build or maintain satisfactory interpersonal relationships with peers and teachers. (C) Inappropriate types of behavior or feelings under normal circumstances. (D) A general pervasive mood of unhappiness or depression. (E) A tendency to develop physical symptoms or fears associated with personal or school problems. The term includes schizophrenia, but does not apply to children who are socially maladjusted, unless it is determined that they have an emotional disturbance."

Hearing impairment: "An impairment in hearing, whether permanent or fluctuating, that adversely affects a child's educational performance but that is not included under the definition of deafness."

Mental retardation: "Significantly subaverage general intellectual functioning existing concurrently with deficits in adaptive behavior and manifested during the developmental period that adversely affects a child's educational performance."

Multiple disabilities: "Concomitant impairments (e.g., mental retardation-blindness, mental retardation-orthopedic impairment) the combination of which causes such severe educational needs that they cannot be accommodated in special education programs solely for one of the impairments. The term does not include deaf-blindness."

Orthopedic impairment: "A severe orthopedic impairment that adversely affects a child's educational performance. The term includes impairments caused by congenital anomaly (e.g., clubfoot, absence of some member), impairments caused by disease (e.g., poliomyelitis, bone tuber-culosis, etc.), and impairments from other causes (e.g., cerebral palsy, amputations, and fractures or burns that cause contractures)."

Other health impairment: "Having limited strength, vitality, or alertness, including a heightened alertness to environmental stimuli, that results in limited alertness with respect to the educational environment, that is due to chronic or acute health problems such as asthma, attention deficit disorder or attention deficit hyperactivity disorder, diabetes, epilepsy, a heart condition, hemophilia, lead poisoning, leukemia, nephritis, rheumatic fever, and sickle cell anemia; and adversely affects a child's educational performance."

Specific learning disability: "A disorder in one or more of the basic psychologic processes involved in understanding or in using language, spoken or written, that may manifest as an imperfect ability to listen, think, speak, read, write, spell, or do mathematical calculations, including such conditions as perceptual disabilities, brain injury, minimal brain dysfunction, dyslexia, and developmental aphasia. The term does not include learning problems that are primarily the result of visual, hearing, or motor disabilities, of mental retardation, of emotional disturbance, or of environmental, cultural, or economic disadvantage."

Speech and language impairment: "A communication disorder such as stuttering, impaired articulation, a language impairment, or a voice impairment that adversely affects a child's educational performance."

Traumatic brain injury: "An acquired injury to the brain caused by an external physical force, resulting in total or partial functional disability or psychosocial impairment, or both, that adversely affects a child's educational performance. The term applies to open or closed head injuries resulting in impairments in one or more areas, such as cognition; language; memory; attention; reasoning; abstract thinking; judgment; problem-solving; sensory, perceptual, and motor abilities; psychosocial behavior; physical functions; information processing; and speech. The term does not apply to brain injuries that are congenital or degenerative or brain injuries induced by birth trauma."

Visual impairment including blindness: "An impairment in vision including blindness means an impairment in vision that, even with correction, adversely affects a child's educational performance. The term includes both partial sight and blindness."

Source [*Federal Register* 34 CFR §300.7(b), (c)]

recommendations for the intervention plan. All of the areas of physical therapy examination discussed throughout this text must be considered for each individual child, although an examination and evaluation of each system might not be indicated. As outlined in Chapter 1, Table 1.3, the *Pediatric Physical Therapy Evaluation and Plan of Care* might be followed. What is included in any specific examination will depend on the child's age, diagnosis, and level of cognitive functioning, as well as the specific purpose of the examination and evaluation. Screening or eligibility evaluations are different from the initial examination for services.

Frequently, the therapist will want to administer a standardized test of motor performance to document present level of performance. Unlike the tests in EI, this evaluation of physical performance is not required to determine eligibility. Commonly used tests include the Peabody Developmental Motor Scales (Folio & Fewell, 2000) for younger children and older children with significant motor skill restrictions; and the Bruininks Oseretsky Test of Motor Proficiency (Bruininks, 1978) for children who are ambulatory but have some movement limitations or restrictions in activities. For children with cerebral palsy (CP), the Gross Motor Function Measure is a very useful tool. In addition to standardized tests of motor performance, tests of functional ability are frequently indicated; these include the Pediatric Evaluation of Disability Inventory (PEDI) (Haley, Coster, Ludlow, Haltiwanger, & Andrellos, 1992) and the School Function Assessment (SFA) (Coster, Deeney, Haltiwanger, & Haley, 1998). The SFA is used to determine the student's current level of participation in the school setting, performance of functional activities, and the supports needed to perform those functional tasks at school. The SFA is a judgment-based questionnaire, which is completed by one or more school professionals who have observed the student performing typical school tasks. The items are written in measurable, behavioral terms that can easily be used in the later writing of the child's IEP. This assessment helps to highlight problems the child might be having in performing common functional tasks at school that are frequently overlooked in measurements of standard motor performance. The sections of the SFA, outlined in Table 11.1, indicate its suitability for assessing common school tasks. This assessment is especially helpful to therapists who are new to educational settings because it highlights the areas of importance to school functioning and assists the therapist in planning appropriate school-based programs. The School Outcomes Measure is a more minimal data set to measure groups of students' performance in school-based therapy that is

now under development (McEwen, Arnold, Hansen, & Johnson, 2003).

Classroom observation should be part of the assessment of all children being considered for services. This naturalis-

Table 11.1 Sections of the School Function Assessment

Part I Participation
Playground/Recess
Transportation
Bathroom/Toileting
Transitions
Mealtime/Snack Time
Part II Task Supports: Physical Tasks
Travel
Maintaining and Changing Positions
Recreational Movement
Manipulation With Movement
Using Materials
Set-up and Clean-up
Eating and Drinking
Hygiene
Clothing Management
Part II Task Supports: Behavioral Tasks
Functional Communication
Memory and Understanding
Following Social Conventions
Compliance With Adult Directives and School Rules
Task Behavior/Completion
Positive Interaction
Behavior Regulation
Personal Care Awareness
Safety

(Continued)

Table 11.1 Sections of the School Function Assessment *(Continued)*

Part III Activity Performance: Physical Tasks
Travel
Maintaining and Changing Positions
Recreational Movement
Manipulation With Movement
Using Materials
Set-up and Clean-up
Eating and Drinking
Hygiene
Clothing Management
Up/Down Stairs
Written Work
Computer and Equipment Use

Part III Activity Performance: Cognitive/ Behavioral Tasks
Functional Communication
Memory and Understanding
Following Social Conventions
Compliance With Adult Directives and School Rules
Task Behavior/Completion
Positive Interaction
Behavior Regulation
Personal Care Awareness
Safety

Adaptations Checklist: Adaptations Routinely Used
Activities of Daily Living
Architectural
Behavioral
Classroom Work
Cognitive

Communication
Computer
Seating/Mobility/Transportation
Other Adaptations

Source: Coster, W., Deeney, T., Haltiwanger, J., & Haley, S. (1998). *School Function Assessment Materials*. San Antonio, TX: The Psychological Corporation.

tic observation is critical to understanding the child's true abilities in a natural setting. Although a physical therapist is not required by law to conduct a classroom observation, this observation can be critical in determining the limitations in the child's activities and also assist in clarifying any questions the therapist might have regarding the scoring of the SFA by other school personnel. For example, knowing the type of stairs in the school, how many children are generally in the hallway, and how far away the school buses park is important in determining realistic goals for stair climbing and getting through the school to the bus.

The examination of a preschooler might take place in the classroom, whereas the examination of a school-aged child might be better in a private setting where other children cannot observe. The examination might also be done as an arena assessment with other professionals, as discussed in Chapters 1 and 10. An arena assessment decreases the amount of handling of the child and allows the professionals to problem-solve together and easily share information.

The actual write-up of the evaluation might be done as suggested in Table 1.3 or will follow the conventions of the LEA. The report is written in **lay language** so that the family and other team members can understand the report. Any "medical terms" that the therapist believes must be used should be explained carefully. Using lay language is no excuse for an incomplete report. Proper documentation of the child's status is critical in determining change in status over time and the outcomes of intervention. The school-based evaluation report does *not* include specific goals and objectives for the child. Goals and objectives are determined with the entire IEP team at the IEP meeting.

IEP Meeting

Once all the necessary examinations and evaluations are performed and the child's eligibility for special education is determined, the IEP team meets. The team includes the parents; a regular education teacher; a representative from the public agency who is knowledgeable and qualified to provide specially designed instruction; an individual who can interpret the instructional implications of the evaluation results; at the discretion of the parent or agency, other knowledgeable individuals, including related service personnel; and, if appropriate, the child [*Federal Register*, 34 CRF §300.344(a)]. This is a very important meeting in planning the child's program, and physical therapists should participate to the fullest extent possible. Some LEAs welcome and expect therapist participation, whereas others consider the participation of therapists to be expensive and attempt to restrict participation to a limited number of people. If the child requires physical therapy to succeed in school, the therapist must be there to advocate for the child and to educate the team as to how the therapist might assist the child and teachers in helping the child achieve his or her individual educational goals. Our role as consultant is critical during the IEP process, and if we are not there, we cannot assist.

The content of the IEP is dictated by IDEA. The IEP must include the following (excerpt, *Federal Register*, 34 CFR §300.347):

(1) A statement of the child's present levels of educational performance, including:
   (i) How the child's disability affects the child's involvement and progress in the general curriculum. …
   (ii) For preschool children, as appropriate, how the disability affects the child's participation in appropriate activities.

(2) A statement of measurable annual goals, including benchmarks or short-term objectives, related to:
   (i) Meeting the child's needs that result from the child's disability to enable the child to be involved in and progress in the general curriculum…or for preschool children, as appropriate, to participate in appropriate activities; and
   (ii) Meeting each of the child's other educational needs that result from the child's disability;

(3) A statement of the special education and related services and supplementary aids and services to be provided to the child, or on behalf of the child, and a statement of the program modification or supports for school personnel that will be provided for the child—
   (i) To advance appropriately toward attaining the annual goals;
   (ii) To be involved and progress in the general curriculum…and to participate in extracurricular and other nonacademic activities; and
   (iii) To be educated and participate with other children with disabilities and nondisabled children in the activities described in this section;

(4) An explanation of the extent, if any, to which the child will not participate with nondisabled children in the regular class and in the activities… .

(5) (i) A statement of any individual modifications in the State or district-wide assessments… .

(6) The projected date for the beginning of services and modifications…and the anticipated frequency, location, and duration of those services and modifications; and

(7) A statement of—
   (i) How the child's progress toward the annual goals…will be measured; and
   (ii) How the child's parents will be regularly informed (through such means as periodic report cards), at least as often as parents are informed of their nondisabled children's progress, of—
      (a) Their child's progress toward the annual goals; and
      (b) The extent to which that progress is sufficient to enable the child to achieve the goals by the end of the year.

How all of the preceding information is written up varies from LEA to LEA. The physical therapist should be involved in the IEP meeting to determine the child's measurable annual goals, including benchmarks or short-term objectives for the year. These goals are *not* discipline specific, and relate to the overall educational needs of the child. They are child goals and, as appropriate, should include goals in the motor domain. Consensus among experts in pediatric occupational and physical therapy indicates that objectives should relate to functional skills and activities, should enhance the child's performance in school, should be understood easily by all individuals, should be free of professional jargon, and should be realistic and achievable within the typical IEP time frame (Dole, Arvidson, Byrne, Robbins, & Schasberger, 2003). These experts suggest that if a skill or an activity cannot be observed or measured during the child's normal school day, then it might not be relevant to the child's educational needs. They also note, although there is no consensus, that generalization of skills across settings is important.

The IEP team then decides the frequency and intensity of participation by various related service personnel and the location of services. These decisions should be based on what is best for the child and not what is convenient for the LEA or service providers. In the past, all too often, children were sent to a special school away from the local school they would have otherwise attended because therapy services were offered only at that special school. That is unfortunate because the location of services should be based on what is best for the individual child. Some children might be best served in a somewhat restrictive environment for certain aspects of their education, whereas other children can function in the general education environment with supports provided from special education and related service personnel. The decision about location of services is a critical component of the IEP meeting. We should always strive for services in the least restrictive and least intrusive environment; however, we must also be aware that "it is important to consider the student's privacy, dignity, and the perceptions of peers when selecting both where services will be provided and what strategies will be used" (Giangreco, 1995, p. 62). Some interventions are best provided in a private area, although there should be frequent re-evaluation to determine the continued need for an isolated environment.

While the IEP meeting is progressing, the decisions are written down and the team and parents agree in writing to the recommendations. If the parents do not agree, they have the right to appeal the decisions and to have a due process hearing. The rights of the parents and child are well defined in IDEA. Related services have been the focal point of many disputes between parents and school districts. These disputes usually involve (1) adequacy of physical therapy services, (2) qualifications of the service providers, (3) the need for physical therapy during the extended school year (summer), and (4) compensatory physical therapy (Rapport & Jones, 2000).

During the due process procedures, the child will continue his or her current educational services and placement, unless everyone agrees otherwise. This is termed "stay put." For a child new to the special education system, this might mean no services. On the other hand, for a child already in the system where fewer services are perhaps being recommended or a change of environment that the parent does not desire, the ability to "stay put" while the plan is appealed might be attractive to the child and family.

Once the IEP is accepted, the services should be provided as stated. This is a time when physical therapy, if indicated, is most important. The therapist needs to consult with the child's teachers regarding their needs, check for accommodations the child might need to fully participate in the classroom, have equipment needs determined, ordered or constructed, and, if indicated, instruct all personnel working with the child in proper positioning and lifting techniques. In addition, safe positioning while traveling on the school bus and management of architectural barriers need to be addressed, as does a safe evacuation from the building if there is a fire or other emergency.

Intervention

As already noted, school-based intervention must focus on the educational needs of the child as determined by the IEP team. Some LEAs are very liberal in that they consider educational benefit and openly accept that the purpose of an education is to prepare individuals for "employment and independent living." Other systems take a very strict view of educational relevance and attempt to limit education to traditional academic skills and severely restrict intervention focused on life skills and achieving independent living. A child might be eligible for physical therapy in one LEA and not be eligible in another LEA just several miles away. There is even greater variation in service provision from state to state.

Some children might clearly require physical therapy intervention but might not be eligible for that intervention because it is not needed for them to benefit from education. In those situations, the therapist must explain to the parents why physical therapy is not indicated in the school setting and perhaps assist the parents in obtaining physical therapy services through another setting. We have a professional obligation to inform the parents of the need for physical therapy; however, we do not have an obligation to provide that therapy through the school system if it is not required for the child to benefit from education. An example of this situation is a child with mild CP who is fully ambulatory and functions well with classroom supports. Physical therapy intervention might help the child achieve a more efficient, attractive gait pattern. Some might say that a more efficient gait pattern will assist the child in navigating the school environment and therefore might improve his or her educational performance and employment outlook. Physical therapy might be provided in that LEA; however, the therapist must be careful about providing therapy that is not clearly educationally relevant and not absolutely required by the child. Remember that time used for physical therapy means time away from other academic tasks. This can be a critical loss of academic time, especially for that child with mild CP, who might be preparing for college and for whom time out of physics class can be very detrimental to educational performance. On the other hand, for a preschooler, increased intervention now might be very appropriate to perhaps lessen the amount of intervention required later. Unfortunately, there is a lack of research on the most sensitive and effective times and ages for intervention, although there is agreement that in general, the earlier the intervention, the better (Harris, 1997).

Coordination, Communication, and Documentation

The *Guide for physical therapist practice* (APTA, 2001) indicates that major areas of intervention are coordination, communication, and documentation. These are very critical areas for school-based practice. As part of a team, the physical therapist must coordinate intervention with the other professionals in the school system and professionals serving the child in the community. Many children also receive therapy outside of the school setting, and the therapists must work together and coordinate their intervention efforts. This, of course, includes communication, both verbal and written.

The LEA, in response to state and federal rules and regulations, generally determines the format of the documentation in school-based settings; however, the therapist must still comply with the state physical therapy practice acts, which might have more extensive requirements for documentation than required by the LEA. The documentation template suggested in the *Guide* (APTA, 2001) has limited applicability in pediatric practice. Use of more traditional methods of pediatric physical therapy documentation has now been reinstated in many LEAs because of the increasing trend of seeking reimbursement from Medicaid or through the family's health insurance in school settings. As therapists work on the goals and objectives written in the child's IEP, they must break down those generic educational goals and objectives into the specific components that the therapist will address. For example, the goal for the child in school might be to independently select and get his or her lunch in the cafeteria. One of many related physical therapy goals might be that the child be able to carry the lunch tray from the food service line to a table without dropping it. To achieve this goal, the therapist might have specific objectives related to improving the child's balance while walking, increasing upper extremity strength to hold a full tray, and improving coordination. These goals and objectives are not part of the IEP; however, they are clearly related to the IEP goal and might be necessary as documentation of physical therapy intervention for reimbursement.

Child-Related Instruction

A priority area of intervention in school settings is child, family, and team **instruction**. Some therapists might rarely actually touch a child, yet they are providing appropriate intervention if they are serving the child through instruction and consultation in the school setting. A consultative service delivery model (see Chapter 1) might be the most appropriate model, whereas other children might require consultation plus direct service and a collaborative model.

The potential areas of child-related instructions are extensive. For example, not only must the child be instructed in how to use a power wheelchair, but so must the parents, teachers, teachers' aides, bus drivers, and so on. In addition to the instruction related to the child, there is school-wide instruction and consultation that is necessary for successful operation of the power wheelchair in this example. Perhaps new ramps must be installed to meet the size and weight requirements of a power wheelchair; perhaps there is a need to modify the bathroom and rearrange the classroom sitting arrangement to accommodate the radius required to maneuver the wheelchair.

Instruction is a team effort. The physical therapist not only provides instruction but also receives instruction from the other disciplines serving the child. In one setting, the physical therapist might provide expert education in power wheelchairs, but in another setting, it might be the occupational therapist who provides the instruction to the team. In school settings there is rarely a strict line of professional demarcation, and therapists must be prepared for role release as required under a transdisciplinary model of service delivery (Rainforth, 1997).

Procedural Interventions

As noted in the *Guide* (APTA, 2001), the physical therapist selects, applies, or modifies the procedural interventions that will be provided to a child in a school setting. The therapist applies therapeutic exercise that includes conditioning, self-care, and functional training for home, school, and play. These would not be referred to as "procedural interventions" in an educational setting: "strategies," or perhaps "interventions," would be more appropriate terminology.

Physical therapy interventions available to the child in special education are diverse. Each IEP team determines the extent and type of services based on the evaluation findings and the team's recommendations. The physical therapist does not independently determine the extent, type, and frequency of physical therapy services in a school setting. There is a trend away from one-to-one service delivery, yet the importance of more than just consultation cannot be overstated. The use of flexible service delivery models that may combine different frequency and intensity options are probably best suited for achieving specific goals and objectives (Hanft & Place, 1996; Swinth & Hanft, 2002; Trahan & Malouin, 2002)). The traditional model of one-to-one service for a certain number of minutes per week should be reconsidered. Perhaps, for a certain child, daily intervention for the first few weeks of school can best meet his or her needs, followed by only monitoring for the remainder of the school year. For other children, group intervention can be the most effective, or at least as effective as one-to-one intervention (Deneka, 1995). The IEP goals, objectives, and frequency of services cannot be changed without another IEP meeting; however, as long as there is no change in the objectives and overall amount of time, adjustments in scheduling of services is possible without another IEP meeting (*Federal Register*, 1992, p. 44839). This decision should be based on professional judgment.

There are school systems in the United States that are willing and able to provide all recommended physical therapy services, including aquatics and therapeutic riding for their children with special needs. On the other hand, some school systems rebel at the thought of putting in ramps for wheelchairs and see no need for the physical therapist to teach a child stair climbing. Therapists must educate administrators regarding the services a physical therapist can offer and the most appropriate degree of service delivery in their community. Mature therapists who are members of the APTA, Section on Pediatrics, do not appear to have problems with overinvolvement or influence from administration (Effgen, 2000), although many therapists, perhaps not as experienced and professionally involved, have noted that their administrations often interfere with professional decision making.

The specific interventions to be used by the physical therapist might be discussed at the IEP meeting, but they, along with educational strategies to be used, are not part of the IEP. The physical therapists' major intervention in school settings was found to be teaching/learning techniques, followed by handling/physical interventions (McDougall et al., 1999). The interventions a therapist uses will vary according to the needs of the individual child, the age of the child, placement of the child, the policies of the LEA regarding degree of intervention, parental input, team opinion, therapist experience, and numerous other factors. The service delivery model used will also vary according to the preceding factors. Initially, the therapist should consult with the classroom teachers to see what their needs are regarding the child. The therapist will frequently need to provide coordination, communication, documentation, and child-related instruction first, followed by some specific procedural interventions. For example a child might walk most safely with a walker (Figure 11–1), but the child has only crutches. The therapist might have to obtain a walker through the school system and then make certain that the child is safe with the walker by providing some intervention and establishing the parameters of safe use of the walker within the school. The therapist would then consult with and instruct classroom teachers, aides, and physical therapist assistants (PTAs) in how the child may safely walk with the walker throughout the building. In the meantime, the therapist or PTA might still be providing direct interventions on the use of crutches in the school building, meeting the IEP objective of being able to safely walk with crutches to the cafeteria when other children are in the halls.

The physical therapist, along with other team members, will decide on the assistive technology, adaptive equipment, and augmentative and alternative communication needs of the child, as discussed in Chapters 16 and 17. IDEA makes it very clear that the assistive technology needs of the child will be met to allow the child to benefit from a free and appropriate public education. How supportive an LEA is in meeting these needs varies greatly and is a reflection of the financial resources of that LEA.

Re-examination

The frequency of re-examination should be based on the individual needs of the child and the child's response to intervention. Unfortunately, additional time for a complete re-examination is rarely provided in an educational setting. IEP meetings are held at least annually (the option of triannual IEP meetings is recommended in the IDEA 2004 reauthorization), and the therapist should perform a re-examination at least that often to assist in determining the program for the following year. An official, *complete* re-examination is required only every 3 years (the triannual evaluation), although even that evaluation can be waived if considered unnecessary by the entire IEP team that includes the family. More frequent re-examination might be required by individual state physical therapy practice acts.

Discharge

The termination of physical therapy services is not a unilateral decision made by the physical therapist in an educa-

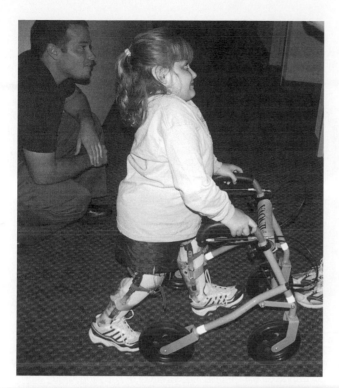

Figure 11-1 Child walking safely with walker at school.

tional setting. The team, during the IEP meeting, decides on the services that will or will not be provided for the child during the next school year. In a recent study (Effgen, 2000), the most important factor in terminating services was the child's attainment of the functional goals. This is in keeping with accepted professional practice. The severity of the child's disability also influenced continuation of services, as did the input of parents and caretakers. As already noted in this study, the mature, professionally active respondents were not unduly influenced by administration in their decisions regarding termination of service delivery.

Least Restrictive Environment

As already mentioned, the location of the child's education and all service delivery should be in schools with children who are not disabled. "Each public agency shall ensure that to the maximum extent appropriate, children with disabilities, including children in public or private institutions or other care facilities, are educated with children who are nondisabled; and that special classes, separate schooling or other removal of children with disabilities from the regular education environment occurs only if the nature or severity

of the disability is such that education in regular classes with the use of supplementary aids and services cannot be achieved satisfactorily" (*Federal Register*, 34 CFR §300.550). It is believed that the majority of children who are eligible for special education and related services are able to participate in the general education curriculum with some adaptations and modifications. This provision of IDEA is intended to "ensure that children's special education and related services are in addition to and are affected by the general education curriculum, not separate from it."

The concept of LRE involves much more than mere physical location of services. There are four key elements to inclusion (Turnbull, Turnbull, Shank, & Smith, 2004):

- Students receive their education in the school they would have attended if they did not have a disability.

- Students are placed in classrooms according to the natural proportion of the exceptionality to the general population. This suggests that because about 10% of the general school population has disabilities, no more than 10% of the children in a classroom should have a disability.

- Teaching and learning for all students should be restructured so that special education and related services can support the general education classroom. Curriculum, instruction, and evaluation should be universally designed.

- School and general education placements should be age and grade appropriate.

Meeting the mandate for inclusive education has not been easy. Initially, when PL 94–142 was enacted in 1975, the concept of a continuum of placement options was encouraged. Taylor (1988), however, eloquently noted that children with disabilities were "caught in the continuum" and had to earn their way out. The inclusion movement has now tried to limit the use of more restrictive settings by creating partnerships between special education and general education (Turnbull et al., 2004). Many schools now have separate spaces for all children to use for different purposes as a way to facilitate learning for everyone. Children with disabilities are now placed much more frequently in general classroom settings. In Figure 11–2, the change in educational placement for children with orthopedic disabilities is indicated for 1990 and 2000. Major decreases in the restrictive environments of special schools and residential facilities have been replaced with increasing percentages of time spent in the general education classroom (U.S. Department of Education, 2002).

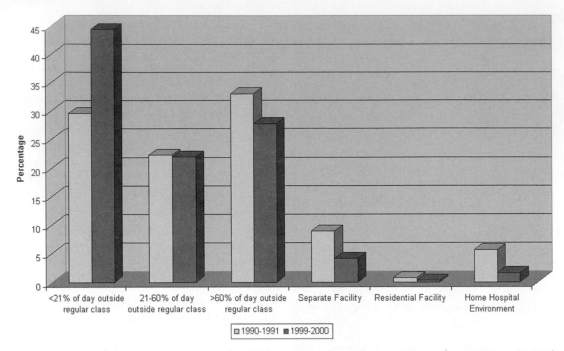

Figure 11-2 Change in educational environment for children with orthopedic impairments from 1990 to 2000. (U.S. Department of Education [2002]. *Twenty-fourth annual report to Congress on the implementation of the Individuals with Disabilities Education Act, p. A-231.* Washington, DC: Author.)

As physical therapists, we must determine how we can best meet the physical therapy needs of the child to allow the child's full participation in the general education curriculum. Our involvement in LRE occurs on at least three levels. First, there are the *architectural considerations*. Perhaps merely adding a ramp or railing to the front stairs of the school would allow the child direct access to the school like all other children. Perhaps push doors or enlarged knobs would allow all children to open doors more easily. Lockers in middle and high schools can be difficult or inconvenient for any child, and care should be taken to make certain that the child's locker is in an easily accessible location and can easily be locked and unlocked.

Consultation with all teachers is another critical component, as discussed under the intervention process. Physical therapists have always worked closely with special education teachers; however, to truly assist in optimizing an inclusive educational environment, we must anticipate the needs of general education teachers. The general education teacher might never have had a child with a disability or with this disability in the classroom. The therapist might be the only health-care professional available to provide information regarding the child's diagnosis and specific needs. Nurses can provide this information, but not all states or LEAs have school nurses. Will the teachers need to be instructed in proper positioning for the child? Will they need to learn proper body mechanics to avoid injury to themselves and the child? Who will check for pressure sores? How does the adaptive equipment work? Who gets called if equipment breaks? What are the physical limitations and expectations for the child? What can and should the child do? How can learned helplessness be prevented? How can obesity be prevented in all children in the classroom? Is the child safely positioned on the school bus? These are just a few of the questions the general education teacher might have for the therapist.

The final area that the therapist must address regarding LRE and full inclusion is the *specific needs of the individual child*. Besides consultation with the special education and general education teachers, does the child require direct services (procedural interventions)? If direct services are indicated, where and when will those services be provided to be the least obtrusive to the child's daily educational routine? There is a growing body of evidence that functional physical therapy (Ketelaar, Mermeer, 't Hart, van

Petegem-van Beek, & Helders, 2001) and therapy provided in natural education settings might result in superior skill acquisition (Karnish, Bruder, & Rainforth, 1995). The location of direct services is significantly influenced by the child's age, classroom placement, cooperation of the teachers, and degree of disability. Providing direct services in a preschool classroom is generally accomplished quite easily, even for a child with significant disabilities (Guralnick, 2001). However, for a high-school child, even a simple activity, such as adjusting a wheelchair seat or desk height, cannot be accomplished easily during the regular classroom routine without calling attention to the child and disrupting the class. The child's dignity must be maintained (Giangreco, 1995). Different service delivery models are discussed in Chapter 1. No one service delivery model should be considered "best practice," and it is unlikely that any one model is adequate to meet the complex needs of all children (Massey Sekerak, Kirkpatrick, Nelson, & Propes, 2003). The LRE for service delivery will depend on each individual child and is likely to change during the years of the child's education.

Working in the general education environment does place some burdens on therapists, which can be overcome with planning and administrative support. Therapists need to travel to schools. This takes time and requires increased staff. The therapist must also bring equipment to the schools, or have duplicate equipment available at each location. Again, this can be costly if the equipment is used for only one child. If there is only one related service provided in a school setting at any one time, there is professional isolation. Therapists are not able to speak with other therapists within and outside their discipline while they are seeing a child, and this isolation means that there is little peer review of the performance of therapists in school settings. School administrations must be sensitive to this isolation and allow therapists to meet frequently to discuss the children they serve and coordinate intervention. In addition, therapists should set up journal clubs and special-interest groups where they can meet with colleagues to seek advanced knowledge and skills.

Transition Services

Transitions, whether they are from EI to preschool, from preschool to elementary school, from elementary school to middle and high school, or from school to the adult community, are all critical periods in the life of any child and family. These periods of transition are especially complex and frequently quite difficult for a child with a disability. The child must leave a familiar setting where he or she knows everyone and is familiar with the physical environment. The child must now go to a new setting where the people, the environment, and even the adaptive equipment might be new. In some small LEAs, the therapist will transition with the child, but in larger systems, the child will have an entirely new team of professionals to work with in the new setting. The degree of adjustment will, of course, depend on the child and the setting, and in no small part on appropriate transition planning by all team members.

The transition from EI, which is covered under Part C of IDEA, to preschool, which is Part B of IDEA, can be particularly difficult for parents. Families must adjust to the different rules and regulations; different levels of service delivery, specifically the shift in focus from development of all developmental skills to only those that are educationally relevant; new service delivery models; new personnel and philosophies; and usually different lead agencies (Hanson et al., 2000). The child goes from receiving home-based services to preschool classrooms with new caregivers and new equipment. A transition plan should have been started between 90 days to 6 months before the child's third birthday to make the transition as "seamless" as possible. The transitions from preschool to kindergarten and then to primary school, middle school, and high school are equally important and complex, but specific planning for these transitions is not required or outlined in IDEA.

When transitioning during the school years, just the change in equipment can be devastating for a child who, for example, uses a power wheelchair and an augmentative communication system. The physical and occupational therapists must plan ahead to make certain the child has the same type of access to the power drive on the wheelchair and the same access to the computer, and the teachers need to make certain the computer programs are the same. If they are to be different, exposure to the new equipment or systems should have occurred long before the transition to the new school. It can take months to receive new equipment in a school setting, and the planning for transition must be started long before the actual event.

One of the most significant transitions in the life of a child and the family is when he or she leaves school. This is especially complicated for a child with significant disabilities who has limited options. Therefore, transition planning and services are required leading to postschool activities. Under IDEA 97, **transition services** are "a coordinated set of activities for a student, designed within an outcome-oriented process which promotes movement from school to postschool activities including postsecondary education, vocational training, integrated employment (including supported employment), continuing and adult education, adult services, independent living, or community participation" [*Federal Register,* 34 CFR §300.29(a)]. Transition planning must begin at age 14 years (earlier if the IEP team determines it is appropriate), and transition services should start at age 16 years. The Tri-Alliance of the American Occupational Therapy Association, the American Speech-Hearing-Language Association, and APTA worked together to have related services included in the IEP team for transition planning for children with disabilities in IDEA 97 [*Federal Register*, 34 CFR §300.29(a), (b)]. In addition to the usual members of the IEP team, transition service participants should also include representatives of agencies likely to be responsible for providing transition services or paying for those services [*Federal Register*, §300.344 (b)] and related service providers as appropriate. Once the child is 16 years of age, other agencies that might be involved in transition are to be included in the transition planning and services.

Transition services should focus on personal/social skills, daily living skills, and occupational/vocational skills so that the young adult may have a meaningful postsecondary school career and positive life outcomes. Consideration must be given to the child's long-term goals and needs. Therapists must help in determining what physical skills the child must have in multiple environments to achieve his or her goals and be successful in the community.

Common themes in "best" practice in transition, according to Flexer, McMahan, & Baer (2001, pp. 57–68), include the following:

- Student self-determination (social skills training and self-advocacy)
- Ecological approaches (assessing and training opportunities in a variety of environments)
- Individualized person-centered planning process (starts with the student's future goals and works backward to the present situation)
- Service coordination and interagency collaboration
- Community experiences (community experiences and exposure to social situations are critical elements in transition)
- Access and accommodation technologies and related services (requires appropriate assessment and selection of technologies)

- Postsecondary educational supports
- Systems change strategies (vocational career education, secondary curricular reform and inclusion)
- Family involvement

The issues involving transitions at each stage are complex, and require the full participation of a dedicated team of professionals along with the child and the parents. Physical therapists have the skills and background to assist in making transitions go more smoothly for children with physical disabilities.

Who Receives School-Based Physical Therapy?

IDEA

The vast majority of children who receive school-based physical therapy services do so under IDEA, based on the deliberations of the IEP team. Ideally, the physical therapist would have performed an examination, written up an evaluation, and attended the IEP meeting to assist in determining goals, objectives, and services. The physical therapist may attend the IEP meeting at the recommendation of the LEA, or at the request of the parents. We are not required to attend all IEP meetings, nor are we barred from attending meetings. During the meeting, we should indicate in what areas physical therapy services might help the child to benefit from his or her education. Then the team decides if physical therapy services are needed, and if so, the frequency, duration, and location of services.

Although any child eligible for special education might also be eligible for physical therapy as a related service, we tend to serve children with restrictions in motor activities: those with the federal classifications (see Box 11.1) of developmental delay, mental retardation, multiple disabilities, orthopedic impairment, other health impairment, and traumatic brain injury. Children who have problems in locomotion, walking, climbing stairs, or using wheelchairs and who have restrictions in activities of daily living will make up the majority of the therapist's caseload. The diagnoses of the children commonly served include CP, myelomeningocele, Down syndrome (especially in preschool and high school), Duchenne muscular dystrophy, osteogenesis imperfecta, arthrogryposis, mental retardation, and general developmental delay (in children up to age 9 years of age). Therapists might also assist in meeting the needs of children with autism, pervasive developmental disorder (PDD), and developmental coordination disorder (DCD). An example of the team approach to meeting the complex needs of a child with autism is in Case Example 11–1 (pages 392–393). Autism is a developmental disability that affects the child's verbal and nonverbal communication and social interaction. Children with autism are likely to have restricted, repetitive, and stereotyped patterns of behavior, interests, and activities. Although gross and fine motor skills generally are achieved, there are frequently problems with sensory motor processing. Meeting the educational and related service needs of the child with autism requires a team approach. Although initially the child might require physical therapy, as the case scenario demonstrates, the need for our involvement decreases as the child progresses through school.

Section 504 of the Rehabilitation Act

Children with diagnoses such as cystic fibrosis (CF) or juvenile rheumatoid arthritis (JRA) might also be served by a physical therapist in a school *if* they qualify for special education. If they do *not* qualify for special education under the rules and regulations of IDEA, they cannot receive related services, including physical therapy under IDEA. They might, however, qualify for services under **Section 504 of the Rehabilitation Act of 1973** (PL 93–112). Section 504 is an antidiscrimination statute designed to ensure that federal funding recipients, such as public schools, treat individuals with disabilities fairly. School systems that receive federal funds are not allowed to exclude qualified individuals with a disability from participation in programs offered by the school. The definition of "qualified handicapped person" under Section 504 is broader than under IDEA and includes any individual who "has a physical or mental impairment which substantially limits one or more major life activities" (*Federal Register*, 1988). Life activities "means functions such as caring for one's self, performing manual tasks, walking, seeing, hearing, speaking, breathing, learning and working." Therefore, a child with a diagnosis such as CF or JRA, who does not require special education but who has physical impairments that substantially limit life activities, such as breathing or walking, could qualify for physical therapy services in the school setting. These services do not follow the strict rules and regulations of IDEA, and there is great variability of services under Section 504 across the nation.

Athletics in Schools

Adaptive physical education for children with disabilities is required under IDEA. Some very large or affluent school systems have athletic trainers and physical therapists on their staffs to meet the needs of school athletes, but there is generally no mandate for such services. This is a specialized area of practice and is discussed in Chapter 12.

What Do Other Disciplines Expect of the Physical Therapist in the Team Setting?

As in EI, team involvement is critical for successful service delivery in school settings. You will be expected to share your expertise, as will other members of the team. Time should be set aside for team meetings and communication. All too often, the only team member who is in the child's school consistently is the teacher. Other team members usually have to serve several schools, especially when children are in general education classrooms. Unfortunately, telephone communication is difficult in school settings, and you do not want cell phones ringing in classrooms. One large city school system has tried to facilitate team communication by providing each therapist with a laptop computer for e-mail correspondence. This will hopefully expand professional communication and could increase communication with parents who also have computer access. We must consistently strive to determine the best ways of communicating with other team members and parents. The traditional small spiral notebook that went home with the child every day and was where teachers, therapists, and parents wrote, might still be the best means of communication in many situations.

Unlike EI, in which any discipline might have primary responsibility for the child and might serve as case manager, once the child reaches school age (3 years of age), the teacher(s) become(s) the primary service provider and coordinator of services. All team members must work closely with teachers to help meet their needs and to see that they are interested and able to assist in carrying out the activities the therapist recommends for the child. If the child needs to practice stair climbing and the teacher has arthritis and does not climb stairs, alternative arrangements must be made to assist the child in practicing stair climbing. Always taking the elevator to the second floor art class does not allow the child practice time in stair climbing or time transitioning from class to class with peers on the stairwell.

Speech-language pathologists and others need input for children with multiple disabilities or severe physical disabilities on positioning for feeding, functional activities, and access to communication systems. Therapists also assist teachers and others in determining alternative positions to decrease the child's pain, maintain range of motion, and prevent skin breakdown.

Professional Development

As in all areas of practice, the therapist must have a plan for professional development. The educational environment is unique and advanced competencies should be obtained (Chiarello, Effgen, Milbourne, & Campbell, 2003; Rapport, & Effgen, 2004). Some states, such as Washington, Colorado, and New Jersey, require special certification to work in school settings. This certification has not been difficult to obtain, but as practice becomes more specialized and the legal requirements more complex, additional states might start to require certification and additional competencies. Another way of providing evidence of clinical competence is certification as a pediatric clinical specialist (PCS) by the American Board of Physical Therapy Specialties. This general pediatric certification provides evidence of a board base of knowledge in pediatrics including school-based therapy. Because there are fewer postprofessional academic specialty programs in pediatrics as a result of the Doctor of Physical Therapy becoming the entry-level degree, the PCS will become the primary way to document competence in pediatric physical therapy.

An unfortunate problem in school-based settings is professional isolation, in which the therapist is not challenged, does not observe state-of-the-art practice, and has no role models from whom to learn or receive evaluation. School systems offer continuing education/in-service programs, but rarely do these programs address issues specific to the professional development needs of the therapists. School-based therapists need to determine their own professional development plan, either with the support and assistance of the school system or independently to guarantee their continued professional competence.

CASE EXAMPLE 11–1 . . . .

Preschool Child With Autism

Developed by
Deborah Widelo,
MSPT, PCS

Parents' Concerns

Chris's parents want him to socialize with peers, be more cooperative, and perform on an age-appropriate level.

Child's History

Chris is 4 years 4 months old and attends preschool in the public school system. He was evaluated last year as he turned 3 years old and transitioned from the home-based Early Intervention (EI) Program to a school-based preschool program. At that time, Chris did not have a specific medical diagnosis, but qualified for EI based on developmental delay. He had a past medical history significant for ear infections. Areas of concern based on the initial preschool screening include language, behavior, vision, hearing, articulation, self-help, and social skills. Chris did not and does not take medication.

Examination and Evaluation

The physical therapy examination and evaluation included parent interview, one-on-one examination of the neuromusculoskeletal system at the preschool, and administration of the Peabody Developmental Motor Scales, Second Edition (PDMS) for standardized assessment of gross motor skills.

Chris was 41 months old at the time of the examination and was well developed physically. He communicated with sounds, imitating some words. He used facial expressions and body language to effectively make his wants and needs known. Vision and hearing were within normal limits. Chris did not make eye contact with other children or adults. He was tactilely defensive and responded with an emotional outburst when he spilled a drink on his clothing. When presented with an unfamiliar task, Chris began to line objects up on the table top, and required 30 minutes of redirection and sensory activities to disrupt that pattern of behavior. ROM and strength were within normal limits; Chris was able to move his extremities and trunk through full joint exertions and against gravity in all planes of motion. Muscle tone was normal. Chris demonstrated symmetrical head, trunk, and hip alignment in sitting and standing.

Chris demonstrated protective extension responses in all planes of movement and had quick protective (parachute) reactions. Equilibrium reactions were present in hands/knees position, tall kneeling, and standing. Static and dynamic sitting and standing balance were normal. He was able to stand on either foot for 2 to 3 seconds as he kicked his opposite foot to hip level. His father studies martial arts, and Chris was able to mimic many of his postures, positions, and activities, but was not able to motor plan to perform these tasks upon request.

Chris was independent and safe walking on level surfaces and on uneven surfaces. He used a handrail to walk up and down steps with a reciprocal gait pattern. He was independent in transferring between level surfaces and uneven surfaces.

Chris demonstrated the following gross motor skills: hop with two feet 17 consecutive times; jump forward 12 inches and down from an object 12 inches high; jump over a hurdle 2 inches high; stand on either leg for 2 to 3 seconds; walk tandem on a visual line for 6 feet; walk on tiptoes with arms overhead with motivation; somersault; throw a large ball 6 feet with directionality; throw a tennis ball 5 feet with two hands, catch a large ball from a distance of 5 feet clasping it to his chest; and catch a tennis ball from 4 feet, clasping it to his chest.

On the PDMS, Chris demonstrated an age equivalent of 35 months (25th percentile, Z-score of −0.67) for stationary skills; an age equivalent of 32 months (16th percentile, Z-score of −1.00) for locomotion; and an age equivalent of 36 months (37th percentile, Z-score of −0.33) for object manipulation. His gross motor quotient was 87 (19th percentile, Z-score of −0.87).

Summary of Findings

Strengths included independent mobility, good ball-throwing skills, and some advanced gross motor skills (such as the somersault). Areas of concern included behavioral breakdown with structured tasks, transitions between activities, and difficulty following directions for task completion. No physical impairment of body structure or function that would affect Chris in the preschool environment was identified, although his behavior affected numerous activities.

IEP/Admissions and Release Committee Meeting

The IEP Team/Admissions and Release Committee (ARC) met to discuss the evaluation results. The data from the Physical Therapy Evaluation were combined with information gathered from the occupational therapist, speech-language pathologist, and psychologist. (The physical therapist and occupational therapist performed their evaluation jointly, as did the speech-language pathologist and psychologist.)

Chris's present level of educational performance indicated a need for physical therapy in his initial preschool years to address following directions and attention to tasks during gross motor activities, per IEP/ARC consensus. An IEP was developed and physical therapy was recommended for the following academic objectives:

1. Chris will be able to transition from one activity to another when given a visual/verbal directive with no disruptive behavior.

2. Chris will participate in a small-group activity with emphasis on interactive play for 1 minute without leaving the group area.

Based on the recommendations of the team, which included his parents, Chris was placed in special education, with related services, for developmental delay and speech and language impairment. He was scheduled for ten 20-minute sessions of physical therapy for his first year of preschool. Modifications in the school environment, recommended by the physical therapist and occupational therapist included adaptive seating on a disc seat for visual and tactile cues during sitting activities. He was to use a rocker board during circle time for vestibular stimulation within his personal space. Physical therapy was integrated in the regular classroom program with demonstration of sensory diet activities before structured task activities individually and with his peers, to provide models of successful interaction for the preschool staff. The occupational therapist provided a visual schedule, visual timers, and behavior modification strategies.

Re-examination

During his first 6 months of preschool, Chris made 10% progress on his first objective and 20% progress on his second objective. This means that he still required maximal physical assistance to transition between activities while he demonstrated tantrum behavior. He would stand with his peers at the water table or art table for 10 to 20 seconds but with no interactive play.

Further Testing

Chris's mother pursued further medical and psychological testing, and Chris was diagnosed with autism by the end of his first year of preschool.

Autism is identified when a child exhibits a cluster of the following characteristics, across a range of severity from mild to profound, and collected across multiple settings:

- Deficits in developing and using verbal or nonverbal communication for receptive or expressive language
- Deficits in social interactions, including social cues, emotion expression, personal relationships, and reciprocal interaction
- Repetitive ritualistic behaviors, including insistence on following routines and persistent preoccupation and attachment to objects
- Abnormal response to environmental stimuli.

Follow-up

Chris received occupational therapy over the summer through an outpatient agency. When he returned for his second year of preschool, his previous educational objectives remained in place because he did not master those objectives during the last school year. Modifications and strategies within the classroom included use of a mini-trampoline for proprioceptive input, a sit and spin, and a rocking chair for vestibular input. The occupational therapist instituted a bear hug vest for deep pressure during transitions, a visual schedule, visual time lines, and a visual timer to help him self-organize.

At this time, 2 months into his second year of preschool, Chris is able to transition between activities and play areas with verbal and tactile cues 80% of the time. Tantrums and verbal outbursts occur with disruptions in the "normal" preschool routine and requirements for task completion.

Chris continues to play independently, with no peer interaction. Physical therapy continues for only eight 20-minute sessions for this school year, and he will be followed as he transitions into kindergarten next year. At that time, he will be due for re-evaluation and will probably be discharged from physical therapy because other professionals might better be able to meet his needs. Occupational therapy will continue to work with the regular education teachers and resource room special educators to facilitate meeting his sensory needs, especially during transitions, in addition to visual cues/prompts to assist him with on-task activities and following directions.

Physical Therapy for Children With Autism

For students with the diagnosis of autism in the school system, physical therapy is indicated on an individual basis to reinforce attention to task and following directions during gross motor activities. As the student progresses through the educational levels, physical therapy is less important as most students with autism have competent mobility and motor skills. Occupational therapy is most effective in providing input for tailoring activities to meet the student's sensory needs for self-organization and time management for long term success.

Summary

School-based practice offers many rewards for the physical therapist. Unlike many other settings, the school gives the therapist the opportunity to follow the child for many years, sometimes throughout the child's entire education. The therapist gets to observe the natural progression of a disability, the immediate and long-term impact of interventions, the effectiveness or lack of effectiveness of interventions, and the implications of their work on the child's functioning in real life situations. The therapist also gets to work with and learn from members of other disciplines. For many therapists, the opportunity to work in their own local school system and to support their community is an added advantage to school-based employment. Therapists must, however, make certain that they continuously update their professional knowledge and skills because working in isolation can restrict their professional development and might impede the progress of the children they serve.

DISCUSSION QUESTIONS

1. Discuss how determining goals and objectives differs in a school setting compared with other settings in which physical therapists practice.

2. Why is eligibility for special education so important for provision of physical therapy in school settings?

3. What is the difference in eligibility requirements under IDEA versus Section 504 of the Rehabilitation Act?

4. Discuss ways of making intervention in a general education classroom successful.

RECOMMENDED READINGS

ASPIIRE/ILIAD IDEA Partnership Projects (2003). *Discover IDEA: Supporting achievement for children with disabilities: An IDEA practices resource guide (pathway guide).* Arlington, VA: Council for Exceptional Children.

Federal Register 34 CFR 111 §300 and §301, 7–1–02 Edition. Part II, Department of Education, Assistance to States for the Education of Children with Disabilities Program and Preschool Grants for Children with Disabilities. (IDEA 97). In print and available at *http://www.access.gpo.gov/nara/cfr/waisidx_02/34cfrv 2_02.html*

Hanft, B.E., & Place, P.A. (1996). *The consulting therapist: A guide for OTs and PTs in schools.* St. Louis, MO: Elsevier Science & Technology Books.

IDEA Practices (2004). Information available from the *www.ideapractices.org.* Web site. Excellent source of information on the laws, regulations, and implementation issues.

McEwen, I. (Ed.) (2000). *Providing physical therapy services under Parts B & C of the Individuals with Disabilities Education Act (IDEA).* Alexandria, VA: Section on Pediatrics, American Physical Therapy Association.

McEwen, I.R., & Sheldon, M.L. (1995). Pediatric therapy in the 1990s: The demise of the educational versus medical dichotomy. *Physical and Occupational Therapy in Pediatrics, 15*(2), 33–45.

REFERENCES

American Physical Therapy Association (APTA) (2001). *Guide for physical therapist practice.*

Bruininks, R.H. (1978). *Bruininks Oseretsky Test of Motor Proficiency.* Circle Pines, MN: American Guidance Service.

Chiarello, L., Effgen, S., Milbourne, S., & Campbell, P. (2003). Specialty certification program in early intervention and school-based therapy. *Pediatric Physical Therapy, 15,* 52–53.

Coster, W., Deeney, T., Haltiwanger, J., & Haley, S. (1998). *School function assessment Materials.* San Antonio, TX: The Psychological Corporation.

Deneka, D.M. (1995). Effects of individual and group treatment settings on increasing duration of head control in young children with severe physical disabilities. Unpublished master's thesis, MCP Hahnemann University, Philadelphia, PA.

Dole, R.L., Arvidson, K., Byrne, E., Robbins, J., & Schasberger, B. (2003). Consensus among experts in pediatric occupational and physical therapy on elements of Individualized Education Programs. *Pediatric Physical Therapy, 15*(3), 159–166.

Effgen, S.K. (2000). Factors affecting the termination of physical therapy services for children in school settings. *Pediatric Physical Therapy, 12*(3), 121–126.

Federal Register (1988). Section 104, 3(j), June 22, p. 26313.

Federal Register (1992). September 29, Part II, Department of Education, 34 CFR Parts §300 and §301, Assistance to States for the Education of Children with Disabilities Program and Preschool Grants for Children with Disabilities, Final Rule, Vol. 57, No. 189, p. 44839.

Federal Register (1997). 34 CFR 111, Parts §300 and §301, 7–1–02 Edition. Part II, Department of Education, Assistance to States for the Education of Children with Disabilities Program and Preschool Grants for Children with Disabilities (IDEA 97). In print and available at *http://www.access.gpo.gov/ nara/cfr/waisidx_02/34cfrv2_02.html*

Fischer, J.L. (1994). Physical therapy in educational environments: Moving through time with reflections and visions. *Pediatric Physical Therapy, 6*(3), 144–147.

Flexer, R.W., McMahan, R.K., & Baer, R. (2001). Transition models and best practices. In R.W. Flexer, T.J. Simmons, P. Luft, & R.M. Baer (Eds.), *Transition planning for secondary students with disabilities* (pp. 38–68). Upper Saddle River, NJ: Prentice-Hall, Inc.

Folio, M.R., & Fewell, R.R. (2000). *Peabody developmental motor scales* (2nd ed.). Austin, TX: Pro-ed.

Giangreco, M.F. (1995). Related services decision-making: A foundational component of effective education for students with disabilities. *Occupational and Physical Therapy in Educational Environments, 15,* 47–67.

Guralnick, M.J. (Ed.) (2001). *Early inclusion: Focus on change.* Baltimore: Paul Brookes.

Haley, S.M., Coster, W.J., Ludlow, L.H., Haltiwanger, J.T., & Andrellos, P.J. (1992). *Pediatric evaluation of disability inventory.* San Antonio, TX: The Psychological Corporation.

Hanft, B.E., & Place, P.A. (1996). *The consulting therapist: A guide for OTs and PTs in schools.* St. Louis, MO: Elsevier Science & Technology Books.

Hanson, M.J., Beckman, P.J., Horn, E., Marquart, J., Sandall, S.R., Greig, D., & Brennan, E. (2000). Entering preschool: Family and professional experiences in this transition process. *Journal of Early Intervention, 23,* 279–293.

Harris, S.R. (1997). The effectiveness of early intervention for children with cerebral palsy and related motor disabilities. In M.J. Guralnick (Ed.), *The effectiveness of early intervention* (pp. 327–347). Baltimore: Paul H. Brookes.

Karnish, K., Bruder, M.B., & Rainforth, B. (1995). A comparison of physical therapy in two school based treatment contexts. *Physical and Occupational Therapy in Pediatrics, 15*(4), 1–25.

Ketelaar, M., Mermeer, A., 't Hart, H., van Petegem-van Beek, E., & Helders, P.J.M. (2001). Effects of a functional therapy program on motor abilities of children with cerebral palsy. *Physical Therapy, 81*(9), 1534–1545.

Massey Sekerak, D., Kirkpatrick, D.B., Nelson, K.C., & Propes, J.H. (2003). Physical therapy in preschool classrooms: Successful integration of therapy into classroom routines. *Pediatric Physical Therapy, 15*(2), 93–103.

McDougall, J., King, G.A., Malloy-Miller, T., Gritzan, J., Tucker, M., & Evans, J. (1999). A checklist to determine the methods of intervention used in school-based therapy: Development and pilot testing. *Physical and Occupational Therapy in Pediatrics, 19*(2), 53–77.

McEwen, I.R., Arnold, S.H., Hansen, L.H., & Johnson, D. (2003). Interrater reliability and content validity of a minimal data set to measure outcomes of students receiving school-based occupational therapy and physical therapy. *Physical and Occupational Therapy in Pediatrics, 23*(2), 77–95.

Rainforth, B. (1997). Analysis of physical therapy practice acts: Implications for role release in educational environments. *Pediatric Physical Therapy, 9*, 54–61.

Rapport, M.J.K., & Effgen, S.K. (2004). Personnel issues in school-based physical therapy. *Journal of Special Education Leadership, 17*(1), 7–15.

Rapport, M.J.K., & Jones, M. (2000). Section III: Federal and State Court decisions, State Education Agency hearings, and letters of inquiry, policy interpretation, and investigations by Federal agencies. In I. McEwen (Ed.), *Providing physical therapy services under Parts B & C of the Individuals with Disabilities Education Act (IDEA)*. Alexandria, VA: Section on Pediatrics, American Physical Therapy Association.

Swinth, Y., & Hanft, B. (2002). School-based practice: Moving beyond 1:1 service delivery. *OT Practice*, September 16.

Taylor, S. (1988). Caught in the continuum: A critical analysis of the principle of least restrictive environment. *Journal of the Association for Persons with Severe Handicaps, 13*(1), 41–53.

Trahan, J., & Malouin, F. (2002). Intermittent intensive physiotherapy in children with cerebral palsy: A pilot study. *Developmental Medicine and Child Neurology, 44*, 233–239.

Turnbull, R., Turnbull, A., Shank, M., & Smith, S.J. (2004). *Exceptional lives: Special education in today's schools* (4th ed., pp. 61–76). Upper Saddle River, NJ: Pearson Prentice Hall.

United States Department of Education (2002). *Twenty-fourth annual report to Congress on the implementation of the Individuals with Disabilities Education Act*. Washington, DC: Author.

Vacha, V.B. (1933). History of the development of special schools and classes for crippled children in Chicago. *Physical Therapy Review, 13*, 21–26.

Chapter *12*

Sports Settings for the School-Aged Child

— Donna Bernhardt Bainbridge, PT, EdD, ATC

National interest in the reduction of risk factors for disease, *especially overweight and obesity*, has focused on the promotion of exercise and fitness (United States Department of Health and Human Services, 2001). Children are encouraged to become involved in recreational and sport activities at a much younger age. Although physical activity by high school students is still below the levels set in *Healthy people 2010*, Heath, Pratt, Warren, and Kann (1994) reported that approximately 37% of all students in grades 9 through 12 engaged in vigorous physical activity for at least 20 minutes 3 or more times per week according to the 1990 Youth Risk Behavior Survey. By the 1997 survey, the percentage of participation had increased to 63.8% (Pratt, Macera, & Blanton, 1999). Participation was higher for males than females (72.3% versus 53.5%) and demonstrated differences in ethnic and racial groups. These rates, however, did not consider the elementary ages or community programs. Current estimates suggest that between 20 and 30 million youth aged 5 to 17 years participate in community-sponsored athletic programs (Adirim & Cheng, 2003; Patel & Nelson, 2000). These participation rates may not be consistent for all living environments; Damore (2002) suggests that suburban preschool and school-aged children are more active than urban children in the same age groups.

Early participation in exercise and sports extends athletic life over many decades. Exposure to sports during significant years of mental and physical development establishes the foundation for future exercise beliefs and training habits. The increase in years of athletic participation can also increase total time exposure and thus the potential for injury. The physical therapist is uniquely qualified to promote and restore wellness, fitness, and health in the physically active child/adolescent in a variety of settings.

The purpose of this chapter is to introduce the physical therapist to the risk of injury in the physically active child and to highlight the differences in injury patterns in children. Two currently established models—the in-school athletic wellness model and the community-based Special Olympics model—will detail the role and involvement of the physical therapist in sports programs for both the normally abled child and the school-aged child/adolescent with disabilities.

Risk of Injury

Children and Adolescents With No Disabilities

Several studies have reported either the number or the percentage of injuries in children and adolescents. A 1988 National Center for Health Statistics survey of 11,840 participants aged 5 to 17 years estimated that 4,379,000 injuries occurred annually from sports and recreation (36% of all reported injuries) (Bijur et al., 1995). Beachy, Akau, Martinson, and Olderr (1997) noted similar rates of injury (35%). The European Home- and Leisure- Accident

Surveillance System recorded an incidence of 73.3 injuries per 1000 children aged 6 to 17 years annually (Sorensen, Larsen, & Rock, 1996). Types of injuries included contusions (37%), fractures (22%), sprains (24.8%), and strains (5%).

Backx, Beijer, Bol, and Erich (1991) reported 399 sports injuries in a population of 1818 children aged 8 to 17 years (22%). The most common injuries were contusions (43%) and sprains (21%). Physical contact, a high rate of jumping, and indoor play accounted for 78% of the total variance. Watkins and Peabody (1996) concur, demonstrating that 62% of injuries were a result of sprains, strains, or contusions. They also note that high or explosive speed and physical contact were responsible for the majority of injuries. Injuries have been reported in both organized and individual sports, notably football, wrestling, soccer, basketball, equestrian, trampoline, bicycling, and skiing (Axe, Newcomb, & Warner, 1991; Campbell-Hewson, Robinson, & Egleston, 1999; Deibert, Aronsson, Johnson, Ettlinger, & Shealy, 1998; Furnival, Street, & Schunk, 1999; Messina, Farney, & DeLee, 1999; Puranik, Long, & Coffman, 1998; Tenvergert, Ten Duis, & Klasen, 1992).

Taylor and Attia (2000) reviewed all sports-related (SR) injuries in children between 5 and 18 years seen in the emergency department over a 2-year period. They noted 677 injuries, with 71% occurring in males. Sports that were most commonly implicated were basketball (19.5%), football (17.1%), baseball/softball (14.9%), soccer (14.2%), in-line skating (5.7%), and hockey (4.6%). Sprains/strains were most frequent, followed by fractures, contusions, and lacerations; these accounted for 90% of all injuries. Conn, Annest, and Gilchrist (2003) evaluated SR injury events in the National Health Interview Survey for 1997–1999. They reported that the estimates for SR injuries were about 42% higher for 5- to 24-year-olds than shown in emergency department data. The highest average annual rates were for children aged 5 to 14 years (59.3 per 1000) and 15 to 24 years (56.4 per 1000). Injury rates were twice as high in males.

A recent study conducted by Radelet, Lephart, Rubenstein, and Myers (2002) observed 1659 children aged 7 to 13 years during two seasons of community baseball, softball, indoor and outdoor soccer, and football. Their definition of injury, broader than the accepted definition, included any injury that the coach examined on field, any injury requiring first aid, as well as any injury preventing participation. They noted injury rates of 1.7 for baseball, 1.0 for softball, 2.1 for soccer, and 1.5 for football per 100 athlete exposures. Rates were significantly higher for games versus practice for all sports except softball. However, the frequency of injury per team per season was

4 to 7 times higher in football, with more severe injuries. The types of injuries were consistent with other studies. Contact was a leading cause for severe injury in baseball (contact with ball) and football (contact with player). Interestingly, children between the ages of 8 and 10 years were more frequently injured than were younger or older children, perhaps because of their transition to more advanced levels of play. Brown, Brunn, and Garcia (2001) noted that 27% of cervical injuries seen in a trauma center were related to sports, and football accounted for 29% of the injuries.

Children and adolescents are becoming more involved in extreme variations of sports, as well as in increased risk taking with everyday sports. Various authors have noted significant injury rates during cycling (Gerstenbluth, Spirnak, & Elder, 2002; Winston et al., 2002); exercycling (Benson, Waters, Meier, Visotsky, & Williams, 2000); all-terrain vehicle use (Brown, Koepplinger, Mehlman, Gittelman, & Garcia 2002); snowboarding and skiing (Drkulec & Letts, 2001; Shorter, Mooney, & Harmon, 1999; Skokan, Junkins, & Kadish, 2003); and inline skate, skateboard, and scooter use (Kubiak & Slongo, 2003; Mankovsky, Mendoza-Sagaon, Cardinaux, Hohlfeld, & Reinberg, 2002; Nguyen & Letts, 2001; Osberg, Schneps, DiScala, & Li, 1998; Powell & Tanz, 2000a, 2000b). Although many of these injuries are contusions, fractures, and sprains/strains, these authors noted significant numbers of renal injuries, head and neck injuries, and hand trauma.

Children and Adolescents With Disabilities

Minimal data have been collected on the incidence and type of sports injuries that occur in persons with disabilities. In a 1981 survey of 102 athletes in a regional wheelchair competition, 72% sustained at least one injury. The majority of injuries occurred in the upper extremity; 33% were soft tissue injuries. Track accounted for 26% of the injuries, whereas basketball caused 24%, and road racing 22% (Curtis, 1982). A 1995 study by Taylor and Williams in the United Kingdom reports the same overall rate of injury. A survey of the 1990 Junior National Wheelchair Games demonstrated injury rates of 97% in track, 22% in field events, and 91% in swimming among 83 athletes (Wilson & Washington, 1993). Among the 20 medical problems noted in 19 athletes in the International Flower Marathon, 13 were injuries: 8 soft tissue injuries and 5 abrasions/ulcers (Hoeberigs, Deberts-Eggen, & Deberts, 1990).

A retrospective study of 426 athletes who participated in the 1989 competitions of the National Wheelchair Athletic Association (NWAA), the United States Association for Blind Athletes (USABA), and the United States Cerebral Palsy Association (USCPA) demonstrated at least one time-loss injury in 32% of all respondents. The NWAA had 26% of all injuries, with 57% of these involving the shoulder and elbow; 53% of USABA injuries involved the lower extremity, whereas injuries in USCPA athletes occurred in all areas equally (Ferrara et al., 1992). A survey of 46 female wheelchair basketball players confirmed a 52% increase in shoulder pain since playing wheelchair basketball (Curtis & Black, 1999).

A Special Olympics injury report documented that 3.5% of all athletes required illness or injury management. The highest injury rate was in track and field (McCormick, Niebiehr, & Risser, 1990). The Connecticut State Special Olympics Games in 1994–1996 noted that the most frequent injuries were sprains/strains to the lower extremities, followed by fractures and dislocations. They also noted a 600-fold increase in heat-related dehydration in 1996 (Galena, Epstein, & Lourie, 1998). Data from the 2001 Special Olympics World Winter Games documented 1081 total incidents (58% mild to moderate and 41% moderate to severe). These injuries were 49.5% orthopedic and 49.8% medical, with a 6% hospital visit rate and 2% hospital admission rate (Special Olympics International, 2001).

Injury Types Specific to Children and Adolescents

Although children and adolescents can sustain many of the same injuries as adults, they are more susceptible to unique injuries related to psychological, developmental, and physiological components. Lack of psychological and developmental maturity for an activity can predispose a child to injury. Tanner scales and psychological attributes, such as attention and ability to follow directions, are often used to assess developmental and psychological readiness.

Evidence from clinical and biomechanical studies suggests that growing articular cartilage has a lower resistance to repetitive loading that may result in microtrauma to the cartilage or to the underlying growth plate. This tissue damage can lead to early onset of osteoarthritis or to asymmetry in growth (Maffulli & Bruns, 2000; Micheli, 1995). The repetitive loading of distance running or jumping might lead to knee osteoarthritis or growth plate disturbance *with subsequent permanent alteration of growth.*

Another weakness of growing articular cartilage is shear stress, especially at the elbow, knee, and ankle (Omey & Micheli, 1999). Research suggests that a segment of the subchondral bone becomes avascular, separates from the articular cartilage, and becomes a loose body known as osteochondritis dissicans (Maffulli, 1990). This repetitive shear is implicated in osteochondritis dissicans of the talus in runners, of the capitellum in "Little League" elbow, and in epiphyseal displacement (Gill & Micheli, 1996; Micheli, 1995).

The third area of weakness in growing cartilage is the apophysis. Evidence suggests that overuse stresses the apophyseal growth center, especially if it is an insertion point for the musculotendinous unit, and causes microavulsion fractures. This process is implicated in Osgood-Schlatter's disease, Sever's disease, and ischial or anterior-superior iliac spine apophysitis (Maffulli, 1990; Micheli & Fehlandt, 1992; Outerbridge & Micheli, 1995; Patel & Nelson, 2000).

The biomechanical properties of bone also alter with growth. As bone becomes less cartilaginous and stiffer, the resistance to impact decreases. Sudden overload may cause the bone to bow or buckle. The epiphysis, the area of growth in the long bones, is more susceptible and may shear or fracture. Examples of this process include avulsion-fracture of the anterior cruciate ligament, avulsion-fracture of the ankle ligament, or growth plate fractures. Because of the difficulty of radiographic analysis, any injury to the epiphyseal area is considered a fracture and treated as such to avoid potential growth disturbance (Coady & Micheli, 1997; Maffulli & Bruns, 2000; Micheli & Wood, 1995).

A final issue of concern is the longitudinal growth of bones, often in spurts, with slower secondary elongation of soft tissue. This process causes periods of loss of relative musculotendinous flexibility during periods of rapid bone growth. A coincident occurrence of bone growth and overuse injury has been noted (Gerrard, 1993; Micheli, 1995; Thabit & Micheli, 1992). Physical therapy prevention focuses on reducing the occurrence, severity, and duration of overuse injuries. These roles are defined more thoroughly in the following models of prevention and management.

Many physiological differences distinguish children from adults and and affect performance. Children have smaller hearts and lower blood volume; this results in a lower stroke volume with compensatory higher heart rate. Children also have a lower glycolytic capacity, limiting anaerobic performance, and a slowly maturing nervous system with incomplete myelination of nerve fibers. Improvements in balance, agility, coordination, and speed will parallel maturation of this system. This neural maturation also affects gains in muscle strength and neuromuscular control (Malina, 1994; Rowland, 1996; Turley, 1997).

Setting-Based Service Delivery Models

The physical therapist is involved in prevention and wellness activities, screening, and the promotion of fitness and positive health behaviors, such as avoidance of smoking, drugs, and alcohol. These goals are directed toward the **prevention** or **reduction of risk** for injury. Primary prevention is focused toward prevention of disease or injury in a potentially susceptible population. Secondary prevention focuses on decreasing the duration, severity, or sequelae of injury/illness through early diagnosis and prompt intervention. Tertiary prevention limits the degree of disability and promotes restoration of function in those with chronic or irreversible diseases. These roles can be defined in the following multidisciplinary models of service delivery.

School-Based Model

The school-based model, one that is funded in whole or part by the school district, has been instituted successfully in many high schools (Bernhardt-Bainbridge, 2000; Swenson, 1991). School personnel may include coaches, school nurses, health educators, and nutritionists. Personnel usually retained on contract are a physician and physical therapist, both preferably with expertise in sports medicine, and possibly a certified athletic trainer (ATC). These programs are designed to provide education in positive health behaviors, promote wellness, reduce the risk of injury, and provide early management of injuries.

The components of the prevention model include a **preparticipation examination**, development of an appropriate training and conditioning program, proper supervision and protection during practice and events, and environmental control. The physical therapist can play an integral part in most of these components.

Preparticipation Screening Examination

The purposes of the preparticipation screening are to determine general health, detect any conditions that might limit participation or predispose to injury, assess maturity and fitness levels, identify sports that may be played safely, and

educate the athlete and his or her family (Bar-Or, 1995; Bernhardt-Bainbridge, 2000). The usefulness of these screenings has been demonstrated in several studies (Bratton, 1997; Drezner, 2000; Fuller et al., 2000; Glover & Maron, 1998; Kurowski & Chandran, 2000; Lyznicki, Nielsen, & Schneider, 2000; Maron, 2002; Rifat, Ruffin, & Gorenflo, 1995). Most states require a preparticipation screening to meet legal and insurance requirements. Although an individual examination is most commonly performed, the multistation examination that objectively screens not only the general health but also aerobic conditioning, strength, flexibility, balance, and power is more cost and time efficient. A complete entry-level examination and evaluation and an annual re-evaluation that includes a brief physical examination, a physical maturity assessment, and an examination of all new problems are the current recommendations (Bratton, 1997). More recently, the state of North Carolina has adopted a preparticipation examination for their specific needs, based on the questions that have shown significant yield (Fields, 1994). One report of a Web-based examination was also noted (Peltz, Haskell, & Matheson, 1999).

The components of the preparticipation examination are a medical history; a physical examination, including cardiovascular and eye examinations; a musculoskeletal examination; body composition assessment; physical maturity evaluation; and sports-specific functional tests (Bernhardt-Bainbridge, 2000; Lombardo, 1991). A standard preparticipation medical questionnaire and examination has been created by several medical professional organizations, and can be obtained from the American Academy of Family Physicians (*www.aafp.org*).

The physician must perform and sign off on the physical examination and systems testing. The physician or nurse should assess physical maturity. As a specialist in the neuromusculoskeletal system, the physical therapist can perform the history and musculoskeletal examination (American Physical Therapy Association, 2002). Several personnel, including the physical therapist, ATC, or coach, can perform the standardized functional testing.

The physical therapist, ATC, or nurse can assess body composition with one of several field tests: body mass index (BMI) (Tables 12.1 and 12.2), skinfold assessment using age-and population-specific equations, or anthropometric measures. Desirable body fat is 10% to 15% for adolescent males and 20% to 25% for adolescent females (Bar-Or, Lombardo, & Rowland, 1988). Percentages have not been well standardized for younger athletes (Klish, 1995).

The preparticipation examination guides the team physician in determining the level of athletic clearance (Tables 12.3 and 12.4 and Appendix 12.A). The examination also

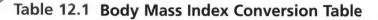

Table 12.1 Body Mass Index Conversion Table

How do you find your BMI risk level?*			

1. Use a weight scale on a hard, flat, uncarpeted surface. Wear very little clothing and no shoes.
2. Weigh yourself to the nearest pound.
3. With your eyes facing forward and your heels together, stand very straight against a wall. Your buttocks, shoulders, and the back of your head should be touching the wall.
4. Mark your height at the highest point of your head. Then measure your height in feet and inches to the nearest $1/4$ inch. Also figure your height in inches only.
5. Find your height in feet and inches in the first column of the Body Mass Index Risk Levels table. The ranges of weight that correspond to minimal risk, moderate risk (overweight), and high risk (obese) are shown in the three columns for each height.

Height	Minimal Risk (BMI <25)	Moderate Risk (BMI 25–29.9): Overweight	High Risk (BMI ≥30): Obese
4'10"	118 lb. or less	119–142 lb.	143 lb. or more
4'11"	123 lb. or less	124–147 lb.	148 lb. or more
5'0	127 lb. or less	128–152 lb.	153 lb. or more
5'1"	131 lb. or less	132–157 lb.	158 lb. or more
5'2"	135 lb. or less	136–163 lb.	164 lb. or more
5'3"	140 lb. or less	141–168 lb.	169 lb. or more
5'4"	144 lb. or less	145–173 lb.	174 lb. or more
5'5"	149 lb. or less	150–179 lb.	180 lb. or more
5'6"	154 lb. or less	155–185 lb.	186 lb. or more
5'7"	158 lb. or less	159–190 lb.	191 lb. or more
5'8"	163 lb. or less	164–196 lb.	197 lb. or more
5'9"	168 lb. or less	169–202 lb.	203 lb. or more
5'10"	173 lb. or less	174–208 lb.	209 lb. or more
5'11"	178 lb. or less	179–214 lb.	215 lb. or more
6'0"	183 lb. or less	184–220 lb.	221 lb. or more
6'1"	188 lb. or less	189–226 lb.	227 lb. or more
6'2"	193 lb. or less	194–232 lb.	233 lb. or more
6'3"	199 lb. or less	200–239 lb.	240 lb. or more
6'4"	204 lb. or less	205–245 lb.	246 lb. or more

*To calculate your exact BMI value, multiply your weight in pounds by 705, divide by your height in inches, then divide again by your height in inches.

Source: Adapted from National Institutes of Health, National Heart, Lung, and Blood Institute (1998). Obesity Education Initiative: Clinical guidelines on the identification, evaluation, and treatment of overweight and obesity in adults. *Obesity Research 6*(suppl 2), 51S–209S; American Heart Association (2003). Body composition tests. Retrieved September 13, 2003, from: *http://www.american-heart.org.presenter.jhtml?identifier=4489*

Table 12.2 Body Mass Index Percentiles for Underweight, at Risk for Overweight, and Overweight* in Children and Adolescents (Ages 2–20 Years)

Underweight	BMI-for-age <5th percentile
At risk of overweight	BMI-for-age = 85th percentile to <95th percentile
Overweight	BMI-for-age ≥95th percentile

*Charts for Stature for Age and Weight for boys and girls can be found in Figure 2.3.

Source: Centers for Disease Control, National Center for Chronic Disease Prevention and Health Promotion (2003, April). *Nutrition & physical activity.* Retrieved July 15, 2004, from Website: *http://www.cdc.gov/nccdphp/dnpa/bmi-for-age.htm*

defines each athlete's strengths and limitations. These levels are the foundation for an individualized training and conditioning program with the following elements: energy training, strength and endurance training, speed work, and nutritional counseling (Birrer & Brecher, 1987).

The preparticipation examination can also be used to screen youth and adolescents for involvement in risky health behaviors, such as tobacco and alcohol use, use of recreational drugs or ergogenic aids (Iven, 1998), and unsafe sexual practices (American Medical Association [AMA], 1993; Nsuami et al., 2003). In addition to actual questions, the examiner can be alert for reported changes in behavior, poor grades, loss of attention, irritability, and weight changes (AMA, 1993).

A review of the literature documented a 3% to 5% overall doping prevalence among children, making this issue a public health problem (Laure, 1997). Risk factors for substance abuse include poor or single parent family situation, poor health perception, other drug consumption,

Table 12.3 Athletic Fitness Scorecards

Athletic Fitness Scorecard for Boys					
Test	0 Below average	1 Above average	2 Good	3 Very good	4 Excellent
Strength Pull-ups (no)	Fewer than 7	7 to 9	10 to 12	13 to 14	15 or more
Power Long jump (in)	Fewer than 85	85 to 88	89 to 91	92 to 94	95 or more
Speed 50-yd dash (sec)	Slower than 6.7	6.7 to 6.4	6.3 to 6.0	5.9 to 5.6	5.5 or less
Agility 6-c agility (c)	Fewer than 5–5	5–5 to 6–3	6–4 to 7–2	7–3 to 8–1	8–2 or more
Flexibility Forward flexion (in)	Not reach ruler	1 to 2	3 to 5	6 to 8	9 or more
Muscular endurance Sit-ups (no)	Fewer than 38	38 to 45	46 to 52	53 to 59	60 or more
Cardiorespiratory endurance 12-min run (mi)	Fewer than $1\frac{1}{2}$	$1\frac{1}{2}$	$1\frac{3}{4}$	2	$2\frac{1}{4}$ or more

Athletic Fitness Scoredcard for Girls					
Test	0 Below average	1 Above average	2 Good	3 Very good	4 Excellent
Strength Pull-ups (no)	Fewer than 2	2 to 3	4 to 5	6 to 7	8 or more
Power Long jump (in)	Fewer than 63	63 to 65	66 to 68	69 to 71	72 or more
Speed 50-yd dash (sec)	Slower than 8.2	8.2 to 7.9	7.8 to 7.1	6.9 to 6.0	5.9 or less
Agility 6-c agility (c)	Fewer than 3–5	3–5 to 4–3	4–4 to 5–2	5–3 to 6–2	6–3 or more
Flexibility Forward flexion (in)	Fewer than 3	3 to 5	6 to 8	9 to 11	12 or more
Muscular endurance Sit-ups (no)	Fewer than 26	26 to 31	32 to 38	39 to 45	46 or more
Cardiorespiratory endurance 12-min run (mi)	Fewer than $1\frac{1}{4}$	$1\frac{1}{4}$	$1\frac{1}{2}$	$1\frac{3}{4}$	2 or more

Your Score							
	Strength	Power	Speed	Agility	Flexibility	Muscular endurance	Cardiorespiratory endurance
Your Score							
Rating (0–4)							

Source: Athletic fitness scorecards (1988). *Patient Care, October 30*, Montvale, NJ: Medical Economics Publishing.

Table 12.4 Sports Classification System

Classification of Sports by Contact		
Contact or Collision	Limited Contact	Noncontact
Basketball	Baseball	Archery
Boxing*	Bicycling	Badminton
Diving	Cheerleading	Body building

(Continued)

Table 12.4 Sports Classification System *(Continued)*

Classification of Sports by Contact		
Contact or Collision	**Limited Contact**	**Noncontact**
Field hockey	Canoeing or kayaking	Bowling
Football	(white water)	Canoeing or kayaking
Tackle	Fencing	(flat water)
Ice hockey†	Field events	Crew or rowing
Lacrosse	High jump	Curling
Martial arts	Pole vault	Dancing §
Rodeo	Floor hockey	Ballet
Rugby	Football	Modern
Ski jumping	Flag	Jazz
Soccer	Gymnastics	Field events
Team handball	Handball	Discus
Water polo	Horseback riding	Javelin
Wrestling	Racquetball	Shot put
	Skating	Golf
	Ice	Orienteering ‖
	In-line	Power lifting
	Roller	Race walking
	Skiing	Riflery
	Cross-country	Rope jumping
	Downhill	Running
	Water	Sailing
	Skateboarding	Scuba diving
	Snowboarding‡	Swimming
	Softball	Table tennis
	Squash	Tennis
	Ultimate frisbee	Track
	Volleyball	Weight lifting
	Windsurfing or surfing	

Classification of Sports by Strenuousness		
High to Moderate Intensity		
High to Moderate Dynamic and Static Demands	**High to Moderate Dynamic and Low Static Demands**	**High to Moderate Static and Low Dynamic Demands**
Boxing*	Badminton	Archery
Crew or rowing	Baseball	Auto racing
Cross-country skiing	Basketball	Diving
Cycling	Field hockey	Horseback riding (jumping)
Downhill skiing	Lacrosse	Field events (throwing)
Fencing	Orienteering	Gymnastics
Football	Race walking	Karate or judo
Ice hockey	Racquetball	Motorcycling
Rugby	Soccer	Rodeo
Running (sprint)	Squash	Sailing
Speed skating	Swimming	Ski jumping
Water polo	Table tennis	Water skiing
Wrestling	Tennis	Weight lifting
	Volleyball	
Low Intensity (Low Dynamic and Low Static Demands)		
	Bowling	
	Cricket	
	Curling	
	Golf	
	Riflery	

* Participation not recommended by the American Academy of Pediatrics.

† The American Academy of Pediatrics recommends limiting the amount of body checking allowed for hockey players 15 years and younger to reduce injuries.

‡ Snowboarding has been added since previous statement was published.

§ Dancing has been further classified into ballet, modern, and jazz since previous statement was published

‖ A race (contest) in which competitors use a map and compass to find their way through unfamiliar territory.

Source: American Academy of Pediatrics. Committee on Sports Medicine and Fitness (2001). Medical conditions affecting sports participation. *Pediatrics, 107*, 1205–1209.

antisocial behavior, depression, and clumsiness. Good communication with a parent, academic achievement, regular sports participation, serious and organized personality, and mother at home were cited as protective factors (Challier, Chau, Predine, Choquet, & Legras, 2000; Stronski, Ireland, Michaud, Narring, & Resnick, 2000).

Research reports that 3% to 12% of adolescent boys and 1% to 2% of girls report having used steroids (Bahrke, Yesalis, & Brower, 1998; Yesalis & Bahrke, 2000). In addition to the risk factors noted for general use of drugs, strength training added another risk for the use of steroids (DuRant, Escobedo, & Heath, 1995; Forman, Dekker, Javors, & Davison, 1995). Other substances that have been used to increase muscle performance include DHEA, branched chain and essential amino acids, creatine, growth hormone, and dietary supplements containing nandrolone and testosterone (Armsey & Green, 1997; Balsom, Soderlund, & Ekblom, 1994; Davis, 1995; Kreider et al., 1998; Kreider, Miriel, & Bertun, 1993; van Hall, Raaymakers, Saris, & Wagenmakers, 1995). Dietary substances including ephedra and carnitine have been used to increase energy and endurance, suppress appetite, and promote weight loss (Bell, McLellan, & Sabiston, 2002; Haller & Benowitz, 2000; Heinonen, 1996).

With the exception of studies of the effect of creatine on muscle during resistance training, research has not supported the efficacy of these substances for performance enhancement. The little research that exists has examined these substances in adults; no research yet exists on the population under the age of 21 years. In addition, research has reported potential risk and harm with ingestion of substantial amounts of several substances, including steroids, nandrolone, ephedra, and branched amino acids. The use of ephedrine-containing compounds has been banned by most professional and collegiate sports organizations, as well as the National Federation of State High School Associations (2003).

Dietary supplements are not approved by the Food and Drug Administration, so actual ingredients are not listed on the bottle, nor are safety and effectiveness validated. The few protections offered to the consumer include a USP label, a nationally known manufacturer, and appropriate and accurate claims supported by research.

Training and Conditioning

Fitness should be a year-round endeavor for the child and youth. The athletic child can develop a fitness program that also trains him or her for improved performance in the activity of choice. Because the body does not respond in a linear manner across all physiological systems, and to maintain interest in the program, a training program is organized into components: off-season, preseason, in-season, and after season. For the child and youth, these programs should emphasize fun, cooperation, team play, and learning.

The focus of off-season energy training is development of an aerobic-based, long-duration activity with low- to moderate-intensity work. A general base of muscular endurance and strength is also developed to balance the body and to reduce risk of activity-related injuries to the musculoskeletal system.

The goals of preseason training are more focused preparation for activity related to strength, balance, and the cardiovascular demands of the activity. Anaerobic efficiency (higher intensity for shorter duration) may be developed in the preseason period, as well as focused strength and speed (Figure 12–1) (Bernhardt-Bainbridge, 2000; Falkel, 1986).

The in-season period is the time for maintenance of condition. The program focuses on specific areas that might be more at risk for injury or limitation. The postseason is a short period designed to allow the body to rest and recuperate. Child athletes should perform activities that they enjoy but that are not their usual choices. For example, the soccer player might choose to swim or cycle.

Strength training for prepubescent and pubescent athletes has been demonstrated to increase strength without alteration of muscle mass (Bernhardt et al., 2001; Blimkie, 1993; Falk & Tenenbaum, 1996; Faigenbaum, Loud, O'Connell, Glover, & Westcott, 2001; Guy & Micheli, 2001; Ramsey et al., 1990). Training has several parameters that make it safe for the youth. Instruction in proper technique with constant supervision is necessary. Activities should be nonballistic and performed through full range of motion with no, or very light, weight. An emphasis on negative or eccentric work should be avoided. Apparatus must also be scaled to the size of the youth (Kraemer & Fleck, 1993). Many examples of sports-specific strength programs exist in the literature (Kraemer & Fleck, 1993). The physical therapist or ATC can design these programs for either the individual athlete or the team. All programs should be coordinated with the coach and performed under direct supervision of an adult.

Proper training requires good nutrition as the fuel for energy production. Nutritional requirements for the younger athlete have been documented (Clark, 1991; Maughan, 2002; Peterson & Peterson, 1988) (Appendix 12.B). Attention should also be directed to adequate caloric intake, as active children burn more calories and can have a balanced diet that has too few calories. Education of youth

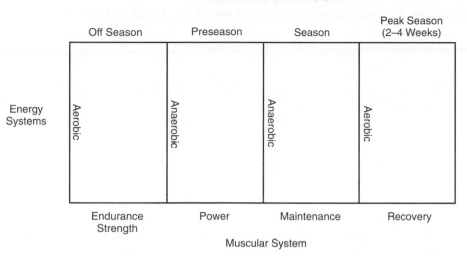

Figure 12-1 Strength-endurance training continuum.

and families should be a part of any training program. This education should be reinforced by both the family and the coach. Youth may have problems with either excess weight and/or excess body fat. If a youth has excess body fat, exercise may convert some fat weight to lean mass. Difficulties with excess leanness and eating disorders are being identified more frequently in the preadolescent population. If a special nutrition program and counseling for weight loss or gain is indicated, it should be supervised by a nutritionist and/or nurse.

Hydration is an important issue with children because they require more liquid per proportional weight than adults. Children also have more difficulty dealing with thermal stress than do adults. Their greater surface area-to-body mass ratio facilitates greater heat gain on hot days and greater heat loss on colder days. Children produce less sweat, and less total evaporative heat loss, and more metabolic heat per pound of body weight during exercises such as walking and running. Finally, although children can acclimatize, they do so at a slower rate than adults (Armstrong & Maresh, 1995; Bar-Or, 1995; Falk, 1998).

Thus, the physical therapist or ATC must closely monitor environmental temperature and humidity. Field precautions and practice recommendations are noted in Table 12.5. Recommendations for hydration include prehydration of 3 to 12 ounces (3 to 6 ounces for less than 90 pounds weight; 6 to 12 ounces for more than 90 pounds weight) 1 hour before activity and 3 to 6 ounces just before activity. During activity, 3 to 9 ounces (3 to 5 ounces for less than 90 pounds and 6 to 9 ounces for more than 90

pounds) should be ingested every 10 to 20 minutes relative to the temperature and humidity. Then 8 to 12 ounces should be consumed for each $^1/_2$ pound of weight lost in 2 to 4 hours after activity (Casa et al., 2000).

Significant research has evaluated the type of fluid to be ingested by children. Children will not ingest enough water to remain hydrated or to rehydrate after activity. However, if flavor is added to the water, the volume of intake is improved substantially (Iuliano, Naughton, Collier, & Carlson, 1998; Passe, Horn, & Murray, 2000). Sports drinks have been shown to improve energy in both intensive and endurance exercise (Below, Mora-Rodriquez, Gonzalez-Alonso, & Coyle, 1995; Davis, Welsh, & Alerson, 2000; Galloway & Maughan, 2000; Utter, Kang, Nieman, & Warren, 1997; Wilk & Bar-Or, 1996). In addition to flavor, well-constituted sports drinks have a simple low-carbohydrate content that provides energy and speeds fluid absorption and sodium to stimulate the thirst mechanism (Passe et al., 2000; Rivera-Brown, Gutierrez, Gutierrez, Frontera, & Bar-Or, 1999; Shi et al., 1995).

Successive hydration programs involve not only fluid intake but also fluid availability. Cool fluids infuse into the system more readily, so accessible liquids should be chilled, or ice should be provided (Greydanus & Patel, 2002; Squire, 1990). Education of everyone involved with the activity is of paramount importance to ensure continued compliance. Knowledge of the common signs of dehydration—irritability, headache, nausea, dizziness, weakness, cramps, abdominal distress, and decreased performance—assist those involved with early recognition and intervention (Casa et al., 2000).

Table 12.5 Restraints on Activities at Different Levels of Heat Stress

WBGT*		Restraints on Activities
°C	°F	
<24	<75	All activities allowed, but be alert for prodromes (symptoms) of heat-related illness in prolonged events
24.0–25.9	75.0–78.6	Longer rest periods in the shade; enforce drinking every 15 minutes
26–29	79–84	Stop activity of unacclimatized persons and other persons with high risk; limit activities of all others (disallow long-distance races, cut down further duration of other activities)
>29	>85	Cancel all athletic activities

*WBGT is *not* air temperature. It indicates wet bulb globe temperature, an index of climatic heat stress that can be measured on the field by the use of a psychrometer. This apparatus, available commercially, is composed of 3 thermometers. One (wet bulb [WB]) has a wet wick around it to monitor humidity. Another is inside a hollow black ball (globe [G]) to monitor radiation. The third is a simple thermometer (temperature [T] to measure air temperature. The heat stress index is calculated as WBGT = 0.7 WB temp + 0.2 G temp + 0.1 T temp. It is noteworthy that 70% of the stress is due to humidity, 20% to radiation, and only 10% to air temperature.

Source: American Academy of Pediatrics. Committee on Sports Medicine and Fitness (2000). Climatic heat stress and the exercising child and adolescent. *Pediatrics, 106,* 158–159, with permission.

Supervision and Protection

The coach is the primary supervisor of the athlete. The American Academy of Pediatrics (1989) recommends that all coaching staff members complete a certification course. Coverage of practices and competitions by qualified medical personnel (physician, physical therapist, or ATC) is a second level of supervision. These individuals provide immediate containment and correct management of injury or illness.

Providing the young athlete with high-quality equipment that is correctly fitted should be mandatory for safe participation (Castaldi, 1986; Kerr, 1986; Napier, Baker, Sanford, & Easterbrook, 1996). This equipment includes footwear, head and eye protection, padding, and mouth guards. Although the coaching staff is responsible for provision of appropriate equipment, it is often the physical therapist or athletic trainer who fits or modifies the equipment to the size or physical needs of the athlete. Physical therapists may also fabricate specialized equipment such as orthotics, soft casts or splints, and braces for athletes who are injured.

Playing areas should be well lit and free from obstacles and possess shock-absorbing qualities. Equipment modifications known to decrease injury (e.g., breakaway bases) should be used, and equipment and playing areas should be scaled to the size of the athletes (Stanitski, 1989). The knowledge of the physical therapist can be vital to correct choice or alteration of surface and equipment for safety of the athletes (i.e., wooden floors for dance activities).

CASE EXAMPLE 12–1 . . . .

A School Model

J.B. is a 14-year-old boy attending his preparticipation screening for high school junior varsity football. The physical therapist documents a right knee injury in middle-school football last year. J.B. reports that he had pain on the inside of his knee with minimal swelling. His knee was not examined by any medical personnel and the injury caused him to lose 2 weeks of play.

Examination by the physical therapist reveals no tenderness over the knee joint line. However, J.B. has tenderness at the origin of the infrapatellar tendon. Stability testing reveals no laxity of the anterior or posterior cruciate or lateral collateral ligaments. Slight laxity of the medial collateral ligament is noted. The physical therapist further documents that girth of the right thigh is decreased by 1 inch. Hip and knee range of motion is normal, but right hamstring flexibility is 15° less than the left side. Single-leg standing balance with eyes open is reduced by 15 seconds on the right lower extremity. Dynamic balance is decreased by 10 seconds on the right side.

The coach notes that timed single leg squats on the right leg are 50% of the left. Controlled lateral step-ups can be performed on a 12-inch step with the left leg but only a 6-inch step with the right. Cutting to the right is more cautious.

J.B. is referred to the physical therapist for development of a preseason training program to increase strength, balance, and power of the right lower extremity. His coach and parents are informed of the situation. The coach will supervise his program at school. He will be re-examined by the physical therapist every 2 weeks. When the strength and balance of the right side are 85% of the left, the physical therapist will release J.B. for play.

Community-Based Model

Many community-based models of sports participation exist for normally abled children and children with disabilities. Peewee Football and Little League are two well-known examples of programs for children with no disabilities. **Special Olympics** is one of the best-developed integrative models for children and adults with intellectual and/or developmental disabilities and will be used as an example of a community-based model.

The Kennedy Foundation spearheaded years of research and development of models and materials for sport skill assessment and programming, which has culminated in an adaptation of the President's Physical Fitness Test for skill evaluation of persons with mental retardation. The merger of testing and need for sports opportunity resulted in the first Special Olympics Games in 1968. The success of these games led to the establishment of Special Olympics, Inc., in 1969, and the subsequent development of accredited National and International Special Olympics Programs in 160 countries. The mission of the Special Olympics is similar to that of the school model: "to provide year-round sports training and athletic competition in a variety of Olympic-type sports for children and adults with mental retardation, giving them continuing opportunities to develop physical fitness, demonstrate courage, experience joy, and participate in a sharing of gifts, skills, and friendship with their families, other Special Olympics athletes,

and the community" (Special Olympics International, 2003).

The components of this model are similar to those of the school model. Physical therapists have participated in the primary care of these individuals to prepare them for participation and to manage their ongoing physical needs. In the fitness and wellness model, the physical therapist has an integral role in prevention through the screening of flexibility, functional strength, balance, and aerobic conditioning in FUNfitness, the physical therapy component of the *Healthy Athlete* (see later paragraph). Physical therapists are the ideal professionals to develop year-round fitness and health promotion programs for these individuals to promote wellness and reduce the occurrence and impact of secondary conditions, such as overweight and obesity, poor nutrition, and poor physical condition.

Preparticipation Screening Examination

The Special Olympics preparticipation screening is an individual physician examination. Persons must have a diagnosis of mental retardation, cognitive delay (I.Q. less than or equal to 80), or significant adaptive or learning problems secondary to the cognitive delay and requiring specially designed instruction to be eligible. The athlete must be at least 5 years of age to participate but more than 8 years of age to compete; no upper age limit for competition exists. An athlete must present an Athlete Registration Packet, which contains a medical examination signed by a physician who is familiar with the athlete. An athlete must submit a new medical application every 3 years unless a significant change in health occurs, necessitating a new medical examination. Any athlete with a diagnosis of Down syndrome must obtain a full radiological examination for atlantoaxial instability and be examined for cardiac anomalies. Jacob and Hutzler (1998) have reported successful use of the Sports-Medicine Assessment Protocol in athletes with neurological disorders as an additional tool to assess neurological function.

The Special Olympics, recognizing the disparity in health care for their members and the need to address routine health care, has developed the *Healthy Athlete* program. This program is a series of health services and education that address the most significant areas of disparity. Current venues include visual examination and eyeglass prescription; hearing examination and referral; dental examination; education and mouth guard fabrication; podiatric evaluation and education in foot and shoe care; education in areas of health promotion including nutrition, skin protection, substance avoidance, and ongoing fitness; and fitness screening and education (FUNfitness). Developed by the American Physical Therapy Association, FUNfitness is a fitness screening in which physical therapists screen athletes for selected flexibility, functional strength, balance, and aerobic conditioning. Based on the results of the screening, physical therapists educate athletes, parents, and coaches about correct and safe methods for improvement. Data collected at state, regional, and world games are being entered into an international database on the athletes.

Training and Conditioning

After athletes have been cleared to participate, they may choose any of 23 summer or winter sports. Each sport has a specific Sports Skills Assessment designed to determine the athlete's present level of function and to monitor training progress. Once a level of function (Level I or Level II) is determined, the athlete follows a specific training and conditioning program outlined in the Sports Skills Program (Special Olympics International, 2001).

These sports-specific program booklets contain sections on coaching techniques, warm-up, clothing, equipment, sportsmanship, and rules, as well as specific pathways for developing strength, flexibility, fitness, and power. The final sections address the development of specific skills for the sport. Each skill is broken down into sequential task progression with a complete task performance analysis and coaching suggestions. The specific training is designed for 8-week sessions before the competition, but longer training and year-round conditioning are encouraged. This expanded training can be performed in community organizations, in special adapted physical education programs, or with special coaches individually or in groups. Physical therapists should be involved in development of these programs in either the schools or the community.

Supervision and Participant Safety

The Special Olympics recommends that all coaches participate in the Coaches Training Program. Three levels of coaching education are available: The Volunteer Coach Certification Course, The Principles of Coaching Course, and The Advanced Coach Certification Course (Special Olympics International, 1994a). Those wishing to become officials must participate in an orientation and must learn specific Special Olympics sport rules. (Also available at *http://www.specialolympics.org/Special+ Olympics+Public+ Website/English/Coach/Training_Opportunities/default.htm)*

Physicians, physical therapists, ATCs, and emergency medical services personnel provide medical coverage at game events. They maintain adequate hydration for the environment and manage injury and illness related to participation. They also monitor the use and need for special equipment or orthotics secondary to physical disability or injury.

Several levels of competition and participation have been designed for athletes based on age, gender, and ability to ensure safe participation. Competitive divisions are established so that each participant has an equal chance of winning based on performance scores. Divisions are structured so that the difference between the best and the worst scores is only 10%.

Levels of competition were developed to ensure fair play. The Motor Activities Training Program (MATP) was designed to provide comprehensive motor activity and recreation training for people with severe mental retardation or multiple disabilities. The emphasis of MATP is on training in motor skill and dexterity and on participation rather than competition. After an 8-week training program, participants may take part in a Training Day to demonstrate a "personal best" (Special Olympics International, 1994b).

The Unified Sports R Program, launched in 1989, is also an option. This pioneer program brings together equal numbers of athletes with and without mental retardation, of similar age and ability, on competitive teams.

Each state holds at least one annual competition for qualifying athletes from each town, city, or area. The states then send representative athletes to the World Games, which are held every other year in the same manner as the Olympic Games. Beginning in 2004, the United States will initiate Regional Games, held annually for athletes from each state in the North American region.

CASE EXAMPLE 12–2. . . .

Community Model

K.T. is a 10-year-old girl who has mild mental retardation and myelomeningocele at T12/L1. She is wheelchair independent. Her physical therapist introduces K.T. and her family to the local Special Olympics coordinator. A physical examination is arranged with a local pediatrician, who clears her to participate. A physical therapist performs an examination and evaluation of her strength, mobility, and endurance. K.T. decides to participate in wheelchair running and is introduced to the local coach, who places her in the appropriate competition level for her age and skill.

The coach and physical therapist modify the Special Olympics training program. K.T. begins training twice weekly, once with her coach and once with her parents. She is re-examined by her physical therapist every 2 weeks for re-evaluation and progression of her program. The physical therapist modifies her wheelchair and her seating for more efficient and safe function during sport. K.T. trains for 12 weeks before she is ready to compete in a state Special Olympics Games. In discussion with her coach and physical therapist, K.T. decides that at the age of 14 years, she will enter a Unified Sports R Wheelchair Running Team for racing and relay.

Summary

Participation in sports and recreation is a vital part of the life of both children and young adults. The elements of safe and successful participation are similar for children with or without a disability. The two models described differ primarily in location, cost, and base of support. Both can apply to all athletes regardless of ability.

The physical therapist has an important role in each model, both in prevention and wellness and in primary care for the management of the athlete. The prevention role encompasses musculoskeletal screening with tests and measurements, formulation of intervention to increase sports function and overall fitness, and education in injury risk prevention. The primary care management might consist of intervention to manage an injury, modification of equipment, or fabrication of special orthotics, prosthetics, or other devices. The broad scientific and medical knowledge of physical therapists makes them integral and vital members of the prevention and management team.

Acknowledgment: Special thanks to Lori Bolgla, PT, ATC, for her thoughtful comments and revisions to this chapter.

DISCUSSION QUESTIONS

1. Describe the research knowledge of types and incidence of injuries in children and youth during sports and recreation.

2. Discuss the unique developmental and physiological characteristics of children that distinguish them from adults.

3. Outline several of the unique injuries incurred by children.

4. Discuss the primary components of any sports model for children and youth.

5. Outline the similarities and differences in models for normally abled children and children with disabilities.

RECOMMENDED READINGS

ACSM's Guidelines for exercise testing and prescription (6th ed.). (2000). Hagerstown, MD: Lippincott Williams & Wilkins.

Anderson, S., & Sullivan, J.A. (Eds.). (2000). *Care of the young athlete.* Rosemont, IL: American Academy of Pediatrics, American Academy of Orthopaedic Surgeons.

Anderson, B. (2000). *Stretching.* Bolinas, CA: Shelter Publishing.

American College of Sports Medicine. Website: *http://www.acsm.org*

American Physical Therapy Association. Website: *http://www.apta.org*

Baechle, T., & Earle, R. (Eds.). (2000). *Essentials of strength training* (2nd ed.). Champaign, IL: Human Kinetics.

Docherty, D. (Ed.). (1996). *Measurement in paediatric exercise science.* Champaign, IL: Human Kinetics.

Durstine, J.L., & Moore, G. (2000). *ACSM's Exercise management for persons with chronic disease and disabilities.* Champaign, IL: Human Kinetics.

Gisolfi, C., & Lamb, D. (Eds). (2001). *Perspectives in exercise science and sports medicine. Volume 2: Youth, exercise, and sports.* New Haven, CT: Cooper Publishers.

Horowicz, S., Kerker, B., Ownes, P., & Zigler, E. (2001). *The health status and needs of individuals with mental retardation.* Washington, DC: Special Olympics, Inc.

Kraemer, W., & Fleck, S. (1992). *Strength training for young athletes.* Champaign, IL: Human Kinetics.

McArdle, W., Katch, F., & Katch, V. (2001). *Exercise physiology: Energy, nutrition, and human performance.* Hagerstown, MD: Lippincott Williams & Wilkins.

McArdle, W., Katch, F., & Katch, V. (1999). *Sports and exercise nutrition.* Philadelphia: Lippincott Williams & Wilkins.

National Athletic Training Association. Website: *http://www.nata.org*

Nicole, N., Barry, M., Dillingham, J., & McGuire, M. (2002). *Nonsurgical sports medicine: Preparticipation exam through rehabilitation.* Baltimore: Johns Hopkins University Press.

Rowland, T. (1996). *Developmental exercise physiology.* Champaign, IL: Human Kinetics.

Special Olympics, Inc. *Website: http://www.specialolympics.org*

Westcott, W., & Faigenbaum, A. (2000). *Strength and power for young athletes.* Champaign, IL: Human Kinetics.

REFERENCES

Adirim, T.A., & Cheng, T.L. (2003). Overview of injuries in the young athlete. *Sports Medicine, 33,* 75–81.

American Academy of Family Physicians, American Academy of Pediatrics, American Medical Society for Sports Medicine, American Orthopedic Society for Sports Medicine, and American Osteopathic Academy of Sports Medicine (1997). *Preparticipation physical examination.* Available from *http://www.aafp.org*

American Academy of Pediatrics, Committee on Sports Medicine and Fitness (1988). Recommendations for participation in competitive sports. *Pediatrics, 81,* 737.

American Academy of Pediatrics (1989). Organized athletics for preadolescent children. *Pediatrics, 84,* 583–584.

American Academy of Pediatrics, Committee on Sports Medicine and Fitness (2000). Climatic heat stress and the exercising child and adolescent. *Pediatrics, 106,* 158–159.

American Academy of Pediatrics, Committee on Sports Medicine and Fitness (2001). Medical conditions affecting sports participation. *Pediatrics, 107,* 1205–1209.

American Heart Association (2003). Body composition tests. Retrieved September 13, 2003, from *http://www.americanheart. org.presenter.jhtml?identifier=4489*

American Medical Association, Council on Scientific Affairs (1993). Ensuring the health of the adolescent athlete. *Archives of Family Medicine, 2,* 446–448.

American Physical Therapy Association (2002). *Guide to physical therapist practice.* CD-ROM, v 1.1. Alexandria, VA: Author.

American Physical Therapy Association (2003). *FUNfitness.* Retrieved September 4, 2003, from *http://www.apta.org/PT_Practice/prevention_wellness/FUNfitness/*

Armsey, T.D., & Green, G.A. (1997). Nutrition supplements: Science vs. hype. *Physician and Sports Medicine, 25,* 77–92.

Armstrong, L.E., & Maresh, C.M. (1995). Exercise-heat tolerance of children and adolescents. *Exercise Science, 7,* 239–252.

Athletic Fitness Scorecards (1988). *Patient care,* October 30. Montvale, NJ: Medical Economics Publishing.

Axe, M.J., Newcomb, W.A., & Warner, D. (1991). Sports injuries and adolescent athletes. *Developmental Medicine Journal, 63,* 359–363.

Backx, F.J., Beijer, H.J., Bol, E., & Erich, W.B. (1991). Injuries in high-risk persons and high-risk sports: A longitudinal study of 1818 school children. *American Journal of Sports Medicine, 19,* 124–130.

Bahrke, M.S., Yesalis, C.E., & Brower, K.J. (1998). Anabolic-androgenic steroid abuse and performance-enhancing drugs among adolescents. *Child and Adolescent Psychiatric Clinics of North America, 7,* 821–838.

Balsom, P.D., Soderlund, K., & Ekblom, B. (1994). Creatine in humans with special reference to creatine supplementation. *Sports Medicine, 18,* 268–280.

Bar-Or, O. (1995). The young athlete: Some physiological considerations. *Journal of Sports Sciences, 13,* S31–S33.

Bar-Or, O., Lombardo, J.A., & Rowland, T.W. (1988). The preparticipation sports exam. *Patient Care,* October, 75–102.

Bar-Or, O., & Unnithan, V.B. (1994). Nutritional requirements of young soccer players. *Journal of Sports Sciences, 12,* S39–S42.

Beachy, G., Akau, C.K., Martinson, M., & Olderr, T.F. (1997). High school sports injuries. A longitudinal study at Punahou School: 1988 to 1996. *American Journal of Sports Medicine, 25,* 675–681.

Bell, D.G., McLellan, T.M., & Sabiston, C.M. (2002). Effect of ingesting caffeine and ephedrine on performance. *Medicine and Science in Sports and Exercise, 34,* 344–349.

Below, P.R., Mora-Rodriquez, R., Gonzalez-Alonso, J., & Coyle, E.F. (1995). Fluid and carbohydrate ingestion independently improve performance during 1 h of intense exercise. *Medicine and Science in Sports and Exercise, 27,* 200–210.

Benson, L.S., Waters, P.M., Meier, S.W., Visotsky, J.L., & Williams, C.S. (2000). Pediatric hand injuries due to home exercycles. *Journal of Pediatric Orthopedics, 20,* 34–39.

Bernhardt-Bainbridge, D. (2000). Sports injuries in children. In S.K. Campbell, D.W. VanderLinden, & R.J. Palisano (Eds.), *Physical therapy for children* (2nd ed., pp. 429–467). Philadelphia: W.B. Saunders.

Bernhardt, D.T., Gomez, J., Johnson, M.D., Martin, T.J., Rowland, T.W., Small, E., et al. (2001). Strength training by children and adolescents. *Pediatrics, 107,* 1470–1472.

Bijur, P.E., Trumble, A., Harel, Y., Overpeck, M.D., Jones, D., & Scheidt, P.C. (1995). Sports and recreation injuries in US children and adolescents. *Archives of Pediatric and Adolescent Medicine, 149,* 1009–1016.

Birrer, R.B., & Brecher, D.B. (1987*). Common sports injuries in youngsters.* Los Angeles: PMIC.

Blimkie, C.J.R. (1993). Resistance training during preadolescence. *Issues in Controversial Medicine, 15,* 389–407.

Bratton, R.L. (1997). Preparticipation screening of children for sports. Current recommendations. *Sports Medicine, 24,* 300–307.

Brown, R.L., Brunn, M.A., & Garcia, V.F. (2001). Cervical spine injuries in children: A review of 103 patients treated consecutively at a level 1 pediatric trauma center. *Journal of Pediatric Surgery, 36,* 1107–1114.

Brown, R.L., Koepplinger, M.E., Mehlman, C.T., Gittelman, M., & Garcia, V.F. (2002). All-terrain vehicle and bicycle crashes in children: Epidemiology and comparison of injury severity. *Journal of Pediatric Surgery, 37,* 375–380.

Campbell-Hewson, G.L., Robinson, S.M., & Egleston, C.V. (1999). Equestrian injuries in the paediatric age group: A two centre study. *European Journal of Emergency Medicine, 6,* 37–40.

Casa, D.J., Armstrong, L.E., Hillman, S.K., Montain, S.J., Reiff, R.V., Rich, B.S.E., Roberts, W.O., & Stone, J.A. (2000). National Athletic Trainers' Association position: Fluid replacement for athletes. *Journal of Athletic Training, 35,* 212–224.

Castaldi, C.R. (1986). Sports related oral and facial injuries in the young athlete: A new challenge for the pediatric dentist. *Pediatric Dentistry, 8,* 311–316.

Challier, B., Chau, N., Predine, R., Choquet, M., & Legras, B. (2000). Associations of family environment and individual factors with tobacco, alcohol, and illicit drug use in adolescents. *European Journal of Epidemiology, 16,* 33–42.

Clark, N. (1991). Nutrition: Pre-, intra-, and postcompetition. In R.C. Cantu & L.J. Micheli (Eds.), *ACSM's guidelines for the team physician* (pp. 58–65). Philadelphia: Lea & Febiger.

Coady, C.M., & Micheli, L.J. (1997). Stress fractures in the pediatric athlete. *Clinics in Sports Medicine, 16,* 225–238.

Conn, J.M., Annest, J.L., & Gilchrist, J. (2003). Sports and recreation related injury episodes in the US populations, 1997–99. *Injury Prevention, 9,* 117–123.

Curtis, K.A. (1982). Wheelchair sports medicine: IV. Athletic injuries. *Sports n' Spokes, January/February,* 20–24.

Curtis, K.A., & Black, K. (1999). Shoulder pain in female wheelchair basketball players. *Journal of Orthopedic and Sports Physical Therapy, 29,* 225–231.

Damore, D.T. (2002). Preschool and school age activities: Comparison of urban and suburban populations. *Journal of Community Health, 27,* 203–211.

Davis, J.M. (1995). Carbohydrates, branched-chain amino acids, and endurance: Influence of HCO_2. *International Journal of Sports Nutrition, 5,* S29–S38.

Davis, J.M., Welsh, R.S., & Alerson, N.A. (2000). Effects of carbohydrate and chromium ingestion during intermittent high intensity exercise to fatigue. *International Journal of Sport Nutrition and Exercise Metabolism, 10,* 476–485.

Deibert, M.C., Aronsson, D.D., Johnson, R.J., Ettlinger, C.F., & Shealy, J.E. (1998). Skiing injuries in children, adolescents, and adults. *Journal of Bone and Joint Surgery (American), 80,* 25–32.

Drezner, J.A. (2000). Sudden cardiac death in young athletes. Causes, athlete's heart, and screening guidelines. *Postgraduate Medicine, 108,* 37–44, 47–50.

Drkulec, J.A., & Letts, M. (2001). Snowboarding injuries in children. *Canadian Journal of Surgery, 44,* 435–439.

DuRant, R.H., Escobedo, L.G., & Heath, G.W. (1995). Anabolic-steroid use, strength training, and multiple drug use among adolescents in the United States. *Pediatrics, 96,* 23–28.

Faigenbaum, A.D., Loud, R.L., O'Connell, J., Glover, S., & Westcott, W.L. (2001). Effects of different resistance training protocols on upper-body strength and endurance development in children. *Journal of Strength and Conditioning Research, 15,* 459–465.

Falk, B. (1998). Effects of thermal stress during rest and exercise in the paediatric population. *Sports Medicine, 25,* 221–240.

Falk, B., & Tenenbaum, G. (1996). The effectiveness of resistance training in children. A meta-analysis. *Sports Medicine, 3,* 176–186.

Falkel, J. (1986). Methods of training. In D.B. Bernhardt (Ed.), *Sports physical therapy* (pp. 55–79). New York: Churchill Livingstone.

Ferrara, M.S., Buckley, W.E., McCann, B.C., Limbird, T.J.,

Powell, J.W., & Robl, R. (1992). The injury experience of a competitive athlete with a disability: Prevention implications. *Medicine and Science in Sports and Exercise, 24,* 184–188.

Fields, K.B. (1994). Clearing athletes for participation in sports. The North Carolina Medical Society Sports Medicine Committee's recommended examination. *North Carolina Medical Journal, 55,* 116–121.

Forman, E.S., Dekker, A.H., Javors, J.R., & Davison, D.T. (1995). High-risk behaviors in teenage male athletes. *Clinical Journal of Sport Medicine, 5,* 36–42.

Fuller, C.M., McNulty, C.M., Spring, D.A., Arger, K.M., Bruce, S.S., Chryssos, B.E., Drummer, E.M., Kelley, F.P., Newmark, M.J., & Whipple, G.H. (2000). Prospective screening of 5,615 high school athletes for risk of sudden cardiac death. *Medicine and Science in Sports and Exercise, 32,* 1809–1811.

Furnival, R.A., Street, K.A., & Schunk, J.E. (1999). Too many pediatric trampoline injuries. *Pediatrics, 103,* e57.

Galena, H.J., Epstein, C.R., & Lourie, R.J. (1998). Connecticut State Special Olympics: Observations and recommendations. *Connecticut Medicine, 62,* 33–37.

Galloway, S.D., & Maughan, R.J. (2000). The effects of substrate and fluid provision on thermoregulatory and metabolic responses to prolonged exercise in a hot environment. *Journal of Sports Science, 18,* 339–351.

Gerstenbluth, R.E., Spirnak, J.P., & Elder, J.S. (2002). Sports participation and high grade renal injuries in children. *Journal of Urology, 168,* 2575–2578.

Gerrard, D.F. (1993). Overuse injury and growing bones: The young athlete at risk. *British Journal of Sports Medicine, 27,* 14–18.

Gill, T.J., & Micheli, L.J. (1996). The immature athlete. Common injuries and overuse syndromes of the elbow and wrist. *Clinics in Sports Medicine, 15,* 401–423.

Glover, D.W., & Maron, B.J. (1998). Profile of preparticipation cardiovascular screening for high school athletes. *Journal of the American Medical Association, 279,* 1817–1819.

Greydanus, D.E., & Patel, D.R. (2002). Sports doping in the adolescent athlete: The hope, hype and hyperbole. *Pediatric Clinics of North America, 49,* 829–855.

Guy, J.A., & Micheli, L.J. (2001). Strength training for children and adolescents. *Journal of the American Academy of Orthpaedic Surgery, 9,* 29–36.

Haller, C.A., & Benowitz, N.L. (2000). Adverse cardiovascular and central nervous system events associated with dietary supplements containing ephedra alkaloids. *New England Journal of Medicine, 343,* 1833–1838.

Heath, G.W., Pratt, M., Warren, C.W., & Kann, L. (1994). Physical activity patterns in American high school students. Results from the 1990 Youth Risk Behavior Survey. *Archives of Pediatric and Adolescent Medicine, 148,* 1131–1136.

Heinonen, O.J. (1996). Carnitine and physical exercise. *Sports Medicine, 22,* 109–132.

Heyward, V. (2001). ASEP Methods recommendation: Body composition assessment. *Journal of Exercise Physiology, 4,* 1–12.

Hoeberigs, J.H., Deberts-Eggen, H.B., & Deberts, P.M. (1990). Sports medical experience from the International Flower Marathon for disabled wheelers. *American Journal of Sports Medicine, 18,* 418–421.

Iuliano, S., Naughton, G., Collier, G., & Carlson, J. (1998). Examination of the self-selected fluid intake practices by junior athletes during a simulated duathlon event. *International Journal of Sport Nutrition, 8,* 10–23.

Iven, V.G. (1998). Recreational drugs. *Clinics in Sports Medicine, 17,* 245–259.

Jacob, T., & Hutzler, Y. (1998). Sports-medical assessment for athletes with a disability. *Disability Rehabilitation, 20,* 116–119.

Kerr, I.L. (1986). Mouth guards for the prevention of injuries in contact sports. *Sports Medicine, 5,* 415–427.

Klish, W.J. (1995). Childhood obesity: Pathophysiology and treatment. *Acta Paediatrica Japonica, 37,* 1–6.

Kraemer, W.J., & Fleck, S. (1993). *Strength training for young athletes.* Champaign, IL: Human Kinetics.

Kreider, R.B., Ferriera, M., Wilson, M, Grindstaff, P., Plisk, S., Reinardy, J., Cantler, E., & Almada, A.L. (1998). Effects of creatine supplementation on body composition, strength, and sprint performance. *Medicine and Science in Sports and Exercise, 30,* 73–82.

Kreider, R.B., Miriel, V., & Bertun, E. (1993). Amino acid supplementation and exercise performance: Analysis of the proposed ergogenic value. *Sports Medicine, 16,* 190–209.

Kubiak, R., & Slongo, T. (2003). Unpowered scooter injuries in children. *Acta Pediatrica, 92,* 50–54.

Kurowski, K., & Chandran, S. (2000). The preparticipation athletic evaluation. *American Family Physician, 61,* 2683–2690, 2696–2698.

Laure, P. (1997). Epidemiological approach of doping in sport. A review. *Journal of Sports Medicine and Physical Fitness, 37,* 218–224.

Lombardo, J.A. (1991). Preparticipation examination. In R.C. Cantu & L.J. Micheli (Eds), *ACSM's guidelines for the team physician.* (pp. 71–94). Philadelphia: Lea & Febiger.

Lyznicki, J.M, Nielsen, N.H., & Schneider, J.F. (2000). Cardiovascular screening of student athletes. *American Family Physician, 15,* 2332.

Maffulli, N. (1990). Intensive training in young athletes. *Sports Medicine, 9,* 229–243.

Maffulli, N., & Bruns, W. (2000). Injuries in young athletes. *European Journal of Pediatrics, 159,* 59–63.

Malina, R.M. (1994). Physical growth and biological maturation of young athletes. *Exercise and Sport Sciences Review, 22,* 389–433.

Mankovsky, A.B., Mendoza-Sagaon, M., Cardinaux, C., Hohlfeld, J., & Reinberg, O. (2002). Evaluation of scooter-related injuries in children. *Journal of Pediatric Surgery, 37,* 755–759.

Maron, B.J. (2002). The young competitive athlete with cardiovascular abnormalities: Causes of sudden death, detection by preparticipation screening, and standards for disqualification. *Cardiac Electrophysiology Review, 6,* 100–103.

Maughan, R. (2002). The athlete's diet: Nutritional goals and dietary strategies. *Proceedings of the Nutrition Society, 61,* 87–96.

McCormick, D.P., Niebiehr, V.N., & Risser, W.L. (1990). Injury and illness surveillance at local Special Olympic Games. *British Journal of Sports Medicine, 24,* 221–224.

Messina, D.F., Farney, W.C., & DeLee, J.C. (1999). The incidence of injury in Texas high school basketball. A prospective study among male and female athletes. *American Journal of Sports Medicine, 27,* 294–299.

Metzl, J.D. (1999). Strength training and nutritional supplement use in adolescents. *Current Opinion in Pediatrics, 11,* 292–296.

Micheli, L.J. (1995). Sports injuries in children and adolescents. Questions and controversies. *Clinics in Sports Medicine, 143,* 727–745.

Micheli, L.J., & Fehlandt, A.F. (1992). Overuse injuries to tendons and apophyses in children and adolescents. *Clinics in Sports Medicine, 11,* 713–726.

Micheli, L.J., & Wood, R. (1995). Back pain in young athletes. Significant differences from adults in causes and patterns. *Archives of Pediatric and Adolescent Medicine, 149,* 15–18.

Napier, S.M., Baker, R.S., Sanford, D.G., & Easterbrook, M. (1996). Eye injuries in athletics and recreation. *Surgical Ophthalmology, 41,* 229–244.

National Federation of State High School Associations (2003). *Heat stress and athletic participation.* Position paper. Indianapolis, IN: Author.

Nguyen, D., & Letts, M. (2001). In-line skating injuries in children: A 10-year review. *Journal of Pediatric Orthopedics, 21,* 612–618.

Nsuami, M., Elie, M., Brooks, B.N., Sanders, L.S., Nash, T.D., Makonnen, F., Taylor, S.N., & Cohen, D.A. (2003). Screening for sexually transmitted diseases during preparticipation sports examination of high school adolescents. *Journal of Adolescent Health, 32,* 336–339.

Omey, M.L., & Micheli, L.J. (1999). Foot and ankle problems in the young athlete. *Medicine and Science in Sports and Exercise, 31,* S470–S486.

Osberg, J.S., Schneps, S.E., DiScala, C., & Li, G. (1998). Skateboarding: More dangerous than roller skating or in-line skating. *Archives of Pediatric and Adolescent Medicine, 152,* 985–991.

Outerbridge, A.R., & Micheli, L.J. (1995). Overuse injuries in the young athlete. *Clinics in Sports Medicine, 14,* 503–516.

Passe, D., Horn, M., & Murray, R. (2000). Impact of beverage acceptability on fluid intake during exercise. *Appetite, 35,* 219–225.

Patel, D.R., & Nelson, T.L. (2000). Sports injuries in children. *Medical Clinics of North America, 844,* 983–1007.

Peltz, J.E., Haskell, W.L., & Matheson, G.O. (1999). A comprehensive and cost-effective preparticipation exam implemented on the World Wide Web. *Medicine and Science in Sports and Exercise, 31,* 1727–1740.

Peterson, M., & Peterson, K. (1988). *Eat to compete: A guide to sports nutrition.* Chicago: Year Book Medical Publishers.

Powell, E.C., & Tanz, R.R. (2000a). Cycling injuries treated in emergency departments: Need for bicycle helmets among preschoolers. *Archives of Pediatric and Adolescent Medicine, 154,* 1096–1100.

Powell, E.C., & Tanz, R.R. (2000b). Tykes and bikes: Injuries associated with bicycle-towed child trailers and bicycle-mounted child seats. *Archives of Pediatric and Adolescent Medicine, 154,* 352–353.

Pratt, M., Macera, C.A., & Blanton, C. (1999). Levels of physical activity and inactivity in children and adults in the United States: Current evidence and research issues. *Medicine and Science in Sports and Exercise, 31,* S526–S533.

Puranik, S., Long, J., & Coffman, S. (1998). Profile of pediatric bicycle injuries. *Southern Medical Journal, 91,* 1033–1037.

Radelet, M.A., Lephart, S.M., Rubenstein, E.N., & Mayers, J.B. (2002). Survey of the injury rate for children in community sports. *Pediatrics, 110,* e28.

Ramsey, J.A., Blunkie, C., Smith, K., Garner, S., MacDougall, J.D., & Digby, G.S. (1990). Strength training effects in prepubescent boys. *Medicine and Science in Sports and Exercise, 22,* 605–614.

Rifat, S.F., Ruffin, M.T., & Gorenflo, D.W. (1995). Disqualifying criteria in a preparticipation sports evaluation. *Journal of Family Practice, 41,* 42–50.

Rivera-Brown, A., Gutierrez, R., Gutierrez, J.C., Frontera, W.R., & Bar-Or, O. (1999). Drink composition, voluntary drinking and fluid balance in exercising. *Journal of Applied Physiology, 86,* 78–84.

Rowland, T.W. (1996). *Developmental exercise physiology.* Champaign, IL: Human Kinetics.

Shi, X., Summers, R.W., Schedl, H.P., Flanagan, S.W., Chang, R., & Gisolfi, C.V. (1995). Effects of carbohydrate type and concentration and solution osmolality on water absorption. *Medicine and Science in Sports and Exercise, 27,* 1607–1615.

Shorter, N.A., Mooney, D.P., & Harmon, B.J. (1999). Snowboarding injuries in children and adolescents. *American Journal of Emergency Medicine, 17,* 261–263.

Skokan, E.G., Junkins, E.P., & Kadish, H. (2003). Serious winter sport injuries in children and adolescents requiring hospitalization. *American Journal of Emergency Medicine, 21,* 95–99.

Sorensen, L., Larsen, S.E., & Rock, N.D. (1996). The epidemiology of sports injuries in school-aged children. *Scandinavian Journal of Medicine and Science in Sports, 6,* 281–286.

Special Olympics International (1994a). *Special Olympics general session information pamphlet.* Washington, DC: Author.

Special Olympics International (1994b). *Special Olympics fact sheet.* Washington, DC: Author.

Special Olympics International (2001). *Special Olympics Winter World Games medical data.* Washington, DC: Author.

Special Olympics International (2003). *The mission of the Special Olympics.* Retrieved September 4, 2003, from *http://www.specialolympics.org*

Squire, D.L. (1990). Heat illness: Fluid and electrolyte issues for pediatric and adolescent athletes. *Pediatric Clinics of North America, 37,* 1085–1109.

Stanitski, C. (1989). Common injuries in preadolescent athletes. *Sports Medicine, 7,* 32–41.

Stronski, S.M., Ireland, M., Michaud, P., Narring, F., & Resnick, M.D. (2000). Protective correlates of stages in adolescent substance use: A Swiss national study. *Journal of Adolescent Health, 26,* 420–427.

Swenson, E.J. (1991). Setting up a high school sports medicine program. *Journal of Musculoskeletal Medicine,* September, 14–28.

Taylor, B.L., & Attia, M.W. (2000). Sports-related injuries in children. *Academy of Emergency Medicine, 7,* 1376–1382.

Taylor, D., & Williams, T. (1995). Sports injuries in athletes with disabilities: Wheelchair racing. *Paraplegia, 33,* 296–299.

Tenvergert, E.M., Ten Duis, H.J., & Klasen, H.J. (1992). Trends in sports injuries, 1982–1988: An in-depth study on four types of sports. *Journal of Sports Medicine and Physical Fitness, 32,* 214–220.

Thabit, G., & Micheli, L.J. (1992). Patellofemoral pain in the pediatric patient. *Orthopedic Clinics of North America, 23,* 567–585.

Turley, K.R. (1997). Cardiovascular responses to exercise in children. *Sports Medicine, 24,* 241–257.

United States Department of Health and Human Services (2001). *Surgeon General's call to action to prevent and decrease overweight and obesity.* Washington, DC: Author.

Utter, A., Kang, J., Nieman, D., & Warren, B. (1997). Effect of carbohydrate substrate availability on ratings of perceived exertion during prolonged running. *International Journal of Sport Nutrition, 7,* 274–285.

van Hall, G., Raaymakers, J.S.H., Saris, W.H.M., & Wagenmakers, A.J.M. (1995). Ingestion of branched-chain amino acids and tryptophan during sustained exercise in man: Failure to affect performance. *Journal of Physiology, 486,* 789–794.

Watkins, J., & Peabody, P. (1996). Sports injuries in children and adolescents treated at a sports injury clinic. *Journal of Sports Medicine and Physical Fitness, 36,* 43–48.

Wilk, B., & Bar-Or, O. (1996). Effect of drink flavor and NaCl on voluntary drinking and hydration in boys exercising in the heat. *Journal of Applied Physiology, 80,* 1112–1117.

Wilson, P.E., & Washington, R.L. (1993). Pediatric wheelchair athletes: Sports injuries and prevention. *Paraplegia, 31,* 330–337.

Winston, F.K., Weiss, H.B., Nance, M.L., Vivarelli-O'Neill, C., Strotmeyer, S., Lawrence, B.A., & Miller, T.R. (2002). Estimates of the incidence and costs associated with handlebar-related injuries in children. *Archives of Pediatric and Adolescent Medicine, 156,* 922–928.

Yesalis, C.E., & Bahrke, M.S. (2000). Doping among adolescent athletes. *Baillieres Best Practice and Research in Clinical Endocrinology and Metabolism, 14,* 25–35.

Appendix *12.A*

Recommendations for Participation in Competitive Sports

	Contact/Collision	Noncontact			
		Limited Contact/Impact	Strenuous	Moderately Strenuous	Nonstrenuous
Atlantoaxial Instability * Swimming: no butterfly, breast stroke, or diving starts	No	No	Yes*	Yes	Yes
Acute Illnesses * Needs individual assessment, e.g., contagiousness to others, risk of worsening illness	*	*	*	*	*

Cardiovascular
  Carditis*
  Hypertension
    Mild
    Moderate
    Severe
  Congenital heart disease
* Needs individual assessment
† Patients with mild forms can be allowed a full range of physical activities; patients with moderate or severe forms, or who are post-operative, should be evaluated by a cardiologist before athletic participation.
	No
	
	Yes
	*
	*
	†
		No
		
		Yes
		*
		*
		†
			No
			
			Yes
			*
			*
			†
				No
				
				Yes
				*
				*
				†
					No
					
					Yes
					*
					*
					†

Eyes
  Absence or loss of function of one eye
  Detached retina
* Availability of American Society for Testing and Materials (ASTM)-approved eye guards may allow competitor to participate in most sports, but this must be judged on an individual basis.
† Consult ophthalmologist
	*
	
	†
		*
		
		†
			*
			
			†
				*
				
				†
					*
					
					†

Inguinal hernia Kidney: Absence of one Liver: Enlarged Musculoskeletal disorders * Needs individual assessment	Yes No No *	Yes Yes No *	Yes Yes Yes *	Yes Yes Yes *	Yes Yes Yes *

	Contact/ Collision	Limited Contact/Impact	Strenuous	Moderately Strenuous	Nonstrenuous
Neurologic					
History of serious head or spine trauma, repeated concussions, or craniotomy	*	*	Yes	Yes	Yes
Convulsive disorder					
Well controlled	Yes	Yes	Yes	Yes	Yes
Poorly controlled	No	No	Yes†	Yes	Yes‡
* Needs individual assessment					
† No swimming or weight lifting					
‡ No archery or riflery					
Ovary: Absence of one	Yes	Yes	Yes	Yes	Yes
Respiratory					
Pulmonary insufficiency	*	*	*	*	Yes
Asthma	Yes	Yes	Yes	Yes	Yes
* May be allowed to compete if oxygenation remains satisfactory during a graded stress test					
Sickle cell trait	Yes	Yes	Yes	Yes	Yes
Skin: Boils, herpes, impetigo, scabies	*	*	Yes	Yes	Yes
* No gymnastics with mats, martial arts, wrestling, or contact sports until not contagious					
Spleen: Enlarged	No	No	No	Yes	Yes
Testicle: Absent or undescended	Yes*	Yes*	Yes	Yes	Yes
* Certain sports may require protective cup					

Source: American Academy of Pediatrics Committee on Sports Medicine and Fitness (1988). Recommendations for participation in competitive sports. *Pediatrics, 81,* 737.

Appendix *12.B*

RECOMMENDED DIETARY ALLOWANCES FOR THE GROWING CHILD

Nutrient Requirements by Age						
Nutrient	**Daily Value**	**1–3 years**	**4–8 years**	**9–13 years**	**Girls 14–18 years**	**Boys 14–18 years**
Protein (grams)	50	16	28	46	55	66
Iron (mg)	18	7	10	8	15	11
Calcium (mg)	1000	500	800	1300	1300	1300
Vitamin A (IU)	5000	1000	1333	2000	2333	3000
Vitamin C (mg)	60	15	25	45	65	75
Fiber	23	6–8	9–13	14–18	19–24	19–24
Sodium (mg)	2400	600 to 1300	1200 to 2000	1900 to 3000	3000	2400 to 2700
Cholesterol (mg)	300	<300	<300	<300	<300	<300
Saturated Fat (g)	20	14	20 to 22	24 to 27	24	33
Total Fat (g)	65	43	60 to 67	73 to 83	73	about 100
Calories	2000	1300	1800 to 2000	2200 to 2500	2200	3000

Source: United States Department of Agriculture/Agricultural Research Service (2003). Children's Nutrition Research Center, Baylor College of Medicine.

Chapter 13

The Pediatric Acute-Care Hospital

— Pamela Girvin Hackett, MPT

The pediatric acute-care hospital presents a unique and challenging environment in which to practice physical therapy. The therapist is required to provide intervention in the context of the child's medical goals with a heightened concern for the individual's physiological stability and tolerance. The wide variety of diagnoses and impairments encountered provides an opportunity to gain more advanced knowledge of physiology, pharmacology, medical technology, and contemporary surgical techniques. In this setting, the physical therapist is a member of a diverse team of medical professionals who must work together to provide a comprehensive intervention program. The fast pace and ever-changing schedule demand both flexibility and strong communication skills because the physical therapist must coordinate intervention around a host of tests, procedures, physician rounds, family visits, and the child's ever-changing medical status.

Within the pediatric acute-care hospital exists a variety of specialized areas of practice, including the intensive care unit (ICU), cardiac ICU (CICU), neonatal ICU (NICU) (see Chapter 14), medical-surgical units, burn units, oncology, and a wide range of outpatient clinics. In this chapter, we will look at the role of the physical therapist in several

of these settings through the clinical management of some common diagnoses.

Pediatric Intensive Care Unit

The **pediatric ICU** provides intensive, close monitoring and intervention for critically ill or injured children, as well as for those at high risk for respiratory, neurological, or cardiovascular failure. This includes children who are in the fragile postoperative period, children or infants requiring mechanical ventilation, children with sepsis or multisystem organ failure, and victims of acute trauma. The ICU is a technology-rich environment that requires the therapist to receive ongoing learning and orientation from nursing, physician, and respiratory therapy staff members. In return, the physical therapist is able to act as a resource for early positioning, mobility, and appropriate stimulation as the rehabilitation process begins. The ICU is a very dynamic place that requires a great deal of flexibility on the part of the rehabilitation team. The children's unstable medical status requires frequent and open communication with the medical staff regarding physician orders and precautions.

Children With Acute Head Trauma

With the regionalization of trauma care for children, the intervention for children with head trauma plays an important part in the therapist's practice in a children's hospital. Traumatic brain injury (TBI) is the most common cause of traumatic death in both children and adults (Ward, 1995). Typical methods of injury vary by age, with falls accounting for most head trauma and deaths in children under age 5, and motor vehicle-related injuries most common among 5- to 55-year-olds (Luerssen & Klauber, 1998). Victims of trauma, as a result of the severity and complexity of their injuries, can require the services of a comprehensive team of medical professionals. The **trauma team** may include representatives from the following services: Trauma Surgery, Neurosurgery, Critical Care, Social Work, Occupational Therapy, Physical Therapy, Speech-Language Pathology, Physiatry, Orthopedics, and Plastic Surgery, as well as a highly skilled nursing staff.

Examination and Evaluation

Physical therapy is generally consulted as soon as the child is no longer in critical condition. Examination and intervention may remain limited as a result of increased intracranial pressure (normal is 10 mm Hg for a person lying flat), spinal precautions, fractures, and general medical instability. Consequently, it is imperative to coordinate the timing and extent of the physical therapy examination and intervention with the nursing and medical staff. In the initial stages, it is often best for the therapy/rehabilitation team to assess the child as a group to minimize duplication of testing and reduce stress.

The process of rehabilitation for both the child and family begins with the initial neuro-rehabilitation examination in the ICU (see Chapters 2 and 6). A thorough reading of the history and physical should precede the initiation of the examination because trauma cases tend to be among the most medically complex that a therapist will encounter. The physical therapy examination should ultimately include an assessment of basic cognitive orientation (see Table 6.4 for Rancho Los Amigos Pediatric Levels of Consciousness), range of motion (ROM), active movement, gross strength and quality of movement, muscle tone or stiffness, postural stability, sensation, and functional mobility. However, in many cases the initial examination is based on observation only because the child often cannot tolerate handling or follow commands. In the ICU, the primary goal of the therapist and trauma team is the child's survival, not the completion of a rehabilitation examination. During the examination, the therapist should carefully monitor the child's physiological responses, including heart rate, respiratory rate, blood oxygen saturation (SaO_2), intracranial pressure, and level of agitation. Dividing the examination into two or three shorter sessions can help modulate the amount of stimulation the child receives at one time.

As the child begins the progression out of coma, it is important to monitor and document improvement in the response to stimulation. For example, are the child's responses generalized or specific? Is there movement? Are the movements purposeful, spontaneous, or random? On what level is the child able to communicate, and can he or she follow simple instructions? Is the child agitated? What increases or decreases agitation? As the child becomes more alert and more medically stable, the therapist is able to assess postural stability. Is the head erect? Are the arms used for support when the child is upright? Can the child sit or stand safely? The rate of improvement provides valuable information to the team as the plan for future rehabilitation needs begins to come together.

Age, mechanism of the injury, severity, multiple trauma, secondary insults, and the extent of other injuries all affect the final outcome. "Interestingly, very young and preschool children have worse outcomes both in mortality and long-term disability than older children and adolescents" (Adelson, 2000). Although a child's initial medical status in the field or the emergency room has been associated with predicting survival, the Glasgow Coma Scale (GCS) (see Chapter 6), particularly the motor component, has been shown to be a better predictor of functional outcome and future disability when performed approximately 72 hours after injury (Michaud, 1992). The lower the child's GCS score, the greater is the chance of significant disability.

Physical Therapy Intervention

Initial physical therapy intervention for children with TBI should include positioning recommendations with the goals of decreasing abnormal posturing, maintaining ROM, and promoting child comfort and safety. For example, sidelying is often used to decrease the stiffness in extensor muscles for children with decerebrate posturing, in which the arms are flexed and the neck, trunk, and lower extremities are extended. Blanket rolls and pillows can provide support to help keep the child in a more flexed position (Figure 13–1). Children with increased stiffness in their plantar flexors may require a custom or prefabricated ankle splint to prevent contracture. Frequently, low-temperature, moldable plastic ankle-foot orthoses (MAFOs), which can be made by the physical therapist at bedside, are an excellent option because they can be refitted easily by the therapist if the child's tone or condition changes (Figure 13–2). When making splinting decisions in the ICU, it is important to consider the need for quick intravenous line access and the child's overall level of agitation or involuntary movement. Also, the amount of stiffness in a child's muscles and joints needs to be assessed over time because it will change according to the amount of medication received, baseline level of arousal, and response to external stimulation. An illustrated bedside program that includes positioning suggestions, schedule for wearing splints, and suggestions for modifying the amount of stimulation the child receives can be an excellent way to facilitate communication with the nursing staff across shifts, as well as involve the family in the child's care.

Out-of-Bed Transfers

The physical therapist is often the first individual to get the child out of bed and into a chair. It is critical to make sure that the child has been cleared for out-of-bed transfers by all of the primary treating services because there may be orthopedic or weight-bearing precautions or neurological concerns in addition to overall medical stability concerns. It is also important to plan ahead for any postural supports the child might need for safe positioning, as well as any additional staff members who might be needed to ensure a safe, smooth transfer. This is especially important when multiple intravenous lines are in place. Before

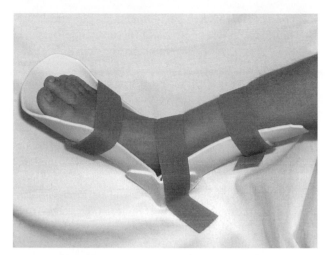

Figure 13-2 Molded ankle-foot orthosis.

initiating the transfer, it is a good rule of thumb to trace each line from the child to the bag to see exactly how much slack is available, and where each intravenous pole should be positioned. Transition to an upright position is done very slowly by first raising the head of the bed a few degrees at a time to assess tolerance because the child may experience a drop in blood pressure, called orthostatic hypotension. Once the transfer is completed, it is important to monitor and document the child's physiological responses to being upright over time. Careful documentation of how the transfer was performed, including any special instructions, will allow other staff to better follow your recommendations for having the child up and out of bed on a regular basis.

After the Intensive Care Unit

Once a child is transferred from the ICU, a more thorough examination of his or her mobility, balance, coordination, and need for assistive devices can be made. In some cases, a child will be moved directly to an inpatient rehabilitation facility as soon as he or she is medically stable. The decision to refer a child for inpatient rehabilitation requires careful examination, evaluation, and documentation. The physical therapist provides important input to the rehabilitation and medical team throughout this process by providing careful documentation of the child's impairments in body functions and structures, and limitations in activities. Ultimately, the decision to transfer a child to a rehabilitation facility is determined by the physicians and the

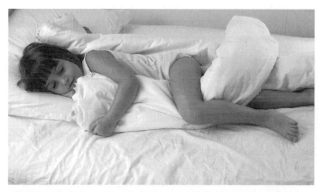

Figure 13-1 Use of pillows to maintain flexed position.

insurance company. In this era of managed care and restrictive insurance coverage, approval of such a transfer for a child with even moderate impairment cannot be taken for granted.

When a child is not transferred to a rehabilitation facility right away, more intensive therapy will be initiated in the acute-care setting. After the physical therapy re-examination, intervention could include working on basic head and trunk control, gait training, or stair climbing, based on the severity of the TBI and the child's functional limitations and needs at that time. Cases in which splinting is indicated and medically possible can be ideal opportunities to fabricate MAFOs. For more severe cases, total contact casting of the feet and ankles may help prevent contracture and reduce stiffness. If the child may be discharged directly to the home, the process of ordering assistive devices, such as a walker or wheelchair, may be initiated in the acute-care setting.

In many cases, children regain their postural control and functional mobility before they have the cognitive skills or judgment to be truly safe and independent. This can make gait training especially challenging, particularly when there are weight-bearing precautions as a result of a fracture. For example, a child who was struck by a car may be referred to physical therapy for crutch training with a diagnosis of tibial/fibular fracture. Even a mild head injury from such an accident could affect your selection of an assistive device because the child may lack the ability to recall basic instructions, such as keeping one foot elevated; to follow multistep commands; or to sequence an activity, such as descending stairs. The child may also be impulsive and lack the judgment to assess whether or not a situation is safe. When this is the case, it is vital that this potential danger be communicated to the family so that they can provide an appropriate level of supervision. Communicating these issues to the family, as well as the rest of the trauma team, is needed to ensure a safe discharge.

Whether a child is going directly to a rehabilitation hospital or home to receive intervention on an outpatient basis, a well-written discharge summary can help ensure a smooth transition from acute care. The discharge summary should include the child's history and a summary of current musculoskeletal, neurological, cognitive, and functional status. Any equipment or orthotics that were ordered or fabricated should also be listed, along with instructions for their use. Listing techniques that have been effective and ineffective in working with the child can help the next therapist begin his or her intervention with the greatest opportunity for success.

Cardiac Intensive Care Unit

In recent years there have been tremendous advancements in the area of pediatric cardiac care, including organ transplants. Physical therapists can play an especially important role in the preparation for and rehabilitation of transplant recipients by helping children maintain an optimum level of physical conditioning preoperatively and by helping to counteract the sequelae of postoperative immunosuppression (Sadowsky, 1996). During the preoperative phase, physical therapists are more involved with children needing heart transplants than with those needing lung transplants. Children with pulmonary involvement generally have pulmonary hypertension, which prohibits physical therapy until after surgery.

Many children awaiting organ transplants are hospitalized for an extended period of time until an organ becomes available. Although many of them have conditions that would normally preclude physical therapy, it is vital that they stay in as good a physical condition as possible. Because these children's conditions change hourly, clear, constant communication among team members is vital. As in the ICU, it is imperative that therapists speak with the children's primary nurse before initiating a direct treatment session, to gain a clear picture of their stability over the course of the day.

Children With a Heart Transplant

Initial Examination and Evaluation

Before initiating the physical examination, a detailed chart review is required, as well as an understanding of the child's level of activity before admission. At the initial contact, the therapist must obtain and document baseline vital signs and underlying rhythm and common arrhythmias. The examination and the intervention program should focus on the child's primary goals, which should incorporate the concerns of the child, family, and medical team. With a child receiving a transplant, the initial focus is on the child's medical goals, such as basic conditioning, rather than functional goals such as mobility.

During examination, the therapist should have a clear, unobstructed view of the cardiorespiratory/electrocardiograph (ECG) monitor. It is also vital that the therapist watch carefully for subtle signs of stress from the child, including color changes (especially around the lips), changes in facial expression, diaphoresis (sweating or clamminess), decreased verbalization, or changes in the child's respiratory pattern. Children who are able to communicate should be encouraged to provide the therapist with feedback about how they feel during the examination. It is often helpful to have the child's nurse and/or parent standing by because they will be most familiar with a child's early warning signs.

The initial preoperative examination of a heart transplant candidate includes many of the components of a standard physical therapy examination, such as active and passive ROM, coordination, and functional mobility. However, it is vital that the examination be performed within the physiological tolerance of the child. This is particularly important when assessing strength because having the child strain during a simple manual muscle test may be contraindicated. A thorough observation of the child should precede the physical examination. Mobility assessments may also be limited because the child may not be allowed to go up or down stairs or even get out of bed. Any medical supports should be noted, including supplemental oxygen, intravenous or arterial line access, and baseline vital signs. Peripheral edema, cyanosis, and any signs of respiratory distress should be documented. A thorough postural assessment can reveal asymmetries, structural deformities, or other musculoskeletal restrictions on respiratory capacity and trunk mobility. Children who have had multiple open heart surgeries may have such significant rib cage tightness that they are unable to rotate their trunk to transition in or out of a sitting position.

A baseline neurological examination is also important because children may have some neurological changes caused by previous episodes of hypoxia or cardiac arrest or as a complication of cardiac procedures. This examination should include assessment of reflexes, coordination, sensation, strength, and muscle tone. A developmental assessment should be performed because young children who have had complex medical histories, such as a major cardiac defect, often present with delays in gross motor skills. These delays may arise from previous neurological complications, prolonged restrictions on activity or movement, or simple musculoskeletal issues; or may be related to a more global syndrome, of which the cardiac defect is only a part.

Physical Therapy Intervention Plan: Pretransplantation

The amount of time during which a child is hospitalized before transplantation can vary dramatically, based on the availability of a suitable donor. During hospitalization, a child's condition continues to deteriorate as the heart fails. This can create tremendous stress on both the child and family and requires a great deal of sensitivity on the part of the entire team. Intervention plans for the child awaiting heart transplantation must be developed individually and may change on a daily or even hourly basis. The primary goals of physical therapy at this time are to maintain optimum conditioning and function within the child's tolerance. This includes the facilitation of appropriate developmental skills.

An infant is generally seen at bedside in the NICU or CICU. Physical therapy may be limited to simple positioning to optimize respiration, facilitate symmetry and normal muscle tone, and promote behavioral organization. A medically unstable infant may be placed in supine position because of the need for accessibility for medical procedures. Small blanket rolls at the infant's sides and under the knees can help encourage flexion and midline orientation (see Figure 13–1). An illustrated bedside program can encourage participation by the family and nursing staff.

With a toddler or school-aged child, conditioning is incorporated into developmentally appropriate play activities. Unless cleared by the physician, the child should be treated while on a monitor for safety so that the therapist can respond quickly to any changes in heart function. Depending on the child's physiological stability, intervention may be limited to transferring out of bed and playing in a supported sitting position, or simply reaching against gravity for toys. Many children need to be encouraged simply to get out of bed during the day. Active movement, ambulation, and being upright are challenging in themselves. In addition, making recommendations for appropriate activities to parents, nursing, and child-life staff can help ensure that a safe but beneficial level of activity is incorporated throughout the child's day.

Developmental or gross motor skill intervention should be provided, based on the outcome of the child's assessment and tolerance for intervention. Providing the family with play activities and a general stretching program to maintain flexibility is an excellent way to ensure carryover throughout the child's day.

Adolescents are often the most challenging to treat because the psychosocial issues that face anyone undergoing a transplant come to the forefront. Hospitalization for an extended period of time is very confining. As the teenager's condition deteriorates, activity becomes more and more restricted, and the question of whether a donor will be found in time becomes more pressing. Because so much of the adolescent's daily life is dictated by others (many are not even allowed to have a bowel movement in private), it is important to provide a choice of activities to regain some sense of control. Because of the varying degree of medical instability of the adolescent, each transplant program has its own protocol for where and when an individual child can receive therapy. During the hospital course, a number of problems may occur that will require the child's physical therapy to be altered, including procedures, new medication, seizure activity, fluid balance problems, behavioral concerns, new arrhythmias, and changes in coagulation times.

If cleared by the medical team, ambulatory children may be seen in the gym as long as certain precautions are carefully followed, such as using a cardiac monitor or making sure the heart rate stays below a certain maximum value. The central intravenous lines through which many children receive their medication also require a safety protocol. These special intravenous lines are inserted in the chest wall or can be fed up through an extremity directly into one of the large veins to the heart. If a central line becomes dislodged, there is the risk of an air bubble going through the heart and into the lungs, which can be fatal. Should a central line become cracked or broken, a clamp should be placed immediately between the break and the child. If it is broken or dislodged, the child should be placed on his or her left side, preferably with the head lower than the feet (Virtual Children's Hospital, 2001). Children should always have their code medications with them, so that if they go into cardiac distress or arrest the medications will be readily available for the code team.

Aerobic activity, such as an exercise bike or treadmill, should be strictly monitored and maintained within recommended parameters for SaO_2 and maximum heart rate. Children should be progressed very gradually when using exercise equipment until they are able to demonstrate a consistent response to activity. Activities in the gym may include warm-up stretching exercises, approximately 30 minutes of mild exercise activities, or games, such as shooting a basketball or Koosh tennis. The child should be observed carefully for fatigue, dizziness, shortness of breath, mental status changes, arrhythmia (heart racing or pounding), or a 10% decrease in SaO_2. Arrhythmias should be reported immediately to the child's nurse and physician (Beaudet, 1996). Ten to 15 minutes (approximately half the length of the exercise portion of the session) should be reserved for cooling down because of the increased risk for arrhythmias during that time. If a child is not able to come to the gym, many of these activities can be performed in the CICU in coordination with the nursing staff. Other preoperative interventions may include deep-breathing exercises and assisted-coughing techniques, which can be beneficial in improving respiratory function and comfort after surgery.

Postoperative Precautions

After transplant surgery of any kind, a child is severely immunocompromised from the medications that must be taken to minimize the risk of organ rejection. This places the child at risk for severe infection from bacteria and viruses that healthy people are exposed to on a daily basis. The physical therapist and all family members and staff must therefore don a mask, gown, and gloves before entering the room. If there is any reason to believe that the therapist is developing an infection or viral illness, it is best to transfer the child to another therapist. For added protection, the child is generally expected to wear a mask whenever he or she is out of the isolation room. This can be quite challenging to enforce because the mask can be unpleasant to wear when doing physical activity. All toys or other equipment, such as walkers or wheelchairs, should be disinfected before being brought into the child's room. If a child is brought to the physical therapy gym, there should not be any other children in the gym, especially those with active respiratory illnesses. This helps minimize the risk of infection. All equipment or toys that the child will use should be thoroughly disinfected.

After transplant surgery, the heart is totally denervated, which results in a blunted heart rate response to increased activity. The donor heart is still able to produce a slower but adequate response to exercise through the mechanical effect of stretching of the heart muscle from increased blood flow, and from circulating catecholamines from the sympathoadrenal system (Shephard, 1992). These delayed-response mechanisms make a prolonged warm-up and cool-down period a must for these children because time is needed for these slower mechanisms to take effect. Children should be carefully monitored for blood pressure, SaO_2 (should be at greater than 95%), and heart rate (generally kept at no more than 50% of age-predicted HR) to ensure that the new heart is able to keep up with the body's demands (Beaudet, 1996).

Physical Therapy Intervention After Transplantation

In most cases, physical therapy must be reordered by the attending physician after surgery, once the child has been extubated and is no longer on bed rest. Postoperatively, the child is in extreme discomfort, with multiple chest tubes, arterial and venous lines, and a large midsternal incision. The child is generally cleared for out-of-bed transfers once the arterial lines and chest tubes have been removed. A full physical therapy re-examination is required and should include baseline vital signs, heart rhythm, any changes in neurological status, and a functional mobility assessment when tolerated. Physical therapy goals and intervention will generally be similar to those before transplantation, including positioning, increasing functional mobility and endurance, developmental intervention when appropriate, and family education. Initial intervention may be limited to simple passive ROM, bed mobility, and slowly increasing tolerance to being upright by elevating the head of the bed. In general, the child is encouraged to be out of bed and mobile as soon as possible and may be discharged as early as 2 to 3 weeks after transplantation. Breathing exercises and assisted coughing techniques may also be reviewed because the cracking of the chest wall during heart transplant surgery has a significant effect on respiratory capacity, initially because of pain and later as a result of scarring. It is also essential that planning for outpatient therapy and adaptive equipment be addressed as early as possible.

Discharge Planning

The medical team, including the physical therapist, will decide if ongoing physical therapy is needed. When setting up outpatient therapy, it is important to remember the precautions necessary to keep the child healthy. For example, you may not want to refer the child to a pediatric therapy setting with a large, open gym and many other children because of the risk of infection. The need for monitoring equipment and the possible need for an emergency response should also be considered.

For families who have children with chronic illness, the process of returning home without the full-time support of a medical staff can be quite intimidating. The physical therapist can help encourage families to maximize their child's independence within clear, safe parameters for activity, based on team recommendations. Adaptive equipment, such as a shower chair or a wheelchair for long-distance ambulation, should be addressed early to make the transition to home as smooth as possible. In setting up outpatient therapy, inconvenience to the family should be minimized. Coordinating therapy with other medical appointments or visits to the hospital can be very helpful to a family that is already feeling overwhelmed. For the child who is returning to school, the physical therapist can provide a helpful summary of the child's mobility restrictions in advance so that the school can make safe, appropriate accommodations. The amount of time a child needs to continue therapy postoperatively varies greatly, depending on his or

her condition before transplantation and medical stability postoperatively.

Medical-Surgical Units

Medical-surgical units in pediatric hospitals serve children of many ages and with a vast array of diagnoses and impairments. Although your role as a physical therapist will vary, certain responsibilities in regard to facilitating the transition to home or rehabilitation facilities are universal.

As hospital stays become shorter, it is important to remember that discharge planning begins at the initial evaluation. As a physical therapist, your primary focus when preparing a child for discharge can be summarized by the following:

- Identifying levels of functioning
- Identifying factors that limit a child's mobility, safety, independence, and activities, and clearly documenting those concerns for other team members
- Prescribing and/or ordering the equipment necessary to allow a safe transition to home, such as wheelchairs, walkers, and other assistive devices
- Providing family education to ensure that the child can be appropriately cared for in a home environment
- Referring the child for outpatient services after discharge, when necessary

In this era of managed care, the physical therapist is often required to interface directly with insurance carriers to make sure that a child has what is needed for discharge from the hospital. This frequently requires multiple telephone calls, writing letters of medical necessity, obtaining prescriptions from the child's physician, and coordinating delivery of equipment. The sooner the child's needs can be identified, the sooner the process can begin.

Children With Orthopedic Problems Status Post Tibial/ Fibular Fracture in Long Leg Cast

One of the more frequent consultations that physical therapists receive in an inpatient setting is for crutch training in children with a leg fracture. This often occurs just before discharge, which may be the same day as the injury. Although a physical therapist must perform an initial examination, the crutch training itself can be delegated to a qualified physical therapist assistant. The family should attend physical therapy sessions because they will need to guard the child independently for safety, particularly on the stairs.

Examination and Evaluation

The initial examination for a child with a tibial/fibular fracture is often quite brief and straightforward because many of these children are otherwise healthy and normally functioning. The examination should include:

- Verify the weight-bearing precautions as written in the chart and on the consult to make sure they are consistent.

- General strength assessment: Assess uninvolved extremities through manual muscle testing or observation, depending on the age of the child. Resistance testing is not recommended for the involved limb. A child will need at least a fair muscle grade in the involved extremity with the cast on in order to keep it elevated off the floor during gait.

- Perform an abbreviated ROM assessment by observing active ROM. Any visible limitations require a more detailed passive ROM examination.

- Perform a brief cognitive assessment, particularly when the injury was traumatic in nature, or when the child is still heavily medicated.

- Identify other injuries, such as lacerations or other fractures, which may limit the child's ability to safely use an assistive device.

- Assess safety during transfers and recommendations regarding an appropriate assistive device.

- Ask the family about the home environment, such as access into and out of the house, stairs, proximity of bedroom to bathroom, and flooring surfaces. Help the family plan to make the home as safe and accessible as possible.

- Assess sensation and adequate perfusion with a new cast because the child's leg may swell when in a dependent position

Physical Therapy Intervention

Gait training is best initiated on the parallel bars, which provide maximum stability for the child. This is a good place to assess the child's tolerance for standing and to instruct the child in the concepts of partial, toe-touch, or non–weight-bearing movements. Select an appropriate

assistive device based on the stability of the child, ability to keep the cast off the floor, and how well movements are sequenced. After this initial examination and evaluation is complete, and there are no outstanding concerns regarding the child's ability to successfully complete crutch training, it is appropriate to transfer the child to a physical therapist assistant for repetitive practice.

Choosing an Assistive Device

There are no hard-and-fast rules dictating the appropriate assistive device for ambulation because each child and each injury is so different (Table 13.1). In general, a child under the age of 5 years has a very difficult time with crutches, particularly when there is a restriction on weight-bearing status. The motor planning and sequencing involved in crutch training further complicate the matter. Many 3- to 4-year-olds can be taught to use a walker safely on level surfaces and to bump up and down the stairs on their bottoms.

With an older child, the ability to use crutches safely depends on general physical condition, strength, weight, cognitive status, presence of an intravenous line (especially in an upper extremity), and other related injuries. A child who is very obese may need to use a walker simply because he or she does not have the strength to stabilize adequately on the tips of two crutches. A child who has postconcussive syndrome, significant attention deficit/hyperactivity disorder, or mental retardation may have such a hard time following instructions and obeying precautions that he or she will need constant adult supervision, at least initially. Given the limited time that a child is in the hospital, the goal for most crutch training is that the child will be independent on level surfaces and on stairs with assistance. To become safe and independent on crutches can take several days of practice, especially with a younger child. A handout with step-by-step instructions for specific weight-bearing status and gait pattern can be a helpful reference for the child and family after discharge. If appropriate, instructions for a home exercise program to maintain strength or ROM should be provided.

Role of the Physical Therapist in Outpatient Clinics

After discharge from the hospital, many children return to outpatient follow-up clinics for ongoing monitoring of their condition. Children with chronic conditions, such as

Table 13.1 Choosing an Assistive Mobility Device

Device	Advantages	Disadvantages
Crutches	Allow fast movement Able to go up and down stairs Allows non–weight bearing (NWB) and partial weight bearing (PWB) Inexpensive Very maneuverable	Small base of support Require sequencing Require use of both hands Require good balance Require good strength in arms and uninvolved leg Require at least fair strength in involved leg
Walker	Very stable Minimal sequencing needed Will work for young child Allows NWB and PWB Can add wheels so that child does not need to lift it Good for impulsive children Good for obese children	Slower moving Not safe on stairs Larger and more cumbersome than crutches
Canes	Small Require use of only one hand Can use quad base to increase stability Good for decreasing pain with weight bearing	Small base of support Safe for weight bearing as tolerated only Requires sequencing

Wheelchair	Good for very young children
	Good for children who cannot maintain
	  weight-bearing precautions because of arm
	  injury or cognitive impairment
	Good for long distances
	Can be rented
		Cumbersome
		Hard to transport in car or public transportation
		Hard to maneuver in home
		Hard to get up and down stairs
		Costly to purchase

cerebral palsy, myopathies, cystic fibrosis, cardiac or pulmonary conditions, myelomeningocele, or a history of prematurity, are usually seen in the clinic on a yearly or biannual basis. Many hospitals also have a neonatal follow-up clinic, which tracks and monitors the progress of premature and high-risk infants. A **clinic team** is made up of a variety of physicians, therapists, and clinical nurse specialists who work together to address the complex needs of these children. Physical therapists are frequently members of the clinic team, providing ongoing examination of children's developmental, functional, and musculoskeletal status, as well as their need for adaptive equipment, exercise programs, and additional physical therapy intervention. Working in a clinic gives the therapist the opportunity to gain a longitudinal perspective of a disorder. It is an excellent opportunity to develop more concentrated expertise in the intervention for a given diagnosis because of the sheer volume of children seen.

Clinics are generally held on a weekly or biweekly basis and may last for a morning or an entire day. Some clinics require the physical therapist to be on call so that the therapist comes to the clinic area only when needed. Other clinics require the therapist to be present for the entire time. When working in a clinic setting, physical therapists must learn to juggle their day-to-day schedule to make sure their regular children are covered while they are attending clinic. Because the clinic therapist is the most familiar with the clinic children, he or she will often see those children when they are admitted to the hospital, to provide better continuity of care.

Children With Cystic Fibrosis: Outpatient Pulmonary Clinic

Cystic fibrosis (CF) is a genetically transmitted disease of the exocrine system (see Chapters 8 and 19). Although it is most commonly associated with the pulmonary system, it actually affects nearly every system in the body. Most pediatric hospitals have outpatient CF programs because children with CF require regular monitoring of their pulmonary status, medications, and home management program. Physical therapists have an especially important role in CF because they are often responsible for teaching children and families about sputum clearance techniques, the importance of exercise, and the use of new devices.

Physical therapists, either individually or as part of a multidisciplinary team, perform an initial examination on new children to get a baseline assessment of their status. This baseline data can be compared with data from periodic re-evaluations during clinic visits.

The physical therapy examination in a clinic setting is usually abbreviated because of the large numbers of children who must be seen in a day. It is important for the therapist to focus on the most critical needs of each individual child. Because the child will be seen by a number of other medical specialists in the clinic, the baseline information on the child's present pulmonary status is often taken by someone else on the team and does not need to be duplicated by everyone. A complete physical therapy examination of a child with CF must be performed. In the clinic, the team must decide which portion of the examination the physical therapist is primarily responsible for in that setting, such as performing a musculoskeletal and exercise examination, and teaching various secretion clearance techniques. The physical therapist's focus will vary from clinic to clinic.

One of the primary roles of the physical therapist in the CF clinic is to make any necessary changes to the method or methods being used for sputum clearance. There are a host of sputum clearance devices and techniques now on the market. Many of these have been found to be clinically effective, but few have well-documented studies to back up their effectiveness. Most pulmonology departments have a repertoire of "preferred" techniques or devices that are recommended to children and their families. However, it is good to become familiar with everything that is available so that you can be a better resource for the children (Table 13.2) (see Chapters 8 and 19).

Part of the physical therapist's evaluation in the clinic should include a discussion of what the child is presently doing at home for secretion clearance: Is it the most effective method for the child? Does the present regimen need to be adjusted to be more appropriate for the child's age? Is the family or child interested in doing something new? As children age, there is a need for more independent means of sputum clearance. If an adolescent is going to college next

Table 13.2 Options for Increasing Sputum Clearance in Children With Cystic Fibrosis

Device	Equipment	Age	Advantages	Disadvantages
Chest physical therapy (PT)	Postural drainage board	All ages	No child participation required	Passive aspiration/reflux precautions Ineffective with unstable airway May cause bronchospasm Need compliance
Chest PT with mechanical percussor	Mechanical percussor	Not for infants	Independence	Expensive Same as chest PT
Percussion vest	Vest Postural drainage board	Ages 4 years and above	As with chest PT	As with chest PT
PEP mask	Mask	Generally 4 years and above	Independence Compliance Active technique	Effectiveness not well documented
Flutter	Flutter device	Ages 6 years and above	Independence Active technique Small Portable	

Device	Equipment	Age	Advantages	Disadvantages
Active cycle of breathing	None	Ages 4 years and above	Child directed Active technique Can be used with percussion Independence	Requires extensive teaching and regular review of technique
Autogenic drainage	None	Ages 12 years and above	Independence Child directed Active	Difficult to learn Requires extensive teaching and practice

year, parents will not be available to perform percussion twice per day, and subsequently he or she will need to try devices such as mechanical percussors, autogenic drainage, or the flutter.

The role of the physical therapist in the ongoing intervention for the child with CF is constantly changing and evolving from one of a direct service provider to a consultant to the young adult. Nowhere is this more apparent than the clinic setting, where the therapist must "change gears" from one minute to the next as he or she moves quickly from one child to another.

Summary

The pediatric acute-care hospital is one of the most diverse and challenging environments in which to practice physical therapy. The sheer variety of children, from the NICU to the ever-changing populations of the medical floors, is endlessly stimulating and provides a tremendous opportunity for learning and professional growth. This was by no means a comprehensive view of the populations seen in this setting; however, the intention was to provide the reader with a view of what the role of the physical therapist is like in this type of service delivery setting.

DISCUSSION QUESTIONS

1. Discuss the signs of stress in a child who is hospitalized.

2. Discuss situations in which using the physical therapy gym might be detrimental for a child who is hospitalized.

3. What discharge issues should be considered during the initial evaluation?

REFERENCES

Adelson, P.D. (2000). Pediatric trauma made simple. *Clinical Neurosurgery, 47,* 319–335.

Beaudet, N. (1996). Children's Hospital of Philadelphia and Children's Seashore House Interdisciplinary Care Guidelines: CICU Heart Lung Transplant Program. (Available from the Children's Hospital of Philadelphia, 3405 Civic Center Blvd., Philadelphia, PA 19104.)

Luerssen, T.G., & Klauber, M.R.. (1998). Outcome from head injury related to patient's age. *Journal of Neurosurgery, 68,* 409–416.

Michaud, L. (1992). Predictors of survival and severity of disability after severe traumatic brain injury. *Neurosurgery, 31*(2), 254–264.

Sadowsky, H. (1996). Cardiac transplant: A review. *Physical Therapy, 76*(5), 498–515.

Shephard, R.J. (1992). Responses of the cardiac transplant patient to exercise and training. *Exercise and Sport Sciences Reviews, 20,* 297–320.

Virtual Children's Hospital (October 2001). Available at *http://www.vh.org/Misc/Search.html*

Ward, J. (1995). Pediatric issues in head trauma. *New Horizons, 3*(3), 539–545.

Chapter *14*

The Neonatal Intensive Care Unit

— Sharon White, PT, MS

The **neonatal intensive care unit** (NICU) is a unique setting serving a highly specialized population. Infants in the NICU are medically and developmentally fragile and require a multidisciplinary team of caregivers. The physical therapist provides examination, evaluation, and a wide scope of interventions in the NICU. A major focus of the intervention is consultation and family education. Because complex problems make infants in the NICU vulnerable to developmental and medical complications, NICU care involves a different approach than that used in other types of pediatric settings. The physiological, medical, and developmental issues facing infants in the NICU require that the physical therapist have advanced training (Sweeney, Heriza, Reilly, Smith, & VanSant, 1999). This chapter therefore provides a basic overview of service delivery in the NICU, and further study is required if you are going to work in the NICU, especially in the most intensive level III nursery.

lems are often referred for physical therapy in the NICU (McCarton, Wallace, Divon, & Vaughan, 1996; Taylor, Klein, Schatschneider, & Hack, 1998) (Box 14.1).

Infants with very low scores on assessment of physiological function, called **Apgar scores** (Table 14.1), require close monitoring and possibly admission to the NICU for observation. Apgar scores are routinely assigned to all infants born in the United States, at 1 and 5 minutes after birth. When low scores are assigned at 1 and 5 minutes, an additional score at 10 minutes may be given. Scores of 8 to 10 at 1 minute after birth are normal. If Apgar scores at both 1 and 5 minutes are 0 to 3, the infant requires resuscitation and there is a risk of neonatal death. The possibility of the infant developing a neurological complication is also associated with extremely low Apgar scores, and particularly with a low score assigned at 10 minutes (Moster, Lie, Irgens, Bjerkedal, & Markestad, 2001). These infants are generally admitted to the NICU and may require physical therapy.

Infants Served

Infants with a variety of diagnoses are served in the NICU. Infants born prematurely or at full term showing signs of central nervous system (CNS) impairment, specific neuromuscular or orthopedic problems, multiple medical or genetic problems, abnormal feeding behaviors, or other symptoms that put infants at risk for developmental prob-

Premature Birth

Infants born between 38 and 40 weeks gestation (postconception) are considered full term. Infants born before 38 weeks gestation are considered **premature** and are at higher risk for medical complications and developmental disabilities than infants born at full term (Bennett & Scott, 1997). Outcomes of preterm birth may lead to visual impair-

430

> ### BOX 14.1 Common Diagnoses of Infants in the Neonatal Intensive Care Unit
>
> Premature birth: Less than 38 weeks' gestation
>
> Low birth weight: Less than 2500 grams
>
> Very low birth weight: Less than 1500 grams
>
> Small for gestational age (SGA): Less than the 10th percentile
>
> Large for gestational age (LGA): Greater than the 90th percentile
>
> Microcephaly: Occipital frontal head circumference of less than the third percentile for the infant's gestational age at birth
>
> Hypoxic ischemic encephalopathy: Full-term infant who has had a significant episode of intrapartum asphyxia
>
> Genetic syndromes/diseases: Chromosomal abnormalities, gene disorders, unusual patterns of inheritance
>
> Compromised respiration: Infant requires medical or mechanical assistance to achieve functional respiration
>
> Persistent feeding problems: Infant is unable to take in adequate calories orally without special assistance
>
> Seizure disorder: Neonatal seizures identified at or shortly following birth
>
> Amniotic band syndrome: Intrauterine development of amniochorionic strands leading to limb and digital amputations/constrictions and other deformities
>
> Myelomeningocele: Malformation of the spinal cord resulting from defective closure of the neural tube

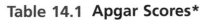

Table 14.1 Apgar Scores*

	Apgar Score		
Sign	**0**	**1**	**2**
Heart rate	Absent	Below 100 bpm	Over 100 bpm
Respiration	Absent	Slow, irregular	Good, crying
Muscle tone	Limp	Some flexion	Active movement
Grimace (reflex irritability)	No response	Grimace	Cough or sneeze
Color (appearance)	Blue, pale	Body pink, extremities blue	Completely pink

*Note: 0, 1, or 2 points are given for each sign based on observation of the infant at 1, 5, and sometimes 10 minutes after birth.

ments, sensorineural hearing loss, learning disabilities, attention deficit/hyperactivity disorder, and other developmental and neurological problems (Kilbride & Daily, 1998; McGrath, Sullivan, Lester, & Oh, 2000). Cerebral palsy (CP) is the most prevalent developmental disability related to premature birth, with approximately 40% of children with CP having been born prematurely (Bennett, 1999). Infants born either at full term or prematurely are also classified by their weight. Those who are tiny (less than the 10th percentile of published norms) for gestational age are referred to as **small for gestational age (SGA)**, and those who are large (greater than 90th percentile of published norms) for gestational age are referred to as **large for gesta**-tional age **(LGA)** (see charts in Figure 2.3). Infants who are SGA or LGA are at greater risk for problems than those whose weights are average for gestational age. Infants born very preterm and those weighing less than 1000 grams at birth have been at the greatest risk for CP and other motor, cognitive, and behavioral disorders (Foulder-Hughes & Cooke, 2003); however, there has been continued improvement in the outcomes of even the smallest infants (Surman, Newdick, & Johnson, 2003).

One CNS complication that is often associated with premature birth is intracranial or **intraventricular hemorrhage (IVH)**. Prematurity puts the infant at risk for IVH because of the vulnerability and vascularity of the infant brain before 38 to 40 weeks gestation (Volpe, 1989). IVH (bleeding in the ventricles of the brain) is detected on cranial ultrasonography. Because IVH is seen in preterm infants, cranial ultrasonography to check for IVH is a routine part of medical treatment in the NICU. When detected, IVH is defined by grades 1 to 4, with grade 1 being the least severe and grade 4 being the most severe. Approximately 35% to 50% of infants born before 32 weeks gestation or with birth weights of less than 1500 grams are diagnosed with IVH (Duncan & Ment, 1993; Volpe, 1998). IVH can become progressively more complicated and may lead to hydrocephalus.

Periventricular leukomalacia (PVL) is another CNS complication that is linked to premature birth. PVL is an ischemic infarction of the white matter adjacent to the lateral ventricles. As white matter damage increases, the risk of poor neurological outcome also increases. PVL is commonly diagnosed by magnetic resonance imaging (MRI) of the brain done months after the infant is discharged home from the NICU. PVL is almost always found in premature infants who have CP (Bennett, 1999).

Infants born prematurely are at risk for many other medical complications, including chronic respiratory disease, hearing loss, anemia, retinopathy of prematurity, feeding difficulties, and other conditions that impair general health (Weisglas-Kuperus, Baerts, Smrkovsky, & Sauer, 1993). **Retinopathy of prematurity (ROP)** causes abnormal development of vascularization in the retina. Progression of ROP can lead to severe visual impairments despite the use of medical treatment such as cryotherapy and laser surgery (Hussain, Clive, & Bhandari, 1999). ROP screening is done routinely in the NICU at various gestational ages, with the first examination usually at 4 to 6 weeks after birth.

Infants born prematurely are at risk for developmental problems, and their development should continue to be monitored after they go home from the NICU. When assessing the development of an infant born prematurely, the corrected age (adjusted age) is used. This refers to the infant's age from the time he or she is at 40 weeks gestation. In other words, an infant born 2 months prematurely, who is chronologically 6 months old, would have a corrected age of 4 months. In this way, the infant is given credit, in the assessment scores, for the true period of time allowed for his or her physiological development since conception. The practice of using the infant's corrected age in monitoring overall development should be done until the child is 3 years old (Bennett, 1999).

Specific Diagnoses

Infants born at full term with conditions requiring NICU care may also be referred for physical therapy; this includes infants with CNS impairments such as microcephaly, hypoxic ischemic encephalopathy, neuromuscular diseases, myelomeningocele, genetic syndromes, or other abnormalities. Additional conditions that might indicate the need for physical therapy are birth-related Erb's palsy (a brachial plexus injury), torticollis (contraction of the sternocleidomastoid muscle of the neck with the head laterally flexed to one side and rotated to the opposite side), positional deformities, amniotic band syndrome, feeding abnormalities,

arthrogryposis, and other conditions causing movement abnormalities or impairment. These diagnoses usually indicate a need for physical therapy in the NICU and for follow-up care after the infant has been discharged to the home. Early physical therapy involvement, while the infant is in the NICU, allows the therapist to determine the infant's baseline level of functional movement and to assist the family and caregivers in addressing known limitations in body structures and functions and restrictions in activities normally expected of an infant.

Infants with severe respiratory disease are at risk for developmental problems regardless of gestational age at birth. Severe respiratory disease may require aggressive medical treatment to ensure survival, such as high-frequency ventilation and extracorporeal membrane oxygenation (ECMO). ECMO uses a modified heart and lung machine to allow nearly total rest of damaged lungs for up to 10 days, allowing time for lung healing to occur. It is used in cases of severe persistent pulmonary hypertension, meconium aspiration syndrome, sepsis, and pneumonia. ECMO is an extreme, life-saving procedure, but it increases the infant's risk for neurological problems (Hunter, Zwischenberger, & Bhatia, 1992). Complications from ECMO may include seizures, IVH, cortical atrophy, muscle tone abnormalities, feeding difficulties, and others problems (Lowes & Palisano, 1995). Neonatal chronic lung disease is sometimes treated with systemic dexamethasone therapy, a drug successful in the management of lung disease in preterm infants. Infants born prematurely who are treated with dexamethasone have been shown to have a decrease in total cerebral tissue volume compared with similar infants not treated with dexamethasone (Murphy et al., 2001). This finding suggests that infants who require dexamethasone might have a need for closer monitoring of their early development.

Neonatal Intensive Care Unit Environment

Levels of Care

Newborn nurseries are defined by the levels of care provided. A level I nursery provides routine maternal and newborn well-baby care. A level II nursery is more specialized, providing some additional care, such as short-term ventilation and neonatal monitoring with some medical interventions. A level III nursery is an NICU that is equipped for the smallest and most ill infants (Kahn-

D'Angelo & Unanue, 2000). The level III NICU is prepared for complicated neonatal issues and has a neonatologist on staff (Figures 14–1 and 14–2). The physical therapist may be involved in care of infants from all three levels.

Sensory Stimulation

The NICU is an overwhelming environment for the infant and his or her family. Light and sound levels are variable and are often high (Gretebeck, Shaffer, & Bishop-Kurylo, 1998). The number of infants in each room, the medical procedures and interventions being done, and the behaviors of the adults present affect the environment. Because infants needing intensive care are sensitive to stimulation, light and noise levels should be kept as minimal as possible. Handling of the infant is best done when care is clustered. This means that procedures requiring handling are grouped together to minimize the frequency of disturbances to the infant, allowing adequate rest. The infant's ability to cope with sensory stimulation and activity is affected by his or her gestational age and physiological stability. Infants who are at 32 weeks gestation or younger and those who are physiologically impaired have difficulty coping with exposure to light and noise. After 32 weeks, limited and cautious

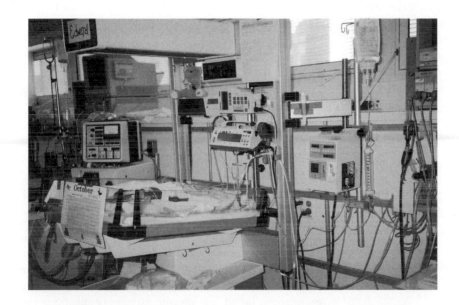

Figure 14-1 Infant in typical technologically rich NICU.

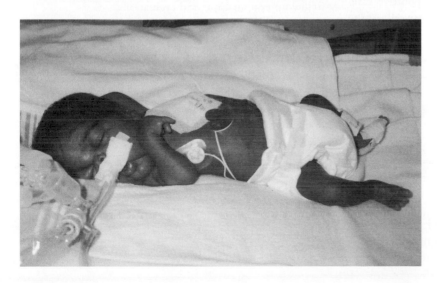

Figure 14-2 Closer view of the infant, who is intubated and connected to cardiac, respiratory, and temperature monitors.

exposure to light and noise can be beneficial (Gretebeck et al., 1998).

Developmentally Supportive Care

Developmentally supportive care is individualized caregiving guided by the infant's physiological reactions, behavioral cues, and signs of stress in response to the immediate environment (VandenBerg, 1997). This method of care encourages the infant's optimal recovery and rest and supports the infant in achieving developmental tasks. It ensures an active, reciprocal relationship between the infant and caregivers. Specific care recommendations may include cycled or dimmed lighting, clustered care, decreased stimulation, decreased noise levels, minimal handling, and specific handling techniques. Developmentally supportive care has been shown to be effective in promoting the infant's general heath, resulting in decreased morbidity, decreased days of hospitalization, and favorable developmental outcome (Als et al., 1986; Als & Gilkerson, 1997; The Infant Health and Development Program, 1990).

The **Neonatal Individualized Developmental Care and Assessment Program** (**NIDCAP**) is an approach used in many NICUs. This approach is based on observation of the infant's behavior, with individualized recommendations for handling and care based on the infant's specific responses. The NIDCAP model and developmentally supportive care planning help the infant in achieving stability both physiologically and behaviorally (Als & Gilkerson, 1997). Many nurseries have a developmental specialist who might be a nurse, physical or occupational therapist, or other professional who works with the infants in the NICU and who has specific training in developmentally supportive care. This person may conduct individualized assessments of the infants and provide recommendations to parents and other NICU staff. The developmental specialist is involved in training NICU staff in this important method of providing care.

Kangaroo care, or skin-to-skin contact, is encouraged and practiced in many NICUs. When the infant is stable enough to allow holding, the mother or father is encouraged to hold the infant skin-to-skin for a period of time several times a day. This skin-to-skin contact was first used in Bogotá, Colombia, as a method to provide heat to infants when incubators were not available (Sloan, Camacho, & Rojas, 1994). Infants who experience kangaroo care in the NICU have a more rapid maturation of vagal tone (indicating more mature responses to internal and external stresses), more rapid improvement in behav-

ioral state organization, longer periods of quiet sleep and alert wakefulness, and shorter periods of active sleep (Feldman & Eidelman, 2003). The physical therapist may consult with parents and caregivers in facilitating kangaroo care as part of the developmental care plan.

Developmentally supportive care is a best practice and is the standard of care for level III NICUs. When the infant's care plan is responsive to signs of stress and cues, the caregivers are able to design the individual infant's environment to provide for optimal growth and development. By using a caregiving approach based on developmentally supportive care, the NICU environment can address the changing and varied needs of the neonate.

Role of Physical Therapy

The physical therapist is a member of a team of caregivers and professionals providing medical and developmental care to the infant in intensive care. A large part of physical therapy intervention is consultation with the family and the medical staff. The infant will have multiple nurses and physicians providing daily care. Through consultation, the physical therapist assists in establishing consistent positioning and handling, individualized caregiving, and any specific therapeutic interventions as needed.

Some infants will have a specific bedside intervention program designed to meet specific goals. Multiple caregivers may carry out this program with instruction from the physical therapist. Physical therapy consultation with the neonatologist and the NICU team involves providing information found during the baseline evaluation and follow-up examinations and evaluations.

Examination and Evaluation

The infant is usually referred for physical therapy by the neonatologist or pediatrician. The initial examination and evaluation is done when the infant is medically stable and shows signs of developmental readiness. The evaluation of the infant begins with chart review, discussion with the family and the NICU team, and observation of the infant. The baseline physical therapy evaluation should include the following information:

- History: birth and medical
- Current medical status

- Precautions/contraindications
- Behavioral state and alertness
- Active movements/strength
- Muscle tone/reflexes
- Feeding
- Positioning and handling recommendations
- Recommendations for follow-up care
- Discharge recommendations

History

The birth history and medical history are reviewed and documented in the evaluation. This assists the therapist in determining when to initiate the examination. The infant's **current gestational age** (number of weeks of gestation plus weeks postdelivery) is noted because it is critical; infants present differently at varying gestational ages. Medical complications and ongoing medical problems may indicate and explain functional limitations. Ongoing medical issues will influence caregiving and therapeutic interventions as well as expected outcomes.

Precautions and Contraindications

Throughout the examination, it is crucial to monitor the infant's tolerance to handling using both physiological and behavioral signs of stress. The physical therapist watches the infant's responses to handling, such as changes in oxygen saturation, respiratory rate, heart rate, and blood pressure. The effects of any current medications on these measurements should be known. Adverse physiological responses are a contraindication to handling, and the examination must be modified or stopped if there are signs of physiological instability.

Physically the infant may respond to handling with skin color changes, hiccups, finger splays, lower extremity stiffening and extension, frowning, or turning away from a noise or a face. These behavioral signs indicate the infant is avoiding being handled. An infant's individual responses to handling can be identified before the examination by observing the infant during a typical caregiving activity. After the physical therapy examination is started, it may be stopped, modified, or shortened as indicated by the infant's behavioral responses and **signs of stress** (Table 14.2). An infant who shows continued signs of stress with handling may be experiencing medical complications, showing signs of CNS dysfunction, or simply not be developmentally ready to tolerate even gentle handling. Basic handling and

Table 14.2 Neonatal Signs of Stress

Physiological	Behavioral
Increased heart rate	Gaze aversion
Decreased heart rate	Finger splays
Decreased respiratory rate	Trunk extension
Increased blood pressure	Facial grimace
Decreased oxygen saturation	Leg extension
Apnea	Tuning out/drowsiness
Bradycardia	Hyperalertness
Skin color changes	Arm salute

Source: Kahn-D'Angelo, L. (1995). The special care nursery. In S.K. Campbell (Ed.), *Physical therapy for children* (pp. 787–822). Philadelphia: W.B. Saunders, with permission.

position changes used in neurological assessments have been shown to cause physiological and behavioral signs of stress in premature infants (Sweeny, 1986, 1989). Because of the potential harm to the infant with handling and position changes, the NICU physical therapist should follow a conservative approach in examination and intervention of infants.

Behavioral State and Alertness

Attention to the infant's behavioral state throughout the examination provides important information and guides the therapist in the process. All infants have states of alertness, drowsiness, and sleep. The infant's ability to move through a variety of behavioral states and to maintain a state of alertness indicates CNS maturity. It also affects the validity of the examination. An infant who is drowsy throughout the examination may appear to be weak or have low muscle tone by simply being unable to maintain the state of alertness needed to respond to handling and position changes. Within several minutes, an infant may move between the behavioral states of deep sleep, light sleep, drowsiness, quiet alertness, and crying (Table 14.3) (Brazelton, 1984). It is not unusual for an infant born prematurely to move erratically from one state to the next and to spend little time in the quiet alert state (Kahn-D'Angelo & Unanue, 2000). Behavioral signs of stress commonly seen in infants are listed in Table 14.2. To cope with stimulation, an infant will use self-calming behaviors or may be assisted in calming as noted in Box 14.2.

Throughout the examination, the infant's visual and auditory reactions are observed. An infant may open the eyes briefly or not at all. Eye opening can be facilitated by shading the infant's eyes with the therapist's hand or by examining the infant in a dimly lit room. Eye contact is possible when the infant is in a quiet alert state and positioned approximately 10 inches from the examiner's face. Horizontal visual tracking may be elicited by having the infant track the slow movement of the examiner's face. An infant in the NICU should respond to the examiner's voice with movement, quieting to the voice, and may turn

---

BOX 14.2 Neonatal Methods of Coping With Stimulation

Self-Calming
- Hand to face or mouth
- Sucking on hand, fingers, thumb, pacifier
- Maintaining flexed posture
- Hands or feet to midline
- Closing eyes, gaze aversion
- Drowsy state to control stimulation

Assisted Calming
- Nesting, positioning in flexion
- Holding in flexion
- Slow rocking
- Swaddling
- Quiet voice

Table 14.3 Behavioral States of Sleep and Arousal

Deep sleep	No movement of body or eyes. Optimal for growth and recovery.
Light sleep	Body jerks and eye movements seen. Heart and respiratory rate responses to noise and lights noted on bedside monitors.
Drowsiness	Transitional state between sleep and wakefulness. Eyes may open briefly. Little spontaneous movement. Behavioral signs of stress often present.
Quiet alertness	Eyes open and eye contact made. Relaxed face and facial expressions. Movements smooth. Ready for interaction.
Active alertness	Eyes open or closed. Facial grimace or hyperalert appearance common. Large-ranged, constant movements of extremities seen. Trunk extension often seen. Behavioral signs of stress present. Increased heart and respiratory rates.
Crying	Eyes closed. Crying. Stressed facial expression. Extremity and trunk movements seen. Increased heart and respiratory rates.

Source: Brazelton, T.B. (1984). Neonatal Behavioral Assessment Scale (2nd ed.). *Clinics in Developmental Medicine, No. 88.* Philadelphia: J.B. Lippincott, with permission.

---

toward the voice. The physical therapist documents the infant's behavioral states throughout the examination, as well as visual and auditory responses, signs of stress, and coping behaviors.

Active Movement and Strength

Active movements and strength are first evaluated by general observation when the infant is awake and alert. Spontaneous movements of the extremities should be smooth and symmetrical in range. The amount of antigravity movements seen will vary depending on the infant's gestational age at the time of the examination. Some jittery movements may be present but should not persist unless they are caused by medication or withdrawal secondary to the mother's drug use. Some active movements seen in the neonate include bringing hands together in midline, hands to face or mouth, pulling at a tube, and lower extremity extension to push against bedding. Infants born prematurely do not have the flexor muscle tone seen in healthy infants born at full term and need assistance to achieve a flexed posture. They also have more difficulty moving against gravity. Some full-term infants who are ill and in intensive care may also lack the ability to maintain flexor muscle tone. Infants who do not have natural flexor muscle tone have more difficulty moving in antigravity directions. They may appear very relaxed in general, with full contact of the body on the bed regardless of how they are positioned. They may also show decreased movement in general while in an alert state.

Strength is evaluated by observing as the infant moves the head, neck, trunk, and extremities against gravity. Head control is normally poor in neonates, but some attempts at controlling head position should be seen. When placed prone in a face-down position, the infant should be able to turn, or to lift and turn the head, to move out of the face-down position. In supported sitting, the infant may briefly extend the neck, holding the head upright for several seconds. Excessive or persistent extension of the neck or trunk in any position is a sign of increased muscle tone. Movements and strength of head, neck, trunk, and extremities should be documented.

Muscle Tone and Reflexes

Muscle tone is evaluated through the assessment of resistance to passive movement, primitive reflex testing, and observation of movements. Resistance to passive movement and, particularly, recoil of the arms and legs gives the examiner information about the infant's resting muscle tone. Muscle tone may be generally decreased in infants born prematurely and in infants born at full term who are ill. They will assume an extensor posture, being unable to overcome the effects of gravity. Primitive reflex development and the symmetry of responses to reflex testing provide information about the infant's neuromotor system. Optimal responses to reflex testing are seen when the infant is in a quiet alert state. Repetitive testing typically causes the infant to accommodate to the stimulus, showing a decreased or an absent response. If repeated examinations show asymmetries, inability to accommodate to testing, or other abnormal responses, these may be warning signs of movement impairment.

Primitive reflex testing usually includes evaluation of the Moro reflex, rooting, palmar grasp and traction, trunk incurvation (Galant reflex), plantar grasp, placing, and stepping reflexes (see Chapter 2, Table 2.7). The Moro reflex should not be tested if the infant is fragile because this may be particularly stressful for the infant. Deep tendon reflexes may be included in the examination and are helpful in identifying asymmetries and increased or decreased muscle tone. They also provide a baseline to use in comparing with future examinations.

Feeding

Feeding by mouth is a landmark skill for the infant in intensive care. Feeding helps determine when the infant will be discharged from the NICU to home. Learning to suck and swallow can be a difficult and long process for the infant and family. The physical therapist may be involved in the evaluation of feeding skills, along with the speech-language pathologist and occupational therapist. The infant's ability to feed by mouth should be considered as part of the examination. Problems seen with feeding may include discoordination or disorganization of sucking, swallowing, and breathing; difficulty in maintaining an alert state to eat; or abnormalities in oral motor skills interfering with the infant's ability to feed. Infants who are unable to feed orally may be fed by an orogastric, nasogastric, or gastrostomy tube.

Positioning and Handling

The infant's ability to maintain a flexed posture in supine, prone, and sidelying positions is noted. The amount of assistance needed to maintain a flexed posture by the caregiver's hands or by using blanket rolls or buntings is described. The infant's responses to handling and tolerance to stimulation are also noted and will influence the intervention plan.

Follow-up Care

The physical therapist makes recommendations for follow-up care as part of the initial evaluation. This may include outpatient physical therapy, early intervention services, and specialist care such as pediatric neurology or orthopedics. In some settings the physical therapist evaluating the infant in the NICU may also provide intervention to the infant in the outpatient or early intervention setting. Follow-up recommendations are modified as needed when the infant is ready for discharge from the NICU.

Intervention

Physical therapy in the NICU varies depending on which disciplines are part of the NICU team. The physical therapist in the NICU provides examination and evaluation of infants, and interventions consist primarily of family and staff education and consultation. Direct hands-on intervention occurs to a lesser extent. Because of the skills required, it is not recommended that physical therapy assistants and aides be used in the NICU (Sweeney et al., 1999). The physical therapy plan of care is individualized for the infant and changes as the infant grows, develops, and stabilizes.

Positioning

The physical therapist instructs others in **proper positioning** of the infant to encourage flexion, symmetrical neck movement, and symmetrical head shape and to promote the ease of breathing (Figure 14–3). These positioning techniques are usually done by nurses, parents, and other caregivers. This is accomplished by positioning the infant with arms and legs close to the body. Blanket rolls and specialized buntings around the infant's head, shoulder girdle, trunk, and legs are used to promote flexion and rest. This nesting effect is best when it is close enough to the infant's body to prevent shoulder and hip abduction. Arms should be positioned with elbows flexed and hands together, assisting in bringing the hands to midline, face, or mouth. Legs should be positioned with hips and knees flexed with a blanket roll at the feet to create a boundary for the infant to push against.

The prone position provides maximal support to the chest wall. This anchors the respiratory muscles and part of the ribcage, helping to ease breathing (Bjornson et al., 1992). Most neonates beyond 34 weeks are able to lift and turn their heads in prone. This aids in development of the postural muscles, including those in the back of the neck and along the spine. This activity also aids in development of head control. Infants who are positioned prone should have both legs flexed with knees under their bodies. Arms should be next to the head with elbows flexed. This allows easy access for bringing the hands to the face or mouth for self-comfort. The prone position is not, however, recommended for sleeping (Gibson, Cullen, Spinner, Rankin, &

Spitzer, 1995), especially when the infant is not on a monitor or is nearing discharge.

The supine position is often used for fragile infants. This allows maximal observation of the infant's face and chest. While the infant is lying supine, support is given to the postural muscles in the back and along the spine. The effects of gravity in the supine position may cause the infant to move out of flexion and into an extended posture. The postures that tend to be assumed are scapular retraction, elbow extension, shoulder extension and abduction, hip abduction, and spinal extension. This position discourages many **self-calming behaviors,** such as hands to midline, face, or mouth; lower extremity flexion; and trunk flexion. Added support of blanket rolls and buntings placed closely to the trunk and hips can help to minimize scapular retraction and hip abduction in supine. Although the supine position allows the caregiver close visual observation of the infant's breathing pattern, it requires the infant to use the respiratory muscles against gravity and may make breathing more difficult.

The sidelying position assists the infant in maintaining hands together and lower extremities flexed. The sidelying position provides some support to the rib cage, assisting in the ease of respiration. The infant should be nested with blanket rolls or a bunting to encourage trunk flexion. It is essential to alternate between both left and right sidelying positions. If one side is used more than the other, the infant may develop an asymmetrical head shape and possibly torticollis.

Infants who require more specific positioning benefit from a customized positioning program. That program can be posted at the bedside. All caregivers carry out this program across different staff shifts with instruction from the physical therapist. The program would typically include drawings or photographs and specific instructions indicating which positions to use and for how long. A need for a customized positioning program is common in infants having the following diagnoses: Erb's palsy, torticollis, myelomeningocele, arthrogryposis, or extreme hypotonia or hypertonia.

Sleep Position Recommendations

The American Academy of Pediatrics currently recommends that infants sleep in the supine position (Gibson et al., 1995). The prone position is not recommended because of the correlations found between infants sleeping prone and sudden infant death syndrome (SIDS). Sidelying is not recommended because infants are generally able to move from sidelying to prone and are therefore at risk of SIDS (Li

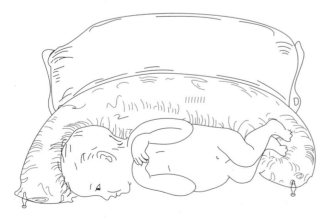

Figure 14-3 Proper positioning of the infant in the NICU.

et al., 2003). Parents are instructed to follow these guidelines and to position their infants in the supine position to sleep. Because infants in the NICU are placed in a variety of positions, including prone, it is recommended that they begin sleeping supine before going home. The physical therapist may make specific recommendations to the family if the infant needs additional hip or shoulder support in the supine position.

Parents need to be educated on the importance of the prone position for the infant's motor development (Davis, Moon, Sachs, & Ottolini, 1998; Jantz, Blosser, & Fruechting, 1997). The infant should spend time each day in the prone position when awake. This is needed for development of neck and trunk muscles and assists in the development of rolling, sitting, and crawling.

Active Movement

Some infants need a program for maintaining or increasing active movement and range of motion (ROM). This is commonly needed for infants with brachial plexus injuries, arthrogryposis, torticollis, amniotic band syndrome, or positional deformities. A ROM program is developed by physical and occupational therapists and can be implemented by all caregivers following careful instruction.

The physical therapist also assists infants in developing active movement. Peripheral nerve injury, myelomeningocele, decreased arousal for age, and extreme hypotonia are some conditions in which movement training is likely. Techniques that will assist a newborn in developing active movement might include assistance in achieving self-calming movements, such as hands to mouth or midline; use of positioning to promote antigravity movements; and use of tactile stimulation to elicit movement. In cases of peripheral nerve injuries and positional deformities, the physical and occupational therapist may fabricate a temporary positioning device such as a splint in order to preserve or increase ROM while allowing recovery to occur and active movement to develop.

Physical Therapy Plan of Care

Each contact that the physical therapist has with the infant is part of the ongoing examination and evaluation. Because the infant develops and changes during the NICU stay, the plan of care is dynamic. Physical therapy often continues after the infant is discharged from the NICU. Information from the physical therapy examination, evaluation, and interventions provides a valuable history of the infant's development. This information is used to help determine the need for ongoing intervention and assists the family in decisions regarding the infant's follow-up care. Many infants discharged from the NICU are eligible for early intervention services under Part C of the Individuals with Disabilities Education Act (see Chapter 10). Referral to the appropriate follow-up programs/services and monitoring of the infant's ongoing development ensure the best developmental outcome for the infant.

Summary and Conclusions

The NICU is a very specialized and continually evolving setting for all health professionals. Medical interventions have become very sophisticated, ensuring survival of very small and fragile infants. Furthermore, infants born at less than 26 weeks gestation are showing consistently increasing rates of survival and less complications (Kilbride & Daily, 1998; Surman et al., 2003). The use of various medications has assisted infants in achieving a generally shorter course of mechanical ventilation, and in achieving medical stability at earlier ages (Kilbride & Daily, 1998). Severity of illness is somewhat predictive of the infant's length of stay in the NICU (Escobar, Fischer, Li, Kremers, & Armstrong, 1995). As neonatal intensive care becomes more complex, physical therapists are becoming more involved with these infants. The physical therapist must use caution to ensure that the timing of the physical therapy examination and handling is appropriate. A typical NICU case is briefly outlined in Case Example 14.1.

Infants discharged from intensive care nurseries are a developmentally at-risk population. These infants require more frequent follow-up care including rehospitalization, outpatient visits to the pediatrician, and specialist visits (Cavalier, Escobar, Fernbach, Quesenberry, & Chellino, 1996). Infants with low birth weights needing NICU care show more problems with neurocognitive and school performance at ages up to 8 years old than infants born at full term with age-appropriate birth weights (McGrath et al., 2000). Physical therapists are involved in the follow-up of these infants as well as referrals to needed community agencies and programs.

The physical therapist is an active member of the NICU team. Physical therapy provides an individualized and developmental approach for infants in intensive care. This is important because much of the infant's care is centered around medical needs. Family education and involvement are essential, and the physical therapist provides valuable information and instruction to families, directly affecting the infant's care. Physical therapists practicing in the NICU need specialized knowledge and training in order to build on their baseline scope of practice and provide safe and effective care.

CASE EXAMPLE 14–1 . . . .

NICU

History

Baby boy James M. was born at 27 weeks' gestation by emergency cesarean section attributable to fetal distress. Apgar scores were 3 at 1 minute, 5 at 5 minutes, and 8 at 10 minutes. James was intubated at birth and remained on the ventilator for 10 days. He received two doses of surfactant and was also treated with Decadron (dexamethasone). James received nutrition through his central umbilical line. At 30 weeks' gestation, he began oral gavage feedings of fortified breast milk. He tolerated feeds and began to breast or bottle feed once daily at 31 weeks' gestational age.

Examination and Evaluation

At 31 weeks, James was medically stable and was ready for a physical therapy examination. The physical therapy examination occurred over two sessions and included observation during caregiving procedures that included feeding and handling. During the initial observation and examination, James was drowsy during most caregiving procedures, including measuring of vital signs, diaper changes, and feedings. He maintained a quiet alert state for approximately 30 seconds and made eye contact. James showed several signs of stress, including hiccups, finger splays, grimace, and trunk arching. He showed self-comforting signs and coped with handling and stimulation by bringing his hands to his face and maintaining a flexed posture with assistance given by the examiner.

Spontaneous movements showed large range movements of all extremities. Movements were symmetrical and lower extremity movements were jittery. When positioned prone, James lifted and turned his head to the left. He showed a preference for cervical rotation to the left in general.

Primitive reflex testing in the quiet alert state showed normal symmetrical responses for the following reflexes: palmar and plantar grasp, trunk incurvation, flexor withdrawal, and crossed extension. The rooting and upper extremity traction reflexes were present bilaterally but were difficult to elicit. Several beats of ankle clonus were present bilaterally. The Moro reflex was not tested because it requires posterior displacement of the head, which can be potentially harmful at 31 weeks' gestation.

Passive ROM indicated tightness in end-range cervical rotation to the right and tightness in end-range cervical lateral flexion to the left. Passive ROM was otherwise within normal limits and symmetrical.

Feeding assessment showed that James remained calm during oral gavage feedings and would suck on a regular pacifier during these feedings. Nipple feeding was done using a bottle with a regular nipple. James showed fair suck and good ability to grip the nipple with his tongue. James consistently showed a decrease in oxygen saturation below 90% with nipple feedings, which resolved by removing the bottle and resting for approximately 30 seconds before reintroducing the bottle.

The family situation included a stable family environment. James's parents were married and had two other children at home. The parents visited twice daily and were available for feeding James during their visits. It was anticipated that he would be discharged to home.

Summary

- Strengths: Spontaneous movements and muscle tone were within normal limits for 31 weeks gestation. Nipple feedings showed age-appropriate difficulty in coordinating suck, swallow, and breathe.

- Limitations in body structure: Mild right torticollis.

- Limitations in activities: Fair tolerance to handling and stimulation with signs of stress including hiccups, finger splaying, grimace, and trunk arching. James coped with stimulation by bringing hands to face and maintaining a flexed posture.

Physical Therapy Plan of Care

- Family instruction: Parents will be instructed in the interventions described below with modifications ongoing to allow for changes in James's status.

- Education/positioning program: Position James in flexion using blanket rolls or buntings to maintain arms and legs close to midline and to assist with hands to midline and hands to face. Alternate positions between right and left sidelying and prone. The supine position should be used more as James approaches discharge to home. Position his head turned to the right whenever possible to decrease tightness in the right sternocleidomastoid and to prevent worsening of the right torticollis. Encourage active flexion during caregiving procedures and holding by (1) assisting in bringing hands and feet to midline and (2) holding and positioning with arms and legs close to his body.

- Feeding: Continue to feed James with a regular-sized nipple. Hold him in a flexed position during feeding. Assist James during nipple feedings by helping him pace the feeding. Count the number of times he sucks by watching his chin move and remove the nipple briefly after 12 sucks. This will help James in coordinating suck, swallow, and breathe.

Physical Therapy Re-examination

As James develops and grows, physical therapy interventions and recommendations will change according to his development. Re-examination will occur on a weekly basis.

Discharge Plan

At the time of discharge, James will be referred to the High-Risk Infant Follow-up Program. This will include a physical therapy re-examination at approximately 1 month after his discharge to home. He may be scheduled for an earlier follow-up appointment if indicated at the time of discharge. He will receive a home health nurse visit after discharge to assess feeding and weight gain. He will also be referred to the community early intervention program for further developmental evaluation and follow-up care.

DISCUSSION QUESTIONS

1. Why is correcting for gestational age important? Until what age do you continue to correct for gestational age?
2. What is the recommended position for the infant while he or she is sleeping? How might this position for sleeping affect the infant's motor development?
3. Explain the importance of flexor muscle tone in the neonate. Why is positioning the infant in flexion important for development of movement?
4. What are some behavioral and physiological signs of stress used by the infant? Why is it important for the physical therapist and other caregivers to adapt the infant's care plan to minimize stress?
5. What is developmentally supportive care in the NICU? How does developmentally supportive care promote neonatal recovery?
6. What is periventricular leukomalacia? Discuss the correlation between the incidence of premature birth and periventricular leukomalacia with the outcome of cerebral palsy.

RECOMMENDED READINGS

Als, H., & Gilkerson, L. (1997). The role of relationship-based developmentally supportive newborn intensive care in strengthening outcome of preterm infants. *Seminars in Perinatology, 21*(3), 178–189.

Kahn-D'Angelo, L., & Unanue, R.A. (2000). The special care nursery. In S.K. Campbell, D.W. Vander Linden & R.J. Palisano (Eds.). *Physical therapy for children* (2nd ed.) (pp. 840–880). Philadelphia: W.B. Saunders.

Neonatology on the Web. Available from *http://www.neonatology.org/index.html*

Sweeny, J.K., Heriza, C.B., Reilly, M.A., Smith, C.S., & VanSant, A.F. (1999). Practice guidelines for the physical therapist in the neonatal intensive care unit (NICU). *Pediatric Physical Therapy, 11*, 119–132.

Sweeny, J.K., & Swanson, M.W. (2001). Low birth weight infants: Neonatal care and follow-up. In D.A. Umphred (Ed.). *Neurological rehabilitation* (4th ed., pp. 205–258). St. Louis, MO: Mosby.

Wolf, L.S., & Glass, R.P. *Feeding and swallowing disorders in infancy: Assessment and management.* San Antonio, TX: Therapy Skill Builders.

REFERENCES

Als, H., & Gilkerson, L. (1997). The role of relationship-based developmentally supportive newborn intensive care in strengthening outcome of preterm infants. *Seminars in Perinatology, 21*(3), 178–189.

Als, H., Lawhorn, G., Brown, E., Gibes, R., Duffy, F.H., McAnulty, G., & Blickman, J.G. (1986). Individualized behavioral and environmental care for the very low birthweight preterm infant at high risk for bronchopulmonary dysplasia: Neonatal intensive care unit and developmental outcome. *Pediatrics, 78*, 1123–1132.

Bennett, F.C. (1999). Developmental outcome. In G.B. Avery, M. Fletcher, & M.G. MacDonald (Eds.), *Neonatology: Pathophysiology and management of the newborn* (pp. 1479–1497). Philadelphia: Lippincott Williams & Wilkins.

Bennett, F.C., & Scott, D.T. (1997). Long term perspective on premature infant outcome and contemporary intervention issues. *Seminars in Perinatology, 21*(3), 190–201.

Bjornson, K.F., Deitz, J.C., Blackburn, S.T., Billingsley, F., Garcia, J., & Hays, R. (1992). The effect of body position on the oxygen saturation of ventilated preterm infants. *Pediatric Physical Therapy, 4*, 109–115.

Brazelton, T.B. (1984). Neonatal Behavioral Assessment Scale (2nd ed.). *Clinics in Developmental Medicine, No. 88.* Philadelphia: J.B. Lippincott.

Cavalier, S., Escobar, G.J., Fernbach, S.A., Quesenberry, C.P., & Chellino, M. (1996). Postdischarge utilization of medical service by high-risk infants: Experience in a large managed care organization. *Pediatrics, 97*(5), 693–699.

Davis, B.E., Moon, R.Y., Sachs, H.C., & Ottolini, M.C. (1998). Effects of sleep position on infant motor development. *Pediatrics, 102*(5), 1135–1140.

Duncan, C.C., & Ment, L.R. (1993). Intraventricular hemorrhage and prematurity. *Neurosurgical Clinics of North America, 4*, 727–734.

Escobar, G.J., Fischer, A., Li, D.K., Kremers, R., & Armstrong, M.A. (1995). Score for neonatal acute physiology: Validation in three Kaiser Permanente neonatal intensive care units. *Pediatrics, 96*(5), 918–922.

Feldman, R., & Eidelman, A.I. (2003). Skin-to-skin contact (kangaroo care) accelerates autonomic and neurobehavioral maturation in preterm infants. *Developmental Medicine and Child Neurology, 45*, 274–281.

Foulder-Hughes, L.A., & Cooke, R.W.I. (2003). Motor, cognitive and behavioral disorders in children born very preterm. *Developmental Medicine and Child Neurology, 45*, 97–103.

Gibson, E., Cullen, J.A., Spinner, S., Rankin, K., & Spitzer, A.R. (1995). Infant sleep position following new AAP guidelines. *Pediatrics, 96*(1), 69–72.

Gretebeck, R.J., Shaffer, D., & Bishop-Kurylo, D. (1998). Clinical pathways for family oriented developmental care in the intensive care nursery. *Journal of Perinatal Nursing, 12*(1), 70–80.

Hunter, J.G., Zwischenberger, J.B., & Bhatia, J. (1992). Neonatal extracorporeal membrane oxygenation: Neurodevelopmental outcome of survivors. *Infants and Young Children, 4*(4), 63–76.

Hussain, N., Clive, J., & Bhandari, V. (1999). Current incidence of retinopathy of prematurity, 1989–1997. *Pediatrics, 104*, e26.

Jantz, J.W., Blosser, C.D., & Fruechting, L.A. (1997). A motor milestone change noted with a change in sleep position. *Archives of Pediatrics and Adolescent Medicine, 151*, 565–568.

Kahn-D'Angelo, L. (1995). The special care nursery. In S.K. Campbell (Ed.), *Physical therapy for children* (pp. 787–822). Philadelphia: W.B. Saunders.

Kahn-D'Angelo, L., & Unanue, R.A. (2000). The special care nursery. In S.K. Campbell, D.W. Vander Linden, & R.J. Palisano (Eds.), *Physical therapy for children* (2nd ed., pp. 840–880). Philadelphia: W.B. Saunders.

Kilbride, H.W., & Daily, D.K. (1998). Survival and subsequent outcome to five years of age for infants with birth weights less than 801 grams born from 1983 to 1989. *Journal of Perinatology, 18*(2), 102–106.

Li, D.K., Petitti, D.B., Willinger, J., McMahon, R., Odouli, R., Vu, H., & Hoffman, H.J. (2003). Infant sleeping position and the risk of sudden infant death syndrome in California, 1997–2000. *American Journal of Epidemiology, 157*(5), 446–455.

Lowes, L.P., & Palisano, R.J. (1995). Review of medical and developmental outcomes of neonates who received extracorporeal membrane oxygenation. *Pediatric Physical Therapy, 7*, 15–22.

McCarton, C.M., Wallace, I.F., Divon, M., & Vaughan, H.G. (1996). Cognitive and neurologic development of the premature, small for gestational age infant through age 6: Comparison by birth weight and gestational age. *Pediatrics, 98*(6), 1167–1178.

McGrath, M.M., Sullivan, M.C., Lester, B.M., & Oh, W. (2000). Longitudinal neurologic follow-up in neonatal intensive care unit survivors with various neonatal morbidities. *Pediatrics, 106*(6), 1397–1405.

Moster, D., Lie, R.T., Irgens, L.M., Bjerkedal, T., & Markestad, T. (2001). The association of Apgar score with subsequent death and cerebral palsy: A population-based study in term infants. *Journal of Pediatrics, 138*(6), 798–803.

Murphy, B., Inder, T.E., Huppi, P.S., Warfield, S., Zientra, G.P., Kilkinis, R., Jolesz, F.A., & Volpe, J.J. (2001). Impaired cerebral cortical gray matter growth after treatment with dexamethasone for neonatal chronic lung disease. *Pediatrics, 107*(2), 217–221.

Sloan, N., Camacho, L.W.L., Rojas, E.P., Maternidad Isidro Ayor Study Team (1994). Kangaroo mother method: Randomised controlled trial of an alternative method of care for stabilized low-birth weight infants. *Lancet, 344*, 782–785.

Surman, G., Newdick, H., & Johnson, A. (2003). Cerebral palsy rates among low-birthweight infants fell in the 1990s. *Developmental Medicine and Child Neurology, 45*, 456–462.

Sweeney, J.K. (1986). Physiologic adaptation of neonates to

neurological assessment. *Physical and Occupational Therapy in Pediatrics, 6*(3/4), 155–169.

Sweeney, J.K. (1989). Physiological and behavioral effects of neurological assessment in preterm and full-term neonates (abstract). *Physical and Occupational Therapy in Pediatrics, 9*(3), 144–146.

Sweeney, J.K., Heriza, C.B., Reilly, M.A., Smith, C.S., & VanSant, A.F. (1999). Practice guidelines for the physical therapist in the neonatal intensive care unit (NICU). *Pediatric Physical Therapy, 11*, 119–132.

Taylor, H.G., Klein, N., Schatschneider, C., & Hack, M. (1998). Predictors of early school age outcomes in very low birth weight children. *Developmental and Behavioral Pediatrics, 19*(4), 235–243.

The Infant Health and Development Program, A Multisite, Randomized Trial (1990). Enhancing the outcomes of low birth weight, premature infants. *Journal of the American Medical Association, 263*(22), 3035–3042.

VandenBerg, K.A. (1997). Basic principles of developmental caregiving. *Neonatal Network, 16*(7), 129–131.

Volpe, J.J. (1989). Intraventricular hemorrhage and brain injury in the premature infant. *Clinical Perinatology, 16*, 387–411.

Volpe, J.J. (1998). Neurologic outcome of prematurity. *Archives of Neurology, 55*, 297–300.

Weisglas-Kuperus, N., Baerts, W., Smrkovsky, M., & Sauer, P.J.J. (1993). Effects of biological and social factors on the cognitive development of very low birth weight children. *Pediatrics, 92*, 658–665.

Chapter *15*

Rehabilitation Settings

— Shirley Albinson Daniels, PT, MS

Rehabilitation involves the restoration of function after disability resulting from impairments, injury, or disease by use of examination, evaluation, diagnosis, prognosis, and intervention, including plan of care and outcomes. A team of professionals, spanning the domains of mobility, feeding, activities of daily living (ADLs), cognition, language and communication, psychosocial and emotional function, and physiological stability, most often provides care. Children are served within the context of their developmental age, family support network, and cultural values, with the goal of returning them to the least restrictive school and community environment possible.

There are various types of rehabilitation hospitals. Some are free-standing hospitals whose mission focuses exclusively on providing care to children with physical disabilities or chronic health-care needs. Other settings may be specialty units located within an acute-care pediatric setting. The National Association of Children's Hospitals and Related Institutions (NACHRI) includes about 160 members and supporters in the United States and Canada, with some 16 listed as specialty hospitals, mostly rehabilitation (NACHRI, 2004). Some pediatric rehabilitation settings have received accreditation from the Commission on Accreditation and Rehabilitation Facilities (CARF), the same agency that reviews adult rehabilitation hospitals.

Children are cared for on a continuum of services that provide the optimal setting to meet their medical and rehabilitation needs. Children whose physiological condition has not been stabilized medically will be served in an inpatient setting, perhaps in the acute-care environment. Rehabilitation as an inpatient will be needed until the family and child are able to function safely in the home, with the assistance of home-care services if necessary. Skilled nursing care facilities are sometimes required for children whose chronic needs cannot be met in the home setting. A day hospital, an option offered by some agencies, provides intense therapeutic intervention during the day but transports the child home to the family for overnight care. As the child recovers, rehabilitation may be provided in the outpatient setting. Generally, the cost of care declines as the child moves through the continuum of service options. The insurance company will usually seek the least expensive alternative to meet the child's needs.

Children entering the rehabilitation setting come with a specific set of admission goals and an expected length of stay, which has been negotiated by the insurance company with the agency. Although the comprehensive needs of the child may be broad, given the many limitations in body structures and functions and restrictions in activities and participation, each episode of care is planned to focus specifically on the urgent needs that must be met in order to move the child back into the home, school, and community. For example, a child with cerebral palsy (CP) who undergoes selective dorsal rhizotomy to improve gait will receive intensive physical and occupational therapy in a rehabilitation setting. The child may also have communication deficits or a cognitive delay that are addressed during the stay. The goals relating to these domains, however, will be secondary to those associated with the mobility issues, which will drive the discharge plan.

Rehabilitation agencies affiliated with universities are often committed to the three-part mission involving excellence in clinical care, teaching, and research. Such agencies may be involved in training professionals in a variety of disciplines at entry level or offer practica for licensed clinicians who wish to specialize in pediatrics. A comprehensive staff development program using both internal and external resources ensures staff competency to provide high-quality clinical care and foster retention. Staff members may be involved in clinical research and present their findings at national conferences and publish them in professional journals.

A rehabilitation setting is often an excellent place to start a career in pediatrics. Therapists work closely with other members of the health-care team, and there are usually experienced mentors within one discipline to guide a therapist new to pediatrics. Therapists are able to spend a significant amount of time with the child and family, thus establishing rapport and seeing firsthand the outcomes of the interventions.

Common Categories of Children Served

Rehabilitation covers a wide range of disabilities with restrictions in activities and participation. These disabilities and related diagnoses usually fall into one of the four broad categories. These categories—neurorehabilitation, developmental habilitation, musculoskeletal rehabilitation, and behavioral rehabilitation—are not exclusive, and there is frequent overlap. Various agencies specialize in clusters of diagnostic groups, depending on the expertise of their medical staff and overall mission.

Neurorehabilitation

Unintentional injury is the leading cause of death in children under 14 years (NACHRI, 2004). Trauma from falls, recreational activities, and motor vehicle accidents are the leading causes of both brain injury and spinal cord injury in the pediatric population. Other etiologies causing brain damage include infections, brain tumors, and child abuse. A child who was developing typically and becomes injured because of trauma suddenly thrusts the entire family into a crisis. Plans of care must incorporate the child or adolescent within the family unit, and a social worker is often pivotal in this role. An interdisciplinary team of professionals is necessary to provide comprehensive care to children with neurorehabilitation needs in order to help the child to function as independently as possible.

Children with more chronic, non–sudden-onset disabilities, such as CP, muscular dystrophy, or arthrogryposis multiplex congenita, may also need rehabilitation services at various times. For example, children with CP may require rehabilitation after orthopedic surgery. School-aged children with spina bifida may require specialized rehabilitation nursing to achieve independent self-catheterization skills. Although many school-aged children with physical disabilities receive the majority of their therapy services in the school setting, only those goals that are related to their educational needs are provided and funded by the educational system. Children with chronic diagnoses and significant restrictions in activities and participation may require the expertise offered by a hospital-based clinical team to oversee their medical and rehabilitative needs over the years. These teams are often organized around multidisciplinary clinics that provide consultation and rehabilitation management of a specific diagnosis.

Developmental Habilitation

Young children with serious developmental disabilities and medical complications may be provided with a program of **habilitation** in an inpatient setting. The term *habilitation* is used because the child is not relearning or rehabilitating a lost skill but rather is learning new life skills. Developmental habilitation programs usually follow the principles learned from the progression of typically developing children. Inpatient developmental habilitation might be required for children with Down syndrome and other genetic disabilities after an illness or surgery. Often the full extent of limitations in body functions and structures and restrictions in activities and participation are not known for several years in infants who are born prematurely or with congenital anomalies. These children are at risk for developmental delay or CP.

Infants who fail to thrive or to gain weight at home may need comprehensive services to diagnose and manage feeding disorders. Graduates of neonatal intensive care nurseries may be ventilator dependent as a result of bronchopulmonary dysplasia, a common complication of prematurity. The needs of the parents must be incorporated into the plan of care, and parents should be taught a variety of nursing and therapy techniques before taking the infant home.

Musculoskeletal Rehabilitation

Children having musculoskeletal diagnoses and impairments may also be cared for in the rehabilitation setting. This may include children with chronic musculoskeletal disorders, such as rheumatic diseases, muscular dystrophy, or achondroplasia (autosomal dominant disorder resulting in short extremities and relatively large head) or those with recent injury, such as burns or amputations. They may have undergone a specific orthopedic procedure to correct a physical impairment, such as limb lengthening for leg length discrepancy or spinal fusion for idiopathic scoliosis. Children who have undergone orthopedic surgery may require intensive physical or occupational therapy to achieve their functional goals. Specialized programs, including aquatic exercise, may supplement traditional therapy. Orthotic or prosthetic prescription and fitting are also commonly part of the care plan for those with musculoskeletal system impairments.

Behavioral Rehabilitation

Behavioral rehabilitation programs may be available for children with autism, severe self-injurious behavior, and other diagnoses. Not all rehabilitation settings are prepared to deal with the complexities of caring for this specialized group of children, and a team of professionals with strong leadership in psychology is essential for their care. Physical therapists who serve on a behavioral rehabilitation team must learn from and follow the recommendations of those trained in behavioral management. Consistency in the utilization of behavior management techniques is critical and must be learned and used by all staff members.

Scope of Services

Given the complex needs of most children requiring rehabilitation, a team of professionals is essential to provide a comprehensive plan of care. Team membership may vary, but often includes a physical therapist, occupational therapist, speech-language pathologist, psychologist (or neuropsychologist), special educator, social worker, rehabil-

itation nurse, nutritionist, child life specialist, or recreation therapist. Medical leadership varies but may include those with credentials in physiatry, developmental pediatrics, general pediatrics, neurology, orthopedics, and psychiatry. Some physicians are double boarded; for example, they may have completed the requirements for board certification in both pediatrics and physiatry. Agencies must also be prepared to meet the needs of children for orthotics, prosthetics, medical equipment, wheelchairs, and assistive technology. These services may be provided through employment of experts or via liaisons with durable medical equipment vendors, orthotists/prosthetists, or rehabilitation engineers.

Regardless of the exact complement of team members, they will need to assess and develop plans of care to deal with the following domains:

1. Physiological Stability—This includes ongoing or emergent medical problems affecting specific systems, current medications, allergies, health supervision issues (e.g., immunizations), nutrition, pain management, and individual participation in medical management.

2. Mobility and Neuromotor Development—This domain includes fine and gross motor development; movement, including transfers, locomotion, balance, and coordination; flexibility and strength; and community mobility.

3. Feeding—This includes oral motor skills; neuromuscular and respiratory stability; positioning for feeding; and textures, volumes, and routes.

4. Activities of Daily Living—ADLs include toileting; hygiene; dressing; self-feeding; and play, recreation, or leisure activities.

5. Cognitive Status—This includes developmental level, orientation, attention span, ability to learn, memory and sequencing, problem solving, processing information, perception, safety and judgment, and school re-entry.

6. Language and Communication Status—This includes developmental level; prelanguage and language skills; speaking, writing, and reading; augmentative communication; and language barriers.

7. Psychosocial and Emotional Status—This includes social, emotional, and behavioral status; social and emotional status of family, including family strengths and needs; coping with limitations and restrictions and hospitalization; cultural and spiritual issues;

sexuality appropriate for developmental level; and self-determination.

8. Discharge Planning—This includes follow-up appointments; need for continuing rehabilitation services; child and family instruction; home, school, and community re-entry, including evaluation of barriers; ordering of adaptive equipment (especially for mobility and ADLs) or medical supplies; prevention and health promotion; and transportation plan, including a car seat.

The physical therapist provides a leading role in addressing goals relating to mobility and neuromotor development. The physical therapist, along with other members of the health-care team, may also provide care relating to feeding, ADLs, and discharge planning.

Team Function

The degree to which team members collaborate on goal setting and implementation of programs has been described in different team models, discussed in more detail in Chapter 1. In the *multidisciplinary team*, a group of professionals work together to provide care. They agree to report their findings to each other but maintain professional boundaries in programming. In the *interdisciplinary team*, professionals collaborate in providing care by merging goals and care plans into a unified program for the child. Professionals agree to work on all of the child's rehabilitation goals by incorporating suggestions from other professionals into their interventions. In the *transdisciplinary team*, professionals assess the child and then delegate the delivery of care to a few key individuals. There is role release on a transdisciplinary team, and members function in domains outside of their traditional training.

The model of team interaction will differ widely among agencies. It may also be somewhat dependent on the experience of the team members and the length of time they have worked together. Only a very mature team of professionals, with members who are comfortable in their own discipline and have cross-trained in other disciplines, can achieve true transdisciplinary status. Many agencies prefer to foster an interdisciplinary team approach, which follows accepted conventions for reimbursement.

Another model of organization is a **product or service line organization.** In this model, professionals from different disciplines are typically assigned to a specific team, such as the neurorehabilitation unit, and receive supervision from an administrator who may be outside of their disci-

pline. Rather than having separate departments of physical therapy, occupational therapy, nutrition, and psychology, all of the professionals may be grouped into the rehabilitation service line and report to one director. The true service line model includes a continuum of care across a variety of venues from acute care to rehabilitation, to ambulatory to home care, and promotes collaboration among professionals of different disciplines.

A **matrix management model** provides for both service line organization and departmental organization. Matrix organizations involve both hierarchical coordination through departments with a formal chain of command and simultaneously lateral coordination across departments through service lines (Kovner & Neuhauser, 1983). A matrix model allows a combination of reporting relationships to occur, with administrative supervision from the service line manager, and professional supervision through supervisors of the same discipline (Figure 15–1). Excellent communication must exist in order to develop a consensus on policies and procedures.

Coordination of Care

Episodes of rehabilitation services for the child are often coordinated by care managers working within the rehabilitation setting and by case managers employed by insurance companies. At the time when the child's rehabilitation needs are identified, the preliminary goals and plan of care are established to obtain preauthorization for admission. For routine cases, critical paths help to clarify the goals to be achieved in the most cost-effective model possible. Critical paths help to standardize medical care among practitioners and provide a vehicle to assess outcomes. Modifications of the path can be based on objective measurement of ongoing care (Spath, 1994).

Once the child is admitted to the rehabilitation setting, the preliminary goals and plan of care are further refined based on a comprehensive examination and evaluation. Some interdisciplinary teams prefer to conduct an arena examination, as discussed in Chapters 1 and 10, in which all professionals assess the child at the same time. Typically, one or two therapists from different disciplines perform the majority of a child's examination, based on suggestions from those observing in the circle around the child. Arena examinations may be written up in one document that also includes the goals and plan of care, and which represents the child's total needs.

In some rehabilitation settings, the child is seen by professionals from each discipline for examination of

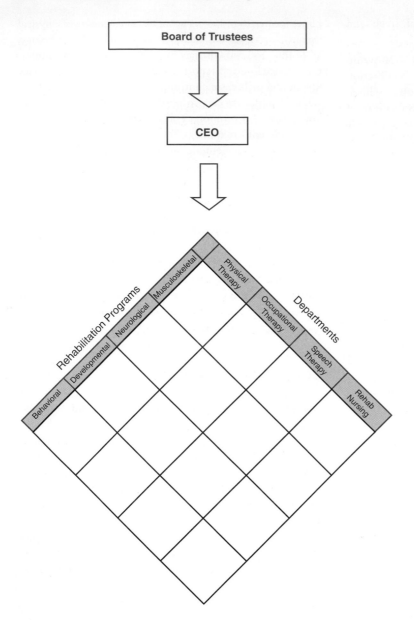

Figure 15-1 Organizational chart for matrix management.

specific domains of function. The findings are written up into separate reports. In either model, the professionals need to come together in a care planning conference to share information that includes the following:

1. Present level of function and problem list

2. Statement of measurable goals, outcomes, and objectives

3. Plan of care and intervention

4. Estimated length of time needed to achieve plan of care

5. Recommendations for additional consultations and tests

6. Considerations for discharge

This initial planning meeting will form the basis for evaluating the child's progress. Future meetings will be scheduled periodically to determine whether the child has achieved the goals in the time frame specified or whether there needs to be an alteration in the plan of care or length of stay. Concurrently, a review of the child's progress will need to be communicated to the insurance company to justify a continued inpatient stay.

Discharge planning begins the moment the child enters the rehabilitative setting. All goals are directed toward helping the child and family achieve functional independence in the next setting, which typically includes home, school, and community. The child and family need to be educated in how to provide any medical care needed at discharge. The physical therapist may teach transfers and safe methods for guarding during ambulation on level surfaces and stairs and provide a home program directed at continuing to work on goals established at discharge. A home exercise program might include improving flexibility, strength, endurance, balance, range of motion, and functional skills. Equipment such as orthotics, ambulation aides, a car seat, a wheelchair with custom modifications, or other durable medical equipment may be acquired before discharge. The physical therapist often is involved in the evaluation and justification for these items, as well as writing the letter describing why they are medically necessary.

A visit to the home and school will assist in identifying architectural barriers and providing guidance in modifications to ensure accessibility. Public buildings, such as schools, should be barrier free, or modifications must be made to the building as required under the Americans with Disabilities Act to meet the needs of the child. Field trips should be incorporated into the rehabilitation stay to assist the child in achieving a smooth re-entry into the community. Teaching skills, such as riding public transportation, shopping, driving, and so on, also helps meet the child's needs for independence.

Other Specialized Rehabilitation Services

In addition to more traditional therapies, other specialty services may be incorporated into the plan of care. For example, aquatic exercise may be used to achieve goals relating to functional mobility. Hippotherapy (therapeutic horseback riding) or dance therapy may be more enjoyable ways to achieve mobility goals. Art or music therapy may be used to identify and address psychosocial problems.

Often educational services can be integrated into the rehabilitation stay so that children can keep pace with their class while they are absent from school. For children with new injuries, especially head trauma, special education along with psychological assessment may be needed to determine what classroom setting will be optimal at discharge.

Orthotics and prosthetic devices are often necessary to achieve the rehabilitation goals. To meet an interim need or to evaluate the effectiveness of a specific prescription, the therapist may fabricate temporary devices. Definitive devices are typically made by the orthotist or prosthetist, who works closely with the team to achieve the mobility goals. Assistive technology can be provided so that the child can achieve full social inclusion, defined as full meaningful inclusion for the child into the social fabric of the culture. Technology can be designed to assist with communication, mobility, cognition, environmental mastery, recreation, and ADLs, as will be discussed in Chapters 16 and 17.

Gait laboratory data may be available to assist in clinical decision making and documentation of outcomes, as well as in clinical research. Objective information about the child's gait characteristics is captured via electromyography, videography, and force plate, for comparison before and after specific interventions.

Adolescents may require services overlapping with those provided in adult rehabilitation. Vocational counseling and rehabilitation can assist teenagers in career selection and preparation of skills for career entry. Individuals with spinal cord injury or neural tube defect must receive age-appropriate counseling regarding their sexuality and life-span issues related to their disability. Teenagers may need a referral for evaluation for driver's training and recommendations for specific adaptations for the car.

Outcomes Measurement

Measuring the rehabilitation outcomes for children and youth with disabilities is very important because future services and interventions for all children are driven by analysis of previous outcomes at the community and clinical levels (Lollar, Simeonsson, & Nanda, 2000). Most hospitals have adopted a standardized functional assessment tool, such as the Functional Independence Measure for Children (WeeFIM) (Granger, Hamilton, & Kayton, 1989) or the Pediatric Evaluation of Disability Inventory (PEDI) (Haley, Coster, Ludlow, Haltiwanger, & Andrellos, 1992) to measure the outcomes of rehabilitation services. The tools are applied at admission and discharge, and changes in the scores are used to demonstrate programmatic outcomes. Less well known in the United States is the Measure of Processes of Care (MPOC), which measures how parents perceive the interpersonal aspects of the care provided by clinicians (King, Rosenbaum, & King, 1995).

Clinical paths or care guidelines can also be used to measure outcome for specific diagnostic groups. Once a detailed path is developed that defines the standard of care to be provided, each child can be compared against the guideline to determine variance. In addition to generalized measures, individualized measures, such as goal attainment scaling (GAS) (Brown, Effgen, & Palisano, 1998; King, McDougall, Palisano, Gritzan, & Tucker, 1999) can be used. GAS is based on the child's individual objectives and is a way of evaluating specific child outcomes. Outcomes measurement in rehabilitation should now also include quality of life and health-related measures (Lollar et al., 2000). A number of measures are available for adults, and now a few measures are beginning to be available for children, as briefly presented in Chapter 2.

Most accrediting bodies, such as the Joint Commission for the Accreditation of Healthcare Organizations (JCAHO), require hospitals to provide objective evidence of patient outcomes. A process that encourages **continuous quality improvement** must be demonstrated in high-volume, problem-prone areas of care. Standards should be written to encourage interdisciplinary team interaction in achieving compliance. Quality improvement activities involve the sequence of planning, designing, measuring, assessing, improving, and repeating the process as necessary (Figure 15–2). Ideally, all members of the care team can participate in the identification of opportunities to improve clinical processes that will improve outcomes. The team generally begins by defining the scope of service and the key processes in providing clinical care. Indicators are then defined, which will measure these key processes, to see if the desired threshold is being achieved. For example, an indicator could be developed around discharge instructions given to families. The indicator might read, "Parents

receive demonstration, practice, and written instruction regarding their child's care before discharge in 95% of cases." Several methods of capturing the information could be considered, such as a parent survey, a chart review, or a specially developed flow sheet kept by team members. The team might also review the written materials it provides and use a computer program to customize home exercise programs. Baseline data can assist in determining if the indicator warrants developing a plan for change, as well as guiding the type of change that would be most likely to improve the process. Maybe the goal would be achieved more consistently if the social worker scheduled a teaching day for the family 1 week before discharge. After implementation of the action plan, data collection is repeated to determine progress toward the goal. Individual outcome data are a high priority in quality improvement and are ideally linked to the clinical paths for specific diagnoses.

Changes That Affect Pediatric Rehabilitation

Managed-care organizations have had a great impact on the health-care environment, and pediatric rehabilitation is not an exception (Wood, 1996). Case managers at these organizations are charged with authorizing whether rehabilitation is necessary, for how long, and at what intensity. Rehabilitation professionals need to communicate clearly with the insurance company regarding the child's problems, goals, and plan of care. To have a comprehensive view of the care needed, most hospitals assign an in-house care manager to be a liaison between the clinical team and the insurance company. Many case managers have a clinical background in nursing, but others may be social workers or even therapists. The case manager must be able to understand the comprehensive rehabilitation needs of the child, and have excellent communication skills.

The physical therapist must also communicate clearly in the child's chart and at planning meetings, to provide the case manager with the information needed to justify an inpatient stay. Emphasis is placed on stating the child's goals in terms that are both functional and measurable. Progress toward the goals should be recorded in the chart daily. At least once a week, a summary note should indicate what care has been provided, what goals have been achieved, what new goals are identified, and how the plan of care will be modified to achieve the new goals. The use of standardized assessments can provide objective evidence of change. Goals relating simply to impairments in body

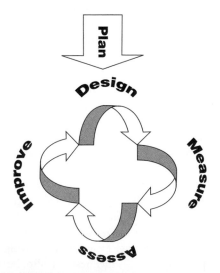

Figure 15-2 Quality improvement process.

structures and function, such as range of motion, are not sufficient to justify continued inpatient rehabilitation.

Many children who used to be admitted for inpatient rehabilitation are now cared for in an outpatient or a school setting. The acuity of needs of the child in the rehabilitation setting is increasing because children are being discharged earlier from the acute care setting. Length of stay is much shorter for those needing inpatient rehabilitation. Care must be focused on the primary reason for admission, and secondary problems may be addressed less thoroughly than in the past. Equipment such as wheelchairs or orthotics may need to be ordered from the vendor specified in the child's insurance network. Managed care has required the health-care team to be accountable for its recommendations and has changed the focus of control on many issues to the case manager, who is charged with providing optimal care for the least amount of money.

Summary

Pediatric rehabilitation is an exciting place to launch a career in pediatric physical therapy. The therapist works closely with other members of the health-care team. The children are often seen twice a day, and the therapist generally develops a close rapport with both the children and their families. Many children make dramatic improvement during their stay, which is always a rewarding experience in rehabilitation. There is generally a wide variety of diagnoses served, which makes it a broad enough first job for those who are clearly committed to the field of pediatrics. Mentorship is typically available from more experienced staff and supervisors in this setting.

There have been, and will continue to be, dramatic changes in the way rehabilitation services are delivered to children as the health-care industry tries to control escalating costs. Therapists must be willing to work toward a cost-effective approach to service delivery.

DISCUSSION QUESTIONS

1. Compare and contrast the role of the physical therapist in a pediatric rehabilitation setting to that in an adult rehabilitation setting. In what ways would it be similar, and in what ways different?

2. Transitions occur as the child moves through a continuum of care from inpatient to outpatient.

How can professionals help to smooth transitions for children and their families?

3. Design a quality improvement study to ensure that care is interdisciplinary.

REFERENCES

Brown, D.A., Effgen, S.K., & Palisano, R.J. (1998). Performance following ability-focused physical therapy intervention in individuals with severely limited physical and cognitive abilities. *Physical Therapy, 78*(9), 934–947.

Granger, C.V., Hamilton, B.B., & Kayton, R. (1989). *Guide for the use of the Functional Independence Measure (WeeFIM) of the uniform data set for medical rehabilitation.* Buffalo: Research Foundation, State University of New York.

Haley, S.M., Coster, W.J., Ludlow, L.H., Haltiwanger, J.T., & Andrellos, P.J. (1992). *The Pediatric Evaluation of Disability Inventory: Developmental standardization, administration manual.* Boston: New England Medical Center Publications.

King, G.A., McDougall, J., Palisano, R.J., Gritzan, J., & Tucker, M.A. (1999). Goal attainment scaling: Its use in evaluating pediatric therapy programs. *Physical and Occupational Therapy in Pediatrics, 19*(2), 31–52.

King, S., Rosenbaum, P., & King, G. (1995). *The Measure of Care: A means to assess family-centered behaviours of health care providers.* Hamilton, Ontario: McMaster University, Neurodevelopmental Clinical Research Unit.

Kovner, A., & Neuhauser, D. (Eds.) (1983). *Health services management: Readings and commentary* (2nd ed.). Ann Arbor, MI: Health Administration Press.

Lollar, D.J., Simeonsson, R.J., & Nanda, U. (2000). Measures of outcomes for children and youth. *Archives of Physical Medicine and Rehabilitation, 81*(12), 46–52.

National Association of Children's Hospitals and Related Institutions (NACHRI) (2004). Retrieved February 8, 2004, from *http://www.childrenshospital.net*

Spath, P.L. (1994). *Clinical paths: Tools for outcomes measurement.* Chicago: American Hospital Publishing.

Wood, E.N. (1996). Kids and managed care. *PT—Magazine of Physical Therapy, 4,* 38–46.

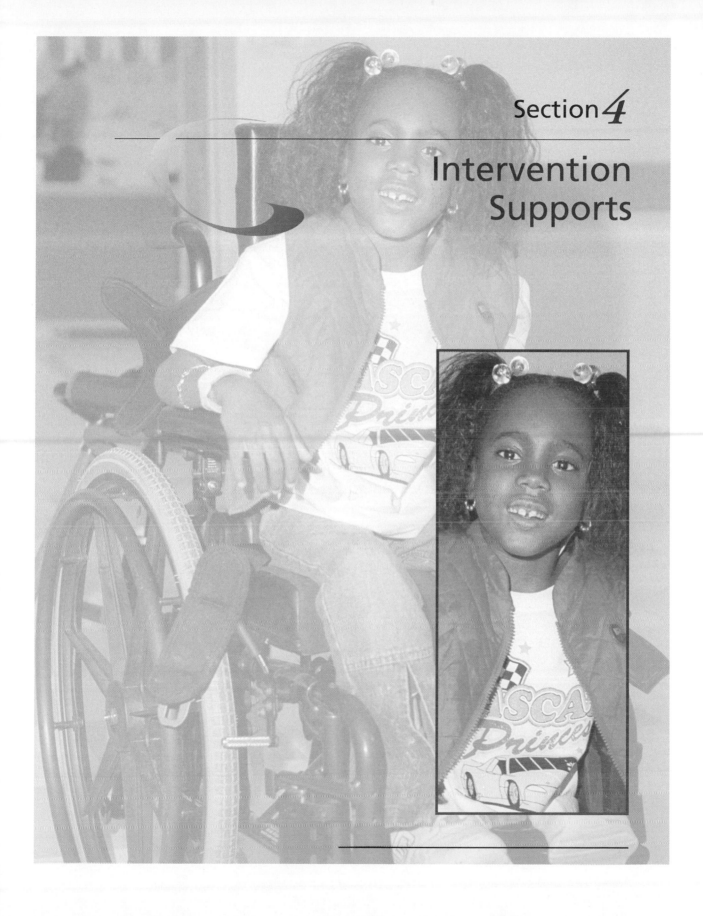

Section 4

Intervention Supports

Chapter *16*

Assistive Technology: Positioning and Mobility

— Maria Jones, PT, PhD, ATP
— Sylvia Gray, MS, ATP

Assistive technology (AT) refers to a wide array of devices and services used to enhance abilities and participation in activities and eliminate functional limitations that arise as a result of impairments commonly seen in children with disabilities. These children are often unable to perform activities in the same manner as their peers. This is attributable to neuromotor or musculoskeletal impairments, including muscle contractures, skeletal deformities, and inadequate balance and control of muscle groups that affect their ability to produce the movement necessary to perform functional skills. Physical therapists, as members of an intervention team, may recommend AT in the areas of positioning, mobility, and communication for children with disabilities to prevent or decrease the influence of neuromotor or musculoskeletal impairments (Bergen, Presperin, & Tallman, 1990; McEwen & Lloyd, 1990; Minkel, 2000; Washington, Deitz, White, & Swartz, 2002). Historically, professionals in rehabilitation and educational environments have used AT to support traditional therapeutic intervention.

With continued advancement of technology and legislation in the United States addressing the provision of AT during the past 20 years, options for devices have grown, and therapists are not limited to using hand-made devices fabricated from low-cost materials. Physical therapists, along with parents and other AT and habilitation service providers, can evaluate a child's need for AT devices and services and make appropriate recommendations to meet those needs (Angelo, 1997; Carlson & Ramsey, 2000; Galvin & Scherer, 1996; Gillen, 2002). The purpose of this chapter is to describe the laws guiding, and processes used to meet, the AT needs of children. The chapter focuses on the role physical therapists play in the selection, acquisition, and implementation of AT.

Assistive Technology Legislation

There are many laws in the United States that address AT and have established a legislative framework designed to ensure that children with disabilities receive the AT services they need. These laws are summarized in Table 16.1 and in Chapter 1.

The Individuals with Disabilities Education Act (IDEA) Amendments of 1997 identify six AT services that may be needed to assist a child in the acquisition or use of AT. Evaluation, the first service identified, may be needed to determine whether a student requires AT and to identify appropriate device(s) or service(s). The second service involves obtaining the device(s) and/or service(s) decided upon by the Individualized Education Plan (IEP) team and included in the IEP as special education, related services, and/or supplementary aids or services. The third service ensures that devices are functional and adapted to the needs and abilities of the student. This includes modifying equipment by mounting switches, customizing a keyboard, or other similar services, all of which should be identified and included in the IEP. In addition, this service ensures

455

Table 16.1 U.S. Federal Laws Related to Assistive Technology

The Rehabilitation Act of 1973 (PL 93–112) and Amendments	Individuals With Disabilities Education Act and Amendments of 1997 (IDEA) (PL 105–17) and Its Precursors	Technology-Related Assistance for Individuals With Disabilities Act of 1988 (PL 100–407) and Amendments	The Americans With Disabilities Act of 1990 (ADA) (PL 101–336)
• Protects civil rights of people with disabilities from discrimination in programs or activities that receive federal financial assistance.	Defines AT device and service.	First legislation to provide the definition of AT device and service.	• Protects civil rights of people with disabilities.
• Definitions of disability are broader than those defined by IDEA.	• Schools must provide AT at no cost to the parent when determined by the IEP team to be needed and addressed in the IEP.	• Provides federal funding for states to establish training and service delivery systems for AT.	• Prevents discrimination in: employment, public services, accommodations, transportation, and telecommunications.
• Some children qualify for services under this definition, although not meeting eligibility criteria of IDEA.	• The need for AT must be considered as part of the IEP process for each child who qualifies for special education.	• Supports the creation of systems change to eliminate barriers to the acquisition of AT.	Includes definitions of AT devices and services.
• AT devices and/or services may be considered reasonable accommodation when needed by children to access and participate in their public education.	• For children birth to 36 months, Part C ensures that the need for AT is addressed in the IFSP.	• Services vary from state to state, but may include information and referral, demonstration, loan libraries of devices, and training.	• Provides for reasonable accommodations, such as AT, to make employment or public services accessible.

that AT is maintained in working order or replaced as necessary. The fourth service required by IDEA addresses the need for coordinated services. If a school pursues other funding sources for the provision of devices and/or services, this should be identified and addressed in the IEP as a service. The process of obtaining funding for AT can be very time consuming. It is beneficial for the team to designate someone to assume responsibility for completing the paperwork and ensuring that the process is moving forward. In the event that no other funding source can be identified or that funding for the requested device or service is denied, the school is still responsible for providing AT identified in the IEP.

The fifth service includes training the child and family and the sixth service addresses training for school personnel and any other significant people in the child's life who support the use of AT in the school, home, vocational, and community environments. These services are of paramount importance to ensure that the child becomes functional in the use of the device(s). The 1997 Amendments to IDEA added the consideration of special factors to the IEP process, and AT is specifically listed as a factor for schools to consider. All IEP teams must determine whether AT devices or services are required by a child to have a free and appropriate public education, as defined by IDEA.

The Process for Providing Assistive Technology Services

Although legislation ensures the provision of AT devices and services, there are few defined processes for therapists to use when making AT decisions. There are, however, critical elements that physical therapists must consider when evaluating, recommending, and implementing AT for children (Angelo, 2000).

Gathering Background Information

The use of a referral form; the review of educational records; and interviews with children, parents, caregivers, or school staff are methods for obtaining background information about children with disabilities. The referral form includes personal information, such as age, medical diagnosis, health information, and potential funding sources. A review of education records yields information about educational performance and the results of educational evaluations, including academic performance, cognitive abilities, strengths, and weaknesses. Interviews with children, parents or caregivers, and important team members, such as teachers, related service providers, and friends, provide not only information regarding abilities and needs but also different perspectives (Reed, 2000).

The AT evaluation team gathers background information regarding the child's abilities. What are the child's motor, sensory, cognitive, language, and social strengths? What are the child's current abilities that allow him or her to use AT today? What improvements can be made to the child's abilities that will result in increased performance? The needs of the child are also important when assessing for AT. What does the child need to do that he or she currently cannot do? Are there activities in which the child is unable to participate, or could perform more independently? The child's history of technology is also important. Has the child tried technology before? If so, what was tried, and were the results successful or unsuccessful? Information should be gathered regarding not only present environments but also future environments. For example, if a child who maneuvers a power wheelchair independently is currently in elementary school but will be transitioning to middle school during the following school year, the physical therapist should evaluate the middle-school environment to ensure that there are no architectural barriers that will prevent the student from being independent.

Gathering Objective Data for Decision Making

One way to gather data is through observation. It is critical to observe children in the context of natural environments

and daily tasks. Observations allow team members to evaluate how children function in different environments and to help identify barriers, which could interfere with the use of AT (Reed, 2000). The identification of barriers is a critical part of the evaluation process. Observing children in the context of familiar activities can provide information about their cognitive, physical, visual, and communication skills. The use of an environmental evaluation tool, such as the Activity/Standards Inventory (Beukelman & Mirenda, 1998), can assist in identifying discrepancies of participation. Beukelman and Mirenda (1998) identify the following opportunity barriers that may be present in the environment and may interfere with the success or use of AT: policy, practice, attitude, knowledge, and skill. When opportunity barriers are present, it is important for the team to propose solutions for addressing them.

Another means for gathering objective data for decision making is the use of formal or informal testing. The team should identify what information is lacking and then select the appropriate tests to gather the needed information. Professionals from the various disciplines should be knowledgeable regarding formal tests related to their areas of expertise.

Assistive Technology Evaluation

To identify and obtain AT for children, service providers, including physical therapists, need to provide an AT evaluation. A systematic evaluation process ensures that AT device selection decisions are based on information regarding the child's abilities, needs, and environments. The AT evaluation is characterized by a team approach, focuses on functional evaluation techniques provided in the natural environment, and is ongoing in nature (Reed, 2000). Although most AT evaluations are not standardized, the evaluation process should be systematic and use a framework for effective decision making.

A team approach is critical in the AT evaluation process. No one professional possesses the knowledge and expertise about all areas of AT. The child's positioning needs, vision, cognitive/linguistic abilities, and computer hardware and software needs are some of the child-oriented areas that the team considers. Children and their parents are essential team members. Other team members may come from a wide range of professions, including physical therapy, occupational therapy, speech-language pathology, education, psychology or psychometry, optometry/ophthalmology, audiology, adaptive physical education, recreation therapy, music therapy, and rehabilitation engineering. It is important that all team members contribute information regarding the child's abilities, needs, environments, and tasks that must be considered in the evaluation and that they actively work together to identify possible AT solutions (Reed, 2000).

AT evaluations should occur in the child's natural environment(s). If the child is in school, the evaluation should occur in the classroom and other environments (cafeteria, playground, rest room, gym, and so on) where the child participates during the school day. For older children and young adults, the evaluation might include school and work environments. Because the evaluation procedures are not standardized, information may be gathered by observing a child in the natural activities of his or her daily routine, such as sitting at the desk, eating in the cafeteria, and playing at centers with other children. The evaluation and recommendations are functional because they remain focused on the child's abilities and needs, not his or her disabilities. For example, even though the child may have limited use of his or her hands to access a communication system, his or her functional abilities could include the use of eye gaze for communication purposes. Identifying and focusing on specific tasks, which are relevant in present and future environments, ensure that the evaluation is functional.

Feature Match With Child's Abilities

Muller and Oberstein (1995) describe **feature match** as the process of AT selection in which the needs of the user are assessed, documented, and then matched to the device that most closely offers the required features. First, the evaluation team identifies the child's needs and abilities. This information is then matched with specific features of AT to develop a list of potential systems for trial purposes. For example, if environmental needs for the user indicate that the system should be portable and easy to support, the team should not consider devices that are not portable or that require extensive support. Using a feature match approach helps narrow the field of options to those that are most relevant for a specific user.

Trial

Once the AT team has proposed a system or systems, a field test is essential in determining the effectiveness of the proposed systems. Field tests are useful if more than one system meets the need, or to document a child's use of the

system to secure funding. The actual trial of the system in the natural environment, and for identified tasks, helps determine if the system will accomplish the identified need. A field test helps children and their families determine if they prefer a specific piece of equipment because they have the opportunity to manage the equipment in the context of their daily routines.

Recommendations

Team members should complete a report that summarizes and synthesizes the information gathered during the evaluation process and provides recommendations for AT devices and services. All team members review the report and reach an agreement regarding implementation of the recommendations. The report includes recommendations for the specific system, including requirements and components, and for AT services needed to support the system (Reed, 2000). If a child, teacher, or caregiver needs training, recommendations should address how much training is required, how team members will provide the training, and who will provide it.

Training and Implementation

Frequently, acquiring AT devices is a preliminary step in the AT process. Team members may believe that a device is the "answer" or "cure" for problems identified in the evaluation process. However, it is increasingly apparent that significant training in the use of a device is necessary for successful generalization across a variety of settings (Behrmann, 1995; Cook & Hussey, 1995; Galvin & Scherer, 1996; McNevin, Wulf, & Carlson, 2000).

When training children to use AT devices, all team members should incorporate motor learning principles. *Motor learning* is defined as processes that lead to relatively permanent changes in a person's ability to produce a skilled action as a result of practice or experience (Schmidt, 1988). As discussed here and in Chapter 7, physical therapists should incorporate concepts, such as transfer of behavior or generalization, practice, and feedback, when training a child to use AT.

Transfer of Behavior

Physical therapists, as well as other AT team members, typically observe children performing skills during therapy sessions but are often frustrated because they do not observe the same skills in other environments or during everyday activities. Children with disabilities often have difficulty transferring behaviors or generalizing skills into new environments or situations (Brown, Effgen, & Palisano, 1998). When training a child to use AT, physical therapists must design practice and provide feedback to ensure the skills performed transfer and generalize across all device use environments (Dunn, 1991; Evans, 1991; Jones, McEwen, & Hansen, 2003; McEwen & Shelden, 1995; McNevin et al., 2000; Reichle & Sigafoos, 1991).

Practice

When providing practice opportunities for children, physical therapists must consider location of practice, organization of practice, and part-whole training. For children to become proficient in the use of AT, they must practice using the specific piece of technology in one or more use environments. For example, if a child is learning to use a powered wheelchair for mobility, practice must include using the wheelchair in places such as the hallways of the child's school, on sidewalks going to the bus, and in the grocery store. Practicing powered mobility in a wide open space, such as a gym, or setting up an obstacle course is less likely to be effective in helping the child to gain independence.

Organization of practice opportunities is another important consideration when designing training in the use of AT. Children with disabilities require more practice opportunities to develop a motor skill than do children without disabilities. All team members must provide an increased number of well-designed practice opportunities within daily activities to assist children in becoming proficient and competent users of AT (Jones et al., 2003; McEwen & Shelden, 1995). When designing practice opportunities for children, therapists can use either blocked practice or random practice. **Blocked practice** involves defining a specific period of time in which a child practices a skill. An example of blocked practice is when a physical therapist sees a child for 30 minutes two times per week to practice powered mobility. **Random practice** involves incorporating numerous opportunities to practice the skill throughout daily activities. An example of random practice is when a student practices powered mobility to and from the bus, transitioning between classes, in physical education class, and during recess. Research indicates that blocked practice may be beneficial for initial skill acquisition, but random practice is necessary for learning, retention, and refinement of a skill (Larin, 2000; Mulligan, Lacy, & Guess, 1982; Reichle & Sigafoos, 1991; Schmidt, 1988).

The final area of practice to consider is **part-whole training**. In traditional therapeutic approaches, a task is broken into smaller component parts, which are practiced during intervention. The whole skill is attempted at the end of the therapy session to determine if the practice worked. In most cases, the child may be able to perform the component skills but cannot put them together to complete the whole task. Studies have shown that tasks can be broken into two categories: serial and continuous. *Serial tasks* are easily broken into component parts and lend themselves to part training. *Continuous tasks* do not break easily into component parts and should be taught as a whole skill through practice and repetition (Larin, 2000; Winstein, 1991).

Feedback

Feedback (i.e., knowledge of results or consequences) refers to use of intrinsic and extrinsic factors to facilitate development of a motor skill. Intrinsic factors include proprioception and kinesthesia. Extrinsic factors include visual, auditory, or tactile cues, which children receive from people and objects within their environment. Research suggests that, although feedback is important and may be provided continuously during initial acquisition of a skill, it must be faded out quickly for actual learning and refinement of the skill to occur. It must be faded out to ensure the child does not become dependent on the feedback to perform the skill (Larin, 2000; McEwen & Shelden, 1995; Reichle & Sigafoos, 1991). (For a more detailed discussion of motor learning, see Chapter 7.)

Categories of Assistive Technology

In 1992, the Rehabilitation Engineering and Assistive Technology Society of North America (RESNA) identified 10 categories of AT for children in educational environments. The categories are as follows:

- Positioning
- Mobility
- Augmentative communication
- Access
- Computer-based instruction
- Environmental control

- Activities of daily living
- Recreation/leisure/play
- Vision technology
- Assistive listening

These categories are the basis of AT intervention and serve as the framework for the following sections and Chapter 17.

Positioning

Positioning children with disabilities plays an important role in their ability to function and participate within the environment. Proper positioning improves head position and control (McEwen & Lloyd, 1990), permits greater control of the arms and head (Myhr & vonWendt, 1991), improves ability to eat, digest, and breathe (Miedaner & Finuf, 1993; Nwaobi & Smith, 1986), improves postural alignment (Washington, et al., 2002), facilitates adult-child interaction (McEwen, 1992), and improves ability to listen and communicate (Bay, 1991).

Positioning refers to the alignment of body parts in relation to one another and to the surrounding environment. For example, children without disabilities may sit while working at the computer, stand while washing dishes, and lie on their stomachs while playing Nintendo. They use various positions throughout the day, depending on the task or skill they need to perform. For children with disabilities, therapists must provide positioning systems that provide proper alignment to promote improved function, movement, and participation in activities.

Positioning Systems

There are two basic categories of positioning systems: recumbent and upright systems. **Recumbent systems** include equipment that provides support in supine, prone, or sidelying positions and are frequently used by children with severe physical disabilities as a means of alternative positioning throughout the day. Recumbent positioning systems (Figure 16–1) include wedges, bolsters, mats, and sidelyers. In general, recumbent positioning systems should not be used during the day because they may have the potential to exclude the child from participating in activities along with his or her peers. Physical therapists must consider the effect recumbent positions have on adult and peer interaction with the child and the movement demands

of the tasks required in that position (Bergen et al., 1990; Carlson & Ramsey, 2000; McEwen, 1992).

In contrast to recumbent positioning systems, **upright positioning** systems support the child in either a seated or standing position. Physical therapists recommend seating systems for children who use wheelchairs as their primary means of mobility, but they may also recommend them for children with less obvious physical disabilities, such as developmental coordination disorders. These children may need seating supports to improve sitting posture in class, especially when doing written work. Physical therapists recommend standing systems to provide alternative positioning throughout the day; allow access to normal work surfaces, such as cabinets and sinks; and provide weight-bearing opportunities for children who are unable to stand independently.

Types of Seating Systems

Seating systems can be divided into four categories: sling, planar, generically contoured, and custom contoured (Bergen et al., 1990; Carlson & Ramsey, 2000; Gilson & Huss, 1995; Kolar, 1996). Each type of support surface has different effects on a child's position. **Sling systems** are the industry standard for mobility bases. Sling systems are usually vinyl or cloth material, which allow folding for transportation. However, they provide little support because the material gives way to the weight and movement of the child, causing a "hammocking effect." Postural deviations commonly caused by sling seating systems include pelvic asymmetries, and adducted and internally rotated hips.

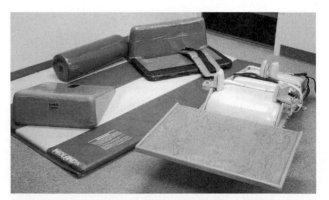

Figure 16-1 Recumbent positioning systems (left to right): Tumble Forms wedge, bolster, and sidelyer and Rifton prone support scooter.

In contrast to sling seating systems, **planar seating systems** provide a more firm base of support for children, preventing the development of common postural deviations. Planar systems are flat seat and back supports, often constructed of a plywood or plastic base with 1 to 2 inches of foam and covered with upholstery. Some pediatric mobility bases, such as the one shown in Figure 16–2, come standard with a planar seating system. Modular components, such as lateral trunk supports, lateral thigh supports, hip guides, and medial thigh supports, are often used in conjunction with planar seating systems to provide the level of support a particular child needs (Bergen et al., 1990; Kolar, 1996; Trefler, Hobson, Taylor, Monahan, & Shaw, 1993). Planar seating systems provide adequate support for children with mild postural problems, symmetrical posture, and no structural deformities.

If planar seating systems do not provide the level of support a child needs to sit upright, cushions that are **contoured** can be considered. Generally, commercially available or off-the-shelf cushions are contoured and approximate the shape of the body in their design and construction (Figure 16–3). Contoured seats provide adequate support for children with moderate postural problems, flexible postural asymmetries, and few, if any, structural deformities (Washington et al., 2002).

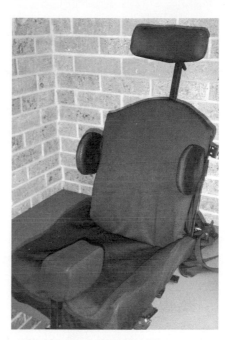

Figure 16-3 Jay Fit Seating System from Sunrise Medical.

For children with the most severe physical disabilities, seating systems in the first three categories often do not provide the level of support needed to enhance function. **Custom-contoured** seating systems are specifically molded to a child's body and are designed to match that child's body contours. Because the seating systems are specifically molded to a child's body, they can accommodate for leg length discrepancies, pelvic asymmetries, and trunk asymmetries. Custom-contoured systems are often used to accommodate fixed structural deformities. With the continued advancement of technology, custom-contoured seating systems, such as those shown in Figure 16–4, are comparable in price with other seating systems and are readily available (Bergen et al., 1990; Carlson & Ramsey, 2000; Gilson & Huss, 1995; Kolar, 1996; Trefler et al., 1993; Washington et al., 2002).

Standing Systems

Therapists most often recommend the use of **standing systems** to provide an alternative position for children who remain in a seated position throughout most of their day. Standing systems are also used as a means of weight-bearing for children who otherwise would be unable to stand.

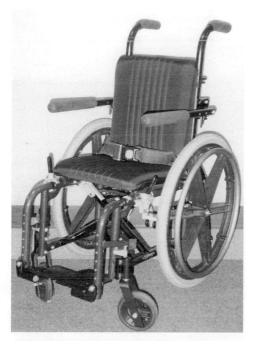

Figure 16-2 Zippie 2 manual wheelchair with planar seating system.

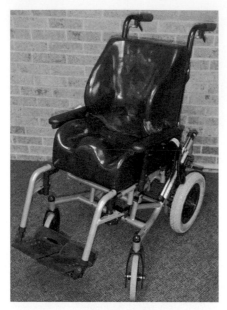

Figure 16-4 Custom-contoured seating system fabricated at the Oklahoma Assistive Technology Center.

Common standing systems include prone, supine, and upright standers (Figure 16–5). Most standers have table or tray attachments that enable the child to play and complete fine motor activities while standing. The benefits of standing include elongation of the knee and hip flexor and ankle plantarflexor musculature; maintenance or improvement in bone mineral density; and facilitation of optimal musculoskeletal development of the hip, knee, and ankle joints (Stuberg, 1992). A child who requires the use of a stander will often have a wheelchair and seating system and a separate standing system. For adults with similar needs, wheelchairs with standing capabilities are available, allowing the same system to serve both functions. Only recently has this technology become available to children (Bergen et al., 1990; Greenstein, 1996).

Benefits of Proper Positioning

Once the child is properly positioned, therapists can begin to assess the impact improved positioning has on the child's overall functional abilities. Bergen and colleagues (1990) identified nine benefits of proper positioning:

1. Normalize or decrease abnormal neurological influence on the body

2. Increase range of motion, maintain neutral skeletal alignment and control, and prevent skeletal deformities and muscle contractures

3. Manage pressure and prevent or decrease the potential for decubitus ulcers

4. Upgrade stability to increase function

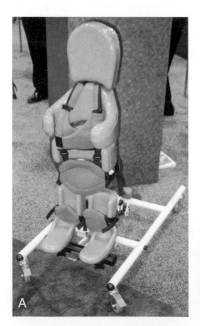
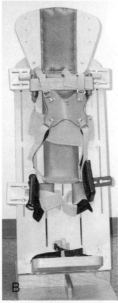
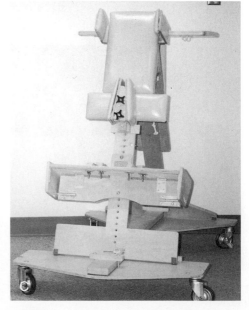

Figure 16-5 *(A)* Tumble Forms TriStander, *(B)* supine stander, and *(C)* Rifton prone stander.

5. Promote increased tolerance of desired position (comfort)

6. Enhance function of autonomic nervous system

7. Decrease fatigue

8. Facilitate components of normal movement

9. Facilitate maximum function with minimal pathology

Physical Examination for Seating Systems

The goal of positioning intervention for a child is to determine the position in which the child has the most control with the least amount of support or restriction. The physical examination should take place in both supine and sitting positions. The supine examination eliminates gravity against the spine and allows examination of passive movement of the pelvis, hips, and knees. The sitting examination provides valuable information about the child's ability to maintain the head and trunk in a neutral and functional position against gravity.

The physical examination is a beginning step to determine the level of support a child needs in a seating system. The primary focus of the physical examination is to determine if a child's postural changes are flexible or fixed.

Flexible deformities can be eliminated or corrected with manual support. Fixed deformities cannot be eliminated or corrected with manual support. When designing a seating system, flexible deformities must be corrected, providing the supports necessary to position a child in neutral alignment. The seating system must accommodate fixed or structural deformities and not apply corrective forces. The goal of providing supports that accommodate existing deformities is to prevent progression of those deformities, while providing a comfortable and functional position for the child (Carlson & Ramsey, 2000; Gilson & Huss, 1995). As part of the physical examination, physical therapists determine the impact of hip and knee movement on the position of the pelvis. With the child in supine position, physical therapists measure hip and knee range of motion, ensuring that the child can flex the hip to at least 90° with the knee positioned at 90° (Figure 16–6). If a child has limited hip or knee movement, adjustments must be made to the seat-to-back angle or knee flexion angle of the wheelchair. In addition, when examining the child's hip flexion, physical therapists must ensure that the lumbar curve does not flatten when bringing the hip to 90° and straightening the knee. If the child has tight hamstring musculature, the lumbar curve may flatten as the hip is flexed to 90° and the knee is extended (Figure 16–7). Additional measurements taken during the physical examination are summarized in Figure 16–8. The examination continues to include the hips, thighs, knees, trunk, head, and arms, but the pelvis

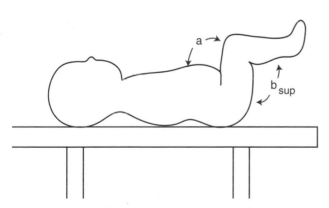

Figure 16-6 In supine, physical therapists measure *(a)* hip and *(b)* knee angles to determine if the child can achieve at least 90° of hip flexion with the knee at 90°. This will determine the seat-to-back angle and footrest angle of the wheelchair. (From Bergen, A.F., Presperin, J., & Tallman, T. [1990]. *Positioning for function: Wheelchairs and other assistive technologies* [p. 15]. Valhalla, NY: Valhalla Rehabilitation Publications. Adapted with permission.)

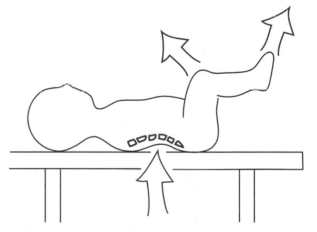

Figure 16-7 While measuring the hip flexion and knee flexion angle, physical therapists must ensure that the lumbar curve does not flatten as a result of hamstring tightness. (From Bergen, A.F., Presperin, J., & Tallman, T. [1990]. *Positioning for function: Wheelchairs and other assistive technologies* [p. 14]. Valhalla, NY: Valhalla Rehabilitation Publications. Adapted with permission.)

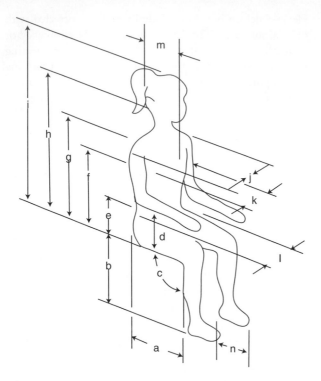

Figure 16-8 Physical therapists take the following measurements in sitting. *(a)* behind hips to popliteal fossa (right and left); *(b)* popliteal fossa to heel (right and left); *(c)* knee flexion angle; *(d)* seat surface to hanging elbow; *(e)* seat surface to pelvic crest; *(f)* seat surface to axilla; *(f)* seat surface to top of shoulder; *(h)* seat surface to occiput; *(i)* seat surface to top of head; *(j)* shoulder width; *(k)* chest width; *(l)* hip width; *(m)* trunk depth; and *(n)* foot length. (From Bergen, A.F., Presperin, J., & Tallman, T. [1990]. *Positioning for function* [p. 16]. Valhalla, NY: Valhalla Rehabilitation Publications. Adapted with permission.)

provides the foundation for postural support (Bergen et al., 1990; Carlson & Ramsey, 2000; Taylor, 1997; Trefler et al., 1993).

Pelvis

The physical evaluation begins by observing if the pelvis is level in sitting. This is done by palpating the anterior superior iliac spines (ASISs) with your thumbs. If the thumbs are level, the child's pelvis is level. If the thumbs are not level, a pelvic obliquity is present. In addition, if one thumb tip is more forward than the other, this detects the presence of pelvic rotation (Figure 16–9). Initially, if thumbs are not level or if one is more forward than the other, the physical therapist should try to reposition the child to see if neutral alignment can be achieved with repositioning. If repositioning does not resolve the identified deviation, the pelvic deformity should be accommodated in the seating system. The position of the ASISs in relation to each other is critical in describing pelvic deformities (Bergen et al., 1990; Carlson & Ramsey, 2000; McEwen, 1997; Taylor, 1997).

Some children are unable to maintain their pelvis in a neutral position without support, so therapists add pelvic supports for stability. The most common support used to stabilize the pelvis in a seated position is a pelvic positioning belt (i.e., seat belt or lap belt). Physical therapists should closely evaluate the angle at which the pelvic belt is placed on a wheelchair and ensure that the belt can be easily removed by the child and caregiver. A general rule is to position the belt at a 45° angle, bisecting the pelvic/femoral angle to maintain a neutral pelvis (Figure 16–10A). In some cases, the child may require additional stability but may also need to shift the pelvis forward to

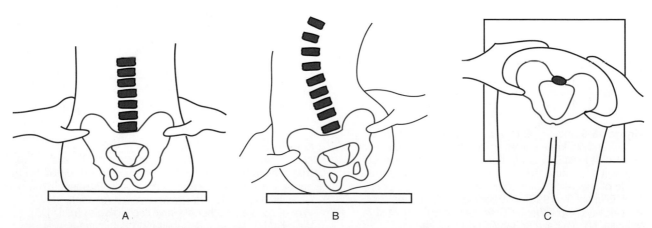

Figure 16-9 Common pelvic positions: *(A)* neutral pelvis, *(B)* pelvic obliquity, and *(C)* pelvic rotation. (Courtesy of Corinne Vance.)

reach. If this is a need, a pelvic belt angle closer to 90° may prove beneficial (Figure 16–10b). Pelvic belts that are positioned too high can cause the child to move into a posterior pelvic tilt (Figure 16–10c) (Bergen et al., 1990). Other pelvic supports include sub-ASIS bars and anterior knee blocks (Rigby, Reid, Schoger, & Ryan, 2001).

Hips

Hip range of motion is critical in determining the seat-to-back angle of a wheelchair. When examining a child's pelvic position in supine, therapists must pay close attention to the effect of hip flexion and knee extension on the position of the pelvis. These factors are used to determine the seat-to-back and knee angle within a mobility base and seating system. A child whose pelvic mobility is not affected by hip flexion or knee extension requires much less support than one who has significant movement limitations. Because children with physical disabilities often present with tight hip flexors, hip extensors, and hamstrings, the pelvis may be fixed in an anterior or a posterior tilt, requiring more extensive levels of support to accommodate the deformities. When examining hip movement, physical therapists should determine if a child can achieve 90° of hip flexion while maintaining neutral pelvic alignment. If a child does not have 90° of hip flexion, then the angle of the back in relationship to the seat (seat-to-back angle) must be reclined to accommodate the lack of hip flexion.

Thighs

For most children, the optimal position of the thighs in sitting is slight abduction. When examining a child's thigh position, therapists should observe whether the child's thighs are too close together or too far apart. Thighs that are too close together indicate a postural deviation commonly caused by muscle imbalance and/or stiffness that pulls the knees together. When a child's thighs are too far apart, it is often indicative of muscle weakness or low muscle tone. Lateral and medial thigh supports (adductor and abductor supports) are designed to control the postural deviations of the thighs. Lateral thigh supports are used to bring a child's legs into adduction, and medial thigh supports separate the legs into a neutral or slightly abducted position. Medial thigh supports are not intended to stretch tight adductors or to prevent the child from sliding forward in the chair. Hip guides are designed to provide lateral control across the greater trochanter to keep the hips from moving laterally in the seating system.

Knee and Foot Supports

When examining a child's knee movement, therapists must consider the impact of tight hamstring musculature on hip movement and pelvic position. Because the hamstring muscles cross both the hip and knee joints, tightness in the hamstrings can cause the hip to extend as the knee is extended, pulling the pelvis into a posterior tilt. The footrest angle should be determined based on a child's knee movement. Footrests that are too far in front of the seating system cause children with tight hamstrings to lose the neutral alignment of their hips and pelvis. In addition, footrests should be adjusted to a height that supports the entire foot while maintaining thigh contact with the seating system.

Most mobility bases include leg and foot support options. Footrest options on wheelchairs include the footrest hanger, footplate, and accessories. The angle of the footrest hanger is critical to proper positioning. Physical therapists should use the child's knee angle to determine the angle of the footrest hanger. The standard footrest hanger is generally angled at 60° or 70°, which is often too far in front of the chair to benefit children with tight hamstring musculature. Most chairs now have other options available, including 80°, 90°, elevating, and contracture platforms.

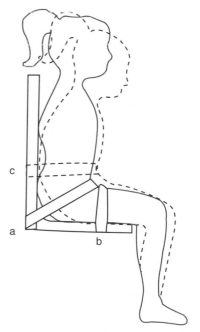

Figure 16-10 Three common seat belt configurations: (a) belt at 45° angle to maintain a neutral pelvis, (b) belt at 90° angle for increased stability and allows forward shift, (c) belt positioned too high causing posterior pelvic tilt. (Courtesy of Corinne Vance.)

The tighter a child's hamstrings, the closer the footrests need to be to the front edge of the chair. In extreme cases, the footrests must angle under the seat to accommodate for tight hamstring musculature (Figure 16–11). Several footplate options are available and can be mounted or attached to the footrest hanger. Options include individual, solid, flip-up, angle adjustable, and dynamic (Figure 16–12). If a child presents with a leg length discrepancy, the therapist should order individual footplates, which allow independent adjustment of each side to accommodate for the difference in length. If a child transfers independently in and out of the wheelchair, flip-up footplates will not interfere with transfers. If a child has structural foot deformities either in plantarflexion or dorsiflexion, angle-adjustable footplates allow therapists to angle the footplate to support the entire length of the child's foot. Other leg/foot support accessories include calf pads, calf straps, heel loops, foot straps, and shoe holders. Most of the leg/foot accessories serve one of two functions: (1) preventing the feet from sliding off the back of the footplates or (2) stabilizing the feet on the footrests.

Trunk

Once a good base of support has been provided at the pelvis and lower body, the position of the trunk, head, and arms can be further examined. When positioning the trunk, physical therapists begin by providing support along the posterior aspect of the child's body, then the lateral aspect, and then the anterior aspect. Posterior support (seat and back cushions) should provide a stable base of support for the pelvis, trunk, and lower body. Lateral trunk supports (scoliosis pads) and anterior trunk supports (chest straps, shoulder harnesses, H-straps) are commonly used supports for the trunk. Lateral trunk supports center the body over the pelvis and correct flexible trunk deformities. Anterior trunk supports facilitate thoracic extension of the spine, allowing the child to rest against the back support (Bergen et al., 1990; Gilson & Huss, 1995; Kolar, 1996).

Head

Frequently, once a child's hips, pelvis, and trunk are well positioned in a seating system, the child's head will often be in a neutral, upright position. However, there are children who require specialized head supports, even after the rest of the body is supported in a neutral position. Head positioning is crucial for children with severe neuromotor impairments because it affects their ability to visually attend to their environment. Specialized head supports are available and should be used much in the same manner as trunk supports (posterior first, followed by lateral, and last anterior). Most headrests provide a combination of posterior head and neck support. The neck support incorporated into many headrests fits below the occiput and supports the cervical spine. Posterior head supports range in size depending on the amount of surface area with which the child needs contact. Children with more significant needs may require the use of lateral and anterior head and neck supports (Figure 16–13). These should be incorporated into a system only when posterior supports do not meet the child's needs because they tend to interfere with peripheral vision (Bergen et al., 1990; Gilson & Huss, 1995; Kolar, 1996; Trefler et al., 1993). Headrests also frequently serve as a control mechanism for a power wheelchair, communication device, and computer controls for children with severe physical disabilities.

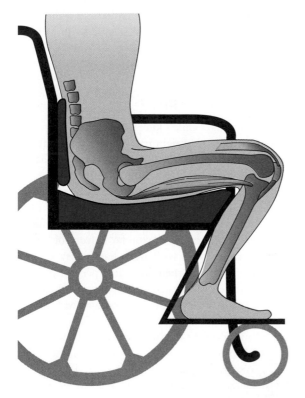

Figure 16-11 When a child has tight hamstring muscles, the footrests must angle under the seat to accommodate for the tightness & allow the pelvis to stay in neutral alignment.

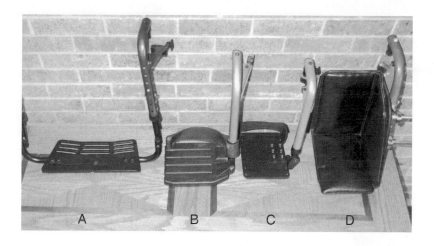

Figure 16-12 Footrest options: (A) 90° hanger with one-piece footplate, (B) 60° hanger with individual composite footplate, (C) 90° hanger with individual angle adjustable footplate, and (D) 70° hanger with Miller solid footbucket.

Arms

The final consideration in the design of a seating system is the position of a child's arms. Physical therapists should support a child's arms in a forward position. The height and angle of armrests and trays have a significant impact on a child's arm position, so careful attention should be given to adjust them appropriately. The most commonly used arm supports for children are armrests and trays. Armrest options on most wheelchairs include desk length, full length, fixed height, height adjustable, fixed, removable, and swing-away; they come in a variety of shapes and styles. Some children who propel their wheelchairs may not require arm supports. Armrests should be omitted from their systems. Armrests are often necessary if the child uses a tray because the tray is generally secured to the armrests for mounting purposes. Trays are commonly recommended for children with limited shoulder movement and upper trunk strength. Trays also provide children a surface from which they can eat, play, and work when they encounter an environment that is not accessible.

Simulation

Based on the findings in the record review, interview with a child and family, and physical examination, the physical therapist can now simulate different seating systems. **Seating simulators** (Figure 16–14) are commercially available and allow easy adjustment of linear components, seating angles, and contouring. Simulators also allow physical therapists to evaluate the effect of recline and tilt-in-space on a child's head position. They are especially useful for examining children with severe physical disabilities.

Simulation may include a process as simple as trying two or three off-the-shelf seating systems with a child. In other situations, it may involve intimate molding around a child's body and adjusting various seating angles, including seat-to-back angle and tilt-in-space, to determine the optimal position. When simulating a seating system, physical therapists should provide as little support as is required for the child to sit upright and participate in activities involved in the environment.

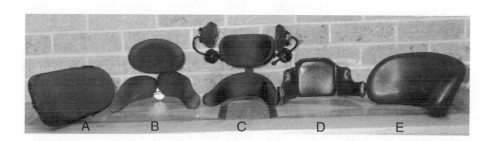

Figure 16-13 Headrest options. (A) Whitmyer Plush 1, (B) Whitmyer SOFT-1, (C) Stealth, (D) AEL Tri Pad Headrest, and (E) OttoBock Combination Head/Neckrest.

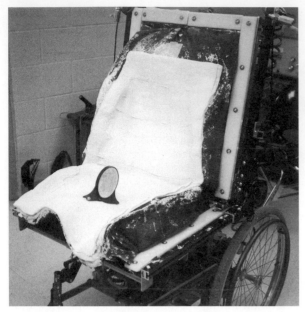

Figure 16-14 The Flamingo Seating Simulator from Tallahassee Therapeutic.

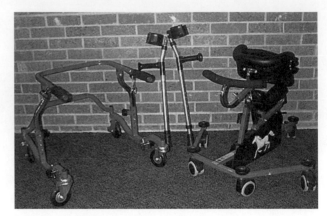

Figure 16-15 Mobility aids. Left to right: Wenzelite reverse walker, Lumex forearm crutches, and Pony prone support walker.

Mobility

Children with disabilities often cannot move freely about their environment. The ultimate goal for mobility is to get from one place to another in a defined period of time and still have the energy necessary to function in the new environment. When considering mobility options for children, team members must consider whether the child can move independently from place to place. Team members must also consider the child's future environments and potential for independence. Mobility aids such as walkers, crutches, canes, and manual and powered wheelchairs can promote independence for children (see Figures 16–2, 16–15, and 16–16). Physical therapists play a significant role in determining the type of mobility aids children need to be as independent and functional as possible.

Children with various disabilities use mobility aids. For example, the use of mobility aids for children with spinal cord injuries and myelodysplasia varies widely depending on the level of lesion and age. Children with injuries from T-11 to L-2 may use knee-ankle-foot orthoses or reciprocating gait orthoses in combination with forearm crutches for indoor mobility only; whereas children whose level of injury is L-3 to S-2 may require only ankle-foot orthoses in combination with forearm crutches or a cane. Lofstrand

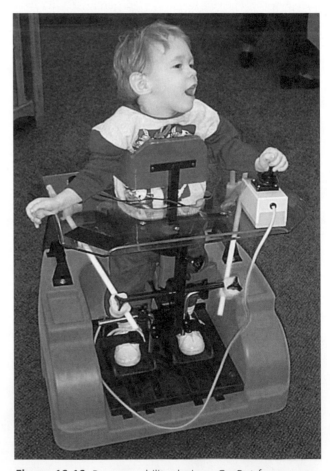

Figure 16-16 Power mobility devices. Go-Bot from Innovative Products, Inc.

crutches or wheeled walkers may be used in a small percentage of children with juvenile rheumatoid arthritis who experience pain, contracture, or weakness in their lower extremities that prevents efficient weight bearing. Children with arthrogryposis multiplex congenita often require the use of a power wheelchair for efficient community mobility. Children with cerebral palsy (CP) often require manual or power wheelchairs to provide efficient mobility. Children with CP or myelomeningocele who are able to walk independently often need an alternative form of mobility, such as a power wheelchair, as they grow and have to travel greater distances at a faster pace to keep up with their peers (Franks, Palisano, & Darbee, 1991).

As previously described, children may use a combination of mobility aids depending on the environmental demands. For example, a child may use a walker in the home and school environments to walk short distances within rooms but may use a power wheelchair for community and outside mobility where longer distances of greater duration are required.

Effects of Mobility on Other Aspects of Development

Children with limited mobility experiences often fall behind in other areas of development because they must rely on others to move them about their environment. Therapists cannot allow years to pass while waiting for a child to walk because motor skills develop rapidly during the first 3 years of life and become the bridge to more advanced learning, socialization, and psychological development (Butler, 1997; Jones et al., 2003; Neely & Neely, 1993).

Therapists must augment a child's mobility to prevent or minimize the detrimental effects caused by immobility. Equipment used to augment mobility includes walkers, canes, crutches, ladder frames, walking frames, splints, orthotics, tricycles, bicycles, and manual and powered wheelchairs. Many children use multiple modes of mobility, depending on the environment in which they need to move. Augmented mobility must be viewed as a tool that promotes independence and continued development rather than a stumbling block that prevents the development of ambulation (Butler, 1997).

Types of Mobility Bases

Children who cannot walk without the assistance of mobility aids rely on a wheelchair to move about in their envi-ronments. Children's needs change over time because of growth and development; therefore there is a crucial need for adaptable systems and/or multiple systems throughout children's lives to ensure that AT promotes and supports their development. Physical therapists work along with families to determine when children need their "first chair." During typical development, most children begin moving independently (in an upright position) between 12 and 15 months of age. If children with disabilities do not have a means of independent, self-produced locomotion by this age, physical therapists assist families in determining the type of mobility base that provides the most independence and function to augment the child's mobility (Jones et al., 2003). Features of a wheelchair that are critical to consider when ordering include method of propulsion (manual or power), frame style (folding or rigid), size, and model. Physical therapists carefully review all the features of a mobility base before ordering a specific chair. They match features of a mobility base with the results from their interview with the child and/or family, record review, and physical examination to ensure that all components of a child's mobility base and seating system are obtained. Team members also ensure that, when delivered, the mobility base and seating system are adjusted to meet the child's needs. Mobility bases can be divided into two basic categories according to the method of propulsion: manual and power. Manual wheelchairs can be further divided into chairs for independent mobility and dependent transport chairs. Children who rely on others to move them from place to place use dependent transport chairs.

Manual Wheelchairs for Independent Mobility

Wheelchairs for independent mobility encompass a wide array of frame styles, sizes, and models. Most fold, allowing the chair to become more compact for transportation. Weight of the wheelchair is an important factor because it affects the ease of propulsion, especially for young children. Chairs are generally classified by their weight and include standard, lightweight, and ultra-lightweight frames.

Standard wheelchairs weigh in excess of 45 pounds and are often difficult for children with disabilities to propel. They generally fold for transportation but have limited adjustability for efficient wheelchair propulsion and growth. **Lightweight chairs** generally weigh between 30 and 36 pounds and have options available that improve their adjustability for wheelchair propulsion and growth. Lightweight chairs usually allow adjustment of the rear wheel position to enable a child to reach the wheels for propulsion. In general, they also allow for adjustment of seat width, seat depth, and back height. The frame adjustability is especially important for children, allowing accommodation of their current size but having versatility to adjust for future growth. **Ultra-lightweight chairs** weigh less than 30 pounds. Chairs in this category can be folding or rigid. Folding frames are beneficial when families must fold the chair for transportation. The folding frame is achieved either with a cross-brace (X-frame) or a folding back (Figure 16–17) (Bergen et al., 1990; Taylor & Kreutz, 1997). *Folding frames*, because of the "flex" in the frame, require more energy to propel than does a rigid frame. *Rigid frames* are more responsive and energy efficient for children to propel independently but often require that families have vans or alternate chairs to use for transportation outside of the school or home (Bergen et al., 1990; Carlson & Ramsey, 2000; Gilson & Huss, 1995; Taylor & Kreutz, 1997).

Manual Wheelchairs for Dependent Mobility

Manual chairs for dependent mobility are most often used for children who are unable to propel their wheelchairs independently. Family members propel the wheelchair, moving the children from place to place. Therefore, when choosing a chair for dependent mobility, the family must also be considered a "user" of the chair. As with manual wheelchairs for independent mobility, various frame styles are available. Manual wheelchairs for dependent mobility can generally be divided into tilt-in-space wheelchairs and strollers (Figure 16–18).

Manual **tilt-in-space wheelchairs** allow adjustment of the frame in relationship to the surrounding environment. Children may require tilt-in-space for position changes throughout the day to prevent the development of pressure ulcers. Children with poor head and trunk control, significant musculoskeletal impairments, and poor endurance may also require tilt-in-space. Team members should consider the child's visual orientation when using tilt-in-space to avoid decreasing a child's visual interaction with people. Adjustments should be made to the seating system or other parts of the frame to limit the degree of tilt-in-space needed as much as possible to facilitate a horizontal eye gaze.

Tilt-in-space wheelchairs are often designed with an adjustable seat-to-back angle. An adjustable seat-to-back angle is important when designing a wheelchair for a child who has limited hip mobility (less than 90° of hip flexion),

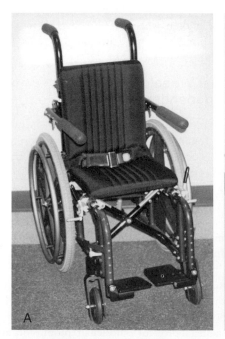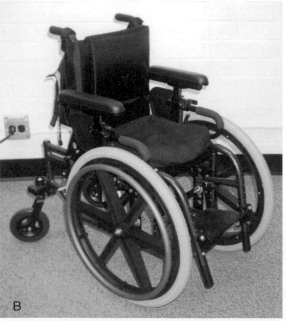

Figure 16-17 *(A)* Zippie 2 manual wheelchair with X-frame and *(B)* Zippie GS manual wheelchair with a folding back.

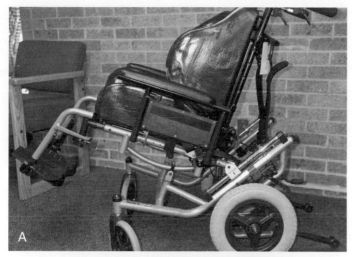

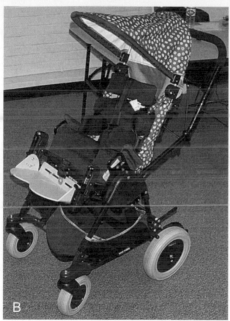

Figure 16-18 (A) Invacare Solara tilt-in-space wheelchair, and (B) KidKart Stroller from Sunrise Medical.

shortened hamstring musculature, or structural kyphosis, or who cannot sit in an upright position because of fatigue or the effects of gravity. Manual chairs with an adjustable seat-to-back angle can generally be adjusted from 90° of hip flexion to a recline angle ranging from 90° to 120° to accommodate a child's structural changes.

Strollers are designed for very young children. Parents of young children who are receiving their first mobility base may be more receptive to a stroller that looks the least like a wheelchair; however, therapists should offer the full range of mobility base options available. Strollers often are easier to fold for transport, making them a preferred option for many parents. Strollers that are easy to fold, however, are not generally designed to provide extensive positioning support, so they may not be beneficial for children with severe physical disabilities. Many of today's commercially available strollers are designed with firm seats and backs and offer the option to add various positioning components. They also can be adapted with custom-contoured seating systems. Strollers are not intended for permanent use by older children, and their use should be limited to young children or as a back-up method of transportation for other children.

Powered Mobility Bases

For children who are unable to maneuver a manual wheelchair independently, but for whom independent mobility is a goal, powered mobility bases are indicated. Recent advancements in the field of powered mobility have made independence a reality for many children with disabilities (Bergen et al., 1990; Carlson & Ramsey, 2000; Jones et al., 2003; Taylor & Kreutz, 1997). Most power wheelchairs for children are direct-drive chairs, which provide a direct connection between the motors and wheels. Direct-drive chairs offer the greatest range of control options. Some powered mobility bases also offer seat height adjustment and standing options. Power tilt and recline systems can be added to these chairs, allowing for position changes throughout the day to prevent the development of ulcers, pain, or fatigue, as well as improve function.

Scooters and add-on battery packs are options available for children, but are less commonly used. Scooters are equipped with either three or four wheels and are controlled with a tiller on which the controls are positioned. Control and positioning/seating options are often limited with scooters, requiring good upper extremity movement and independent sitting balance. Scooters are better suited for indoor than outdoor use. Add-on battery packs fit over the rear wheels of a manual wheelchair and convert it to a powered mobility base. Power packs perform better on level surfaces and are not designed for rigorous outdoor use.

Controls for powered wheelchairs are either *proportional* or *microswitch*. Typical power wheelchairs are controlled through a joystick mechanism, although other electronic control systems also are available. Typically, the joystick is mounted on the armrest and controls the speed and direction of the chair in a 360° arc of movement. Alternate mounting options and joystick sizes are available. For children who are unable to use a proportional control, other electronic controls or microswitches can control a chair for independent mobility. Electronic controls include sip-and-puff options, chin controls, head controls, and foot controls. Microswitch controls consists of four separate switches that control a single direction of the chair (forward, backward, right, left). Figure 16–19 illustrates some popular wheelchair controls (Bergen et al., 1990; Taylor & Kreutz, 1997).

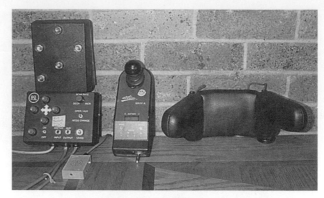

Figure 16-19 Wheelchair control options. Left to right; ASL single switch direction scan, ASL head array, and standard joystick.

Physical therapists, in collaboration with other team members, play a critical role in researching, presenting, trying, and possibly developing appropriate control systems to provide children with a means of independent mobility. The physical therapist's contributions are (1) identifying potential movement patterns that can be reliably and voluntarily controlled, (2) identifying the potential body part that will operate the control mechanism, (3) determining the type of control mechanism that best interfaces with the movement pattern, (4) trying potential options and evaluating a child's ability to activate, control direction, and release the wheelchair control mechanism, and (5) determining how to mount the control mechanism.

Physical therapists, whether recommending a manual or powered wheelchair, work with durable medical equipment vendors to review the finer details of the chair. The wheelchair's overall size and adjustability of component parts, such as seating angles, footrests, armrests, and turning radius, as well as ease of maneuvering, disassembly, and transport, are details physical therapists and durable medical equipment vendors discuss with the child and family. Such details are crucial in making an appropriate, informed recommendation.

Summary

AT devices and services allow children with disabilities to participate in activities alongside their peers. Devices are designed to promote independence, improve activities and participation, and enhance the lives of children with disabilities. AT allows children to overcome neuromotor, musculoskeletal, and sensory impairments and to eliminate secondary limitations in activities and participation that arise as a result of such impairments. Physical therapists play a key role in the selection, acquisition, modification/ customization, and implementation of AT devices, ensuring that children receive, and can effectively use, the technology they need across all environments. AT is an integral part of a child's therapeutic program and cannot be viewed as a separate task for which therapists have no responsibility. Physical therapists work with families and other team members to provide AT evaluations, complete paperwork necessary to apply for funding, incorporate motor learning principles when training children to use AT, and provide ongoing support and follow up to ensure the AT provided continues to meet a child's changing needs. AT devices change rapidly, as do the needs of children. Therefore, physical therapists must stay current on the equipment available to meet the needs of children. As with other areas of practice, continued research evaluating the impact and use of AT is critical.

DISCUSSION QUESTIONS

1. What are the critical elements that provide information as part of the assistive technology decision-making process?

2. What motor learning principles should you use when training children to use assistive technology?

3. What factors should you consider when determining the type of seating system to recommend for a child?

4. What factors should you consider when determining the type of wheelchair to recommend for a child?

RECOMMENDED READINGS

Angelo, J. (1997). *Assistive technology for rehabilitation therapists.* Philadelphia: F.A. Davis.

Furumasu, J. (Ed.). (1997). *Pediatric powered mobility: Developmental perspectives, technical issues, clinical approaches.* Arlington, VA: Rehabilitation Engineering and Assistive Technology Society of North America.

Reed, P. (Ed.). (2000). *Assessing students' needs for assistive technology: A resource manual for school district teams.* Oshkosh, WI: Wisconsin Assistive Technology Initiative.

REFERENCES

Angelo, J. (2000). Factors affecting the use of a single switch with assistive technology devices. *Journal of Rehabilitation Research and Development, 37*(5), 591–598.

Angelo, J. (1997). *Assistive technology for rehabilitation therapists.* Philadelphia: F.A. Davis.

Bay, J.L. (1991). Positioning for head control to access an augmentative communication machine. *The American Journal of Occupational Therapy, 45,* 544–549.

Behrmann, M.M. (1995). Assistive technology training. In K.F. Flippo, K.J. Inge, & J.M. Barcus (Eds.), *Assistive technology: A resource for school, work, and community* (pp. 211–222). Baltimore: Paul H. Brookes.

Bergen, A.F., Presperin, J., & Tallman, T. (1990). *Positioning for function: Wheelchairs and other assistive technologies.* Valhalla, NY: Valhalla Rehabilitation Publications.

Beukelman, D., & Mirenda, P. (1998). *Augmentative and alternative communication: Management of severe communication disorders in children and adults* (2nd ed.). Baltimore: Paul H. Brookes.

Brown, D.A., Effgen, S.K., & Palisano, R.J. (1998). Performance following ability-focused physical therapy intervention in individuals with severely limited physical and cognitive abilities. *Physical Therapy, 78*(9), 934–947.

Butler, C. (1997). Wheelchair toddlers. In J. Furumasu (Ed.), *Pediatric powered mobility: Developmental perspectives, technical issues, clinical approaches* (pp. 1–5). Arlington, VA: Rehabilitation Engineering and Assistive Technology Society of North America.

Carlson, S.J., & Ramsey, C. (2000). Assistive technology. In S.K. Campbell, D.W. Vander Linden, & R.J. Palisano (Eds.), *Physical therapy for children* (2nd ed., pp. 671–708). Philadelphia: W.B. Saunders.

Cook, A.M., & Hussey, S.M. (1995). *Assistive technologies: Principles and practice.* St. Louis, MO: Mosby–Year Book.

Dunn, W. (1991). Integrated related services. In L.H. Meyer, C.A. Peck, & L. Brown (Eds.), *Critical issues in the lives of people with severe disabilities* (pp. 353–377). Baltimore: Paul H. Brookes.

Evans, I.M. (1991). Testing and diagnosis: A review and evaluation. In L.H. Meyer, C.A. Peck, & L. Brown (Eds.), *Critical issues in the lives of people with severe disabilities* (pp. 353–377). Baltimore: Paul H. Brookes.

Franks, C.A., Palisano, R.J., & Darbee, J.C. (1991). The effect of walking with an assistive device and using a wheelchair on school performance in students with myelomeningocele. *Physical Therapy, 71*(8), 570–577.

Galvin, J.C., & Scherer, M.J. (1996). *Evaluating, selecting, and using appropriate assistive technology.* Gaithersburg, MD: Aspen Publishers.

Gillen, G. (2002). Improving mobility and community access in an adult with ataxia. *American Journal of Occupational Therapy, 56*(4), 462–466.

Gilson, B.B., & Huss, D.S. (1995). Mobility: Getting to where you want to go. In K.F. Flippo, K.J. Inge, & J.M. Barcus (Eds.), *Assistive technology: A resource for school, work, and community* (pp. 87–103). Baltimore: Paul H. Brookes.

Greenstein, D.B. (1996). It's child's play. In J.C. Galvin & M.J. Scherer (Eds.), *Evaluating, selecting, and using appropriate assistive technology* (pp. 198–214). Gaithersburg, MD: Aspen Publishers.

Jones, M.A., McEwen, I.R., & Hansen, L. (2003). Use of power mobility for a young child with spinal muscular atrophy. *Physical Therapy, 83,* 253–262.

Kolar, K.A. (1996). Seating and wheeled mobility aids. In J.C. Galvin & M.J. Scherer (Eds.), *Evaluating, selecting, and using appropriate assistive technology* (pp. 61–76). Gaithersburg, MD: Aspen Publishers.

Larin, H.M. (2000). Motor learning: Theories and strategies for the practitioner. In S.K. Campbell, D.W. Vander Linden, & R.J. Palisano (Eds.), *Physical therapy for children* (2nd ed., pp. 170–197). Philadelphia: W.B. Saunders.

Individuals with Disabilities Education Act Amendments of 1997, PL 105–17, 20 U.S.C. §§1400 et seq.

McEwen, I.R. (1992). Assistive positioning as a control parameter of social-communicative interactions between students with profound multiple disabilities and classroom staff. *Physical Therapy, 72*(9), 634–646.

McEwen, I.R., & Lloyd, L.L. (1990). Positioning students with cerebral palsy to use augmentative and alternative communication. *Language, Speech, and Hearing Services in Schools, 21,* 15–21.

McEwen, I.R., & Shelden, M.L. (1995). Pediatric therapy in the 1990s: The demise of the educational versus medical dichotomy. *Occupational and Physical Therapy in Educational Environments, 15*(2), 33–45.

McNevin, N.H., Wulf, G., & Carlson, C. (2000). Effects of attentional focus, self-control, and dyad training on motor learning: Implications for physical rehabilitation. *Physical Therapy, (80)*4, 373–385.

Miedaner, J., & Finuf, L. (1993). Effects of adaptive positioning on psychological test scores for preschool children with cerebral palsy. *Pediatric Physical Therapy, 5,* 177–182.

Minkel, J.L. (2000). Seating and mobility considerations for people with spinal cord injury. *Physical Therapy, 80*(7), 701–709.

Muller, C.A., & Oberstein, J.S. (1995). Selecting augmentative communication devices: A transdisciplinary feature-match process. Paper presented at the American Speech and Hearing Association Convention, Orlando, FL.

Mulligan, M., Lacy, L., & Guess, D. (1982). Effects of massed, distributed or spaced trial sequencing on severely handicapped students' performance. *Journal of the Association of the Severely Handicapped, 7*(2), 48–61.

Myhr, U., & von Wendt, L. (1991). Improvement of functional sitting position for children with cerebral palsy. *Developmental Medicine and Child Neurology, 33*(3), 246–256.

Neely, R.A., & Neely, P.A. (1993). The relationship between powered mobility and early learning in young children with physical disabilities. *Infant-Toddler Intervention, 3* (2), 85–91.

Nwaobi, O.M., & Smith, P.D. (1986). Effect of adaptive seating on pulmonary function of children enhance psychosocial and cognitive development. *Developmental Medicine and Child Neurology, 28,* 351–354.

Reed, P. (Ed.). (2000). *Assessing students' needs for assistive technology: A resource manual for school district teams.* Oshkosh, WI: Wisconsin Assistive Technology Initiative.

Reichle, J., & Sigafoos, J. (1991). Establishing spontaneity and generalization. In J. Reichle, J. York, & J. Sigafoos (Eds.), *Implementing augmentative and alternative communication: Strategies for learners with severe disabilities* (pp. 157–171). Baltimore: Paul H. Brookes.

RESNA Technical Assistance Project (1992). *Assistive technology and the individualized education program* (updated). Washington, DC: RESNA Press.

Rigby, P., Reid, D., Schoger, S., & Ryan, S. (2001). Effects of wheelchair-mounted rigid pelvic stabilizer on caregiver assistance for children with cerebral palsy. *Assistive Technology, 13*(1), 2–11.

Schmidt, R.A. (1988). *Motor control and learning: A behavioral emphasis.* Champaign, IL: Human Kinetics.

Stuberg, W.A. (1992). Considerations related to weight-bearing programs in children with developmental disabilities. *Physical Therapy, 72,* 35–40.

Taylor, S.J. (1997). Evaluation for wheelchair seating. In J. Angelo & S. Lane (Eds.), *Assistive technology for rehabilitation therapists* (pp. 15–42). Philadelphia: F.A. Davis.

Taylor, S.J., & Kreutz, D. (1997). Powered and manual wheelchair mobility. In J. Angelo & S. Lane (Eds.), *Assistive technology for rehabilitation therapists* (pp. 117–158). Philadelphia: F.A. Davis.

Trefler, E., Hobson, D.A., Taylor, S.J., Monahan, L.C., & Shaw, C.G. (1993). *Seating and mobility for persons with physical disabilities.* Tucson, AZ: Communication Skill Builders.

Washington, K., Deitz, J.C., White, O.R., & Schwartz, I.S. (2002). The effects of a contoured foam seat on postural alignment and upper extremity function in infants with neuromotor impairments. *Physical Therapy, 82*(11), 1064–1076.

Winstein, C.J. (1991). Designing practice for motor learning: Clinical implications. In M.J. Lister (Ed.), *Contemporary management of motor control problems: Proceedings of the II STEP Conference* (pp. 65–76). Alexandria, VA: Foundation for Physical Therapy.

Chapter *17*

Assistive Technology: Augmentative Communication and Other Technologies

— Sylvia Gray, MS, ATP
— Maria Jones, PT, PhD, ATP

Children with disabilities often require multiple pieces of equipment to meet their needs across various environments. Physical therapists, in collaboration with other team members, will assess for the other technologies after a child's positioning has been addressed. As discussed in Chapter 16, proper positioning promotes improved function, movement, and participation in activities. Once a child is well positioned and can move about his or her environment independently, the need for communication and other technologies increases. This chapter provides information pertinent to physical therapists working as members of an assistive technology (AT) team when addressing the remaining categories of AT.

Augmentative Communication

Augmentative and alternative communication (AAC) is the use of means other than speech to assist children in communication. The term "augmentative" refers to the use of systems that support existing speech to assist in communicating a message. In essence, all speakers use augmentative techniques from time to time. Speakers often augment their messages with facial expressions and gestures, or by pointing to visual supports in the environment in an effort to make sure the message is understood. "Alternative" communication describes systems that are intended to be the primary communication systems for children who are nonspeaking. AAC systems consist of a wide variety of techniques, systems, and intervention strategies that enable a person to become a functional communicator.

For any given AAC user, a core group of people, including the child, family members, and professionals from two or three disciplines, typically assume the role of AAC team (Reed, 2000). Each person provides essential information. For example, the AAC user or potential user identifies his or her abilities, limitations, needs, and desires. Family members provide information about any pertinent medical and educational history; day-to-day communication needs; family dynamics, strengths, and needs; family resources; and environmental considerations. Educators discuss current and projected educational abilities, learning needs and potential, and use of materials in the classroom. Speech-language pathologists discuss current receptive and expressive communication abilities, current and future communication abilities, needs, opportunities, and barriers and provide communication intervention. When AAC users or potential users also have physical disabilities that limit their motor control, a physical therapist can make a contribution by (1) assessing motor control, (2) identifying body part(s) and movement(s) to control AAC devices, (3) assessing positioning and ensuring that positioning systems promote optimal motor control and use of devices, (4) designing a system that best matches the motor abilities of the child, and (5) designing intervention strategies to promote functional use of the AAC system (McEwen, 1997). AAC systems are broadly categorized as unaided or aided.

Unaided Systems

Unaided systems are systems that are naturally available to us and do not require the addition of something external. Examples of unaided systems are gestures, body language, vocalizations or speech, facial expressions, signals, and manual signs. For some children, behaviors, such as crying, smiling, or tensed or relaxed body tone, may serve as communication systems. Gestures may be conventional or idiosyncratic in nature. Conventional gestures are behavioral postures or movements that are generally interpreted by society as having a specific meaning (e.g., head nod = yes; head shake = no, hand wave = hello/good-bye). Idiosyncratic gestures are those that are unique in production to a child and whose meaning has been assigned by familiar communication partners, limiting the meaning of that gesture to those partners. The use of body language also assists in the expression of a communication message. Moving closer to a person usually indicates interest, whereas moving away generally indicates disinterest or a desire to terminate a conversation.

Even though a person may have limited capabilities for producing speech, vocalizations and word approximations can still be effectively used to augment communication. For example, vocalizations combined with facial expressions can effectively communicate messages, such as accept and protest or yes and no. Vocalizations may also effectively provide a means of gaining someone's attention. Word approximations are often recognized by parents, friends, and caretakers, thus enhancing communication in certain situations.

Manual signs and sign languages are formal systems in which conventionalized gestures are assigned relatively abstract meanings and communication with these gestures is based on specific rules (Blischak, Lloyd, & Fuller, 1997). Just as with spoken language, there are many sign languages. For example, the sign that represents the word "doctor" may not be produced the same way across languages. American Sign Language (ASL) is the language most often used by the deaf community in the United States.

Aided Systems

Aided communication systems are those in which something is added to a person to help with communication. Aided systems may consist of manual communication systems (e.g., communication boards, communication notebooks, or communication wallets) or electronic systems such as voice output communication devices. Walser and Reed (2000b) categorize aided augmentative communication systems as follows: simple communication boards, simple voice output devices, leveling or layering devices, devices using icon sequencing, dynamic display devices, and devices that spell with a speech synthesizer/written text (Figure 17–1).

Communication boards may be designed using objects, photographs, graphic symbols (line drawings), or letters/words to represent messages for communication. Decisions regarding which type of representation to use depend on many factors, such as the child's visual, cognitive-linguistic, and academic abilities. Communication boards can be designed to have any number of symbols accessible to create messages. Communication boards are also designed based on how the child accesses or sends the message to another person, whether it is by eye gaze or by pointing.

Simple voice output devices have single symbol/single message capabilities. A message can be stored in a single location using digitized speech. Digitized speech means that the message is programmed with recorded speech. These devices are easily programmed. Programming consists of pushing down a button and recording the message into the microphone. The message is then retrieved or spoken when the device is activated by touch or through the use of a switch. Simple voice output devices may range in vocabulary capacity from 1 message to more than 100 messages.

Leveling or layering devices operate by storing vocabulary in levels, which are like pages in a book. Level-based systems increase the amount of stored vocabulary or messages without the need for reprogramming and also provide a system for organizing the vocabulary. The vocabulary or message storage capacity depends on the number of levels available on the device, as well as the memory capacity. Some level-based systems use digitized speech and others use synthesized speech. Synthesized speech is computer-generated speech that uses a speech synthesizer and requires less memory than digitized, but programming is not as easy. Level systems allow vocabulary to be stored

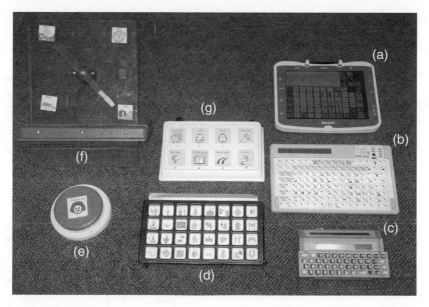

Figure 17-1 Different types of AAC devices. *(a)* Sunrise Medical DynaVox (dynamic display device). *(b)* Prentke Romich DeltaTalker (Minspeak device). *(c)* Zygo LightWriter (text-to-speech device). *(d)* AMDI TechSpeak (leveling device). *(e)* AbleNet Big Mack (single message device). *(f)* Dial Scan. *(g)* Cheap Talk 8 (simple voice output).

based on activities or environments. For example, if a system has the capacity for four levels, vocabulary can be stored as follows: Level 1: Circle time vocabulary; Level 2: Snack time vocabulary; Level 3: Story time vocabulary; and Level 4: Getting ready for bed. Touching a button or turning a dial changes the levels. The display for the vocabulary is usually a paper overlay and has to be physically changed to match the voice messages.

Dynamic display devices automatically change the visual display on the screen of the device based on user input. This feature makes the display or message choices "dynamic" as opposed to "fixed" or "static." Pages or levels of vocabulary are linked through programming the device. Making a choice on one screen links the user to another screen with more vocabulary options. These systems can be designed to use picture symbols, letters for spelling, or word prediction, depending on a child's abilities. To access a message such as "I would like a glass of milk," the child might first select the picture on a screen representing foods. This selection causes a display of food categories to appear, such as drinks, vegetables, fruits, desserts, and so on. The child then chooses "drinks." A display with the following choices might appear: water, milk, juice, coffee, and so on. The child now selects "milk" from the array of choices to indicate the desire for milk. Most dynamic display systems are designed with touch screen capabilities, but other methods of access are available.

Another group of devices uses icon sequencing or Minspeak to store and retrieve messages. When using Minspeak, a message is stored and recalled using a two- or three-picture symbol sequence. Minspeak relies on a child's ability to make multiple associations with a picture and sequence two or three symbols to create a message. With Minspeak, a two-symbol sequence may be used to store the name of a color, such as the rainbow icon + the sun icon = "yellow." The message "What color is it?" might be stored under the question mark icon (?) + the rainbow icon.

For children who have functional literacy skills (at least third-grade level), devices that take advantage of "text-to-speech" capabilities may be considered. These devices operate like a talking keyboard—the user types in a message and the device speaks what has been typed. Some of these devices have rate enhancement strategies to assist with message generation for children with motor control problems. Rate enhancement strategies may include letter prediction, word prediction, or abbreviation/expansion. The letter prediction feature assists by trying to predict the next letter to be typed. Word prediction assists by trying to predict the word a person is typing. After that word is selected, it may predict the next word. Abbreviation/expansion lets the user store or encode a word, phrase, or sentence message by assigning the message a string of letters. When the letter string is typed, the message is expanded to the full text that was stored, saving the user many keystrokes. The user must be able to assign the message a letter code and remember it. For example, NSG might represent "My name is Sylvia Gray."

Access for Communication Systems or Computers

Access refers to how children are going to use or provide input into a device, such as a communication system or computer. Most children turn on a tape recorder by pushing the play button. For children with disabilities this may not be possible; therefore, they need some other means of accessing the devices or tools within their environment. There are two basic forms of access: direct selection or indirect selection (scanning).

Direct Selection

Direct selection describes techniques in which the child can directly interact with the device or system. One example of direct selection is using two hands to access a computer keyboard. Children may also use direct selection with a head pointer, chin pointer, mouthstick, or hand splint. When using these options, children make physical contact with the device or system. They can, however, make a direct selection without making physical contact. For example, children can use their eyes, a light pointer, or their voices to select activities or make choices. New technology continues to develop and makes it easier to find a method of direct selection for accessing a system. Whenever possible, the identification of a method for direct selection is preferred because it is usually faster than indirect selection and less cognitively demanding.

Indirect Selection

Children who are unable to use direct selection must rely on indirect selection to provide input or access to devices or systems. Indirect selection involves the use of a switch in combination with an encoding system, such as scanning or Morse code. Switches provide an interface between the child and the device or system he or she is controlling (Angelo, 2000). They can be interfaced with a communication system, computer, battery-operated device, or control unit to provide another means for using or accessing the device. Scanning provides a child with access to a group of items, such as the alphabet, pictures, or icons on a computer. The system scans through the group of items, making only one item available at a time. For example, if a

student wants to type his name, "Chris," he must activate the switch to begin scanning, wait for the cursor to pass over the "A" and "B," and be ready to activate the switch again when the cursor highlights "C." This process is then repeated for each letter in his name. Scanning is much slower than direct selection but requires only reliable motor control of one movement. Figure 17–2 illustrates movement options available for switch control for AAC or computer access.

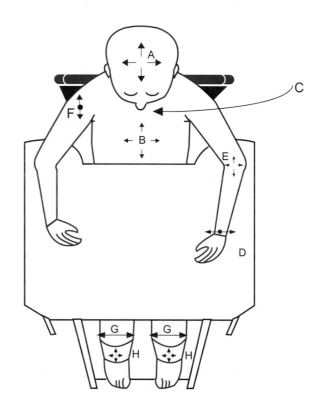

A. Head Control - forward/backward and left/right movement of the head

B. Chin Control - forward/backward and left/right movement of the chin, as with a chin-controlled joystick

C. Mouth/Tongue/Lip or Puff/Sip Control

D. Hand Control - up/down and left/right hand movement

E. Arm/Elbow Control - movement of the elbow outward or sliding the arm forward and backward

F. Shoulder Control - elevation/depression or protraction/retraction of the shoulder

G. Leg/Knee Control - inward/outward movement of the knee

H. Foot Control - left/right and up/down movement of the foot

Figure 17-2 Potential movement and control sites. (From D.M. Bayer, 1984, *DU-IT*, Control Systems Group, Inc. 8755 TR 513, Shreve, OH. Adapted with permission.)

A wide variety of switches are commercially available (Figure 17–3). Categories of switches include pressure, pneumatic, motion, photosensitive, physioelectric, and sound activated (DeCoste, 1997). Applying *pressure* causes activation of pressure switches. *Pneumatic* switches are activated by air, such as sip and puff switches and air cushion switches. The release of air into the switch causes activation to occur. Examples of motion switches are mercury or infrared switches. Examples of photosensitive switches include blink switches. *Physioelectric* switches are those that detect muscle movements such as tension and relaxation for activation. *Sound* switches are activated by the detection of sound. With the wide variety of switches available, it is possible to identify and provide a means of indirect selection for just about any degree of physical ability.

The evaluation process for determining a method of indirect selection involves identifying (1) movement patterns that the child can reliably and voluntarily control, (2) the point or body part that will access the switch, (3) the type of switch that best interfaces with the movement pattern, and (4) how the switch will be mounted. The physical therapist should be an integral part of the evaluation process. The physical therapist's contributions are to (1) determine whether a child has the motor control necessary for unaided AAC, (2) identify body part(s) and movement(s) to control AAC devices, (3) assess positioning and

ensure that positioning systems promote optimal motor control and use of devices, (4) design a system that best matches the motor abilities of the child, and (5) design intervention strategies to promote development of motor control for functional use of the AAC system (Angelo, 2000; McEwen, 1997).

The next phase of this evaluation process involves looking at how the child is able to access the switch. A child's ability to activate and release the switch can be categorized in three ways: (1) the child has timed or controlled initiation/releases, (2) the child has untimed initiation/timed release, or (3) the child has untimed initiation/release. The way the child activates and releases the switch helps determine the type of scan system that is appropriate. Factors to be considered include scan technique and scan pattern.

Types of *scan techniques* include automatic, inverse, and step. *Automatic* means that the child activates the switch and the indicator automatically moves through the scan pattern. When the desired target is lighted, the child again hits the switch to indicate the desired selection. Children need controlled initiation/release activation of the switch for this method. In *inverse* (i.e., directed) scan technique, the child initiates and maintains contact with the switch. As long as the child maintains contact with the switch, the indicator light moves through the scan pattern. Once the indicator is on the desired target, the child releases the switch to make the selection. Children with good ability to maintain contact and perform controlled releases are often matched with this type of scan technique. In *step* scan, there is a one-to-one correspondence between switch activation/release and movement through the scan pattern. Children who have difficulty with timed or controlled movements may be matched with this type of scan technique.

Scan pattern refers to how the indicator moves through the array of choices presented on the communication or computer display. Types of scan patterns include circular, linear, and group item. *Circular* scans move item by item through a circular pattern, like a second hand on a clock face. A dial scan or clock communicator are examples of devices that use a circular scan pattern. This type of scan is useful for a child who can activate and hold a switch but who also has timed release to stop the "scan" on the appropriate choice. *Linear* scans move item by item and line by line from left to right, such as in the CheapTalk 8. *Group-item* scans move through the array of choices first by highlighted groups of choices (i.e., row or quadrant) and then item by item through the options available in that particular group. Row-column, column-row, and quadrant scanning are options of group-item scan patterns. When

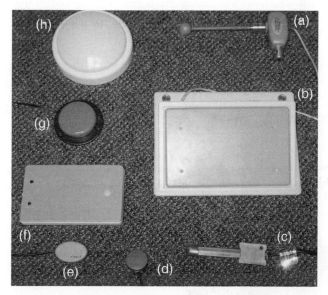

Figure 17-3 Different types of switches. *(a)* Enabling Devices Ultimate Switch. *(b)* Enabling Devices Plate Switch. *(c)* Zygo Leaf Switch. *(d)* Able Net Spec Switch. *(e)* Ellipse Switch. *(f)* Don Johnston Bass Switch. *(g)* Able Net Jellybean Switch. *(h)* WATI Light Switch.

row-column scanning is used, an entire row is highlighted at once. When the row containing the desired choice is lit, the child activates the switch, indicating the item is in that row. The scanning then continues to highlight each item in that row individually. The child then activates the switch a second time when the cursor reaches the desired choice. The child must have quick, controlled activation and release of a switch to use linear or group-item scanning.

Computer-Based Instruction

Children who have physical, sensory, or other disabilities may not be able to access a computer with a standard keyboard or mouse. However, there are many ways in which computers can be adapted to enable children with disabilities to use them (Walser & Reed, 2000a). Currently, both Macintosh and Windows operating systems provide features in the control panels that can make a computer more accessible. Sometimes the use of these features alone may provide sufficient adaptation to make the computer accessible; however, they are usually used in combination with other access methods. Physical therapists should become familiar with these built-in accessibility features when assessing children's needs for adapted computer access. With the constant change in technology, it is important for physical therapists to frequently update their knowledge of available products.

In addition to features that are built into computer oper-

ating systems, there are options for assisting direct selection access to computers. These include keyguards, keycaps, and arm supports. Keyguards fit over the keyboard and are attached using Velcro. They are made of metal or Plexiglas and have holes drilled through them to match the layout of the keyboard. They are helpful for those who have trouble isolating or targeting keys on the keyboard or communication device because they more definitively separate the keys and prevent accidental keystrokes. When selecting a keyguard, make sure the keyguard matches the keyboard or communication device. Keycaps are labels or stickers that can be placed on the keyboard. They provide a greater visual contrast and larger print. Keycaps may be helpful for children who have low vision or visual perceptual difficulties. Arm supports provide forearm stability and assist with movement for children with limited strength.

Children who cannot access a computer when provided with adaptations to a standard keyboard may have to rely on an alternate keyboard for access. Alternative keyboards include those that provide a larger keyboard area for access (expanded keyboards) and those that provide a smaller keyboard area for access (mini-keyboards) (Figure 17–4). Those who have a restricted range of motion may use mini-keyboards. Those who need larger areas to target may use expanded keyboards. Most alternative keyboards are designed to plug directly into the computer.

If children are unable to access a computer using standard, modified, or alternative keyboards, they may access a computer through voice recognition software. Voice recognition software is installed on the computer and

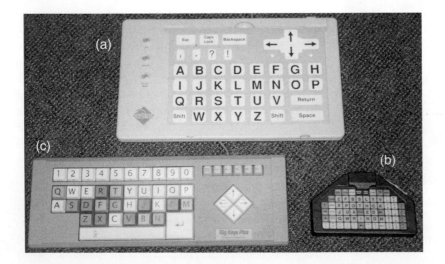

Figure 17-4 Alternate keyboards. *(a)* IntelliKeys by IntelliTools. *(b)* TASH mini keyboard, *(c)* Big Keys Plus Keyboard.

access is provided through voice commands. Children must have fairly good articulation skills and consistent speech patterns to benefit from voice recognition. Voice recognition is often not useful for children with cerebral palsy or traumatic brain injuries who may have problems with articulation and difficulty coordinating phonation with respiration.

Students who need adaptation to a keyboard may also require alternate mouse access. A wide variety of other alternatives are available, including Touch Windows, touchpads, trackballs, different mouse styles, keypad mouse, joysticks, and pointing systems such as those illustrated in Figure 17–5.

Pointing systems allow a user to control the cursor and provide input through head and/or eye movements. In pointing systems, a sensor attached to the computer translates head or eye movements. Once the cursor is in the desired location, mouse clicks may be performed either by "dwelling" on the location for a predetermined length of time or by accessing a separate switch. To provide total "hands-free" computer access, these systems are used in combination with on-screen keyboards. An on-screen keyboard is a software program that, when installed and activated, places a visual keyboard on the computer screen. This allows a person to use a pointing device such as a mouse, touchscreen, or head pointing system to have total keyboard control.

Environmental Control

Environmental control units (ECUs) promote a child's interaction, independence, and control of appliances or devices in the environment. Benefits related to the use of environmental control include improved personal satisfaction, increased participation in daily activities, and possible reduction in cost for personal care attendants (Dickey & Shealy, 1987; Jutai, Rigby, Ryan, & Stickel, 2000). ECUs can allow children to participate in activities that they would otherwise be unable to do. For example, a child can help prepare a snack by turning a blender on and off to make milkshakes.

ECUs consist of three main components: the input device, the control unit, and the appliance. The input device controls the ECU by either direct selection or scanning using switches. The control unit is the "brain" of the appliance, translating the input signal into an output action, giving the appliance a direction. Last, there is an appliance or a piece of electronic equipment. Table 17.1 provides a summary of control strategies for ECUs.

Activities of Daily Living

AT is often used to promote independence in activities of daily living (ADLs). Team members must consider whether a child can manage daily care activities and evaluate how technology can assist the child's performance. Children with disabilities often require equipment in the areas of toileting, grooming/hygiene, and eating. Toileting equipment can be as minor as a footstool to increase sitting stability but includes grab bars, raised toilet seats, and supportive potty chairs. Grooming/hygiene equipment often used by children and their families includes bath or shower chairs and can range from adapted toothbrushes to architectural modifications to a home. Many products are commercially available depending on the needs and age of the child (Figure 17–6). Adaptive eating utensils, such as spoons with built-up handles, cut-out cups, and scoop plates (Figure 17–7), can assist a child in becoming independent in this area. Physical therapists, along with other team members, especially the family and occupational therapist, can improve a child's level of independence by using AT for ADLs.

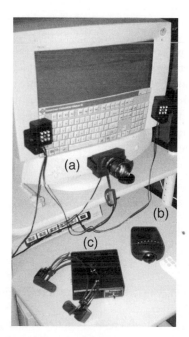

Figure 17-5 Computer control systems. *(a)* Quick Glance by EyeTech Digital Systems. *(b)* Madentec Tracker. *(c)* HeadMaster.

Table 17.1 Advantages and Disadvantages of Various Control Strategies for Environmental Control Units

Type of ECU Control	Advantages	Disadvantages
Ultrasound (uses high-frequency sound waves).	Child does not have to point the control directly at the control box. Systems are wireless, portable, and small.	The transmitter must be in the same room as the control box.
Infrared (activated from a remote control).	Systems are portable.	The child must point the remote directly at the control box with nothing obstructing the signal.
Radio control (translate control codes to appliances).	Transmission cannot be blocked by objects, making it possible to signal an appliance in one room while in another room.	Radio frequencies are limited in the distance they can travel, ranging between 50 and 200 feet. Interference from another control unit is possible.
AC power (uses existing electrical wiring to send input to activate appliances). The input device can be remote or be part of the control unit that is plugged into the wall. The appliances are also plugged into a module that is plugged into an existing electrical outlet.	AC power does not require additional wiring, but modules must be programmed.	These systems require several electrical outlets and older electrical wiring can pose problems.

Recreation/Leisure/Play

The ability to play is an important part of childhood. Play is a child's work. A child who cannot participate in play activities is missing an opportunity to experience normal development. Children with physical disabilities may not be able to manipulate toys independently or move around the environment to explore. Children with sensory impairments may also have reduced opportunities for independent exploration and a need for toys and play materials to be adapted. As a result, the play experiences for children with disabilities may be qualitatively and quantitatively different than play experiences for children who are developing typically. As children become older, the need for recreation/leisure activities becomes important. The area of recreation/leisure should be considered and addressed as part of the intervention program for all children with disabilities.

Therapists should consider the need for AT to facilitate recreation/leisure/play activities whenever a child with a disability is not able to play independently or interact with others during play or other recreation/leisure activities (Besio, 2002; Lane & Mistrett, 2002; Lane & Mistrett, 1996). Given the options that are available today, no child should sit on the sidelines and just "watch" other children play. For some children, toys or materials may need to be stabilized to make them more accessible. Materials such as Velcro, Dycem or other nonslip material, play boards, and C-clamps can be used to help stabilize play materials and toys and promote independent play opportunities. Velcro can be placed on toys or puzzle pieces to help make them easier to handle. When hook Velcro is placed on the play materials, they attach to any Velcro-sensitive surface such as indoor/outdoor carpet, tempo loop fabric, or loop Velcro. Other toys and objects can be adapted by building up handles or adding materials to make them easier to grasp. Beads, blocks, or shower curtain rings can be attached to play items to make them easier to manipulate. The use of a foam grip that increases the diameter of a surface may make it possible for some students to hold materials.

For children who are not able to interact directly with toys and other recreational devices, the use of simple technology components such as switches, battery adapters, ECUs, and latch timers may provide options for play. With the wealth of computer programs, children of all ages and abilities are enjoying video and computer games. Switches

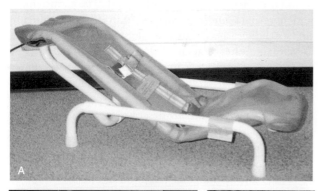

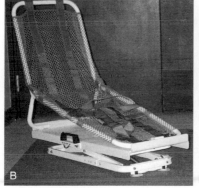

Figure 17-6 *(A)* Columbia reclining bath chair. *(B)* Flipper adjustable bath chair. *(C)* High-back potty chair.

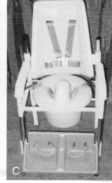

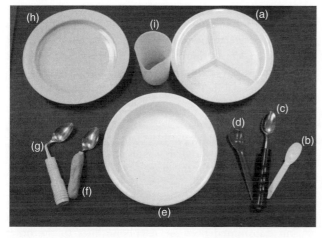

Figure 17-7 Eating/drinking utensils. *(a)* Partitioned scoop plate. *(b)* Child's feeding spoon. *(c)* Weighted handle spoon. *(d)* The maroon spoon. *(e)* Melamine scoop dish. *(f)* Spoon modified with modeling clay. *(g)* Homecraft angled spoon. *(h)* Plate with inside edge. *(i)* Nosey cut-out cup.

provide an alternative means for children with disabilities to access computers, tape recorders, battery-operated toys, or even electrical appliances, as previously discussed. Switches can be purchased commercially or home made. Switches are used in combination with switch interfaces to provide computer access. Likewise, battery adapters are used for battery operated devices and ECUs are used for electrical appliances.

Switches are described in detail in the previous section on AAC. Battery adapters or interrupters can be made simply and inexpensively or can be purchased commercially. The battery adapter is placed between the battery(ies) and a contact terminal to "interrupt" the power to the motor. The switch is then plugged into the battery adapter, and when the device is turned on, it will run when the child activates the switch.

A computer may provide a recreation/leisure activity. Software exists to cover a wide range of personal interests such as music, drawing, and games. Access to the Internet can provide a source of recreation/leisure to those who have an interest in "surfing" the Internet or telecommunicating with others online. As the technology field evolves, computers may change the world of opportunities for children with disabilities more than anything else in the 21st century.

Children in school environments may require specialized equipment to facilitate their access and participation in playground and recess activities. Several companies market adaptive playground equipment. In addition to specialized equipment, therapists can modify games so that all children can participate in these activities. Physical therapists should be active participants in their communities' ADA and playground committees, so that all children can participate in community "play" environments.

Visual Technology

Visual impairments can significantly affect functioning in major areas of life. Depending on the nature and severity of the impairment, a person's ability to be independent in accessing the environment, to use materials and tools of daily activities, and to access a computer may be affected. The use of AT is critical in helping children with visual impairments be as successful and as independent as possible.

Visual impairments significantly affect a person's independent mobility skills. A child's lack of awareness of the environment may contribute to reduced exploration, which affects the developmental process for young children and safety in travel at any age. Services from an orientation and mobility specialist and AT devices can assist a child with visual impairments to be more independent. An orientation and mobility specialist can help the child in navigating environments by using canes, guide dogs, and electronic travel aids.

Visual impairments also significantly affect a person's ability to use the tools and appliances needed in daily life. There are many commercially available devices designed to allow children with visual impairments to be more independent. Commercially available devices include devices that talk or provide audible feedback (e.g., talking thermometers, talking clocks, talking calculators, books on tape), Braille devices (e.g., clock faces with Braille, Braille instruction manuals, and Braille label makers), and large-print items.

Visual impairments also affect reading and writing abilities. For children with low vision, the use of low vision aids such as magnifiers, large print books, closed circuit television systems, larger computer monitors, and computer-based programs that combine optical character recognition, large font, screen magnification, color contrasts, and speech capabilities can make print accessible. For children who are blind, a Braille system or computer-based system that reads the text and graphic information on screen makes print accessible.

To facilitate writing, children with visual impairments may require the use of raised line paper, writing guides, or broad tip felt markers. Children who use Braille as their writing system may rely on the following (1) a slate and stylus, (2) devices such as the Braille N Speak or Type N Speak, or (3) computer-based systems with Braille translation software and a Braille printer.

When working with children with visual impairments, physical therapists need to alter their intervention to make it more meaningful. For example, physical therapists need to have a variety of toys that provide auditory or tactile feedback, not just visual. They also need to talk with the child throughout activities, explaining what they are doing and providing verbal feedback to the child regarding changes in the environment. Physical therapists can also be a valuable team member when children have both sensory and motor disabilities.

Assistive Listening

The terms "hard of hearing" and "deaf" are used to describe children with hearing losses. Hearing loss is often described as mild, moderate, severe, or profound. The terms "mild" and "moderate" indicate that an individual has difficulty understanding speech that is not amplified. The term "severe" indicates that amplification is required to hear speech. "Profound" loss indicates the inability to understand speech that is amplified. Hard of hearing usually describes a person who can understand speech with the ear with difficulty. Deaf usually describes a person who cannot hear or understand speech with amplification.

For children with hearing impairments, the use of AT is needed for communication, environmental control, ADLs, recreation and leisure, and reception of auditory information. Devices such as alarm clocks, door bells, smoke detectors, or telephones are designed to alert people by sending an auditory signal. These devices are also available so that a visual signal such as a strobe light, flash of light, or vibrating signal can be sent instead. Assistive listening devices can aid in the reception of auditory information. Most children with a hearing loss have a personal amplification device, such as a hearing aid, that an audiologist individually prescribes. However, the use of other assistive devices in combination with personal devices may be needed in environments that are very noisy. If a child uses an assistive listening device, physical therapists need to make sure that they use the transmitter during intervention, so that the child can hear auditory cues provided by the therapist. Although there are assistive listening systems that aid in the reception of auditory information, some people require or may prefer the use of sign language to receive information. In most instances, the use of oral interpreters is required.

Captioning is another method for enhancing reception of auditory information. In captioning, text appears at the bottom of a screen and provides a transcription of the aural information. Open captioning does not require the use of a special decoder to access the captioning. Closed captioning requires a special decoder to access the captioned information.

People who are deaf require AT to use the telephone. Since the implementation of the ADA, this technology has become more readily available. A device called the telecommunications device for the deaf (TDD) is used to make the telephone accessible. To use a TDD, both parties must have access to a device. The receiver of the telephone is placed in the coupler of the TDD, and the conversation is typed on it and transmitted over the telephone lines to the other TDD. When both parties do not have access to TDDs, a relay system is needed. Relay services have been established in all states to ensure accessibility. A person at the relay service has a TDD and acts as an interpreter/transcriptionist between the party who has access to the TDD and the party who does not.

The expressive communication of a person may be affected, depending on the onset and severity of the hearing loss. ASL is considered the native language of the people who are deaf, but not all people with a hearing loss rely on sign language for communication. Children who have combined physical and hearing impairments may have difficulty using sign language for communication. Physical therapists play a critical role in determining if a child has the motor control necessary to use sign language as a functional means of expressive communication.

Funding

Funding has long been a barrier to the acquisition of AT devices. As awareness about AT has increased, service providers have led the way in accessing funding sources. As members of the AT team, physical therapists must be familiar with funding options for AT. They must understand the basic differences between funding agencies to ensure technology is paid for by the most appropriate funding source.

Differences Between Funding Sources

Public or private sources of funding may be available to pay for AT devices and services for children. Private sources are not under government control and can be divided into national, statewide, and regional/local programs. Federal or state governments, laws, or acts control public sources of funding. The U.S. government classifies sources under their control as either discretionary or entitlement programs.

Discretionary programs are not required to provide all services to every eligible child under the program. Authorizing personnel within the agency, usually a case manager or counselor, determines whether the agency will provide the service or equipment. Discretionary programs have a limit on the money available to serve children under the program within a given year. Vocational rehabilitation is an example of a discretionary program (Enders, 1993; Wallace, 1995).

Entitlement programs provide all services to every eligible child under the program. In an entitlement program, once children meet eligibility criteria, they are guaranteed all the benefits of the program. Medicaid is an example of an entitlement program. Governments control entitlement programs by either limiting eligibility criteria or narrowing the cost, duration, and scope of services provided under the program (Enders, 1993; Golinker & Mistrett, 1997).

Some of the more common funding sources of payment for AT devices for children are (1) Medicaid (Title XIX of the Social Security Act), including Early, Periodic, Screening, Diagnosis, and Treatment (EPSDT); and state waiver programs; (2) early intervention (birth to 3 years) programs and local school districts, as part of Individuals with Disabilities Education Act (IDEA); (3) private insurance; and (4) service clubs and organizations (Golinker & Mistrett, 1997; Mendelsohn, 1996). Medicaid is a federal/state medical assistance program for selected people with low incomes or children who come from families with low incomes. Medicaid coverage varies from state to state, and therapists should become familiar with Medicaid procedures in their state. Early intervention programs, which serve children from birth to age 3 under IDEA, can pay for AT that is required by the child to achieve his or her Individualized Family Service Plan (IFSP) goals. Local school districts, as part of IDEA, pay for AT that is required by children to benefit from their educational program. A child's Individualized Education Plan (IEP) team determines the AT needs. Private insurance is a contract between the company (or individual) and the insurance provider or carrier. Companies or employers determine the coverage. Private insurance coverage varies widely between and within companies. Two families, who may be covered by the same insurance company, will not necessarily have the same insurance benefits unless their employer is also the same. Many private insurance companies have nurse case managers on staff who can provide assistance when trying to determine what coverage is available to a child. In general, they can also provide information about the medical review process, which is used to determine if equipment will be purchased under a family's policy.

With the funding sources available for payment of AT services and devices, physical therapists must be proficient at completing the paperwork necessary to apply for funding, such as certificates of medical necessity for private insurance and Medicaid or letters of justification for private funding sources. Although there are no "magic words" to ensure a funding agency will approve recommended equipment, physical therapists can use terms that are specific or familiar to the agency. If therapists apply to Medicaid, their justification must be written in terms of "medical necessity." If a child's educational team determines a local school district should purchase the equipment, the justification must demonstrate the impact of the AT on the child's educational performance. If therapists approach vocational rehabilitation, documentation must demonstrate how the technology supports the vocational goals or employment opportunities.

In addition to using specific or familiar terms when completing funding requests, therapists must also include necessary components. Necessary components for a certificate of medical necessity or justification letter include (1) the child's diagnosis and/or general physical condition as it applies to equipment recommendations, (2) a description of limitations in the child's abilities as they relate to the need for the equipment, (3) a description of current equipment, (4) a prognosis relating to how the equipment serves to "resolve" the limitations described previously, (5) a description of critical features needed in the equipment, including the purpose of each feature and how it relates to increased function for the child, and (6) the list of all team members involved in the selection of the piece of equipment. It is also beneficial and sometimes necessary to include pictures and/or videotapes of the child during simulation or while using trial equipment (Taylor & Kreutz, 1997).

Summary

This chapter describes augmentative communication and other technologies that may benefit children with disabilities. Assessment for augmentative communication and other technologies takes place once a child's positioning needs are addressed. The AT described in this chapter allows children with disabilities to accomplish tasks that they would otherwise be unable to do (Hammell, Lai, & Heller, 2002). Whether it is saying "I love you" to a friend or relative, or simply turning the television on or off, AT provides for independence and a sense of control over the environment. Children with AT needs will require ongoing support and intervention from physical therapists and other service providers to ensure that they are successful in obtaining and using technology.

Difficulties in obtaining technological equipment for children can often be a barrier to the use of technology. Funding is a crucial part of the process. Without funding, the technology can never be put into action and the possibilities remain hidden. The information presented in this chapter provides therapists with the basic information needed to approach various funding agencies and access AT for children.

DISCUSSION QUESTIONS

1. What contributions can a physical therapist make when assessing a child with physical disabilities for augmentative communication?

2. What is the difference between direct selection and indirect selection? Give an example of each.

3. Describe different modifications that can be made for a child who needs to use a computer but has limited motor skills.

4. What are the different components of an environmental control unit?

5. Describe the differences between a discretionary program and an entitlement program.

6. How would you justify equipment differently if you were approaching a school system for funding versus an insurance company?

REFERENCES

Angelo, J. (2000). Factors affecting the use of a single switch with assistive technology devices. *Journal of Rehabilitation Research and Development, 37*(5), 591–598.

Besio, S. (2002). An Italian research project to study the play of children with motor disabilities: The first year of activity. *Disability and Rehabilitation, 24*, 72–79.

Blischak, D.M., Lloyd, L.L., & Fuller, D.R. (1997). Terminology issues. In L.L. Lloyd, D.R. Fuller, & H.H. Arvidson (Eds.). *Augmentative and alternative communication: A handbook of principles and practices.* Boston: Allyn & Bacon.

Dickey, R., & Shealy, S.H. (1987). Using technology to control the environment. *American Journal of Occupational Therapy, 41*, 717–721.

DeCoste, D.C. (1997). In S.L. Glennen & D.C. DeCoste (Eds.). *Handbook of augmentative and alternative communication* (pp. 243–282). San Diego, CA: Singular Publishing.

Enders, A. (1993, June). Beyond the ABCs of reimbursement: Development of creative strategies for funding assistive technology. Symposium conducted at the annual meeting of the Rehabilitation Engineering and Assistive Technology Society of North America, Las Vegas, NV.

Golinker, L., & Mistrett, S.G. (1997). Funding. In J. Angelo & S. Lanc (Eds.). *Assistive technology for rehabilitation therapists* (pp. 211–234). Philadelphia: F.A. Davis.

Hammell, J., Lai, J.S., & Heller, T. (2002). The impact of assistive technology and environmental interventions on function and living situation status with people who are aging with developmental disabilities. *Disability and Rehabilitation, 24*, 93–105.

Jutai, J., Rigby, P., Ryan, S., & Stickel, S. (2000). Psychosocial impact of electronic aids to daily living. *Assistive Technology, 12*(2), 123–131.

Lane, S.J., & Mistrett, S. (2002). Let's play! Assistive technology interventions for play. *Young Exceptional Children, 5*(2), 19–27.

Lane, S.J., & Mistrett, S. (1996). Play and assistive technology issues for infants and young children with disabilities: A preliminary examination. *Focus on Autism and Other Developmental Disabilities, 11*(2), 96–104.

McEwen, I.R. (1997). Seating, other positioning, and motor control. In L.L. Lloyd, D.R. Fuller, & H.H. Arvidson (Eds.). *Augmentative and alternative communication: A handbook of principles and practices.* Boston: Allyn & Bacon.

Mendelsohn, S. (1996). Funding assistive technology. In J.C. Galvin & M. Scherer (Eds.). *Evaluating, selecting, and using appropriate assistive technology* (pp. 345–359). Gaithersburg, MD: Aspen Publishers.

Reed, P. (Ed.). (2000). *Assessing students' needs for assistive technology: A resource manual for school district teams.* Oshkosh, WI: Wisconsin Assistive Technology Initiative.

Taylor, S.J., & Krcutz, D. (1997). Powered and manual wheelchair mobility. In J. Angelo & S. Lane (Eds.). *Assistive technology for rehabilitation therapists* (pp. 117–158). Philadelphia: F.A. Davis.

Wallace, J.F. (1995). Creative financing of assistive technology. In K.F. Flippo, K.J. Inge, & J.M. Barcus (Eds.). *Assistive technology: A resource for school, work, and community* (pp. 245–268). Baltimore: Paul H. Brookes.

Walser, P., & Reed, P. (2000a). Assistive technology for writing, including mechanics, computer access, and composing. In P. Reed (Ed.), *Assessing students' need for assistive technology: A resource manual for school district teams* (pp. 57–90). Oshkosh, WI: Wisconsin Assistive Technology Initiative.

Walser, P., & Reed, P. (2000b). Augmentative and alternative communication. In P. Reed (Ed.). *Assessing students' need for assistive technology: A resource manual for school district teams* (pp. 90–109). Oshkosh, WI: Wisconsin Assistive Technology Initiative.

Case Studies

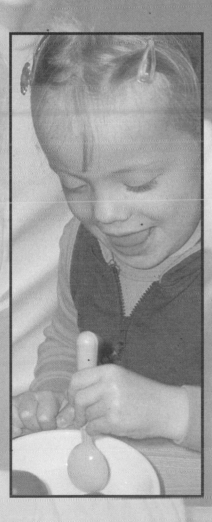

Chapter *18*

Case Study: Cerebral Palsy

— Donna Cech, PT, MS, PCS

This case study focuses on the physical therapy management of Kayla, a teen-aged girl with spastic, diplegic cerebral palsy (CP). Kayla is 13 years old and a seventh grader in the local junior high school. She was born prematurely and has received physical therapy services in a variety of settings since infancy.

Individuals with CP frequently present with impairments of range of motion (ROM), soft tissue mobility, strength, coordination, and balance, resulting in motor control difficulties. CP implies damage to the immature cortex, involving the motor system. Associated problems with vision, seizures, perception, and cognition may be seen if areas of the cortex associated with these functions are also damaged. Although the cortical lesion is nonprogressive, as the infant grows and strives to become more independent, functional limitations become more apparent, as do restrictions in activities and community participation. Secondary impairments, such as ROM limitations, disuse atrophy, and impaired aerobic capacity, may further limit functional motor skills and ability. Multiple episodes of physical therapy management are frequently warranted as the child attempts more complex functional skills and as the risk for secondary impairments increases. Children with CP present with a variety of functional abilities, reflecting the severity of their original neurological insult. The Gross Motor Function Classification System (GMFCS) provides a mechanism to classify these children, based on their gross motor abilities and limitations (Palisano et al., 1997).

Based on the American Physical Therapy Association (APTA)'s *Guide to physical therapist practice* (2001), Kayla's physical therapy needs may best be addressed by Preferred Practice Pattern 5C: Impaired Motor Function and Sensory Integrity Associated with Nonprogressive Disorders of the Central Nervous System—Congenital Origin or Acquired in Infancy or Childhood. This pattern was chosen because the pathology leading to the presenting impairments occurred in the prenatal, neonatal, or infancy period, and therefore involve the immature motor cortex. The resulting impaired motor function will potentially have a negative effect on the developing muscular, skeletal, cardiovascular, and pulmonary systems. The practice pattern chosen should most comprehensively address the developmental issues brought about by abnormal motor control from infancy and throughout childhood and adolescence. Kayla's physical therapy at ages 6 and 13 years is summarized, as well as a discussion of her potential lifelong physical therapy needs. Physical therapy is being provided by therapists working in educational settings and in accordance with the federal Individuals with Disabilities Education Act Amendments of 1997 (IDEA 97) in both episodes of care reported. In the first episode of care, Kayla is also receiving home health physical therapy services because she has recently had orthopedic surgery, and medically oriented physical therapy services are indicated.

◢ EXAMINATION: AGE 6 YEARS

History

Kayla is the youngest of four children. She was born prematurely, at 34 weeks' gestation and, as reported by her mother, had a fairly uneventful neonatal course. She was hospitalized for 2 weeks after birth because she had difficulty sucking and experienced periods of bradycardia. She did not have respiratory problems and was not noted to have had an intraventricular hemorrhage at that time. Her family became concerned when at 10 months of age she could not sit or crawl. When held in standing position, she was very stiff and could not balance. She was diagnosed at that time with spastic, diplegic CP.

Kayla was enrolled at a center-based early intervention program at 1 year of age. She was seen by a physical therapist, an occupational therapist, a speech-language pathologist, and an early childhood educator. Her primary areas of difficulty were gross motor function, fine motor function, and visual perception. At 3 years of age, Kayla began attending an early childhood program in her local school district and has continued in this setting until the present. She is now transitioning into a full-day, first-grade setting. Kayla has also received occupational and physical therapy services outside the school setting, after neurosurgical and orthopedic surgical procedures. Kayla's family has been very active in her intervention program and has strongly advocated for Kayla to be an active participant in community activities for children her age. She has participated in a local preschool at ages 3 and 4 years and in library programs and a park district day camp, and she is now beginning in Brownies.

Medically, Kayla's history includes ocular surgery at 18 months of age to correct a muscular imbalance, a selective dorsal rhizotomy at 4 years of age to decrease spasticity, bilateral derotational femoral osteotomies and medial hamstring release to improve lower extremity alignment at $5\frac{1}{2}$ years of age, and a right tibial plateau fracture at age 5 years after a fall from her swing set. At age $4\frac{1}{2}$ years, she was diagnosed with a mild temporal lobe seizure disorder, which is controlled with medication (Tegretol).

Systems Review

Cardiovascular and Pulmonary

No problems are noted in cardiovascular or pulmonary function. Kayla is very active physically and has good endurance. She does not have problems with respiratory infections. Kayla's blood pressure (100/70 mm Hg) and her heart rate (100 beats per minute) are within normal limits (WNL) for her age (Cech & Martin, 2002).

Integumentary

Kayla wears bilateral hinged ankle-foot orthoses (AFOs), and her parents report that she occasionally has areas of redness and irritation related to them. At this time, however, no problems with skin condition are noted.

Musculoskeletal

Kayla demonstrates muscle atrophy and weakness of her lower extremities, especially distally. Trunk weakness is also noted. The family reports that the weakness is especially noticeable since her recent orthopedic surgery, but has been noted ever since her dorsal rhizotomy. Bilateral hip flexion and knee flexion muscle contractures were reported before the recent orthopedic surgery, but at this time, functional ROM appears to be WNL. Further examination of muscle strength and ROM is warranted.

Neuromuscular

Hypertonicity and increased muscle stiffness are noted in the lower extremities. Some tremor is noted in the upper extremities during reaching and fine manipulative activities. Kayla cannot balance in standing position, does not walk without an assistive device, and has difficulty with coordination. Further examination of gait, motor function, and self-care is needed.

Cognition, Language, and Communication

Kayla's language development and communication skills are good. She may demonstrate a mild cognitive delay, but this might be related to visual perceptual difficulties. These areas will be further evaluated by the educational team and current classroom staff.

Tests and Measures

In completing a physical therapy examination with Kayla at 6 years of age, baseline function was determined in several areas. In the following discussion, areas of function that were found to be normal or identified an impairment that did not strongly affect function are briefly described. Tests and measures for areas that were thought to be affecting motor function are discussed in more detail.

Aerobic Capacity and Endurance

Kayla is able to keep up with her friends on the playground, even though she is using a walker. She does not get short of breath and does not appear to have problems with aerobic capacity or endurance.

Assistive and Adaptive Devices

Kayla uses a variety of assistive devices to aid mobility. She uses a motorized cart for community locomotion, a walker when walking for long distances or in more active environments (i.e., recess), and bilateral quad canes for short distances within her home. All devices currently fit appropriately and are in good repair. Kayla can use the cart and walker very safely in all environments. She can use the quadcanes only for short distances (10 to 15 feet) and with close supervision.

Gait, Locomotion, and Balance

Kayla safely uses a wheeled rear-walker in all terrains and environments (school, home, and community). She has begun to use quad canes, but she fatigues quickly and has difficulty picking her feet up high enough, causing her to trip when using the canes. For community mobility, Kayla uses a motorized cart and safely navigates curb cuts and school hallways. She drives it approximately two blocks to or from school. Before her recent orthopedic surgery, Kayla had a full computerized gait assessment with and without her orthotics. This examination was performed at a gait laboratory affiliated with the hospital where she sees her orthopedic surgeon and had her surgery.

Kayla has difficulty with sitting and standing balance. She cannot stand without support. She can sit on the floor independently, but she does not reach too far outside of her base of support or reach over her head. When sitting on a bench, she cannot reach out of her base of support to the right or the left. She also demonstrates a loss of balance when she reaches above shoulder level. In most sitting positions, Kayla's posture is kyphotic, with rounded shoulders and a forward head position. Her most stable and favored sitting position is W-sitting.

Motor Function

Kayla creeps easily, using a reciprocal lower extremity pattern, and can knee-walk for 3 to 5 feet. She has difficulty grading movements, often initiating the movement quickly. In fine motor activity, she demonstrates fine tremors with both hands when reaching for a target and grasping. She frequently overshoots the target. She uses a pincer grasp to pick up many types of small objects but stabilizes her wrist on the surface for very small objects, such as beads.

In standing, Kayla keeps her weight shifted forward onto the balls of her feet, her lumbar lordosis increased, and her shoulders back. If her weight is shifted onto her full foot and her lordosis is reduced, her lower extremities buckle into flexion and she falls to the floor. When falling forward or to the side from sitting, kneeling, or standing, her protective reactions are good. No protective reactions are seen when she falls backward.

Muscle Performance

Kayla's upper extremity muscular strength is very good. When she stabilizes by stiffly extending or adducting her lower extremities, she can maintain an upright trunk position. Isolated strength of the trunk extensor and flexor muscles is approximately 3/5. Lower extremity hip flexion and quadriceps strength are good (4/5). Hip extension, hip abduction, and knee flexion strength are 2–3/5, whereas distally at the foot, strength in dorsiflexion and plantar flexion are 1–2/5. Functionally, Kayla is able to perform concentric muscle contractions easily, but she has more difficulty with eccentric muscle control. For example, she cannot lower herself slowly from standing back down to sitting.

Neuromotor Development and Sensory Integration

Kayla demonstrates delays in fine motor development, with skills reflective of the 4- to 5-year age level based on the Peabody Developmental Motor Scale (PDMS), Fine Motor subsection (Folio & Fewell, 1983). She has difficulty using scissors with precision, manipulating and controlling a pencil, and manipulating small objects (e.g., coins, small pellets). In the area of gross motor development, Kayla is functioning significantly below her age level because she cannot balance in standing, walk, run, and so on. She has difficulty using her lower extremities reciprocally when she is walking. Based on the PDMS, Gross Motor subsection

(Folio & Fewell, 1983), she is functioning at less than the second percentile compared with age-matched peers. The PDMS was significantly revised and the Peabody Developmental Motor Scale (2nd ed.) (PDMS-2) was published in 2000 (Folio & Fewell, 2000). The newer edition of this standardized test has been normed on a sample reflective of the United States population and stratified to age. Improved scoring criteria better differentiate between possible scores on items; item revision and administration revisions have been made. The PDMS-2 is appropriate for children between birth and 6 years.

Orthotic Devices

Kayla's recent AFOs are hinged with a plantar flexion stop. Before receiving these orthotics, Kayla used a solid ankle AFO. She appears to be able to control the hinged ankle during gait. No knee hyperextension is seen during the stance phase. The orthotics fit well, and Kayla and her family are very good at monitoring skin condition after using the orthotics.

Range of Motion

Hamstring tightness is noted, with a popliteal angle of 15° on the left and 20° on the right. Even though muscle tightness is noted in the hip adductors, hip internal rotators, and plantar flexor muscles, passive ROM is WNL, with the following exceptions. Dorsiflexion is limited to neutral on the right and hip flexion is 5° to 110° bilaterally. Hypermobility is noted in lumbar extension, hip internal rotation, and knee extension.

Reflex Integrity

Muscle tone is increased in the lower extremities, the right greater than the left. The left lower extremity hip adductor, hip internal rotator, quadriceps, and plantarflexor muscle groups were scored at a grade of 2 on the Modified Ashworth Scale (Bohannon & Smith, 1987), indicating motion possible, but resistance noted. The same muscle groups of the right lower extremity were scored at a grade of 1 on the Modified Ashworth Scale, indicating a "catch" of resistance at the initiation of the movement. The Modified Ashworth Scale has been found to be reliable in documenting resistance to passive motion in individuals with a variety of neurological conditions (Gregson et al., 2000; Allison, Abraham, & Petersen, 1996).

Self-Care and Home Management (Including Activities of Daily Living and Instrumental Activities of Daily Living)

Kayla is fairly independent in basic activities of daily living (ADLs) and instrumental activities of daily living (IADLs). She is independent in bathing, toileting, and eating. She needs some assistance with putting on her socks and shoes, but otherwise is independent in dressing. Kayla uses a walker for independent ambulation at school. She is also beginning to use bilateral quad canes for walking short distances in her home. She uses a motorized cart for community mobility. She often "walks" to school with her older brother and safely drives the cart two blocks to and from school. At home, Kayla helps with age-appropriate household chores, such as folding laundry and making her bed. At school, she is able to participate in classroom activities, but her handwriting is slow and requires a lot of concentration. With modified lesson plans and assistance from a classroom aide, Kayla is able to work with her classmates.

When evaluated with the Pediatric Evaluation of Disability Index (PEDI) (Haley, Coster, Ludlow, Haltiwanger, & Andrellos, 1992), Kayla demonstrates age-appropriate skills in social function and independence in all areas of function. Mild difficulty is seen in self-care skills, especially related to precise fine motor control (e.g., buttering bread, parting hair). Significant functional limitations are noted in activities, such as transitioning into or out of sitting without arm support, walking without support, stair climbing, and dynamic balance activities in standing. As a result, her performance in the mobility functional skill domain is well below that in other areas.

EVALUATION, DIAGNOSIS, AND PROGNOSIS (INCLUDING PLAN OF CARE)

In a review of the data collected from the examination, Kayla was found to be an active first grader in her local school program. She successfully uses adaptive equipment to participate in home, school, and community activities. She does present with impaired muscle function (muscle strength, muscle endurance, and muscle tone), motor function (motor control, balance, and coordination), and functional ROM. These impairments contribute to functional limitations in activities, such as ambulation, sitting and standing, posture/control, and fine motor manipulations. Based on her ability to walk with assistive devices and her ability to sit independently, Kayla would be rated at Level III on the GMFCS (Palisano et al., 1997).

Kayla recently underwent bilateral lower extremity orthopedic surgery and subsequent casting for 6 weeks, resulting in increased lower extremity weakness, increased muscle tightness, and decreased endurance. Because of the chronicity of Kayla's condition, she has been followed for physical therapy on a regular basis since she was 1 year old. Services have been provided in school, home, and outpatient settings. She has continued to make functional gains despite her motor limitations. Growth, development, and medical interventions (i.e., selective dorsal rhizotomy, bilateral femoral osteotomies) have affected her ability to function motorically. With periods of growth in height, muscle tightness has increased, affecting her balance and mobility skills. Orthotic needs have become apparent and orthotic modifications have been necessary to accommodate growth. Throughout the course of normal development, she has been encouraged to explore her environment and participate in her community, even though she had gross and fine motor activity restrictions. After surgery, she has participated in intensive physical therapy (at home and at school), both to regain presurgical functional status and to learn to move within the context of altered muscle performance and bony alignment.

Prognosis

It is anticipated that with therapy Kayla will return to presurgical levels of function at home, at school, and in her community. The focus of Kayla's therapy program will be on helping her function as independently as possible in her local school program and at home. As Kayla learns to use less restrictive assistive devices in a more energy-efficient manner, she should be better able to access her school environment. Assistance will still be needed to adapt curriculum and assist with fine manipulative activities. In addition, it is anticipated that Kayla will be able to participate in age-appropriate leisure activities (tricycle/bicycle riding).

Goals

The following goals will be achieved within the current school year (within 8 months), with physical therapy provided twice weekly (30 minutes per session) at school, and 60 minutes per week at home.

- Kayla will use bilateral quad canes to independently walk 20 feet, within her home and classroom environment, in 2/3 trials.

- Kayla will ascend/descend three stairs, using a railing and standby assistance, in 2/3 trials.

- Kayla will independently pedal a tricycle or a bicycle with training wheels for one block in 2/3 trials.

- Kayla will independently put on her socks in 2/3 trials.

INTERVENTION

Coordination, Communication, and Documentation

Frequent communication among Kayla, her family, her physicians, and her therapists is very important. Progress should be communicated to her orthopedic surgeon as she continues to recover from her bilateral femoral osteotomies. In Kayla's case, therapists at both home and school should communicate to coordinate care. The school therapist also needs to communicate with teachers, classroom aides, and other school personnel.

In addition to written physical therapy evaluations and progress notes, therapists will contribute to Kayla's individualized education plan (IEP), daily education plans (e.g., position suggestions) and develop a home program. Collaboration with Kayla and her parents is important to adequately meet their needs with the therapy plan and home program.

Expected outcomes of this comprehensive coordination and communication will include coordination of care between Kayla and her family, school personnel, and physical therapists; collaboration and coordination among school, home, and home-health therapist; and enhanced decision making and case management.

Patient/Client-Related Instruction

Within Kayla's physical therapy management, Kayla and her parents, teachers, classroom aides, and siblings will all benefit from patient/client-related instruction. Instruction strategies must be designed appropriately for each person, focusing on the person's learning style and the activities in which he or she will be assisting Kayla. Instruction strategies for Kayla and her siblings, parents, and classroom staff members may be very different from one another, but all should include an opportunity for the learner to demonstrate what he or she has learned to the therapist.

For caregivers, instructions regarding specific activities, such as putting on AFOs or climbing stairs with a railing, should be presented verbally and reinforced in writing and/or pictures. The therapist should also demonstrate activities and watch the caregiver perform the activity. Feedback can be given to reinforce or revise the caregivers' participation in the activity.

Expected outcomes of this patient/client-related instruction include increased functional independence; improved safety in home, school, and community settings; and improved mobility.

Procedural Interventions

Activities in several direct intervention categories are discussed as follows.

Therapeutic Exercise

The prime focus of Kayla's therapeutic exercise program is on balance and coordination training, lower extremity- and trunk-strengthening activities, and gait training. Balance and coordination activities are done in kneel-standing, sitting on a bench, and standing. Use of these and other functional activities also result in lower extremity and trunk strengthening. As multiple repetitions of activities are completed, muscle endurance is increased. Kayla's family has been encouraged to take her to indoor playgrounds for climbing, pulling, and ambulation activities (Figure 18–1).

When sitting on a bench, Kayla can reach forward but cannot easily reach to the side outside of her base of support. Therapy activities, including having Kayla reach for objects, catch and throw a ball, and throw beanbags at targets in various locations, make therapy sessions fun. When performing these activities, Kayla is challenged to shift her weight and reach just outside her base of support, requiring active trunk control, while the upper extremities are involved in another activity.

Kneel-standing balance activities are included, as well as lower extremity-strengthening exercises, such as lowering to side-sitting and then back up. This activity also improves active control of trunk rotation and ROM (hip internal and external rotation) of the lower extremities. Other functional

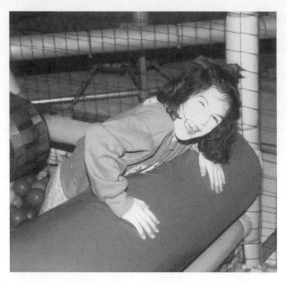

Figure 18-1 Strengthening and coordination emphasized during activities at indoor playground.

activities, such as slowly moving from standing to sitting, are included to improve eccentric muscle control and strengthening.

In the area of gait training, Kayla is learning a 4-point gait with bilateral quad canes. Use of the canes will ultimately allow her greater access at school, at home, and in the community, as she learns to use them on the stairs (which is not possible with the walker). The canes are also less bulky than the walker and will make locomotion around the crowded classroom more effective. The 4-point gait pattern should reinforce more active trunk control during walking and reciprocal upper and lower extremity function.

Functional Training in Self-Care

The areas of focus for Kayla in ADLs and IADLs are lower extremity dressing activities, gait and locomotion training in school and community environments, and age-appropriate play activities (pumping a swing, pedaling a bike). Safety is emphasized as a wide variety of school and community environments are explored.

Taking off shoes, orthotics, and socks is practiced in sitting, both on a bench and on the floor. In bench sitting, Kayla must shift her weight, use both hands in the activity, and actively balance her trunk. This is a challenging activity because of the amount of balance required, and stand-by assistance is needed. For more independent doffing of shoes and socks, Kayla ring-sits on the floor, which requires a lesser amount of trunk control and balance. She is practicing putting on socks in floor sitting and also in supine. These positions require less balance and allow her to practice precision in bimanual activities (placing sock correctly on her foot) while increasing functional ROM in hip flexion and external rotation.

Both pumping a swing and pedaling a tricycle or bicycle are difficult for Kayla because she must activate lower extremity muscles in a different way from the one she usually uses. In tricycle or bicycle riding, her feet frequently push into plantarflexion and off the pedal. When her feet are secured onto the pedals, she actively uses lower-extremity muscles to pedal herself. Kayla has been using a tricycle, but it is becoming too small for her. She is now trying a bicycle with wide-base training wheels. It is hoped that these wheels will provide a more stable base as she turns corners (Figure 18–2).

Manual Therapy/Range of Motion

Therapy sessions are initiated with activities designed to increase soft tissue mobility and ROM of the lower extremities. Not only does this provide increased circulation to the tissues that will be used in functional activities, but also it

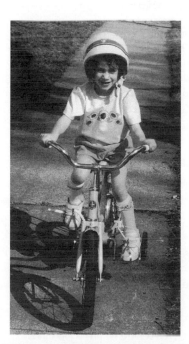

Figure 18-2 Age-appropriate recreational activity (bike riding) contributes to lower extremity strengthening and balance training.

is hoped that increased mobility will improve Kayla's motor control and function. Active and passive ROM activities are included, emphasizing slow, prolonged stretch. Avoiding quick stretch activities will minimize activating the stretch reflex and eliciting spasticity.

Electrotherapy

Even though Kayla is only 6 years old, biofeedback is being used to help her isolate muscle activation in the lower extremities and volitionally relax muscles. Both auditory and visual feedback from the biofeedback unit let Kayla experience actively contracting or relaxing a muscle. Surface electrodes are placed on muscles that initiate knee flexion, knee extension, plantar flexion, and dorsiflexion, and Kayla is asked to focus on which muscles she should make work to complete a motion, as well as which muscles must be quiet during the motion.

Summary of Procedural Interventions

Expected outcomes of procedural interventions include decreased risk of secondary impairments, increased safety, development and improvement of functional motor skills, and independence in these activities. Impaired strength, ROM, and balance should also be improved. Kayla will be able to assume her self-care, home, school, and community roles.

TERMINATION OF EPISODE OF CARE

This episode of care will be terminated when Kayla has achieved the stated goals. Within her school-based setting, it is anticipated that the goals would be achieved during the current school year. If the goals are achieved sooner, the episode of care will be terminated and a new episode of care initiated if new goals are identified.

For children with CP, it is anticipated that they may "require multiple episodes of care over the life span to ensure safety and effective adaptation following changes in physical status, caregivers, environment, or task demands" (APTA, 2001, p. 345). For Kayla, it is anticipated that as musculoskeletal growth occurs; classroom tasks change throughout her elementary school career; teachers and caregivers change; additional medical or surgical issues arise; or level of impairment, functional limitation, or activity restrictions change, additional episodes of physical therapy care will be indicated.

Episodes of physical therapy maintenance (APTA, 2001),

which include a series of occasional clinical, educational, or administrative services necessary to maintain the child's level of function, may be required to monitor fit, repair, and determine the appropriateness of adaptive equipment and orthotics.

Episodes of physical therapy prevention (APTA, 2001) may also be useful to focus on primary and secondary prevention and health promotion. Secondary impairments of ROM, muscle strength/endurance, integumentary integrity, and aerobic conditioning often occur as skeletal growth continues. Not only does increased bone length frequently cause increased muscle tightness, but also increases in extremity and trunk length may biomechanically challenge the child. Larger amounts of weight must be moved or balanced over longer lever arms.

EXAMINATION: AGE 13 YEARS

History

Kayla is now 13 years old and continues to live at home with her parents and three siblings (aged 14 to 18 years). She has been enrolled at her local elementary school in inclusive classroom settings from first through sixth grade. Kayla actively participated in Girl Scouts until she was in the fifth grade and has participated in various clubs at school. This is her first year at the junior high school, where she is a seventh grader. Some adaptations have been made to the curriculum every year to accommodate Kayla's needs, and she has participated in an adaptive physical education class.

Kayla has been relatively healthy over the past 6 years. She has developed some allergies to dust and mold, which have resulted in seasonal sinus infections. At age 10 years, she had increased respiratory difficulty with her allergies and was diagnosed with asthma. In addition to regular allergy medication, Kayla will use breathing treatments when her asthma is triggered. Last year she also underwent a right tibial derotational osteotomy. Respiratory issues and growth have resulted in Kayla adopting a less physically active lifestyle. As she has gotten more homework, she also has less time to actively ride her bike or exercise after school, contributing to a more sedentary lifestyle. She has continued to receive physical and occupational therapy as part of her school program. She has also participated in adapted swimming, aerobic exercise, and karate programs offered in her community. This year she is enrolled to participate in a peer group at a local outpatient center for individuals with disabilities, where she will have a chance to socialize and talk with other teen-age girls with physical disabilities.

Kayla's goals are to transition successfully to junior high school, where she will have to change classrooms every period and carry her books. She is also hoping that she will be able to walk without her AFOs and transition to a less noticeable orthotic. Kayla's parents are concerned about her level of fitness and increased weight gain over the past year. They have noticed that it is harder for her to walk long distances at the shopping mall.

Systems Review

Cardiovascular and Pulmonary

Kayla's heart rate and blood pressure are WNL for her age. Her resting respiratory rate is 25 breaths per minute, but this increases to 32 breaths per minute with moderate amounts of activity (e.g., walking between rooms at school) and Kayla reports that she gets "short of breath" easily. Further examination of aerobic conditioning is indicated, especially with her history of asthma.

Integumentary

Kayla does not demonstrate any areas of redness or skin breakdown under her AFOs.

Musculoskeletal

Kayla's height is within the 30th percentile and her weight is in the 60th percentile for her age. Hip flexion and knee flexion contractures are noted. Kayla also presents with a thoracic kyphosis and increased lumbar lordosis. Muscle strength and endurance of the lower extremities are decreased. More detailed examination of ROM and muscle strength is indicated.

Neuromuscular

Kayla continues to demonstrate impaired motor control with hypertonicity and increased muscle stiffness of the lower extremities. She can balance in standing position for short periods of time (2 to 3 minutes), which is helpful during ADLs, and can walk independently with bilateral forearm crutches. Further examination of motor function and motor control is indicated.

Communication, Affect, Cognition, Language, and Learning Style

Kayla's communication skills are good. She has mild cognitive delays and continues to demonstrate some problems with visual perception. She learns best by demonstration and feedback during task performance.

Tests and Measures

Aerobic Capacity and Endurance

Kayla becomes fatigued and short of breath after walking short distances. Lower-extremity muscle weakness appears to contribute to this problem. After walking for 2 minutes, her heart rate increases to 168 beats per minute, returning to a resting heart rate of 110 beats per minute within 1 minute of rest.

Assistive and Adaptive Devices

Kayla uses forearm crutches when walking in her home and classroom settings (Figure 18–3). She will also use a walker for long distances to increase her speed and decrease her fatigue. For community locomotion, Kayla uses a motorized cart (Figure 18–4). At this time, all adaptive equipment fits well and is in good repair.

Gait, Locomotion, and Balance

Kayla walks with bilateral forearm crutches, using a 4-point gait pattern, within her home and classroom settings. As she

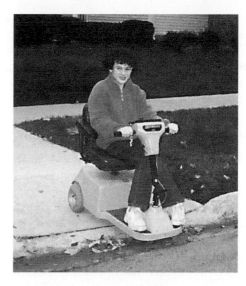

Figure 18-4 Motorized cart provides a mode of age-appropriate community mobility.

becomes fatigued, she begins dragging her right toe and occasionally trips. She safely uses a walker for longer distances but tends to use a swing-to gait pattern and support herself primarily on her upper extremities if she is in a hurry. Kayla safely drives her motorized cart within her community, using curb cuts. Occasionally she will drive off the sidewalk. She usually quickly corrects herself and can get the cart back on the sidewalk, but occasionally her wheel gets stuck in the grass or dirt and she needs assistance.

Kayla can balance in static standing position for 2 to 3 minutes. When participating in dynamic standing activities, she often places her hand on a surface for support or leans against a stable object. This is sufficient for her to participate in ADLs, such as combing her hair and securing fasteners after toileting. She can also independently transition from sitting to standing and back to sitting, using her hands for support. The Berg Balance Test (Berg, Wood-Dauphinée, Williams, & Gayton, 1989), although originally designed as a measure of balance in elderly individuals, has been suggested as a measure of functional balance in children with CP (Kembhavi, Darrah, Magill-Evans, & Loomi, 2002). Kayla's score on the Berg Balance Test was 29 of a possible 56 points.

Motor Function (Motor Control and Motor Learning)

In addition to walking with assistive devices as described above, Kayla moves efficiently through her home by either

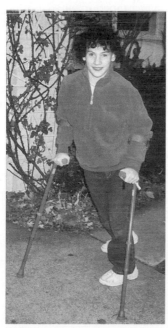

Figure 18-3 Walking with bilateral forearm crutches is functional for short distances.

creeping or cruising holding onto furniture or walls. She can ascend and descend stairs using a railing.

Mild intention tremor persists during activities such as buttoning or putting toothpaste on her toothbrush.

Muscle Performance

Pelvic and lower extremity weakness persists, especially distally (Table 18.1). Manual muscle testing has been chosen as an examination method because no special equipment is needed and it is a well-recognized method of muscle strength examination used by a variety of healthcare providers. Recent literature has suggested that myometry, using a hand-held dynamometer, is more reliable and valid for quantifying the muscle strength of children with a variety of conditions (Sloan, 2002; Stuberg & Metcalf, 1988). Because Kayla's body mass and height have increased, it is more difficult for her to fully extend her lower extremities against gravity and support her body weight. Muscle endurance also is decreased.

Orthotic Devices

Kayla uses bilateral, hinged AFOs with a dorsiflexion stop at 5° and a plantar flexion stop at neutral. The orthotics fit well and appear to be appropriate for her current needs.

Range of Motion

Kayla presents with hip and knee flexion contractures bilaterally; external rotation is also limited. Goniometric measurements are listed in Table 18.2. The reliability of goniometric measurements has been questioned in the literature. It has been suggested that goniometry is most reliable when completed by the same tester in subsequent tests. In this case, because measurements even on repeated tests can vary by several degrees, it is suggested that use of the average score from two consecutive measurements improves reliability (Stuberg, Fuchs, & Miedaner, 1988; Watkins, Darrah, & Pain, 1995).

Reflex Integrity

In standing position and when stabilizing herself during sitting, Kayla demonstrates increased hip adduction and internal rotation. Muscle tone is increased in the bilateral lower extremities, the right greater than the left. During passive abduction and external rotation motion, the left leg has a score of 1 on the Ashworth Scale and the right leg a score of 2. These scores are very similar to the scores recorded when Kayla was 6 years old.

Self-Care and Home Management

Kayla is independent in dressing, bathing, toileting, transferring, and locomotion (using assistive devices). She has difficulty walking and carrying objects, which will be a difficulty in junior high school. She also has difficulty pouring beverages from a container while sitting.

Although she is older than recommended for the PEDI, her level of functional independence was measured using the scaled score for this test. Her skill level still falls within the parameters of the test, and use of the tool allows comparison with earlier performance. Scaled scores in functional skills, self-care, and social function domains have improved from Kayla's performance at 6 years of age. Kayla has achieved all items on the PEDI in these areas. In the area of the functional skills mobility domain, her scaled score has improved from 68.7 at 6 years of age to 75.2 at this time, continuing to reflect difficulty in walking or transferring without hand support, as well as ascending or descending stairs.

Table 18.1 Lower Extremity Muscle Strength as Measured by Manual Muscle Test

Muscle Group	Right	Left
Hip abduction	2/5	2/5
Hip extension	2/5	3/5
Knee extension	3/5	3/5
Knee flexion	3/5	4/5
Dorsiflexion	1/5	2/5

Table 18.2 Lower Extremity Range of Motion

Motion	Right	Left
Hip flexion	15°–120°	10°–120°
Hip external rotation	0°–15°	0°–30°
Knee flexion	5°–120°	5°–120°
Dorsiflexion	0°	0°–3°

Work, Community, and Leisure Integration

Kayla functions well in school and community settings. She is able to participate in karate classes, school clubs, swimming, and so on. She also continues to ride an adult-size three-wheel bike, which provides more stability than her two-wheel bike. This is important because her height and weight have increased, and leisure time physical activity should be a regular part of her day.

EVALUATION, DIAGNOSIS, AND PROGNOSIS (INCLUDING PLAN OF CARE)

Although Kayla functions independently in her home, school, and community settings, she presents with activity and participation restrictions. These restrictions are related to functional limitations in standing balance, walking, and fine motor function. She is able to walk only by holding on to furniture and walls or with an assistive device (bilateral forearm crutches or wheeled walker). The energy cost of balance and ambulation is high. Movement patterns are inefficient, and she requires more time than is typical to complete activities. Her most efficient means of community mobility is with a motorized cart, but she cannot use this in all weather conditions (e.g., snow and ice) or in nonaccessible environments.

Kayla presents with impaired aerobic capacity, muscle performance (strength and endurance), motor function (motor control), and ROM, which interfere with her ability to efficiently complete ADLs.

Prognosis

Kayla is expected to function in the junior high school setting as independently as possible. Improved muscle strength, ROM, and endurance will assist in accomplishing tasks more efficiently, and Kayla will actively participate in her educational experience.

Goals

The following goals will be achieved within the current school year (within 8 months), with physical therapy services provided once weekly (30 minutes per session) at school.

- Kayla will independently open her locker and store or retrieve items from a standing position in 90% of trials.
- Kayla will move between classrooms within the 5-minute changing period, 6 periods per school day.

INTERVENTION

Coordination, Communication, and Documentation

Services between home, school, and community settings should be coordinated. Regular communication must occur with Kayla, school personnel, Kayla's parents, and her physician. As Kayla enters the junior high school setting, coordination and communication with previous elementary school therapy and classroom staff should take place. Personnel at the high school should also be aware of Kayla's programming needs in anticipation of her enrollment 2 years from now.

In addition to written physical therapy evaluation and progress notes, therapists will also contribute to Kayla's IEP and daily education plan and develop a home program with Kayla. Kayla's parents remain an important part of the team; however, at this time Kayla will begin playing a more prominent role and should be encouraged to assume some of the responsibility for her therapy program.

Expected outcomes of this comprehensive coordination and communication will include increased effectiveness of case conferences, coordination of services, development of Kayla's IEP, and effective transition between the elementary and junior high schools.

Patient/Client-Related Instruction

With Kayla's transfer to a new school setting, personnel at the junior high school who will be interacting with Kayla should be instructed in how to assist Kayla in functional mobility within the school setting, positioning requirements (e.g., type and size of classroom chair), and any other elements of her program in which they may be involved.

Kayla and her parents should be well informed in regard to functional expectations and safety in the junior high school setting and any expected developmental changes as Kayla progresses through puberty (impact of growth spurts, importance of continued weight-bearing activities to promote bone growth). Kayla should take a more active role in developing her goals, objectives, and functional mobility program. Increased emphasis on fitness and maintaining an active lifestyle should be included.

Expected outcomes of patient/client-related instruction will include reduced risk of secondary impairments; increased functional independence in home, school, and community settings; and improved safety for Kayla and her caregivers.

Procedural Interventions

Therapeutic Exercise

The prime focus of Kayla's therapeutic exercise program at this time is on improving muscle performance, aerobic capacity/endurance, and ROM. As increasing height and body weight have negatively affected Kayla's ability to efficiently perform ADLs and ambulation, it is important for her to maximize her muscle strength and endurance. Although muscle weakness does limit her activities at this time, her more sedentary lifestyle may also negatively affect aerobic capacity.

Muscle-strengthening activities include weight training with light weights and multiple repetitions. Resistive exercise has been demonstrated to be beneficial and appropriate for children with CP, especially when maximal resistance or overloading of the muscle is avoided (Damiano, Dodd, & Taylor, 2002). At Kayla's age, she is motivated by tracking her progress as she performs more repetitions and uses more weight. The main muscle groups targeted in the weight training program are hip extensors, hip abductors, hip flexors, knee extensors, and knee flexors. Active ROM is used to strengthen musculature at the ankle. Kayla is encouraged to perform both concentric and eccentric muscle contraction. Strengthening programs have been found to contribute to positive outcomes for children with CP. Some of the functional changes seen have been increased gait speed, improved walking/running/jumping skills, and improved endurance (Damiano & Abel, 1998).

Kayla's adaptive physical education program is focused on encouraging development of lifelong physical activity. Presently Kayla is participating in a walking program, with her crutches or walker. With the crutches, she works harder at actively using lower extremity musculature and this reinforces the weight training program. With the walker, Kayla is able to walk longer distances at a faster pace, fostering aerobic conditioning.

Active and passive ROM activities are included at the beginning of each therapy and exercise session to improve alignment during functional mobility and "warm up" the muscle before beginning to exercise it.

Biofeedback

Biofeedback is used to help Kayla actively contract ankle plantar and dorsiflexor muscle groups. Both auditory and visual feedback reinforce correct muscle group contraction.

Functional Training in Work, Community, and Leisure Integration

Kayla will be encouraged to continue in leisure activities, such as swimming, riding her bike, and walking. These activities can be carried on throughout the life span and will encourage a physically active lifestyle.

Summary of Procedural Interventions

Expected outcomes of these procedural interventions are improved muscle strength and endurance; improved ROM; improved balance; increased functional independence in self-care, home, school, and community activities; increased safety during activity; and prevention of secondary impairments. More specifically, improved muscle performance and motor control will help Kayla meet her goals to access her locker and change classes with her peers. Kayla's aerobic capacity should also be improved, and she will assume a role in maintaining a physically active lifestyle.

TERMINATION OF EPISODE OF CARE

The present episode of care will be terminated when Kayla meets the goals/objectives listed previously. If her status changes (e.g., health issues, task demands), the episode of care may be modified. A new episode of care may be initiated as new goals/objectives are written. It is anticipated that additional episodes of physical therapy care will be required until skeletal maturity is reached, when she must transition into the high school setting, and in preparation for work. It is also anticipated that secondary impairments (muscle weakness, ROM limitations, and decreased aerobic capacity) may negatively affect her ability to function optimally and independently in her community.

Kayla will benefit from therapy until she can function efficiently and independently in home, school, and community settings. She is entitled to physical therapy services within her educational program until she is 21 years of age, as long as she has difficulty meeting her educational objectives because of a movement dysfunction. After the age of 21 years, future episodes of physical therapy care, physical therapy maintenance, and physical therapy prevention are likely to be required. Individuals with CP may need multiple episodes of care over their lifetime to ensure safe and optimal functioning as they assume new roles and responsibilities, as caregiver changes occur, and as they function in new environments. Frequently an episode of physical therapy maintenance, consisting of occasional visits to maintain function, is appropriate. Episodes of physical therapy prevention also contribute to improved fitness, wellness, and function. These occasional services may include education regarding prevention of secondary impairments, revision of a fitness program, and monitoring condition and appropriateness of assistive devices and orthotics.

DISCUSSION QUESTIONS

1. Identify potential secondary impairments of body function and structure that Kayla may develop at 6 years and 12 years of age. What possible prevention strategies should be integrated into her therapy program to minimize development of these impairments?

2. Hypothesize potential areas of secondary impairment of body function and structure, and limitations in activities and participation, at 21 years of age and 40 years of age. What aspects of prevention could have been emphasized throughout childhood to minimize these impairments and restrictions in adulthood?

3. What impairments in body functions and structures contribute to Kayla's difficulty with sitting and standing balance?

4. Identify intervention strategies for each impairment that would contribute to improved sitting and standing balance.

REFERENCES

Allison, S.C., Abraham, L.D., & Petersen, C.L. (1996). Reliability of the Modified Ashworth Scale in the assessment of plantar flexor muscle spasticity in patients with traumatic brain injury. *International Journal of Rehabilitation Research, 19*(1), 67–78.

American Physical Therapy Association (APTA) (2001). Guide to physical therapist practice (2nd ed.). *Physical Therapy, 81*, 9–744

Berg, K., Wood-Dauphinée, S.L., Williams, J., & Gayton, D. (1989). Measuring balance in the elderly: Preliminary development of an instrument. *Physiotherapy Canada, 41*, 304–311.

Bohannon, R., & Smith, M. (1987). Interrater reliability of a Modified Ashworth Scale of muscle spasticity. *Physical Therapy, 67*, 206–207.

Cech, D., & Martin, S. (2002). *Functional movement development across the life span.* Philadelphia: W.B. Saunders.

Damiano, D.L., & Abel, M.F. (1998). Functional outcomes of strength training in spastic cerebral palsy. *Archives of Physical Medicine and Rehabilitation, 79*, 119–125.

Damiano, D.L., Dodd, K., & Taylor, N.F. (2002). Should we be testing and training muscle strength in cerebral palsy? *Developmental Medicine and Child Neurology, 44*, 68–72.

Folio, M.R., & Fewell, R.R. (1983). *Peabody Developmental Motor Scales.* Austin, TX: DLM Teaching Resources.

Folio, M.R., & Fewell, R.R. (2000). *Peabody Developmental Motor Scales* (2nd ed.). Austin, TX: Pro-Ed.

Gregson, J.M., Leathley, M.J., Moore, A.P., Smith, T.L., Sharma, A.K., & Watkins, C.L. (2000). Reliability of measurements of muscle tone and muscle power in stroke patients. *Age and Ageing, 29*(3), 223–228.

Haley, S.M., Coster, W.J., Ludlow, L.H., Haltiwanger, J.T., & Andrellos, P.J. (1992). *Pediatric Evaluation of Disability Inventory (PEDI).* Boston: New England Medical Center Hospitals, Inc.

Kembhavi, G., Darrah, J., Magill-Evans, J., & Loomi, J. (2002). Using the Berg Balance Scale to distinguish balance abilities in children with cerebral palsy. *Pediatric Physical Therapy, 14*, 92–99.

Palisano, R., Rosenbaum, P., Walter, S., Russell, D., Wood, E., & Galuppi, B. (1997). Development and reliability of a system to classify gross motor function in children with cerebral palsy. *Developmental Medicine and Child Neurology, 39*, 214–223.

Sloan, C. (2002). Review of the reliability and validity of myometry with children. *Physical and Occupational Therapy in Pediatrics, 22*(2), 79–93.

Stuberg, W.A., & Metcalf, W.K. (1988). Reliability of quantitative muscle testing in healthy children using a hand-held dynamometer. *Physical Therapy, 68*(6), 977–982.

Stuberg, W.A., Fuchs, R.H., & Miedaner, J.A. (1988). Reliability of goniometric measurements of children with cerebral palsy. *Developmental Medicine and Child Neurology, 30*, 657–666.

Watkins, B., Darrah, J., & Pain, K. (1995). Reliability of passive ankle dorsiflexion measurements in children: Comparison of universal and biplane goniometers. *Pediatric Physical Therapy, 7*, 3–8.

Chapter *19*

Case Study: Cystic Fibrosis

— Heather Lever Brossman, DPT, MS, CCS
— Coleen Schrepfer, PT, MS

This case study focuses on the physical therapy management of Jerry, who has cystic fibrosis (CF), at three different ages: 2 months (initial diagnosis), 8 years, and 16 years. For children with a diagnosis of CF, repeated episodes of physical therapy services may be necessary across the life span. Progression of the disease process and increasing independence of the child in his or her physical therapy management indicate a need for repeated episodes of care.

Children with CF generally present with impaired airway clearance, viscous mucus deposition along mucosal linings, recurrent respiratory infections, progressive lung tissue damage, increased work of breathing, postural deformations related to chronic increased work of breathing, decreased cardiorespiratory and muscular endurance, malnutrition, and failure to thrive. The CF gene transcribes an abnormal transmembrane protein, the CF transmembrane regulator (CFTR), which lines the gastrointestinal, respiratory, and reproductive tracts. The CFTR protein blocks chloride ion passage across the cell membrane and disrupts the diffusion of water. Ultimately, viscous mucus accumulates along the tract linings, trapping bacteria and white blood cells. CF is a chronic disorder that requires daily medication and airway clearance techniques for the lifetime of the individual. The most appropriate airway clearance technique is determined by many factors, including the child's age, caregiver involvement, lifestyle, and the manifestation of the disease process determined by chest radiograph, pulmonary function tests, and physical examination. To better delineate the variability of care in children with CF, Jerry's physical therapy examination and intervention during three different acute care hospital admissions are presented in this case study.

Based on the American Physical Therapy Association's *Guide to physical therapist practice* (APTA, 2001), the impairments presented by Jerry throughout his childhood may be best addressed by the physical therapy management described in the Preferred Practice Patterns 6C: Impaired Ventilation, Respiration/Gas Exchange, and Aerobic Capacity/Endurance Associated with Airway Clearance Dysfunction; 6E: Impaired Ventilation and Respiration/Gas Exchange Associated with Ventilatory Pump Dysfunction or Failure; and 6F: Impaired Ventilation and Respiration/Gas Exchange Associated with Respiratory Failure. The practice pattern 6C best represents Jerry's limitations in body structure and function at the ages of 2 months and 8 years. The practice patterns 6E and 6F best address Jerry's limitations at 16 years of age.

EXAMINATION: AGE 2 MONTHS

History

Jerry was referred to the hospital at 2 months of age for work-up related to poor weight gain and reflux since birth. Although he was initially diagnosed with failure to thrive, a positive sweat test ultimately confirmed the diagnosis of

CF. Jerry and his family were immediately referred to physical therapy for family instruction in airway clearance techniques.

General Demographics

Jerry is a 2-month-old white male infant. The family is of Northern European descent and speaks English. Jerry lives with his mother, father, and 8-year-old half-sister. Both parents smoke in the home. Pedigree analysis reveals no family history of CF.

Growth and Development

Jerry was born at full term, with a normal spontaneous vaginal delivery. He weighed 8 pounds ³/₄ ounce at birth. Iron deficiency anemia complicated the pregnancy. He went home on day 2 of life, at which time he experienced emesis after feeding. No weight gain was noted despite various trials on infant formulas, including Enfamil (cow's milk based), Isomil (soy based), and Nutramigen (elemental formula that is more easily absorbed). At 3 weeks of age, he weighed 7 pounds 14 ounces. At 8 weeks of age, he weighed 9 pounds, an increase of only 15.25 ounces since birth, despite a large, voracious appetite. He was also noted to have yellow, greasy stools. A sweat test revealed a sodium level of +150 mg (normal is less than 60 mg), and he was diagnosed with CF.

Medications and Diet

Jerry's medications include Coenzyme-S, Poly-Vi-Sol (a liquid multivitamin), vitamin E, and vitamin K. Both vitamins E and K are fat-soluble vitamins. He is currently fed Similac with iron, a cow's milk-based formula.

Other Tests and Measures

Jerry's chest radiograph displays hyperinflation with mild lower airway disease. Pulmonary markings are slightly prominent. Bowel gas pattern appears normal. His laboratory values are provided in Table 19.1.

Systems Review

A systems review of Jerry's integumentary, neuromotor, and sensory (vision and hearing) systems did not indicate any difficulties. Jerry's gross motor development appears to be age appropriate.

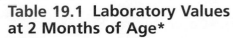

Table 19.1 Laboratory Values at 2 Months of Age*

Laboratory Value	Jerry's Values	Normal Values for Age
Hemoglobin	**8.5 g/dL**	10–13 g/dL
Hematocrit	**25%**	30–40%
White blood cell count	9,500 cells/μL	3,000–10,000 cells/McLl
Sodium	139 mEq/L	135–144 mEq/L
Potassium	5.1 mEq/L	3.6–5.2 mEq/L
Chloride	105 mEq/L	97–106 mEq/L
Bicarbonate	**17 mEq/L**	24–34 mEq/L
Blood urea nitrogen	15 mg/dL	5–18 mg/dL
Creatinine	**0.6 mg/dL**	<0.5 mg/dL
Glucose	**101 mg/dL**	60–100 mg/dL
Prothrombin time	12.1 seconds	11–13 seconds
Partial prothrombin time	25.3 seconds	20–30 seconds

Source: Normal values obtained from Children's Liver Association for Support Services (July 14, 2004).

*Bold indicates abnormal value.

Cardiovascular and Pulmonary

Jerry's cardiovascular and pulmonary systems appear to be functioning within normal limits (WNL) (see Chapter 8, Figure 8–8) at this time, with a pulse of 138 beats per minute (bpm), blood pressure (BP) of 88/63 mm Hg, oxygen saturation (SaO_2) at 95% on room air at rest, and respiratory rate (RR) of 30 breaths per minute. Heart rate (HR) and rhythm are regular and without murmur.

Musculoskeletal

Jerry's length is 57.5 cm (50th percentile of age) and weight is 3.99 kg (10th percentile for age). Head circumference is 37.5 cm (20th percentile for age).

Tests and Measures

Aerobic Capacity and Endurance

Diaphragmatic breathing pattern is notable at all times, which is considered normal. At times his feedings with a bottle take longer than would be expected. He takes long breaks to breathe during bottle feedings. A small increase in HR and mild nasal flaring are seen during sucking, but there is no drop in SaO$_2$. He was evaluated by the speech therapist, who found his ability to bottle feed to be WNL.

Muscle Performance

At this age, muscle performance is evaluated through observation of the infant's movements to determine if the muscles are strong enough to move a joint through its entire range of motion (ROM). Weakness is defined as inability to move the joint through its entire ROM. Jerry moves strongly against gravity, but he appears to be less vigorous than would be expected for a baby his age. This seems to imply age-appropriate muscle strength, but perhaps endurance limits his performance.

Neuromotor Development

Jerry is able to lift and turn his head easily when he is lying in a prone position. In the prone position, he can also lift and hold his head up momentarily to look at a toy. He holds his head in midline when held at the shoulder and will also hold a small rattle placed in his hand. These skills reflect age-appropriate performance on the Peabody Developmental Motor Scales (Folio & Fewell, 2000).

Range of Motion

Jerry's active range of motion (AROM) and passive range of motion (PROM) are WNL for his age.

Ventilation and Respiration/ Gas Exchange

Breath sounds are equal and clear, with no rhonchi, rales, or wheezes. No chest wall retractions or nasal flaring are notable. Jerry is pale, but no mottling or cyanosis is observable. No head bobbing was seen on inspiration or when sucking from his bottle, reflecting that he did not need to use accessory respiratory muscles.

EVALUATION, DIAGNOSIS, AND PROGNOSIS (INCLUDING PLAN OF CARE)

Jerry presents with malabsorption and poor weight gain. Because of his diagnosis of CF, impaired airway clearance and inefficient gas exchange are anticipated. During this episode of care, it is anticipated that his family will become proficient with techniques to maximize airway clearance and gas exchange, thereby enhancing his ability to function within his environment. Jerry will demonstrate optimal ventilation to support developmental skill acquisition and weight gain.

Goals

The following goals, related to Jerry's parents, will be achieved during his hospitalization:

1. Jerry's parents will verbalize understanding of the disease process and verbalize the necessity for daily use of regular airway clearance techniques for prevention of secondary complications.

2. Jerry's parents will independently and appropriately perform non-Trendelenburg postural drainage, percussion, and vibration on all lobes of Jerry's lungs for 1.5 minutes per segment.

3. Jerry's parents will verbally commit to eliminating his exposure to second-hand smoke and identify a location outside of the home for their smoking.

INTERVENTION

Coordination, Communication, and Documentation

Coordination, communication, and documentation of physical therapy management will be directed toward the family and cystic fibrosis clinic personnel. With appropriate communication, coordination of care will be enhanced, risk reduction will be improved, and the family will understand the goals and objectives of the physical therapy management protocol. The family verbalizes knowledge about the hospital's outpatient cystic fibrosis clinic and the medical team members to contact for future needs related to CF.

Patient/Client-Related Instruction

At this time, it is of the utmost importance that the caregivers demonstrate independence with postural drainage, percussion, and vibration (PDPV). The family is given materials with both written descriptions and illustrations delineating the appropriate postural drainage positions and areas for percussion (see Chapter 8). PDPV is to be performed at home two times daily, either before meals or an hour and a half after meals, and increased to three times daily when Jerry is experiencing a pulmonary exacerbation. Secondary to Jerry's history of reflux, the Trendelenburg position is contraindicated. The importance of encouraging play activities after an airway clearance session, to promote further expectoration of mucus in the larger airways, is also discussed. The parents demonstrate independence with the airway clearance techniques and demonstrate a clear understanding of the disease progression and preventive strategies to minimize future complications. The parents verbalize the importance of preventing their son's exposure to second-hand smoke and verbally commit to smoke outside the home only.

Procedural Interventions

As anticipated, postural abnormalities are not observed because Jerry has negligible lung pathology at this time; therefore no specific intervention is indicated. Jerry is also developing appropriately for his age and therefore is not provided with a developmental intervention program, nor is he referred to community-based early intervention services.

Airway Clearance Techniques

Postural drainage with percussion and vibration (PDPV) is performed two times daily, incorporating five alternative positions for each session, without implementation of the Trendelenburg position secondary to reflux. The anticipated outcomes of this intervention are improved airway clearance, prevention of accumulation of mucus, and maximized ventilation/respiration.

TERMINATION OF EPISODE OF CARE

The family achieved all goals during Jerry's first hospitalization, and he was discharged from physical therapy with a daily home program. The parents demonstrated knowledge of the outpatient cystic fibrosis clinic and the medical team members to contact for future needs related to CF. A physical therapist will follow Jerry through the outpatient clinic, which will provide continual family support and will continually screen Jerry's motor development. When Jerry reaches 12 months of age, the physical therapist will progress PDPV instruction to include all 12 positions secondary to his increased chest wall surface area. Factors that would indicate a need for a new episode of physical therapy care include pulmonary exacerbation, delayed acquisition of developmental milestones, and the need to oversee education of additional family members for PDPV.

EXAMINATION: AGE 8 YEARS

Jerry is followed quarterly in the cystic fibrosis clinic. He has had no hospitalizations from the time of his initial diagnosis at 2 months of age until 8 years of age. At this time he presents to clinic with a 1-week history of persistent cough, increased work of breathing, and weight loss. Inpatient physical therapy is consulted secondary to the child's impaired endurance directly related to his first acute pulmonary exacerbation.

History

General Demographics

Jerry is 8 years old and currently in second grade. He lives with his mother, father, and half-sister. Both parents continue to smoke in the home.

Medical/Surgical History

Jerry was diagnosed with asthma at 7 years of age through the outpatient cystic fibrosis clinic.

History of Current Condition

Jerry experienced a recent bout of varicella (chickenpox). Since this exposure, he has had a worsening cough, associated post-tussive emesis, increased volume and thickness of secretions, as well as decreased exercise tolerance. Over the past year, his pulmonary function tests have declined. On admission, he is found to test positive for colonized mucoid and nonmucoid *Pseudomonas aeruginosa* and coagulase-positive *Staphylococcus* bacteria.

Functional Status and Activity Level

Jerry reports independence in all functional activities. He regularly participates in sports activities during gym class, after-school play with friends, and league ice hockey throughout the year. Jerry reports daily physical exercise, which is corroborated by his parents. He reports the ability to keep up with his friends' activity level without compromise.

Medications

Jerry takes several medications on a regular basis to improve absorption of lipids and improve ventilation. Pancrease is a pancreatic enzyme replacement supplement, which helps the child with CF better digest and absorb fats, proteins, and carbohydrates. Mucomyst helps to thin pulmonary secretions to make airway clearance easier. Albuterol (Ventolin) is a bronchodilator that decreases airway resistance. Intal is an antiasthmatic medication that can help prevent bronchospasm. Jerry also regularly takes vitamin E and multivitamin supplements.

During Jerry's hospital admission, antibiotics (tobramycin, oxacillin, and ticarcillin) were prescribed.

Other Tests and Measures

Pulmonary function test results (Table 19.2) reflected small airway involvement with a mildly reduced forced expiratory volume in 1 second (FEV_1), $FEF_{25-75\%}$, and FEV_1/forced vital capacity (FVC). A chest radiograph, taken on admission, displays moderate hyperinflation, increased anterior posterior thoracic diameter, and moderate peribronchial thickening in the central portions of the lungs. No focal atelectasis, infiltrate, or effusion is noted. The soft tissue shadow of the liver is not enlarged. Five days later, a chest radiograph displays mildly hyperinflated lungs with peribronchial thickening. No focal parenchymal infiltrate, pleural effusion, or pneumothorax is noted. No other cystic changes are observed. The radiographs in Figure 19–1 display common findings in children with CF.

Systems Review

Systems review of the integumentary and neuromuscular systems was WNL.

Cardiovascular and Pulmonary

Cardiovascular and pulmonary system functions are an area of concern because Jerry has elevated resting vital signs of HR, 92 bpm; BP, 130/80 mm Hg; and RR, 24 breaths per minute. See Chapter 8, Table 8.8, for a review of normally expected vital sign values in children. HR and rhythm are regular and without murmur. Minimal lateral intercostal and suprasternal retractions are observed at rest. Mild clubbing of the digits is observed, but no cyanosis is noted. Pulses are normal throughout.

Musculoskeletal

Jerry's height is 49 inches (124 cm), falling within the 25th percentile for his age. His weight is 50 pounds (23 kg), falling within the 25th percentile for his age.

Table 19.2 Pulmonary Function Tests*

Age	FEV_1	$FEF_{25-75\%}$	FVC	FEV_1/FVC	PO_2
Admission: 8 years	71	68	110	67	96%
Discharge: 8 years	86	72	117	70	100%
Admission: 16 years	83	49	71	86	95%
Discharge: 16 years	92	54	97	89	98%

*Values are reported as percentage of expected value. Expected values are greater than or equal to 80 for FEV_1, $FEF_{25-75\%}$, FVC, and FEV_1/FVC.

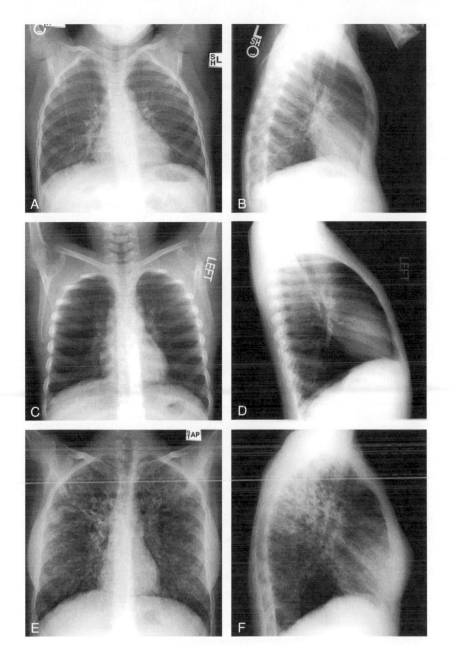

Figure 19-1 Radiographs of lungs of children having cystic fibrosis at different ages. *(A)* Anterior posterior and *(B)* medial lateral radiograph of 3-year-old with cystic fibrosis showing mild interstitial changes. *(C)* Anterior posterior radiograph of 9-year-old with cystic fibrosis with bronchiectatic changes visible. *(D)* Medial lateral radiograph of 9-year-old with cystic fibrosis with infiltrate visible in the upper lobe. *(E)* Anterior posterior and *(F)* medial lateral radiograph of 16-year-old with cystic fibrosis with diffuse infiltrates visible.

Tests and Measures

Aerobic Capacity and Endurance

Jerry is able to ambulate on the treadmill at 2.2 mph for 18 minutes but is limited by shortness of breath. Vital signs during exercise are SaO_2 of 94% to 96%; HR, 110 to 126 bpm; and RR, 32 to 44 breaths per minute. All values return to values equal to or below baseline levels within 9 minutes postexercise (SaO_2 of 98%, HR, 85 bpm, and RR, 15 breaths per minute). Jerry reports a rate of perceived exertion (RPE) of 6/10 on the modified Borg scale (Borg, 1982) (see Chapter 8, Figure 8–11) during exercise with a maximum HR of 126 bpm. The RPE is reported to be a reliable measure of exertion with individuals of any age or gender (American College of Sports Medicine, 1991; Yankaskas & Knowles, 1999).

CYSTIC FIBROSIS

Muscle Performance

Muscle strength appears to be WNL, with strength throughout all extremities graded with a score of 5/5.

Neuromotor Development and Sensory Integration

All neuromotor development areas appear to be WNL.

Posture

No postural deformities are observed.

Range of Motion

Jerry demonstrates full AROM throughout all extremities.

Self-Care and Home Management

Jerry reports a mild increase of his work of breathing related to activities at school and home during the 2 weeks before this admission. He has not participated in ice hockey in the 2 weeks before this admission because of increased coughing and increased work of breathing.

Ventilation and Respiration/ Gas Exchange

Minimal suprasternal and intercostal retractions with some accessory muscle use are noted at rest. On auscultation, good air movement is noted bilaterally, with minimal adventitious sounds including soft rales on the right only. The adventitious sounds clear with a cough. Pulmonary function testing completed at the hospital admission (see Table 19.2) indicates that Jerry has mild small airway disease. Jerry does present with a chronic cough. At this time there is increased congestion and the cough is productive of light yellow sputum.

Work, Community, and Leisure Integration

Jerry has no chronic limitations or restrictions in his activities or participation related to his disease. Outside of his 2-week departure from sport activity immediately before this admission, he has fully participated in all school activities and competitively engaged in extracurricular endeavors with his peers for the past few years.

EVALUATION, DIAGNOSIS, AND PROGNOSIS (INCLUDING PLAN OF CARE)

Since the age of 2 months, Jerry has been followed quarterly in the cystic fibrosis clinic and has not had significant problems related to his chronic disease. This is his first acute pulmonary exacerbation requiring an inpatient admission. Pulmonary function tests have declined slightly over time, indicating mild small airway disease. For this admission, Jerry presents only with impaired pulmonary endurance related to his acute exacerbation. Within this episode of care, it is anticipated that he will demonstrate optimal ventilation, optimal respiration/gas exchange, and optimal aerobic capacity, enabling him to fully participate in school, home, community, and leisure activities. It is also anticipated that he will assume more responsibility for his airway clearance management.

Goals

The following goals will be achieved during his hospitalization.

1. Jerry will perform all bathing, grooming, and dressing independently and without increased work of breathing.

2. Jerry will demonstrate adequate aeration of bilateral lung fields, without adventitious sounds.

3. Jerry's parents will demonstrate independence in postural drainage, percussion, and vibration for all segments for 1.5 minutes each segment.

4. Jerry will demonstrate independence with a daily airway clearance session consisting of five or six sets of peak positive expiratory pressure (PEP) breathing; 8 to 10 breaths per set, followed by cough, with rest periods between sets.

INTERVENTION

Coordination, Communication, and Documentation

Issues discussed during the care conference include the need for Jerry to possess the skills for independence with an airway clearance technique and the need to reinforce with the parents the importance of elimination of second-hand smoke. The physical therapist educated the school nurse on the protocol for use of the PEP device. The nurse was aware that Jerry would use the device in the nurse's office as needed. The case manager is directed to procure a mechanical percussor and PEP device for the home.

Patient/Client-Related Instruction

Jerry is instructed in alternative airway clearance techniques to previously taught PDPV. A hand-held mechanical percussor and sonic percussor are introduced. He elects to use the mechanical percussor and independently manages clearance of his anterior and lateral segments. The family continues to perform manual percussion of his posterior lobes.

Jerry is also instructed to supplement the primary airway clearance technique of manual or mechanical percussion with the use of the PEP or the Flutter device (see Chapter 8, Figures 8–17 and 8–18). The PEP and Flutter devices are easily transportable and enable him to clear his airway immediately before or during a sport or gym activity. In addition, the PEP or Flutter gives him the opportunity to increase the number of daily independent airway clearance sessions, as needed. Jerry chose to use the PEP device.

Previously, in the cystic fibrosis clinic, the family was instructed to implement vibration immediately after percussion to each lung segment while Jerry performed a pursed-lipped, slow, and protracted exhalation. During this admission, the family is instructed in proper use of the mechanical percussor and PEP device. The family prefers manual percussions to mechanical percussion on Jerry's posterior segments to be able to palpate fremitus. All of the techniques are reviewed and the family demonstrates the ability to perform these activities appropriately. Child and family instruction related to the prevention of complications and the impact of smoking on Jerry's pulmonary status are reiterated.

Procedural Interventions

Therapeutic Exercise

Aerobic Capacity/Endurance Training

In light of his failure-to-thrive comorbidity, closed-chain activities, such as ice hockey, are encouraged to promote increased bone density. Physical activity also assists in attaining peak oxygen consumption and aerobic capacity. With physical activity, ventilation will also increase, which could assist in clearing secretions.

Airway Clearance Techniques

Jerry is instructed on how to differentiate diaphragmatic breathing from accessory muscle breathing. Diaphragmatic breathing exercises are performed twice daily when he is at rest and during the vibration portion of his airway clearance protocol.

Jerry is instructed on proper use of the mechanical percussor as a primary airway clearance technique on his anterior and lateral segments, in the respective postural drainage positions. The duration of percussion per segment remains at 1.5 minutes and will be performed twice daily. The family elects to continue to manually percuss and vibrate Jerry's posterior segments. Jerry and the family are instructed how to properly use the PEP device as a supplement to the primary airway clearance technique. The PEP is to be used at school, as well as whenever else Jerry deems it necessary.

EXAMINATION: AGE 16 YEARS

Jerry has had numerous hospitalizations from the age of 8 until the age of 16 because of pulmonary exacerbations and failure to thrive. Over the past year, his pulmonary function tests have showed a progressive decline (see Table 19.2).

History

General Demographics

Jerry is 16 years old and continues to live with his father and half-sister. His parents are now amicably separated. The father works nights. Both the sister and father smoke in the home. He is in the 10th grade and regularly plays organized ice hockey in an after-school league.

Medical/Surgical History

Jerry has had multiple admissions to the hospital for pulmonary exacerbations within the past 8 years. His most recent admission was 3 months before this admission, during which he had a gastrostomy tube placed for overnight feeding because of his continued failure to thrive.

Before the gastrostomy tube, he received night feeding through a nasogastric tube. A high-frequency chest wall oscillator (HFCWO) was also ordered for him, for more independent airway clearance techniques.

History of Current Condition

One month before this admission, Jerry reported symptoms of increased coughing, fever, weight loss, and post-tussive emesis. He was treated with tobramycin, ciprofloxacin, and prednisone over a 4-week period while at home. His pulmonary function tests showed no improvement at home, so he is now admitted to the hospital for more aggressive therapy.

Growth and Development

Jerry is below the fifth percentile for height and weight. His height is 60.12 in (152.7 cm) and weight is 90.7 lbs (37.8 kg).

Living Environment

Discharge to the home is anticipated.

Medications

Jerry continues to take albuterol, Intal, and Mucomyst to assist in control of bronchospasm and improve airway clearance. Other medications that he regularly takes are Sudafed, Flovent, and Claritin, which are sinus and allergy medications; Cisapride, which is used to control reflux; Flonase, for asthma control; Fosamax and calcium carbonate, to minimize bone loss; Pulmozyme, to reduce frequency of respiratory infection and improve pulmonary function; and Ultrase, a pancreatic enzyme supplement. Jerry also continues to take vitamin A, D, E, and K supplements.

During his hospital stay, Jerry is also taking tobramycin, which is an antibiotic used specifically to treat *Pseudomonas* infection. Prolonged use of tobramycin may result in irreversible ototoxicity (dizziness and tinnitus) and neurotoxicity (headache, dizziness, tremors). Although he does not report any of these symptoms at this time, these concerns should be considered during physical therapy re-examination. Other medications taken during admission include prednisone to reduce inflammation and ceftazidime to minimize stomach upset and diarrhea.

Jerry's diet now includes Scandishake (3 times a week) and Nutren (ingested via gastrostomy tube). His total caloric intake per day is 3408 kcal.

Other Tests and Measures

The chest radiograph demonstrated bilateral bronchiectasis, mucus plugging, peribronchial thickening, increased interstitial markings, and flattening of bilateral diaphragms. Pulmonary function tests (see Table 19.2) revealed FEV_1 of 83% and FVC of 71%. Sputum cultures revealed mucoid and nonmucoid *P. aeruginosa* bacteria. Laboratory studies included a DEXA scan, which revealed no change from a scan performed 3 months earlier. Jerry's scores on the scan showed bone mass to be −3.67 SDs below the mean, indicating a 60% predicted bone mass. The DEXA scan revealed a bone age of 13, which is considered a significant delay.

Systems Review

Cardiovascular and Pulmonary

Function of the cardiovascular and pulmonary systems is of concern during this admission attributable to the chest radiographic changes displaying more severe cystic changes and poor pulmonary function tests (see Table 19.2).

Integumentary

The gastrostomy tube site with button is clean and dry.

Musculoskeletal

Musculoskeletal development is an area of concern because of the significantly poor bone density, as well as Jerry's failure to display appropriate weight and height gain. Jerry is 60.12 in (152.7 cm) and weight is 90.7 lbs (37.8 kg), respectively, and both are below the 5th percentile for his age.

Tests and Measures

Aerobic Capacity and Endurance

Jerry's vital signs at rest are HR of 104 bpm; RR, 22 breaths per minute; and BP, 107/76 mm Hg. Based on expected values for his age, HR and RR are slightly increased (see Chapter 8, Table 8.8). SaO_2 is 94% on room air, which is lower than the expected SaO_2 of 97% to 98%. HR is regular, and the rhythm is without murmurs. Jerry is able to ambulate on a treadmill at 2.5 mph with 5% incline for 12 minutes. His exercise vital signs are HR of 120 bpm; RR, 38 breaths per minute; and SaO_2, 97%.

Muscle Performance

Bilateral lower and upper extremities strength is grossly 5–/5 throughout. Decreased trunk strength is also noted.

Range of Motion

Jerry presents with AROM that is within functional limits. Passively, he has decreased hamstring flexibility evidenced with popliteal angles of 55° bilaterally. He has some rounding of the shoulders, but no limitation of functional upper extremity ROM.

Posture

Postural deviations include an increased thoracic kyphosis, forward head, rounded shoulders, winging scapula on the left greater than the right, posterior pelvic tilt, and elevated shoulder girdles with the left greater than the right. Hypertrophied accessory breathing musculature is also evident, with poor thoracic cage mobility and a barrel-shaped chest.

Ventilation and Respiration/ Gas Exchange

Jerry uses his accessory muscles for quiet breathing. On auscultation, he has bilateral rales, which clear with a cough. Rales are especially noted in the right middle lobe, and decreased breath sounds in the right lower lobe. Moderate clubbing of the digits is noted. His pulses are normal throughout.

Work, Community, and Leisure Integration

Jerry continues to participate fully in all school activities and compete in extracurricular endeavors. He has no limitations or restrictions related to CF. He is independent with all his activities of daily living. He does, however, report that during pulmonary exacerbations, he requires a longer time to finish tasks around the house and at school. He will take the elevator at school if he is feeling too fatigued to take the stairs. Jerry reports that he will take longer breaks during his hockey games when he requires longer recovery times.

EVALUATION, DIAGNOSIS, AND PROGNOSIS (INCLUDING PLAN OF CARE)

Jerry's primary areas of concern include impairments in ventilatory capacity, decreased muscular endurance, decreased bone mineralization, and postural deviations with resultant decreased muscular flexibility. In addition, Jerry knows no alternative airway clearance technique to the HFCWO and PDPV. The physical therapy diagnosis is as follows: decreased cardiorespiratory endurance, decreased muscular endurance and strength, decreased muscular flexibility, decreased independence with alternative airway clearance techniques, and postural deviations related to increased work of breathing.

Goals

The following goals will be achieved during six 1-hour-long physical therapy sessions per week for the duration of 2 weeks or until medical discharge.

1. Jerry will demonstrate independence with the PEP device as an alternative airway clearance technique.

2. Jerry will demonstrate independence with monitoring vital signs of HR and RR before, during, and after exercise.

3. Jerry will demonstrate independence with a home exercise program that will include:
   a. Weight-bearing endurance activity 3 to 4 times per week to achieve 60% HR maximum for 20 minutes.
   b. Strengthening protocol throughout all extremities and including spinal extension.

4. Jerry will demonstrate increased muscular endurance and ventilatory capacity in tolerance of treadmill for 25 minutes with 4-minute warm-up and cool-down maintaining SaO_2 of greater than 94%, achieving 60% HR maximum.

INTERVENTION

Patient/Client-Related Instruction

Jerry demonstrates independence with the HFCWO, his primary airway clearance technique. He continues to be quite active in sports in school, especially with his participation in ice hockey. He did, however, complain recently of the inability to participate in a full period of ice hockey because of his poor ventilatory capacity. He will therefore greatly benefit from the implementation of an additional airway clearance technique, such as the PEP, to use independently before and during his sport engagement. His family continues to recognize the benefit of not smoking in the home in order for Jerry to avoid second-hand smoke. They do not, however, cease this activity, and this issue continues to be a focus of the team.

Procedural Interventions

Therapeutic Exercise

Aerobic Capacity/Endurance Training

Jerry is instructed to participate daily in an aerobic activity that is weight bearing in nature for a minimum of 30 minutes. Weight-bearing exercise should also help increase bone mineral density. He is to continue to work on diaphragmatic breathing exercises to minimize accessory muscle use.

Flexibility Exercises

Jerry is given instruction on stretching exercises, including hamstring and thoracic cage stretches. Emphasis is also placed on stretching neck, shoulder girdle, and trunk muscles that contribute to current postural deviations and increase the work of breathing.

Strength, Power, and Endurance Training

Of concern is his recent diagnosis of moderate osteopenia, evidenced on DEXA scans. Jerry's exercise program was modified to implement weight training and continued use of closed chain activities to encourage ossification and increased muscle strength. Breathing exercises for respiratory muscle strengthening is also included in his program.

DISCUSSION

The most important goal when treating a child with CF is to achieve early independent airway clearance strategies. The specific intervention strategies that the therapist and child elect to use are dependent on the age of the child, the caregivers' training, and the manifestation of the disease process. Jerry originally presented at 2 months of age with emesis, voracious appetite, pancreatic dysfunction, and failure to thrive. Deficits that emerged later in his life included osteopenia, asthma, a decline in his ventilatory capacity, and the persistence of failure to thrive, which required the placement of a gastrostomy tube for night feedings.

Because the lungs of an infant with CF are normal at birth, lung pathology will not present until later. Jerry was, in fact, diagnosed with CF secondary to failure to thrive. His therapist performed a developmental evaluation to ensure that he was achieving his developmental milestones despite poor nutritional metabolism and episodes of emesis with feedings. If, at that point, a developmental delay were identified, then an early intervention referral would have been made. The primary goals at 2 months of age are ensuring the family's independence with PDPV and the monitoring of the child's ability to meet developmental milestones.

After Jerry's initial diagnosis, he was followed in the cystic fibrosis clinic regularly through adolescence. The airway clearance techniques were progressed to include percussion of additional lung fields that included the Trendelenburg position and vibration. By the age of 8 years, he was instructed in an alternative airway clearance technique to PDPV. He should have performed at least one of the three required daily airway clearance sessions independently. This could have been with the handheld mechanical percussor or an HFCWO. In addition, by 8 years of age Jerry should be able to demonstrate the ability to supplement the primary airway clearance technique of PDPV, with the use of the PEP or Flutter device. The PEP and Flutter devices are easily transportable and would enable him to clear his airway immediately before or during his sport activity or gym class. In addition, the PEP or Flutter would give him the opportunity to increase the number of airway clearance sessions he could have in a day independently, if the necessity arose.

At 16 years of age, Jerry's DEXA scan revealed a significant decrease in bone mineralization, and that is a concern. He was placed on medication for this condition and also has greatly benefited from the promotion of a rigorous and monitored strengthening program and of closed chain exercises to stimulate the production of bone. A 16-year-old should also be able to monitor his cardio-vascular status during exercise through the use of the Borg perceived exertion scale (Borg, 1982) and by measuring his vital signs to achieve and maintain an optimal aerobic workout.

The intervention strategies used on entering into adulthood do not vary significantly from those mandated in adolescence. It will be important to ensure that he adheres to airway clearance techniques and is offered other strategies to better incorporate airway clearance into his daily routine.

DISCUSSION QUESTIONS

1. What do Jerry's vital signs during his exercise test tell you about his aerobic capacity?

2. What does a muscle strength grade of 3/5 tell you about a 2-month-old?

3. How would you work on the strength of a 2-month-old?

4. What are the purposes of the various medications taken by a child with CF?

5. For what purpose is an HFCWO prescribed? When would you order one?

6. How would you convince this family to provide a smoke-free environment for Jerry?

7. In chronic disease such as CF, what do you see as a barrier to the child's participation in his or her own care?

RECOMMENDED READINGS/RESOURCES

Brannon, F.J., Foley, M.W., Starr, J.A., & Saul, L.M. (1998). *Cardiopulmonary rehabilitation: Basic theory and application* (3rd ed.). Philadelphia: F.A. Davis.

Cystic Fibrosis Foundation, available at *http://www.cff.org*

DeJong, W., vanAalderen, W.M., Kraan, J., Koeter, G.H., & van der Schans, C.P. (2001). Inspiratory muscle training in patients with cystic fibrosis. *Respiratory Medicine, 95*(1), 31–66.

Gondor, M., Nixon, P., Mutich, R., Rebovich, P., & Orenstein, D. (1999). Comparison of flutter device and chest physical therapy in the treatment of cystic fibrosis during pulmonary exacerbation. *Pediatric Pulmonology, 28,* 255–260.

Nixon, P. (2003). Cystic fibrosis. In J.L. Durstine & G.E. Moore (Eds.), *ACSM's exercise management for persons with chronic diseases and disabilities* (pp. 111–116). Champaign, IL: Human Kinetics.

Yankaskas, J.R., & Knowles, M.R. (1999). *Cystic fibrosis in adults.* Philadelphia: Lippincott-Raven.

REFERENCES

American College of Sports Medicine (1991). *Guidelines for exercise testing and prescription* (4th ed.) Philadelphia: Lea & Febiger.

American Physical Therapy Association (APTA) (2001). *Guide to physical therapist practice* (2nd ed.). *Physical Therapy, 81,* 6–746.

Borg, G.V. (1982). Psychophysical basis of perceived exertion. *Medicine and Science in Sports and Exercise, 14,* 377.

Children's Liver Association for Support Services (2004). *Pediatric Lab Values.* Retrieved July 14, 2004 from *www.classkids.org/library/refliverlabs.htm*

Folio, M.R., & Fewell, R.R. (2000). *Peabody Developmental Motor Scales* (2nd ed.). Austin, TX: Pro-Ed.

Yankaskas, J.R., & Knowles, M.R. (1999). *Cystic fibrosis in adults.* Philadelphia: Lippincott-Raven.

Chapter *20*

Case Study: Down Syndrome

— Katie Bergeron, PT, MS

— Carol Gildenberg Dichter, PT, PhD, PCS

This case study focuses on the physical therapy management of Carrie, a teenager with Down syndrome. Carrie is now 16 years old and has received physical therapy services from the age of 4 weeks to the present. For individuals with a diagnosis of Down syndrome, physical therapy services may be necessary across the life span, addressing changing issues as growth occurs, and as the child gains increasing independence in a variety of environments. Functional demands change as the individual moves from infancy, through the school years, and into adulthood.

Individuals with Down syndrome frequently present with impairments in strength (Stemmons-Mercer & Lewis, 2001), range of motion (ROM) (Zausmer & Shea, 1984), tone (Shea, 1991), and balance and coordination (Connolly & Michael, 1986), leading to delay in acquisition of motor skills and to functional limitations. Associated impairments, such as mental retardation, cardiovascular pathology, and frequent middle ear infections, may also have a negative impact on motor skill acquisition and activities.

The impairments of body structure and function and limitations in activities and participation presented by Carrie may be best addressed by the physical therapy management described in Preferred Practice Patterns 5B: Impaired Neuromotor Development, or 4C: Impaired Muscle Performance as outlined in the American Physical Therapy Association's *Guide to physical therapist practice* (2nd ed.) (APTA, 2001). Pattern 5B: Impaired Neuromotor Development was selected because of Carrie's delayed motor skill development, impaired cognition, and sensory integration impairments. Episodes of care at 3

years and 16 years of age will be detailed. Physical therapy services at both ages were provided by therapists working in educational settings in accordance with the federal legislation Individuals with Disabilities Education Act (IDEA).

EXAMINATION: AGE 3 YEARS

History

At Carrie's birth, doctors were suspicious of a potential diagnosis of Down syndrome. She presented with some soft signs, including slanted eyes, poor suck, and hypotonia (Figure 20–1). Carrie was transferred from her local rural hospital to a major urban hospital for genetic testing when she was 2 days old. At this time, a diagnosis of Down syndrome was confirmed. Her parents, Tim and Peggy, were both 35 years old and already had three other children: Wendy, 12 years; Jamie, 9 years; and Thea, 4 years. Tim and Peggy's initial reactions were love for Carrie, fear of the unknown, and uncertainty of their capabilities as parents of a child with special needs. However, they were determined to help Carrie in every way they knew.

When Carrie was 4 weeks old, her family began the process of early intervention (EI) to help them foster Carrie's development. EI services have been continued to the present, and the EI team has included an educator, a speech therapist, and a physical therapist. Carrie has received weekly home visits from a physical therapist to assist the family with facilitating her gross motor development. Throughout Carrie's EI experience, the physical

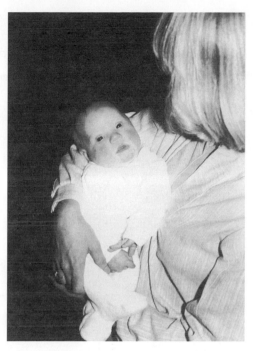

Figure 20-1 Carrie at birth.

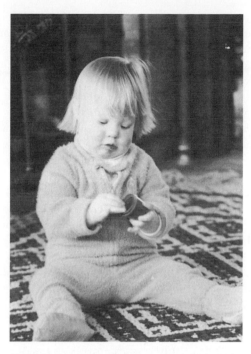

Figure 20-3 Maintaining sitting position during play.

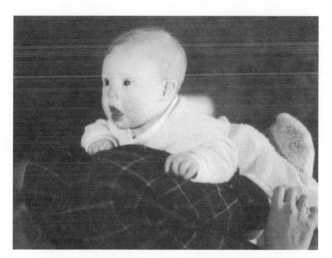

Figure 20-2 Prone position on mother's legs.

therapist has given the family different activities to work on with Carrie, including spending time in the prone position, maintaining her sitting balance while playing with toys, and propelling a ride-on toy (Figures 20–2 through 20–4).

At 2 years of age, Carrie had open-heart surgery to repair a persistent patent ductus arteriosus that never closed on its own when she was an infant. Before the surgery, Carrie was continuously sick. She had frequent ear infections, scarlet

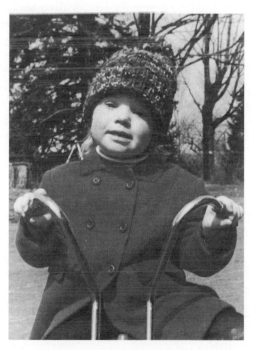

Figure 20-4 Propelling a ride-on toy.

fever (twice), and pneumonia. This hindered some of her progress in the areas of speech, cognition, fine motor, and gross motor development. After the surgery, Peggy and Tim noticed a significant improvement in Carrie's health. She has recovered well from her heart surgery. The ages at which Carrie achieved her gross motor milestones from birth to 29 months are listed in Table 20.1.

Because of the recurrent ear infections, Carrie had tympanostomy tubes put in her ears when she was 30 months old. There is no known hearing loss at this time.

Carrie is starting to attend her Mom's preschool 1 day per week. She also attends Sunday school at church, where she is with peers. After Carrie chooses her own toy, she occasionally plays near the other children at preschool and with her siblings at home. She engages in pretend play at home and at school.

When Carrie becomes 3 years old in a few weeks, she will transfer out of her EI program and into her local school district program. Peggy and Tim want to make sure that they maintain a high level of participation in Carrie's therapy sessions, as well as the design of her Individualized Educational Plan (IEP). They are concerned about Carrie's continued development in all areas. Although she has recovered well from her surgery a year ago, they are still concerned about her health and how it affects her development. Peggy and Tim would like to see Carrie integrated into all areas of their local community, as their other children have been, to the level that Carrie can effectively sustain participation. Their major gross motor concern is related to Carrie's limited ability to participate independently in the community, specifically with endurance, ambulation on uneven surfaces, playground independence, and stair negotiation.

Systems Review

Cardiovascular and Pulmonary

Carrie's cardiovascular and pulmonary systems appear to be functioning within normal limits at this time with a pulse of 76 beats per minute (bpm), blood pressure (BP) of 90/60 mm Hg, and respiratory rate (RR) of 19 breaths per minute. All measurements were taken at rest.

Integumentary

A well-healed scar from the open-heart surgery is noted between ribs 6 and 7, beginning at the anterior portion of the left upper chest and following along the ribs to the

Table 20.1   Age at Which Carrie Achieved Gross Motor Milestones

Gross Motor Milestones	Age Achieved (mo)
Lift head to 90° in prone prop	4.5
Roll from stomach to back	5
Roll from back to stomach	6
Pivot in prone	9
Sit with arms propped for support	9
Sit unsupported	10
Belly crawling	11
Transition from prone to quadruped	12
Pull to stand from sitting	13
Creeping on hands and knees	14
Transition from prone to sitting	15
Transition from supine to sitting	15
Cruise	15
Stand independently for 10 seconds	17
Walk 10 feet with two-hand support	17
Walk 20 feet with a push toy	18
Walk 5 steps without support	20
Creep up stairs independently	22
Independent household ambulation	24
Crawl down stairs independently	25
Walk up stairs with two-hand support	28
Walk down stairs with two-hand support	29

posterior portion of the left upper chest. It measures 7 inches long and 0.25 inch wide.

Musculoskeletal

Height and weight are within the 40th percentile for her age. Joint hypermobility and generalized weakness with hypotonia are noted.

Neuromuscular

Impaired balance and coordination are noted, and development of functional motor skills is delayed.

Cognition

Carrie is typically alert and aware of her surroundings. She manipulates toys to explore their novel features and demonstrates an attention span of at least 15 minutes when playing with one of her favorite toys, especially with anything musical. Carrie demonstrates keen observation skills that allow her to deduct the location of a hidden object and to anticipate the path of a rolling ball.

Carrie's family and therapists have noticed that Carrie is a visual learner. They use pictures to label objects to assist Carrie in learning new words and skills (e.g., brushing teeth, eating, and putting on socks).

Carrie's receptive language is age appropriate, but she has a delay with expressive language and has articulation problems. She uses sign language along with verbal expression to communicate her wants and needs with two-word sentences.

Tests and Measures

Aerobic Capacity and Endurance

Carrie demonstrates enough endurance to walk for at least 300 feet at a time and to "run" stiffly for 50 feet. This is a significant improvement occurring after her recovery from open-heart surgery. Before surgery she was limited to walking 50 feet because of fatigue, shortness of breath (SOB), and generalized muscle weakness.

Gait, Locomotion, and Balance

In standing position, Carrie exhibits a wide base of support, hip external rotation, and flat feet. She ambulates with a heel strike followed by a foot slap because of poor eccentric control of her dorsiflexors. She has a wide base of support and holds her arms at her side. She attempts to "run" stiffly when playing with her siblings and peers. She negotiates up and down stairs with two hands on the railing and placing both feet on each step. Carrie demonstrates delayed equilibrium reactions in sitting and in standing. She demonstrates protective reactions forward and to the sides in sitting and standing. This skill is emerging to the rear. Carrie leads with one foot and needs both hands for support when attempting to jump in place. She balances on one foot for 3 seconds with both hands held. Carrie propels a ride-on toy up to 5 feet at a time independently, on a flat surface.

Motor Function (Motor Control and Motor Learning)

Carrie's resting sitting posture is ring sitting with external hip rotation, flexed spine, and a forward head (Figure 20–5). She can ambulate and climb stairs, as noted previously. She has mastered simple fine motor activities, including using a pincer grasp for small objects, manipulating push/pull levers, and completing a four piece shape puzzle.

Carrie has difficulty developing motor plans for novel, multistep tasks. She needs to have the tasks broken down into steps. After a demonstration of each of the steps, she

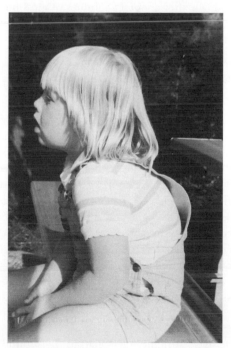

Figure 20-5 Resting posture in sitting.

can put them together once she has mastered the individual steps. Carrie still has difficulty grading the amount of force she needs when performing both fine motor and gross motor tasks.

Muscle Performance

Carrie has low muscle tone throughout her body. This low tone is more prevalent proximally compared with distally. Although she demonstrates enough strength to move her upper and lower extremities through full ROM against gravity, she has poor midrange control. She has difficulty extending her neck and back musculature against gravity for long periods of time (e.g., sitting during circle time). She is unable to sit straight up from a supine position, indicating weak abdominal muscles. This functional, general assessment of muscle strength was chosen because other more standardized methods are difficult to use reliably with children as young as 3 years of age and children who have cognitive impairments.

Carrie's decreased muscle strength and limited midrange motor control limit her abilities to keep up with her peers during gross motor play, including running, climbing on playground equipment, negotiating stairs independently, and propelling a riding toy. In addition to the decreased muscle strength and motor control issues, Carrie's muscle endurance is limited. Her mother reports that Carrie will often sit down after about 15 minutes of gross motor play and remain seated for up to 10 minutes at a time until she returns to the activities with her peers.

Neuromotor Development and Sensory Integration

Carrie's equilibrium is good when she is able to anticipate her environment (e.g., negotiating up a grassy knoll that she is practicing on). However, when surrounded by peers, which alters her ability to predict her environment (e.g., traversing the same grassy knoll with her friends and getting bumped), she will lose her balance 50% of the time.

Carrie seeks out light touch by lightly rubbing her fingers on her palms and forearms, suggesting that this sense is diminished. She demonstrates limitations in activities and participation by getting distracted by her need to provide this sensory feedback for herself. Her mother notes that Carrie's occupational therapist gave them light-touch activities to do before Carrie needs to concentrate on activities.

Carrie has difficulty articulating her sounds when attempting to produce words. It is hard for her to produce the consonant sounds /k/, /t/, /g/, /l/, /tr/, /d/, and /s/. She uses one- to two-word sentences to convey her wants and needs. When she is unable to articulate, she uses Signed English to help others understand her. She knows approximately 90 Signed English words.

Range of Motion

Carrie presents with joint hypermobility, especially proximally, throughout all of her joints. Specific goniometric measurements for these joints are listed in Table 20.2. Because of the concern of atlantoaxial instability in individuals with Down syndrome (see Chapter 5 for a discussion relative to this topic), Carrie had radiographs taken of her atlantoaxial joint, and the results were negative for hypermobility.

Self-Care and Home Management (Including Activities of Daily Living and Instrumental Activities of Daily Living)

Carrie drinks from a cup without assistance and takes a few sips through a straw. She uses a spoon independently with some spilling. She demonstrates a pincer grasp to pick up small objects (e.g., raisins) and uses a palmar grasp with a spoon. She uses the same palmar grasp with crayons to make vertical and circular scribbles on either a flat surface or an easel.

There are measurement instruments readily available today that can be used to test self-help skills: Carolina Curriculum for Infants and Toddlers with Special Needs—

Table 20.2 Goniometry Measurements

Joint motion	Right	Left
Hip flexion	0–136°	0–138°
Hip extension	0–10°	0–8°
Hip external rotation	0–80°	0–86°
Shoulder flexion	0–200°	0–202°
Shoulder extension	0–66°	0–64°
Shoulder external rotation	0–114°	0–110°

Second Edition (Johnson-Martin, Jens, Attermeier, & Hacker, 1991), Functional Independence Measure for Children (Granger et al., 1991), and Pediatric Evaluation of Disability Inventory (Haley, Coster, Ludlow, Haltiwanger, & Andrellos, 1992) (others presented in Chapter 2).

Work (Job, School, Play), Community, and Leisure Integration

Carrie enjoys playing with other children at school, on the playground, and at home. She does her best at keeping up but struggles to do so. At school she needs assistance negotiating the stairs to get in and out of her school, climbing onto various gross motor climbing structures in the gym, and propelling ride-on toys. When on the playground, Carrie falls 50% of the time while transitioning from one surface to another (e.g., pavement, sand, and grass). Because her home environment is more familiar to her, she falls there only 30% of the time. This suggests that Carrie needs repetition to help her generalize gross motor skills to new environments.

EVALUATION, DIAGNOSIS, AND PROGNOSIS (INCLUDING PLAN OF CARE)

Carrie presents with overall developmental delays in the following areas: gross motor, fine motor, cognition, self-help, social/emotional, and language. Her gross motor and fine motor functional limitations yield disabilities in her life role as a family member by limiting her independence.

Diagnosis

Carrie has demonstrated impairments of motor function, balance, motor planning, sensory integration, cognition, and expressive language, decreasing her functional independence and restricting her activities and participation. Specific impairments in muscle strength, low muscle tone, and increased ROM negatively affect mid-range control of the lower extremities during ambulation and limit her ability to use stairs.

Activity Limitations

Carrie's decreased muscle strength and balance are major contributing factors to her gross motor developmental delay, including in the following:

- Independent stair negotiation
- Ambulation on uneven surfaces
- Climbing onto and off of various surface levels
- Independent jumping skills
- Independent propulsion of ride-on toys
- Ball skills

Prognosis

Over the course of 12 months, Carrie will demonstrate an increased level of independent motor function at home, school, and in her community. She will also demonstrate ongoing neuromotor development of gross motor skills typical of preschoolers.

Goals/Objectives

Suggested gross motor goals (Table 20.3) were developed after this evaluation. They are expected to be achieved within 1 year, with the assistance of weekly physical therapy visits. These suggested gross motor goals will be shared at Carrie's upcoming IEP Team Meeting for further discussion and modification by all team members (Peggy, Tim, the physical therapist, speech therapist, occupational therapist, psychologist, educator, and others). The focus and location of service delivery will change as Carrie moves from receiving EI services to school-based services.

INTERVENTION

Coordination, Communication, and Documentation

Carrie will be served by an interdisciplinary team that will have monthly case conferences for all of the therapists and educators involved. In addition, Carrie's family will be able to schedule meetings when they deem it necessary.

Carrie's weekly physical therapy visits will alternate between home and preschool. The physical therapist will have direct communication with Carrie's mother, Peggy, and other caregivers present at the two settings. Written material will be given to Peggy to share with caregivers not present at home visits to ensure maximum carryover. A copy of this material will be placed in Carrie's file for other team members to review. An annual report will be sent to

DOWN SYNDROME

Table 20.3   Suggested Gross Motor Goals for Carrie's IEP at Age 3 Years

	Functional Independence Goals
1	Carrie will negotiate up stairs with alternating feet without support with close supervision 80% of the time.
2	Carrie will negotiate down stairs with alternating feet with one hand on the railing 80% of the time.
3	1. Carrie will ambulate on uneven surfaces independently without falling 80% of the time, including but not limited to: (a) Grass (b) Sand (c) Gravel (d) Sidewalk (e) Soft surface (i.e., mattress or foam)
4	2. Carrie will independently climb onto and off of a variety of surface level heights without falling to increase her independence 80% of the time, including but not limited to: (a) Chair at the kitchen table (b) Step stool at the bathroom sink (c) Family room furniture (d) Toddler playground equipment
	Advanced Motor Skill Goals
1	Carrie will jump off the floor with both feet together with one hand for support to play hopscotch 80% of the time.
2	Carrie will propel a riding toy 50 feet using a reciprocal pattern with her feet on the floor with close supervision 80% of the time.
3	Carrie will negotiate a playground-type ladder up and down with contact guarding 100% of the time.
	Ball Skill Goals
1	Carrie will kick a playground-sized ball at least 5 feet with accuracy 80% of the time.
2	Carrie will throw a playground-sized ball at least 5 feet with accuracy 80% of the time.

Carrie's developmental pediatrician to keep him informed of Carrie's progress and current goals.

Carrie's family will be given information about the National Down Syndrome Congress (NDSC) and a local parent support group for further resources about issues related to Carrie's specific needs.

Expected outcomes of this comprehensive coordination and communication will include the following:

- Collaboration among home, school, and the therapists and educators working with Carrie
- Supplementary information specific to children with Down syndrome for family, therapists, and teachers

available through NDSC and local parent support group

- Referrals to appropriate professionals when necessary

Patient/Client-Related Instruction

During the examination, the physical therapist found it useful to use a variety of instructional methods, including visual cues, verbal cues, and hands-on facilitation, when teaching Carrie new skills. All three methods in combination were necessary to help Carrie gain new skills (Table 20.4).

Table 20.4   Example of Instructional Cues for a New Skill

New skill	Jumping off floor with two feet together
Visual cue	Demonstrate the skill
Verbal cue	"Bend your knees and jump."
Hands-on facilitation	Two-hand support at her hips to facilitate the movement

In addition, the team will provide Carrie's family with information about the differences between EI and school-based services. (See Chapters 10 and 11 for further details regarding the federal regulations governing these services.)

Procedural Interventions

Therapeutic Exercise

Therapeutic exercise focuses on improving aerobic capacity and endurance; balance, coordination, and agility training; neuromotor development training; and muscle strengthening. Table 20.5 includes therapeutic exercises for Carrie to perform in a variety of settings (shown in Figures 20–6 through 20–8).

Expected outcomes of these therapeutic exercises include the following:

- Increased aerobic capacity and endurance
- Increased balance and coordination
- Increased neuromotor development
- Increased strength

Functional Training in Self-Care

A proper seating position for Carrie will be determined for use during mealtimes and fine motor activities to provide the proper support needed to allow the highest level of independent functioning. Appropriate-sized step stools will be placed in front of the bathroom sinks to allow for independence with hand washing and tooth brushing.

To help Carrie become more independent with dressing, the physical therapist will instruct her family and primary caregivers on teaching her to balance on one leg. This will

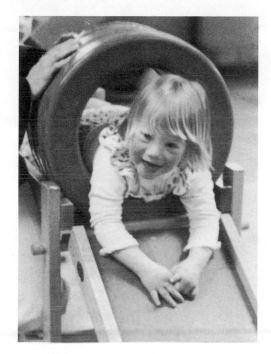

Figure 20 6 Obstacle course.

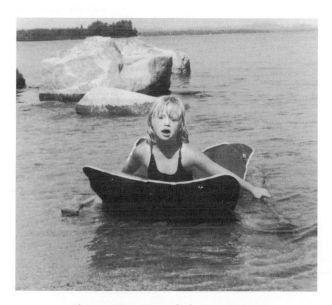

Figure 20-7 Water balance activity.

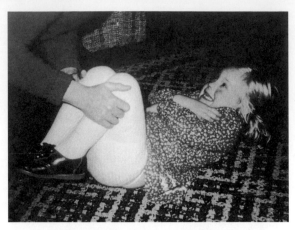

Figure 20-8 Abdominal exercises.

help with putting on her pants and shoes and taking them off while standing.

Another activity to work on with Carrie is the negotiation of stairs and curbs, both up and down, as well as getting on and off various playground equipment and toys. She currently requires assistance, making her dependent on others.

Expected outcomes of this functional training in self-care tasks include the following:

- Increased independence in daily tasks and activities
- Increased balance and coordination
- Increased neuromotor development
- Increased strength

Table 20.5   Therapeutic Exercise

Aerobic Capacity/Endurance Conditioning	
Running	Run in the yard with her siblings to catch bubbles
Swimming	Motor boat—Carrie kicks her legs while she is supported by her arms
Building with blocks	Move building blocks of various sizes and shapes from one corner of her classroom to the other to build a fort
Balance Coordination and Agility Training	
Ball activity	Kick ball at a target
Sitting	Sit on a small ball (kickball-size) during circle time
Obstacle course	Negotiate over, under, up, down, and around through various play structures (see Figure 20–6)
Bean bag toss	Throw bean bags at designated target—Have Carrie stand on a piece of foam as her aim improves to increase the challenge
Water game	Balance while sitting on a small raft in the water (see Figure 20–7)
Neuromotor Development Training	
Jumping	Jump on a small trampoline then on the floor
Stairs	Learn an alternating feet pattern to negotiate stairs
Climbing	Use alternating pattern between feet and hands when climbing on various structures
Strength and Endurance Training	
Abdominal exercises	Sit-ups (see Figure 20–8)
Stairs	Negotiate up and down stairs with the least amount of support
Ride-on toy	Propel ride-on toy between classrooms at school
Walking	Walk home from school and in the grocery store instead of riding in the stroller or shopping cart

TERMINATION OF EPISODE OF CARE

This episode of care will be terminated when Carrie has achieved the stated goals and outcomes. Within the early childhood practice settings goals are anticipated to be achieved in approximately 1 year. If the goals were achieved sooner, the episode of care would be terminated and a new episode of care initiated if new goals were identified by the IEP Team.

It is anticipated that individuals with Down syndrome may "require multiple episodes of care over the lifetime to ensure safety and effective adaptation after changes in physical status, caregivers, environment, or task demands" (APTA, 2001, p. 334). Additional episodes of physical therapy care for Carrie will be indicated as musculoskeletal growth occurs, classroom task requirements change, teachers and caregivers change, medical or surgical issues arise, or level of impairment or physical function changes. As Carrie continues to have educationally relevant needs, as determined under IDEA, related services, including physical therapy, will be provided in the school setting. As Carrie becomes older, her physical therapy may need to be transitioned to an outpatient setting if the goals are no longer educationally based.

EXAMINATION: AGE 16 YEARS

History

Carrie is now 16 years old. She has been relatively healthy medically over the past 13 years. She still struggles with her balance, endurance, strength, and weight control. Carrie has attended her local public school elementary and high school programs in inclusive settings each year. She is now a ninth grader in high school. At 12 years of age, Carrie's IQ was 68 and her educational classification of multiply handicapped (educable mentally retarded and speech impairment) was established. She has received speech therapy and physical therapy services as part of her educational program. Carrie is a member of the high school choir, and in the past, she participated in the elementary and junior high choirs. Carrie will participate in the annual high school musical production this year as a member of the chorus. Her family is very musical, and all of her siblings participated in these activities when they were in high school. Carrie is proud to participate in the same activities as her siblings. Her parents allow her to participate in school activities that are appropriate for her because it helps her interact socially with her peer group.

To help facilitate friendships for Carrie, last year her parents enrolled her in a weekly program for teenagers with disabilities, the Resource Center for Independent Living. This program helps Carrie develop self-esteem, self-advocacy, friendships with others with all types of mental and physical disabilities, and awareness of other disabilities. Interviewing skills, job shadowing, and technology training are also provided through the program. Carrie and her family are also active members of both the NDSC and their local parent-support group. Both organizations have provided information to Carrie's parents and siblings, as well as a support network for the family, but especially for Carrie.

Carrie had several ear infections throughout her early childhood. She had tubes placed in both ears when she was 6 years old; however, they were not effective. Because of her numerous ear infections, her right ossicle was corroded and her right eardrum was perforated, yielding a 60% hearing loss in her right ear. There is no hearing loss in her left ear. Carrie is nearsighted and has astigmatism. She wears glasses to correct these problems.

At the age of 14 years, Carrie developed hand and then full body tremors. She also had a "seizurelike" episode with unconsciousness. She was determined to have Graves' disease (hyperthyroidism), which caused these symptoms. Because children with Down syndrome often have hypothyroidism (Pueschel & Bier, 1992), Carrie's condition is unusual. She initially took medication to decrease her thyroid hormone levels, but then required radioactive iodine treatments to regulate the thyroid hormone levels. She is monitored monthly by an endocrinologist.

Carrie has maintained a physically active lifestyle. She participated in community soccer programs from ages 8 to 10 years and gymnastics from the ages of 9 to 12 years. Her endurance became limited with extreme heat and humidity. In these weather conditions, she had multiple fainting episodes when she pushed herself to continue participating.

Carrie now monitors her heart rate before, during, and after any type of exercise. She has a blue belt in karate and attends karate classes twice weekly. She wants to continue with her karate classes to ultimately achieve her black belt (Figure 20–9). She realizes that she needs to exercise and eat well-balanced meals to continue to develop her endurance, balance skills, and strength and to maintain a healthy weight. She has just started taking kardio-kickboxing, which focuses more specifically on her aerobic endurance.

Functionally, Carrie is able to care for herself independ-

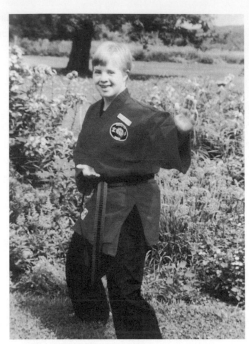

Figure 20-9 Carrie in karate uniform.

ently in the areas of dressing and hygiene. She still needs assistance in making healthy choices for meals. She is also learning a variety of home management skills, such as cooking, housecleaning, and laundry. For the past 2 years, Carrie participated in a county-funded program that provides a one-on-one assistant for adolescents with disabilities to learn life skills. Carrie's assistant comes to her house for 20 hours per week to help Carrie increase her independence with household chores. They focus on cleaning, cooking simple meals, doing laundry, keeping her checkbook updated and balanced, and socialization skills when out in the community. Carrie's mother is especially grateful for this program because she felt that her relationship with Carrie was being strained. Peggy felt that she was always on top of Carrie to do things instead of being a source of encouragement for her.

Carrie's goal is to become a special education teacher's assistant when she graduates from high school. This goal was included in her IEP, and the school set up a special program for Carrie to participate in this school year. She tutors in the elementary school self-contained classroom 3 days per week for 45 minutes. Her responsibilities include tutoring the children in reading and math. This program helps Carrie increase her self-esteem, and it gives her great joy and confidence to help others.

Systems Review

Cardiovascular and Pulmonary

Carrie's cardiovascular and pulmonary systems appear to be functioning within normal limits, with a pulse of 64 bpm, BP of 115/65 mm Hg; and RR of 16 breaths per minute. All measurements were taken at rest. When Carrie has fainting episodes in the heat and humidity, her pulse and blood pressure usually increase.

Integumentary

Carrie's scar from her surgery is well healed and does not present any problems.

Musculoskeletal

Carrie's height and weight are within the 50th percentile for age. Joint hypermobility with hypotonia are still noted.

Neuromuscular

With high-level vestibular activities, such as riding a bicycle, Carrie is unable to balance herself. She feels dizzy, does not know where her body is in space relative to the bicycle, and then gets very anxious about the activity. Even with training wheels attached, she is still afraid of attempting to pedal because of her lack of body-in-space awareness when on the bicycle. Her family and therapists have encouraged her to try again every spring, with no improvement. Carrie still has the desire to ride a bike, so her family purchased an adult-sized tricycle for her last year. The increased base of support of the tricycle (28 inches versus 12 inches with training wheels) provides enough stability for Carrie to be able to negotiate on the pavement (Figure 20–10). She is now learning traffic safety rules for riding on the streets.

Cognition

Carrie requires repetition for learning and does so at a slower pace relative to her peers. She is included in English and science classes with her peers, but needs a self-contained classroom setting for math.

Carrie stopped using Sign Language completely at 5 years of age. She now has difficulties with dysfluency and articulation. However, most people understand her as long as she concentrates on what she is saying and takes her time.

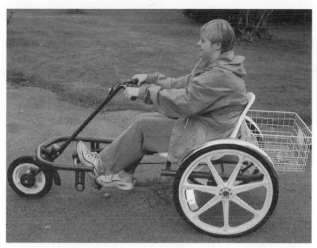

Figure 20-10 Carrie on tricycle.

Tests and Measures

Aerobic Capacity and Endurance

Carrie's involvement in sports over the years has given her a fun and social way to work on increasing her endurance. Currently, as mentioned, she is working toward her black belt in karate. Carrie currently completes a 1-mile walk-run in 14 minutes, which is slightly higher than the average for her age of 10:30 minutes (Ross, Dotson, Gilbert, & Katz, 1985). One of the criteria for achieving her black belt is to complete a 9-minute mile.

Arousal, Attention, and Cognition

Carrie's IQ is 68. She is motivated to do her best in school and in her athletic endeavors. Following auditory multi-step tasks is difficult for Carrie. She can complete the first step but often needs to ask for the latter steps to be repeated.

Circulation

Carrie monitors her pulse during exercise. She understands the need to vary the intensity of her workout to maintain her target heart rate between 65% and 80% (33 and 41 beats per 15 seconds, respectively).

She was also trained to use the Original Borg Scale (Borg, 1982) to track her perceived exertion during her exercise routines. The following are average scores for Carrie over the past year:

- Karate class: Sparring = 15
- Karate class: Kata Demonstrations = 9
- Kardio-kickboxing = 14
- Running = 16
- Weight training = 12

Gait, Locomotion, and Balance

Carrie's equilibrium is good for most basic activities requiring balance. She is able to maintain her balance during walking, running, and karate; however, intricate balancing activities are difficult for Carrie. Her current gait is characterized with excessive foot pronation during the stance phase when walking without shoes. When Carrie ambulates with her inframalleolar orthotic in her shoes, the pronation is significantly reduced. A forward head, rounded shoulders, and a pronounced kyphotic spinal column characterize Carrie's upper body positioning during ambulation and other activities.

Motor Function (Motor Control and Motor Learning)

Carrie is able to demonstrate muscle control throughout her body through extensive strength and coordination training in her karate classes.

Carrie continues to be a visual learner. She masters skills with some type of visual representation coupled with repetition.

Muscle Performance

Carrie's overall muscle strength has improved. She can move against gravity with her whole body. Muscle strength examination with a handheld dynamometer is valid and reliable for use in individuals with Down syndrome (Stemmons-Mercer & Lewis, 2001). Muscle strength for large muscle groups was evaluated with a handheld dynamometer and was as follows:

- Hip extension = 30 pounds
- Hip flexion = 28 pounds
- Hip abduction = 43 pounds
- Hip adduction = 28 pounds
- Knee extension = 56 pounds
- Knee flexion = 45 pounds

DOWN SYNDROME

- Ankle dorsiflexion = 17 pounds
- Ankle plantarflexion = 23 pounds
- Shoulder flexion = 32 pounds
- Shoulder extension = 25 pounds
- Elbow flexion = 27 pounds
- Elbow extension = 24 pounds
- Wrist flexion = 16 pounds
- Wrist extension = 12 pounds

Carrie's muscle endurance has also improved. She is able to participate in karate class for 1 hour without breaks to sit down. Three years ago, she needed to sit and rest 30 minutes into the class. Her 14-minute mile is also an improvement from her 17-minute mile 3 years ago. She walks 3 miles home from school with ease.

Range of Motion

Carrie still presents with hypermobility in her shoulders, but it does not affect her functionally.

Self-Care and Home Management

Carrie is independent with dressing and hygiene. She can cook independently in the microwave but needs supervision when using the stove.

Work, Community, and Leisure Integration

Carrie would like to achieve independent community mobility, including driving. She had difficulty learning to ride a two-wheel bike because of decreased balance and anxiousness about the task. She has an adult-sized tricycle that she rides in the driveway and is learning to ride in the street.

Carrie is aware of basic dangers to the children she tutors. She knows to keep sharp objects away from the children, to use proper body mechanics when assisting with transfers, and never to leave the children unattended.

EVALUATION, DIAGNOSIS, AND PROGNOSIS (INCLUDING PLAN OF CARE)

Carrie remains partially dependent on her family, friends, and home-waiver assistant to participate in the community. She still has difficulties in the areas of gross motor, speech, cognition, and self-help. She will continue to receive physical therapy in school because she has educationally relevant needs; however, she will also be seen in an outpatient setting to address goals that are not related to her educational needs.

Diagnosis

Carrie demonstrates impairments of motor planning attributable to her need for repetitious verbal and visual cues for multistep tasks. Muscle weakness, decreased balance, and decreased endurance make it difficult for her to complete the 9-minute mile required for karate or to ride a bike.

Prognosis

Over the course of this episode of care, it is anticipated that Carrie will demonstrate improved motor planning, balance, strength, and endurance, allowing her to achieve increased levels of independence in work, community, and leisure activities. At Carrie's present age, it is important to strive for maximal independence as she begins to transition from school to work environments.

Goals/Objectives

Carrie receives outpatient physical therapy consultation once per month in a variety of settings (i.e., home, school, recreation/gym facilities) to assist in achieving Goals 1 to 3 listed in Table 20.6. She also receives monthly physical therapy consultation at school to focus on Goal 4.

INTERVENTION

Coordination, Communication, and Documentation

Services are coordinated among home, school, and community recreation settings. Consultation services are provided in all settings to ensure that appropriate supervision can be given and Carrie will safely participate in activities. Direct communication with Carrie, her respective trainers, and school personnel is given at each site. Written material is given to Carrie to share with her parents at each monthly visit.

Table 20.6   Physical Therapy Goals for Carrie at Age 16 years

Functional Independence Goals	
1	Carrie will increase her aerobic endurance in order to run a 9-minute mile, a requirement for her karate classes.
2	Carrie will increase her balance to ride a bicycle independently on the road, following traffic rules.
3	Carrie will maintain high-level balance skills by completing the appropriate Kata for each karate level.
4	Carrie will maintain safety standards during student transfers in the classroom.

Expected outcomes of this comprehensive coordination and communication will include the following:

• Collaboration between Carrie, home, school, and the physical therapist
• Referrals to appropriate professionals when necessary

Patient/Client-Related Instruction

Carrie and her family are already discussing her transition from high school, which is anticipated in 4 years. She would like to get a certificate at the local community college to be a teacher's aide for preschoolers with special needs. She needs to remain healthy and physically fit in order to interact easily with preschoolers.

With Carrie's learning style, visual aids should be used when teaching her new tasks and reviewing learned skills.

Expected outcomes of this patient/client–related instruction will include the following:

• A plan to help her meet her transitioning goals
• Increased ability to learn new skills and tasks

Procedural Interventions

Therapeutic Exercise

Carrie attends karate class 2 to 3 times per week. She works on increasing balance, endurance, strength, and coordina-

tion during her Kata routines. Katas are series of choreographed movements that work on these areas. Sparring (staged offensive and defensive maneuvers) also helps Carrie to develop these skills. Six months ago, Carrie inquired about adding kardio-kickboxing to her regimen to get more endurance training.

Carrie also completes a strength training circuit on machines that use concentric, eccentric, and isometric muscle contractions for her arms, legs, abdominals, and back muscles. She focuses on her weaker muscle groups: triceps, rhomboids, trapezius, latissimus dorsi, deltoid, pectoralis major, rectus abdominis, gluteus maximus, hip adductors, and tibialis anterior. Carrie's trainer at the gym immediately relays any changes in weight, repetitions, or sets of this routine to the physical therapist.

Expected outcomes of these therapeutic exercises are:

• Increased balance and coordination
• Increased neuromotor development
• Increased strength
• Increased endurance
• Maintenance of health and physical condition

Functional Training in Work, Community, and Leisure Integration

Transfer techniques are reviewed with Carrie monthly so that she can assist with transfers in the preschool classroom. Body mechanics, specific scenarios, and emergency procedures are demonstrated to Carrie. She is then required to repeat the specific steps from memory.

Carrie loves water sports. Recommendations will be made that she alternate between kardio-kickboxing and water aerobics for variety.

Expected outcomes of functional training in work, community, and leisure integration are that Carrie will:

• Maintain safety standards during transfers at a preschool work setting
• Vary endurance and strength training activities to keep interest level high

TERMINATION OF EPISODE OF CARE

Carrie will be discharged from outpatient physical therapy when she functions within her home, school, and community in an independent and safe manner, meeting all of her

DOWN SYNDROME

goals. Other situations that may change Carrie's physical therapy episode of care are a change in the status of her Graves' disease, medical complications, a decision by Carrie or her caregiver to terminate services, or Carrie no longer benefitting from the services.

Carrie and her family, along with her medical professionals, will review annually the need for outpatient physical therapy. As Carrie becomes older, her weight and physical endurance will continue to be struggles for her. The physical therapist's role is to help Carrie with prevention activities and continue her exercise programs in a safe manner to address these areas of need.

Carrie has an established diagnosis of Down syndrome and has the right to receive educationally based services from her local school district until the age of 21 years, as long as she has difficulty functioning independently within the education setting.

DISCUSSION QUESTIONS

1. What are some common characteristics of the gait pattern of a child with Down syndrome?

2. At what ages might a child with Down syndrome benefit the most from physical therapy intervention?

3. What might be the role of the physical therapist during transition periods (early intervention to preschool, preschool to school, and high school to work) in the life of a child with Down syndrome?

4. Discuss appropriate recreational activities for children with Down syndrome at different ages.

REFERENCES

American Physical Therapy Association (2001). *Guide to physical therapist practice* (2nd ed). *Physical Therapy, 81*(1), 6–746.

Connolly, B.H., & Michael, B.T. (1986). Performance of retarded children, with and without Down syndrome, on the Bruininks-Oseretsky Test of Motor Proficiency. *Physical Therapy, 66*(3), 344–348.

Borg, G.V. (1982). Psychological basis of perceived exertion. *Medicine and Science in Sports and Exercise, 14*, 377–381.

Granger, C., Braun, S., Griswood, K., Heyer, N., McCabe, M., Msau, M., et al. (1991). *Functional independence measure for children.* Buffalo, NY: Medical Rehabilitation, State University of New York, Research Foundation.

Haley, S.M., Coster, W.J., Ludlow, I.H., Haltiwanger, J.T., & Andrellos, P. (1992). *Pediatric Evaluation of Disability Inventory.* Boston, MA: Department of Rehabilitation Medicine, New England Medical Center Hospital.

Johnson-Martin, N.M., Jens, K.A., Attermeier, S.N., & Hacker, B.J. (1991). *Carolina Curriculum for Infants and Toddlers with Special Needs* (2nd ed.). Baltimore: Paul H. Brookes.

Pueschel, S.M., & Bier, J.A. (1992). Endocrinologic aspects. In S.M. Pueschel & J.K. Pueschel (Eds.), *Biomedical concerns in persons with Down syndrome* (pp. 259–272). Baltimore: Paul H. Brookes.

Ross, J.G., Dotson, C.O., Gilbert, C.G., & Katz, S.J. (1985). The National Youth and Fitness Study. 1: New standards for fitness measurement. *Journal of Physical Education, Recreation and Dance, 56*, 62–66.

Shea, A.M. (1991). Motor attainments in Down syndrome. In M.J. Lister (Ed.), *Contemporary management of motor control problems: Proceeding of the II STEP conference* (pp. 225–236). Alexandria, VA: Foundation for Physical Therapy.

Stemmons-Mercer, V., & Lewis, C.L. (2001). Hip abductor and knee extensor muscle strength of children with and without Down syndrome. *Pediatric Physical Therapy, 13*(1), 18–26.

Zausmer, E., & Shea, A. (1984). Motor development. In S.M. Pueschel (Ed.), *The young child with Down syndrome* (pp. 143–206). New York: Human Sciences Press, Inc.

Chapter *21*

Case Study: Pediatric Leukemia

— Victoria Gocha Marchese, PT, PhD

Each year in the United States, approximately 12,400 children and adolescents younger than 20 years are diagnosed with cancer, and leukemia accounts for 25% of these childhood cancer cases (Ries et al., 1999). The diagnostic groups and specific diagnoses of pediatric leukemia are outlined in Table 21.1.

Medical intervention for children with leukemia varies according to the type of leukemia and the protocol. There are specific protocols that each medical institution uses to guide the drugs and dosages that children will receive. All children with leukemia receive chemotherapy. If a child with acute lymphoblastic leukemia (ALL) has a relapse, meaning that the cancer has returned, a stem cell transplant (SCT) or bone marrow transplant (BMT) is typically administered. Children with acute myeloid leukemia (AML) often receive chemotherapy for a few months and then receive a BMT or SCT. SCT includes only the most immature type of cell, given before the cell has differentiated to a specific type. BMT involves administering marrow, including all types of cells. The protocols for children with leukemia include some or all of the following phases:

1. *Induction,* which lasts approximately 4 to 6 weeks. High doses of a combination of chemotherapy agents are given to eliminate the leukemia cells, with the goal of achieving remission.

2. The *consolidation* and *intensification phases,* which last 1 to 2 months and are periods during which high

doses of chemotherapy are given to eliminate any remaining cancerous cells.

3. *Maintenance therapy,* which for children with ALL lasts approximately 2 calendar years for girls and 3 calendar years for boys. Low doses of chemotherapy are given with the goal of preventing relapse.

4. *BMT* or *SCT,* which is performed after a child has received chemotherapy. Children are admitted to the hospital approximately 1 week before receiving the transplant for what is called *conditioning.* This is the time when children receive chemotherapy agents, such as thiotepa or Cytoxan, and total body irradiation with the goal of depressing their bone marrow. During this period, the children are at risk for infection, bruising, and fatigue.

Certain chemotherapy agents cause secondary complications such as myelosuppression, peripheral neuropathy, myopathy, and osteonecrosis. Myelosuppression is a process in which bone marrow activity is inhibited, resulting in decreased production of platelets, red blood cells (RBCs), and white blood cells (WBCs), thus increasing the risk for bleeding, anemia, and infection. Vincristine is a chemotherapy agent known to cause peripheral neuropathy, affecting primarily ankle dorsiflexion and the intrinsic musculature of the feet and hands (Vanionpaa, 1993). Studies have identified that children who receive vincristine are susceptible to decreased ankle dorsiflexion

TABLE 21.1 Common Types of Pediatric Leukemia

Lymphoid Leukemia	Nonlymphoid Leukemia
• Accounts for 75% of all childhood leukemia cases	• Accounts for 19% of all childhood leukemia cases
Acute lymphoblastic leukemia (ALL) • Accounts for 99% of the lymphoid leukemias • Nearly 80% survival rate for children older than 1 year and younger than 10 years of age. Infant and adolescent survival rates are not as favorable.	Acute myeloid leukemia (AML) • Accounts for 69% of the nonlymphoid leukemias • Approximately 40% survival rate

Source: Ries, L.A.G., Smith, M.A., Gurney, J.G., Linet, M., Tamra, T., Young, J.L., & Bunin, G.R. (Eds). (1999). *Cancer incidence and survival among children and adolescents: United States SEER program 1975–1997.* Bethesda, MD: National Cancer Institute, SEER Program. NIH Pub. No. 99–4649.

active range of motion (AROM) and strength (Marchese, Chiarello, & Lange, 2003; Marchese, Chiarello, & Lange, 2004; Wright, Halton, & Barr, 1999). Dexamethasone and prednisone may cause proximal muscle weakness and osteonecrosis (DeAngelis, Gnecco, Taylor, & Warrell, 1991; Mattano, Sather, Trigg, & Nachman, 2000). Methotrexate is another chemotherapy agent that interferes with skeletal growth and causes osteoporosis and fractures, primarily in the lower extremities (Schwartz & Leonidas, 1984).

Physical therapists receive consultations for children with cancer for many reasons. A child may have decreased active and passive ankle dorsiflexion range of motion (ROM), reduction in muscle strength, pain, delayed gross motor development, limited functional mobility requiring an assistive device such as crutches, and decreased participation in school, social activities, or sports functions because of fatigue. Considering that children with cancer are at risk for blood levels that are below normal, the physical therapist must be cognizant of these numbers and modify the examination and interventions accordingly. See Tables 21.2 and 21.3 for examples of exercise guidelines.

CASE STUDY

This case study focuses on the physical therapy management of a 6-year-old girl, Claire, who has ALL. The medical management of her disease may result in the secondary complications discussed earlier, which may negatively affect her motor function.

Based on the side effects of chemotherapy, deconditioning secondary to several months of chemotherapy, and Claire's inability to keep up with her peers at school, the American Physical Therapy Association's *Guide to physical therapist practice* (APTA, 2001) Preferred Practice Pattern 6B: Impaired Aerobic Capacity/Endurance Associated with Deconditioning was chosen.

EXAMINATION: AGE 6 YEARS

History

Claire was a healthy 6-year-old girl when diagnosed 10 months earlier with ALL. A lumbar puncture identified

TABLE 21.2 Exercise Guidelines Used by the Physical Therapists at The Children's Hospital of Philadelphia for Children Before and After Bone Marrow Transplantation

Platelet Counts	Recommended Activity Level
>50,000/mm^3	Resistive exercises (e.g., weights and exercise bands)
10,000–50,000/mm^3	Active exercise (e.g., riding a stationary bike, walking, and performing squats while playing)
<10,000/mm^3	Active and passive range of motion, gentle stretching, and light exercise (e.g., shooting hoops)

TABLE 21.3 American Physical Therapy Association Acute Care Clinical Practice Section Exercise Guidelines

Parameter	No Exercise	Light Exercise	Resistive Exercise
White blood cells (/mm^3)	<5,000 with fever	>5,000^3	>5,000 (as tolerated)
Platelets (mm^3)	<20,000/mm^3	20,000–50,000	>50,000
Hemoglobin (g/100 mm)	<8	8–10	>10
Hct	<25%	25–30%	>30%

Source: Garritan, S., Jones, P., Kornberg, T., and Parkin, C. (1995). Laboratory values in the intensive care unit. *Acute Care Perspectives, The Newsletter of the Acute Care/Hospital Clinical Practice Section of the American Physical Therapy Association,* p.10. Adapted with permission.

central nervous system (CNS) disease in the cerebrospinal fluid. Claire is receiving medical treatment according to the Children's Cancer Group (CCG) protocol. She is in the maintenance phase of her medical intervention, with 3 months of chemotherapy remaining. Claire has a central line, called a Broviac. The indwelling catheter is under the skin just below the clavicle and enters into a major vein of the heart. Central lines, such as a Port-a-Cath, Hickman, or Broviac, are used for the administration of chemotherapy agents and for withdrawing blood. These catheters are used because they decrease frequent needle sticks and allow large doses of toxic medication to be delivered. However, there are risks of infection and the formation of clots in the line.

Claire's medical treatment has included craniospinal irradiation and a combination of the following chemotherapy agents: vincristine, L-asparaginase, prednisone, mercaptopurine, dexamethasone, doxorubicin, cyclophosphamide, thioguanine, intrathecal (administered directly into the cerebrospinal fluid), cytosine arabinoside (ara-C), and methotrexate.

Claire has no significant past medical history and has achieved age-appropriate motor milestones. She lives with her mother and 8-year-old brother in a two-story home. Her father is involved in Claire's care; however, he lives in another state. Claire is in the first grade and enjoys roller skating, bike riding, coloring, and playing with her friends in the neighborhood.

Claire was referred to outpatient physical therapy because she was tripping at the end of the day and twisted her ankle twice while roller skating. Her mother noticed her daughter not running as smoothly and not keeping up with the other children. Claire's goals were to keep up with her friends and to regain her roller-skating skills. Her mother's goals were for Claire to avoid a serious fall and to return to her previous level of function. She also expressed concern with her daughter's ability to focus on tasks for a long period of time.

Systems Review

Cardiovascular and Pulmonary

Heart rate, respiratory rate, blood pressure, and temperature are all within normal limits (WNL).

Integumentary

The skin around Claire's central line is clean and dry. No other skin problems are noted.

Musculoskeletal

Claire presents with decreased active and passive ROM in her ankles and decreased strength in her lower extremities.

Neuromuscular

Deep tendon reflexes are decreased at the patellar and Achilles tendons. Vision, auditory, and other sensations are WNL.

Communication, Affect, Cognition, Language, and Learning Style

Claire's communication skills are WNL. Cognitive, language, and learning skills were recommended for examination by a psychologist.

Tests and Measures

Before beginning further specific tests and measures in the examination process, it is important to review Claire's blood count levels. The day of the physical therapy examination, Claire's blood counts were WNL (WBCs, 6,000 [normal range, 5,000 to 13,000]; RBCs, 4.2 [normal range, 4.1 to 5.70]; hemoglobin, 13 [normal range, 11.0 to 16.0]; and platelets, 200,000 [normal range, 140,000 to 450,000]).

Aerobic Capacity and Endurance

Claire performed the 9-minute walk-run test, a measure of maximal functional capacity and endurance of the cardiorespiratory system, completing 650 yards. This score places her below the 5th percentile for her age and gender (American Alliance for Health, Physical Education, Recreation, and Dance, 1980). Claire's heart rate was 88 beats per minute (bpm) at rest and ranged from 145 to 160 bpm during the 9-minute walk-run test. Claire did not demonstrate any nasal flaring or increased work of breathing.

Gait, Locomotion, and Balance

Claire walks and runs independently in a variety of environmental settings. Gait was characterized by a mild steppage pattern and flatfoot at initial contact caused by her limitations in ankle dorsiflexion active ROM and strength. While Claire was running, the therapist noted increased upper body rotation and decreased flight phase (time when both feet were off the floor). Within the first 5 minutes of performing the 9-minute walk-run test, Claire caught her left toe on the ground twice. She was able to catch herself independently, thus avoiding a fall to the ground. However, during the final minute of the 9-minute walk-run test, Claire was running and again caught her left toe on the ground and fell without injury.

She can start and stop ambulation on cue without extra steps and perform a dual task, such as walking on grass for 50 feet while answering math problems. She turned 180°

without loss of balance. Claire performed single-limb stance on the left foot for 8 seconds and the right foot for 11 seconds. She was unable to tandem walk on a 3-inch balance beam without loss of balance.

Motor Function

Claire independently transitioned from ring-sitting to standing position and from standing to sitting on the floor, requiring the use of her upper extremities. She independently ascended and descended 12 steps with the use of a rail within 10 seconds, placing one foot on a step at a time.

Muscle Performance

Claire presented with upper extremity strength grossly WNL (5/5) and bilateral lower extremity strength 5/5, except for bilateral hip flexion (4/5), knee flexion and extension (4/5), and bilateral ankle dorsiflexion (3+/5), within Claire's available active ROM. Considering that Claire is 6 years old and follows directions very well, manual muscle testing and hand-held dynamometry measurements were performed. Dynamometry testing in children 6 years of age is a reliable and valid outcome measure (Backman, Odenrick, Henriksson, & Ledin, 1989; Marchese et al., 2003; Stuberg & Metcalf, 1988). Hand-held dynamometer measurements identified that Claire's left ankle dorsiflexion strength was 1.7 kg, and on the right ankle it was 2.2 kg. According to Backman and colleagues (1989), ankle dorsiflexion strength for a girl 5.5 to 7 years of age should be 12.6 kg.

Claire performed 4 sit-ups in 60 seconds, placing her below the 5th percentile for her age (American Alliance for Health, Physical Education, Recreation and Dance, 1980). She performed bilateral heel rises five times in standing position, using her upper extremities to assist with balance.

Pain

The Faces Pain Scale (FPS) was used to document Claire's pain level (Wong & Baker, 1988). This scale has 6 pictures of faces, ranging from 0 with a very happy face to 6 with a crying face. The FPS is typically used for children 3 to 7 years of age. Claire reported a dull ache in her ankles and rated the pain as 4 on the FPS. This pain occurred after Claire walked long distances or played in the yard. She also reported pain of 3 in the proximal muscles in her legs.

Range of Motion

Claire presented with full active ROM in all extremities, except ankle dorsiflexion active and passive ROM. She achieved actively 2° of left ankle dorsiflexion with her knee extended, and 3° on the right. Passive ankle dorsiflexion with her knee extended on the left was 6°, and 8° on the right. With the knee flexed, Claire achieved active dorsiflexion on the left 6° and right 7°; passively, left 7° and right 9°.

Self-Care and Home Management (Including Activities of Daily Living)

Claire is independent with activities of daily living such as brushing her teeth and dressing herself. Claire's mother carries her daughter upstairs (11 stairs) to bed at least 3 nights a week because Claire reports her legs hurt too badly, and she is too tired.

Work, Community, and Leisure

Claire rides the bus to school. She holds the bus driver's hand and a rail while ascending the bus steps. All of Claire's classes are on the first floor except music and art, which are on the second floor. The school's principal has expressed concern about Claire's ability to climb the school steps. On two occasions, Claire tripped while ascending the steps and bruised her knee. The school nurse reported seeing Claire three times this year for falling on the playground. During gym class, the teacher reported that Claire was not included in play activities and cried numerous times because of not keeping up with her friends while running. She also frequently misses school because of physician appointments and not feeling well.

EVALUATION, DIAGNOSIS, AND PROGNOSIS (INCLUDING PLAN OF CARE)

Evaluation

Claire is a cooperative, sociable, and active little girl with great family support. She presents with pain in her proximal and distal lower extremities, decreased active and passive ankle dorsiflexion ROM, decreased lower extremity muscle strength, decreased endurance, decreased high-level gross motor skills, and limitations in participation in school recess, gym class, and neighborhood activities.

Diagnosis

Claire's diagnosis consists of pain, impaired ankle ROM, impaired lower extremity strength, and impaired endurance. These impairments contribute to functional limitations in her gait pattern and ability to participate in school and neighborhood activities.

Prognosis

Claire has a good prognosis from a medical standpoint. Through stretching, strengthening, aerobic conditioning, and family consultation, she has a good prognosis to demonstrate improvements in motor functional activity and participate fully in school and community activities.

The recommended frequency of physical therapy is 3 times per week for the first week, 2 times per week for the second week, and 1 time during the third week, followed by 3 months of monthly physical therapy sessions to advance Claire's home program.

Goals

1. Increase right and left active ankle dorsiflexion ROM to WNL.

2. Increase lower extremity strength to 5/5 so that Claire can ascend and descend the school bus stairs independently without holding the railing.

3. Increase endurance so that Claire is able to keep up with her peers in school and her neighborhood and does not demonstrate signs of fatigue such as sitting down or becoming short of breath.

INTERVENTION

Coordination, Communication, and Documentation

Communication and coordination of activities with Claire and her parents, nurses, physician, schoolteacher, and gym coach are important. Communication with Claire's physician confirmed that she did not have osteonecrosis in the sites where she complained of pain. Frequency and duration of physical therapy services were also discussed with her insurance company. Recommendations were made for referral to a psychologist for further evaluation of Claire's limited attention span.

Clear documentation of Claire's physical therapy management and outcomes is important to measure progress and to assist in modifying the intervention program. A notebook was used to send suggestions to school personnel.

The expected outcomes of effective coordination, communication, and documentation of services are improved collaboration with all individuals working with Claire; coordination of care with Claire, her family, and other health-care professionals; and assurance that appropriate referrals are made to other care providers as necessary.

Patient/Client-Related Instruction

Claire, her parents, and school personnel were informed regarding Claire's present status, including strength and ROM limitations. Common side effects of medications influencing motor performance were discussed, and a plan of care was developed to address impaired strength and ROM. Health, wellness, and fitness programs were also discussed, with emphasis on aerobic activity for someone

with Claire's health problems. The plan of care is summarized in Table 21.4.

The expected outcomes of the patient/client-related instruction are improved physical function and health status; improved safety in home, school, and community settings: and decreased risk of secondary impairments (Figure 21–1).

Procedural Interventions

Therapeutic Exercise

Aerobic capacity/endurance conditioning activities focused on bike riding and roller skating, which were Claire's activity selections. While Claire was in the physical therapy clinic, the therapist assisted her in determining her level of exercise intensity when performing her aerobic activities at home. Heart rate and rate of perceived exertion were monitored during bike riding and roller skating while working at 70% of her maximum heart rate. Claire roller skated with kneepads, elbow pads, and a helmet in the physical therapy clinic and while at home with her mother present. The skates laced up tightly over Claire's ankles, providing stability and deep pressure. She skated continuously for 20 minutes with her heart rate between 65% and 70% of her maximum without complaints of ankle pain.

Strengthening exercises were performed on the lower

TABLE 21.4 Summary of Plan of Care

Area of Focus	Activity	Frequency	Comments
Stretching	• Ankle dorsiflexion stretch with a towel	• 1 repetition holding for 30 seconds, 5 times per week	• This exercise can be performed in standing lunge position with shoes on to support the arch. • Emphasis on form and proper body alignment while stretching to prevent secondary complications.
Strengthening	• Squatting to pick up a large ball and toss overhead/mid-chest/underhand • Ankle pumps in the bathtub • Jumping (like a frog)	• 20 repetitions, 3 sets, 3 times per week • 20 repetitions, 3 sets, 3 times per week • 20 feet, 3 sets, 3 times per week	• Other activities the child enjoys may be performed to accomplish strengthening of the trunk, and upper and lower extremities.
Aerobic exercise	• Bike riding • Roller-skating	• 30 minutes daily	• Perform the aerobic activity continuously even if it requires slowing down.

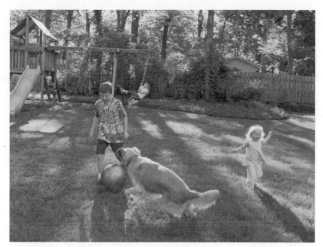

Figure 21-1 After 3 years of long and difficult treatments for acute lymphoblastic leukemia, 10-year-old Devin, who had the same diagnosis and course of treatment as Claire, enjoys a healthy life and playing outside with his sister.

extremities. These exercises included Claire tapping her feet to music, heel walking, and ankle dorsiflexion with resistance (offered by water or the therapist's hand). Outcomes of the flexibility and strengthening program were monitored with goniometric measurements and dynamometry of lower extremity strength.

Manual Therapy

Passive ROM yielded improved ankle joint mobility. This intervention contributed to improved balance and coordination when Claire was walking in the home, school, and community settings.

Gentle massage of Claire's proximal and distal lower extremities was performed to assist with pain relief. It was also recommended that Claire wear sneakers versus sandals to help with foot alignment and support, with the expectation of increasing safety during gait and decreasing pain.

TERMINATION OF EPISODE OF CARE

Claire was discharged after 4 months of physical therapy. Her active ankle dorsiflexion ROM on the left had increased from 2° to 10°, and on the right from 3° to 14°. Her bilateral lower extremity strength was grossly 5/5, except for bilateral ankle dorsiflexion, which was 4/5. She increased the distance traveled on the 9-minute walk-run by 100 yards from 650 to 750 yards, placing her performance in the 5th percentile. Claire also increased her number

of sit-ups performed in 60 seconds from 4 to 6, placing her in the 5th percentile. Claire did not require her mother's assistance to go up the steps in her home. Her teacher reported no incidences of tripping at school. Most important, Claire reported to her mother and teachers that she felt bigger and stronger and that she could keep up with her friends.

With her increased ankle ROM and lower-extremity strength, Claire decreased her chances of falling, thus preventing a possible fracture. Progression of further ROM limitations was prevented, which could have required surgical intervention. Claire's overall physical wellness and her family's awareness of their daughter's general physical abilities increased.

Claire and her family were also made aware of what issues might trigger a need for additional physical therapy services. Long-term side effects from Claire's medical treatment may include the following: a lower-extremity fracture from the radiation and chemotherapy agents, especially methotrexate; osteonecrosis from the steroids; musculoskeletal pain, especially in the ankles from the peripheral neuropathy caused by the chemotherapy agent vincristine; and obesity caused by irradiation. It would not be unusual for Claire to develop a secondary cancer as a progression of her original disease.

DISCUSSION QUESTIONS

1. Explain why Claire is a good candidate for ankle-foot orthoses.

2. What were the possible reasons why the physical therapist did not fit Claire for lower-extremity orthotics?

3. Describe the types of difficulties Claire is at risk for in the future.

4. List three of Claire's physical, family, and environmental characteristics that will guide her into a healthy and happy young-adult life.

5. What are a few questions a physical therapist must consider before providing physical therapy services to a child with cancer?

REFERENCES

American Alliance for Health, Physical Education, Recreation, and Dance (1980). *Health related physical fitness test manual.* Reston, VA: American Alliance for Health, Physical Education, Recreation, and Dance.

PEDIATRIC LEUKEMIA

American Physical Therapy Association (APTA) (2001). *Guide to physical therapist practice* (2nd ed.). *Physical Therapy, 81*, 6–746.

Backman, E., Odenrick, P., Henriksson, K.G., & Ledin, T. (1989). Isometric muscle force and anthropometric values in normal children aged between 3.5 and 15 years. *Scandinavian Journal of Rehabilitation Medicine, 21*, 105–114.

DeAngelis, L.M., Gnecco, C., Taylor, L., & Warrell, R.P. (1991). Evolution of neuropathy and myopathy during intensive vincristine/corticosteroid chemotherapy for non-Hodgkin's lymphoma. *Cancer, 67*, 2241–2246.

Marchese, V.G., Chiarello, L.A., & Lange, B.J. (2003). Strength and functional mobility in children with acute lymphoblastic leukemia. *Medical and Pediatric Oncology, 40*(4), 230–232.

Marchese, V.G., Chiarello, L.A., & Lange, B.J. (2004). Effects of physical therapy intervention for children with acute lymphoblastic leukemia. *Pediatric Blood and Cancer, 42*(2), 127–133.

Mattano, L.A., Sather, H.N., Trigg, M.E., & Nachman, J.B. (2000). Osteonecrosis is a complication of treating acute lymphoblastic leukemia in children: A report from the children's cancer group. *Journal of Clinical Oncology, 18*(18), 3262–3272.

Ries, L.A.G., Smith, M.A., Gurney, J.G., Linet, M., Tamra, T., Young, J.L., & Bunin, G.R. (Eds). (1999). *Cancer incidence and survival among children and adolescents: United States SEER program 1975–1997.* Bethesda, MD: National Cancer Institute, SEER Program. NIH Pub. No. 99–4649.

Schwartz, A.M., & Leonidas, J.C. (1984). Methotrexate osteopathy. *Radiology, 11*, 13–16.

Stuberg, W.A., & Metcalf, W.K. (1988). Reliability of quantitative muscle testing in healthy children and in children with Duchenne muscular dystrophy using a hand-held dynamometer. *Physical Therapy, 68*(6), 977–982.

Vanionpaa, L. (1993). Clinical neurological findings of children with acute lymphoblastic leukemia at diagnosis and during treatment. *European Journal of Pediatrics, 152*, 115–119.

Wong, B.L., & Baker, C.M. (1988). Pain in children: Comparison of assessment scales. *Pediatric Nursing, 14*(1), 9–17.

Wright, M.J., Halton, J.M., & Barr, R.D. (1999). Limitations of ankle range of motion in survivors of acute lymphoblastic leukemia: A cross-sectional study. *Medical and Pediatric Oncology, 32*, 279–282.

Chapter *22*

Case Study: Duchenne Muscular Dystrophy

— Shree Devi Pandya, PT, MS

As physical therapists, we are routinely involved in the care of children with inherited neuromuscular disorders. The most common disorders that we are likely to encounter are Duchenne muscular dystrophy (DMD), a muscle disorder; spinal muscular atrophy (SMA), an anterior horn cell disorder; Charcot-Marie-Tooth disease (CMT), a neuropathic disorder; and many other congenital and/or pediatric forms of muscular dystrophies and neuropathies. There is a wide variation in impairments of body structures and functions, secondary complications, natural history/prognosis, and medical management of these disorders. The common elements among all these disorders are (1) the etiology (they are all genetic/inherited disorders); (2) they are progressive; (3) the primary impairment is muscle weakness, resulting in difficulties with functional activities; and (4) secondary complications resulting in increased morbidity and mortality.

We provide services for children with these disorders in various settings, including home, daycare, school, and outpatient clinics, as well as in the hospital. Our roles and responsibilities vary according to the setting. We may be involved as team members in a multidisciplinary specialty clinic, providing evaluations and recommendations over extended periods of time. As members of the team at school, our main roles may be those of consultant, educator, and coordinator, facilitating the provision of services and transitions within the school system. We may be involved with specific episodes of care after surgical inter-

ventions, or in the provision of and training regarding braces, wheelchairs, and so on.

In this chapter, using a case study of a boy with DMD, the knowledge and processes necessary to arrive at evidence-based treatment decisions and management plans will be illustrated using elements from the American Physical Therapy Association's *Guide to physical therapist practice* (APTA, 2001). The *ICD-9-CM* code for inherited progressive muscular dystrophies is 359; for SMA, it is 335; and for hereditary peripheral neuropathies, it is 356. Practice patterns for examination, evaluation, and intervention can be found in the *Guide* (APTA, 2001) under all four systems to meet the varying needs of these children. Some common examples include 4C, Impaired Muscle Performance; 5G, Impaired Motor Function and Sensory Integrity Associated with Acute or Chronic Polyneuropathies; 6B, Impaired Aerobic Capacity and Endurance Associated with Deconditioning; and 6E, Impaired Ventilation/Respiration Gas Exchange Associated with Ventilatory Pump Dysfunction.

DMD is the most common inherited muscle disease of childhood. It is an **X-linked inherited disorder** with an incidence of 1:3500 male births (Emery, 1991). A third of the cases arise from new mutations and therefore may not have a family history of the disorder. The condition was first described in the late 1800s (Duchenne, 1868; Gowers, 1879), but the gene lesion was discovered in 1985 (Kunkel, Monaco, Middlesworth, Ochs, & Latt, 1985) and the protein product was described in 1987 (Hoffman, Brown,

DUCHENNE MUSCULAR DYSTROPHY

& Kunkel, 1987). The mutation is located on the short arm of the X chromosome in the Xp-21 region, affecting the gene that codes for a protein termed dystrophin. Boys with DMD have an absence of **dystrophin**, a protein normally expressed in skeletal muscle, smooth muscle, and the brain. In the skeletal muscle, dystrophin is located in the sarcolemmal membrane, and is believed to play a role in maintaining the integrity of the muscle fibers. One hypothesis is that the absence of dystrophin and associated structural proteins leads to a breakdown of muscle fibers, resulting in progressive weakness and loss of function.

Even though DMD is an inherited disorder and the gene defect is present from birth, most boys do not come to medical attention until age 3 to 7 years unless there is a family history of the disorder. Early motor milestones, such as rolling, sitting, and walking, are usually achieved at expected ages. The symptoms that cause parents to seek medical attention for their son include difficulty running, jumping, climbing stairs, and keeping up with peers in physical education class or on the playground. The *primary impairment* causing limitations in activities in DMD is weakness. The weakness does not affect all muscles similarly, but has a very specific pattern of distribution and progression. The natural history of progression of weakness in DMD has been well documented by the Clinical Investigation of Duchenne Dystrophy (CIDD) Group (Brooke et al., 1983). More than 100 boys aged 5 to 15 years were followed for longer than a year in this multicenter study. Pertinent findings from this study are described.

Weakness of neck flexors is present very early, and the child has difficulty attempting a sit-up. The next group of muscles to demonstrate weakness are the pelvic girdle muscles (hip extensors and abductors) and the quadriceps, resulting in the need to use **Gowers' maneuver,** or the use of the hands to push up from the floor and onto the legs to get into an upright position (Figure 22–1). Progressive weakness of the lower-limb muscles eventually results in the loss of ability to walk independently by age 12 years. Weakness of the shoulder girdle muscles results in difficulty with overhead activities by the early teens. Eventually distal muscles of the upper extremities are involved, too, leading to difficulty with feeding, grooming, and writing. The muscles that are notably spared are the gastrocsoleus muscles. It should also be noted that the facial and eye muscles, the muscles involved in speech and swallowing, and the sphincters are not involved in DMD.

The early pattern of unequal muscle weakness (extensors worse than flexors) leads to muscle imbalance at a given joint, resulting in the *secondary problem* of the development of tightness and contractures. In the CIDD study, contrac-

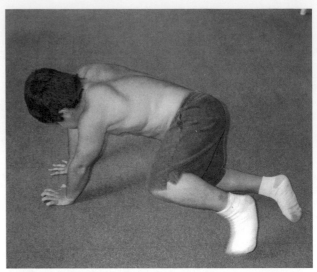

Figure 22-1 Child with Duchenne muscular dystrophy getting up from the floor using Gowers' maneuver.

tures at the ankles and hips attributable to tightness in the gastrocsoleus, the iliotibial band/tensor fasciae latae (ITB/TFL), and the hip flexors were present by age 6 years. Contractures at the knee caused by tightness of the hamstrings and at the elbows and wrists caused by elbow flexor and wrist flexor tightness were present by age 9 years. The contractures at the hips, knees, elbows, and wrists worsen as the child spends increasing amounts of time in a wheelchair. The weakness and the contractures contribute to restrictions in activities and participation. Between the ages of 8 and 10 years, more than 50% of the boys in the CIDD study had lost the ability to get up from the floor or climb stairs. Several worldwide studies have documented loss of independent walking between the ages of 8 and 12 years (Emery, 2003). As the boys start spending an increasing amount of time in a wheelchair, the development of scoliosis becomes a major concern. More than 80% of the boys develop significant scoliosis by their late teens. Several factors are hypothesized to contribute to the development of scoliosis, including unequal trunk muscle involvement, handedness, loss of normal lordosis with increased sitting, and so on. The increasing scoliosis can affect pulmonary function, comfort in sitting, and the use of upper extremities for functional activities. With the loss of standing, the risk of increased osteopenia, especially in the lower extremities, leads to a concern about fractures.

Muscles of respiration and the cardiac muscle are also involved in DMD. Involvement of the respiratory muscles results in lower than normal respiratory function during the first decade and a gradual decline in respiratory function in the second decade (Rideau, Jankowski, & Grellet, 1981). With decreased respiratory reserves, even a simple cold can lead to severe respiratory problems. More than 70% of the boys with DMD die as a result of pulmonary complications (Emery, 2003). Involvement of the cardiac muscle results in cardiomyopathy, and even though almost all boys have a certain amount of cardiac involvement, the severity of the problem varies greatly. Less than 30% of boys die as a result of cardiac complications. In addition to the respiratory and cardiac muscles, the smooth muscle in the gastrointestinal (GI) tract is involved. This causes GI motility problems, especially in the later stages of the disease, resulting in problems with constipation and impaction. The exact role of dystrophin in the brain is not well understood, but almost 30% of boys with DMD have learning problems and require evaluation and related services in the school setting (Dubowitz, 1995).

Over the past two decades, not only have major advances occurred in our understanding of the genetics, pathophysiology, and natural history of DMD, but major advances have also occurred in the medical, surgical, and rehabilitation interventions available for children with DMD. An aggressive program that includes daily stretching, functional activities, swimming, bracing with knee-ankle-foot orthoses (KAFOs), and contracture release surgery helps prolong walking for up to 3 years and standing thereafter for up to another 2 years (Brooke et al., 1989; Harris & Cherry, 1974; Heckmatt, Dubowitz, & Hyde, 1985; Vignos, Wagner, Karlinchak, & Katirji, 1996). Prolonged walking and standing delay the development of contractures and scoliosis. Correction of scoliosis and spinal stabilization with the Luque procedure (Luque, 1982) delays decline in pulmonary function (Galasko, Delaney, & Morris, 1992), improves sitting comfort, and allows continued use of the upper extremities for functional activities (Miller, Moseley, & Koreska, 1992). Greater use of noninvasive mechanical ventilation has had an impact on life expectancy. The mean age of death in the 1960s was 14.4 years; whereas, since the 1990s, it is about 25.3 years for those who chose ventilation (Eagle et al., 2002).

The use of corticosteroids, prednisone and deflazacort, is also changing the natural history/prognosis of DMD. The effects of both medications have been well documented in several short-term, randomized, controlled trials (Angelini et al., 1994; Backman & Henriksson, 1995; Griggs et al., 1991, 1993; Mendell el al., 1989; Mesa, Dubrovsky, Corderi, Maarco, & Flores,1991). Corticosteroids improve muscle mass, strength, and function within the first 6 months of treatment. With continued treatment, the improvement is maintained for up to 18 months (Griggs et al., 1993), and the subsequent decline is slower than predicted (Fenichel et al., 1991). Delays in the loss of independent ambulation and decline in pulmonary function are documented by several open follow-up studies of cohorts (Biggar, Gingras, Feblings, Harris, & Steele, 2001; DeSilva, Drachman, Mellits, & Kunel, 1987; Pandya & Moxley, 2002; Schara, Mortier, & Mortier, 2001). The impact of corticosteroids on the development of scoliosis, progression of cardiomyopathy and on mortality continues to be monitored. Based on the benefits documented to date, corticosteroids are now recommended as a treatment in the management of children with DMD (Manzur, Kuntzer, Pike, & Swan, 2004; Wong & Christopher, 2002). Even though this disorder remains "incurable," the available supportive and symptomatic interventions have had a great impact on the life span and quality of life. These advances are changing the description of this disorder from "fatal" to "chronic."

CASE STUDY

This case study of a boy with DMD illustrates (1) the long-term approach to the management and care of children with inherited neuromuscular disorders; (2) the role of the physical therapist as a member of a multidisciplinary team of care providers; and (3) an evidence-based approach to management and intervention that integrates the best research evidence with clinical expertise and child/family preferences. To give the reader an appreciation of the issues encountered in the long-term management of children, this case covers a follow-up period of almost 15 years. For the sake of brevity, not all encounters are presented, and within the visits described, not all elements from the *Guide* (APTA, 2001) are covered. Only highlights of specific elements pertinent to that encounter are provided.

Sam was referred to a Muscular Dystrophy Association (MDA)-funded clinic in July 1990 at age 5 years. The core team at this clinic included a pediatric neurologist, an orthopedist, a nurse, and a physical therapist. Access to other specialists, such as genetic counselors, dieticians, occupational therapists, orthotists, pulmonologists, respiratory therapists, and cardiologists, was available as necessary. The role of the physical therapist in this specific clinic also included coordination of care for the child among all the providers and with the team at school. Sam has been followed at this clinic for the past 15 years. He has been seen at least yearly. The reason for this schedule of visits is based on the nature of the condition and the changing needs of the child. Synopses of specific visits that highlight essential elements of his examination, interventions, and plan of care are described.

EXAMINATION: AGE 5 YEARS

History

The following is a summary of information from the medical notes accompanying the referral. Sam was brought to medical attention because his family had noticed that he was unable to keep up with his peers in daycare, especially on the playground. He had difficulty running, hopping, and climbing the jungle gym and the steps to the slide. No problems had been noted during pregnancy or childbirth or in development of the early milestones, such as rolling, sitting, walking, and talking. The pediatrician noted the enlarged calf muscles and the difficulty Sam had rising from the floor. Sam used Gowers' maneuver. There was no family history of muscular dystrophy, or more specifically, DMD. The pediatrician ordered a screening blood test. The creatine kinase (CK/CPK) was more than 1000 times normal, and he referred Sam to a pediatric neurologist for further evaluation. The neurologist followed up with a blood test/genetic test for DMD and a muscle biopsy. The genetic test reported a deletion, and the biopsy showed an absence of dystrophin, confirming the diagnosis of DMD. Sam's mother is awaiting results of her genetic tests to see if she is a carrier. Sam has an older sister, and his mother is worried that her daughter might be a carrier. She is also concerned about her two sisters, who are of child-bearing age and planning families.

Parent Interview

Sam is independent in age-appropriate, self-care activities at home. He enjoys books, knows the alphabet, is working on numbers and colors, and looks forward to starting school. Currently Sam is in daycare full time. Except for the problems noted on the playground and the fact that he needs to get up from the floor using his hands, he is able to keep up with his peers.

Systems Review

Growth and Development

Height and weight are within normal limits (WNL).

Cardiovascular and Pulmonary

Sam's cardiovascular and pulmonary system, based on a review of the vital signs, seems WNL. Pulmonary involvement is common in DMD; therefore, Sam will undergo a forced vital capacity (FVC) measurement today. Because of the possibility of cardiac involvement, Sam is also scheduled for a baseline electrocardiogram (ECG).

Integumentary

The integumentary system is WNL.

Musculoskeletal

On musculoskeletal examination, Sam exhibits a lordotic posture with slight winging of the scapula. He also has enlargement of the calf muscles similar to that in the child in Figure 22–2. Given the medical diagnosis, a detailed examination of ROM and muscle strength will be performed.

Neuromuscular

Neuromuscular examination is WNL in terms of motor control, sensory integrity, and tone. Specific functional activities known to be affected will be examined in detail.

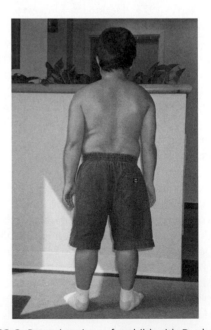

Figure 22-2 Posterior view of a child with Duchenne muscular dystrophy displaying "winging" of the scapula and enlargement of the calf muscles.

Cognition and Communication

Sam is a very friendly and curious 5-year-old who has been very cooperative through all the tests he has undergone today with the various providers. He communicates at age-appropriate level and follows instructions well.

Tests and Measures

Based on Sam's age and diagnosis, the elements for detailed examination were chosen based on the understanding of, and findings from, the natural history studies of DMD. The items included muscle force measurements by manual muscle tests (MMTs) and range of motion (ROM) measurements by goniometric tests, timed function tests, and measurements of FVC. Studies have shown that these items can be reliably documented in children with DMD aged 5 years and older (Florence et al., 1984) and are sensitive to disease progression (Brooke et al., 1983) and therapeutic interventions.

Muscle Performance

Muscle force measurements with MMTs were performed on selective muscles known to show early involvement: neck flexors, hip extensors, abductors, flexors, and knee extensors. The MMT procedures used are those described by Daniels and Worthingham (Hislop & Montgomery, 2002), and the scoring system used is a modification of the Medical Research Council (MRC) scale, as used in the CIDD studies. The intrarater and interrater reliabilities of the procedures and the scoring system have been documented in this population (Florence et al., 1984; Florence et al., 1992).

Range of Motion

ROM tests for ankle dorsiflexion and knee extension, Thomas test for hip flexor tightness, and Ober test for ITB/TFL tightness were performed. Goniometric tests were performed and scored using procedures described by the American Academy of Orthopedic Surgeons and the CIDD study group. Reliability of goniometric measurements in this population is documented (Pandya et al., 1985).

Motor Function

Three timed function tests were performed: (1) time to get up from the floor from a supine position, (2) time to

run 30 feet, and (3) time to climb four steps. Sam was instructed to perform all of these tests "as quickly as you can." The timed function tests are the simplest objective measure of progress that are easy to perform and have relevance for the child and his parents. These tests have also been shown to be reliable and sensitive in this patient population (Brooke et al., 1983; Florence et al., 1984).

Ventilation and Respiration

FVC has been recommended as a simple measure to document respiratory function in the muscular dystrophics (Rideau et al., 1981) and has been shown to be reliable and sensitive in children aged 5 years and older (Brooke et al., 1983; Florence et al., 1984). Results of the MMT, ROM, timed function tests, and FVC are presented in Table 22.1. The findings from these tests allow us to establish a baseline against which progression can be documented in the future.

EVALUATION, DIAGNOSIS, AND PROGNOSIS (INCLUDING PLAN OF CARE)

Evaluation

Sam's height, weight, and vital signs are all WNL. Strength is decreased in the neck flexors, hip flexors, extensors, abductors, and quadriceps. His ROM is WNL, except for the ankle, where he is beginning to show tightness in the gastrocsoleus group. Sam got up from the floor using Gowers' maneuver because of the pelvic girdle weakness. Sam runs with a wide base and a "waddle" attributable to the weakness of the hip abductors. He prefers to use the railing when climbing stairs and is unable to go step over step as would be expected for his age. His FVC is lower than predicted for his age. All these findings are consistent with his medical diagnosis of DMD.

Diagnosis

Physical therapy diagnoses at this stage include impaired posture, ROM, muscle performance, respiratory function, and locomotion.

Table 22.1 Results of Longitudinal Follow-up Examinations

Sam (DOB: 7/85)			Diagnosis: DMD		
	July 1990	**July 1991***	**July 1995**	**July 2000**	**July 2003**
Age (yr)	5	6	10	15	18
Height (cm)	113	115	120	133	157
Weight (kg)	18.6	20.2	33.4	50.9	69.1
Vital Signs	WNL	WNL	WNL	WNL	WNL
Timed Tests (seconds)					
Stand from supine	3	2*	3	7	Unable
Run 30 feet	5	3	3	5 (Walk)	7 (Walk)
Climb 4 stairs	3	2*	3	4	Unable
Neuromuscular (Muscle Performance)					
Neck flexors	2	3*	3	3	3
Hip extensors	4−	4+*	4	4−	3−
Hip abductors	4−	4+*	4	4−	3−
Hip flexors	4	4+*	4+	4	4−
Knee extensors	4	4+*	4	4−	3−
Musculoskeletal (Range of Motion)					
Ankle/dorsiflexion	+10	+10	0	−10	−15
Hip/extension	+20	+20	+10	0	−10
Knee/extension	WNL	WNL	WNL	WNL	−10
ITB/TFL	WNL	WNL	WNL	−10	−20
Pulmonary					
FVC (mL)	600	1000	1600	1900	2600†

*Improvements secondary to initiation of prednisone 6 months ago.

†FVC (forced vital capacity) continues to improve and does not show a plateau yet.

Prognosis

Based on Sam's medical diagnosis, the prognosis for improvement is poor in the long term. In the short term, progressive ROM restrictions can be delayed with a daily program of stretching, positioning, and splinting (Scott, Hyde, Goddard, & Dubowitz, 1981). Muscle performance can be improved with submaximal strengthening exercises (DeLateur & Giaconi, 1979). Unfortunately, long-term studies of effects of strengthening have not been done in this specific population or in other muscular dystrophy populations. Respiratory function, although below age-expected levels, will continue to increase based on natural history information and is not expected to plateau or decline until the teens. Impairments in posture, gait, and functional activities have not been shown to be amenable to physical therapy interventions.

Goals

Given an understanding of the etiology of this condition, the knowledge about its natural history, and the efficacy of various interventions, the following goals were developed after discussion with Sam's parents.

Long-term goals: Maximize Sam's functional abilities within the limitations imposed by a progressive disorder. Delay and/or prevent the loss of strength and ROM.

Short-term goals for this specific visit and episode of care are as follows:

1. Sam's ankle ROM will remain the same through the assistance of his parents correctly performing passive stretching exercises at least once daily.

2. Sam will maintain hip extension by lying prone for at least two 30-minute sessions each day.

3. Sam will maintain present strength and functional status by exercising in a community pool program.

INTERVENTION

Coordination, Communication, and Documentation

A decision was made that, as soon as school started and the personnel working with Sam were identified, we would establish communication with the classroom teacher, physical education teacher, school nurse, and school physical therapist.

Patient/Client-Related Instruction

Sam's parents have been trying to get as much information as possible about DMD from the health-care professionals they have encountered. They have talked with the services coordinator from MDA about the services MDA provides and the child support groups available in their area. We

briefly discussed what could be expected in the short term, given his diagnosis and age. The roles and areas of expertise of the various clinic team members were explained to them. How Sam's care would be coordinated between the clinic team, his pediatrician, and the school was also discussed. Sam would continue to be followed by the pediatrician for his regular needs, such as annual checkups, immunizations, and booster shots.

Procedural Interventions

Sam's parents were given a demonstration on how to perform passive stretching exercises to maintain ROM at the ankle. They were also instructed regarding positioning him in prone when he is watching television to prevent tightness from developing at the hip. Sam's parents were also asked to explore opportunities for swimming or a pool program for Sam. Pool therapy is commonly recommended because it allows a whole-body workout in a fun environment. In addition to providing an exercise option for the musculoskeletal system, it allows the incorporation of a pulmonary program.

TERMINATION OF EPISODE OF CARE

Sam was seen for a regularly scheduled episode of physical therapy prevention (APTA, 2001, p. 679), as part of the MDA clinic in his local community. The purpose of these visits is to support maintenance of optimal function, health, wellness, and fitness. Sam will also be followed by a physical therapist at school, who will develop a specific plan of care for the school setting. Sam's family was advised to contact the clinic if they had any questions or concerns before the next regularly scheduled visit.

EXAMINATION: AGE 6 YEARS

History

Sam has been healthy over the past year. He has completed kindergarten and did well in school. He was mainstreamed and did not require any type of assistance or services in the classroom or in transportation to school. He participated in regular physical education classes. The physical education teacher and the school physical therapist discussed the physical education program and worked out modifications necessary to accommodate limitations in activities secondary to his weakness. They have also incorporated Sam's stretching needs into the physical education program. The family has joined the local YMCA, and they try to go swimming at least twice a week, once during a weeknight and once over the weekend. They continue to perform the stretching exercises and positioning as instructed at least 5 times a week.

Six months ago Sam was started on prednisone 0.75 mg/kg/day as recommended by the pediatric neurologist based on the findings from several randomized, controlled trials. Parents have noticed an improvement in Sam's functional abilities since he started on prednisone. He does not need the railing to climb stairs and goes up alternate steps. He gets up from the floor more easily and seems to be able to run faster. Sam has learned to ride a bike and therefore is able to keep up and socialize with the neighborhood kids. He is hungrier (a known side effect of prednisone), but his parents are encouraging him to eat fruits instead of cookies or chips, and the dietician is pleased with the dietetic control they have been able to maintain in terms of restricting sugar and salt and unnecessary calories.

Systems Review

Growth and Development

Height and weight are WNL. It is extremely important to monitor height and weight, because the major concerns with steroid therapy are weight gain and decreased growth.

Cardiovascular and Pulmonary

Vital signs are WNL. Sam's baseline ECG done last year showed abnormal Q waves and prominent R waves, suggesting ventricular hypertrophy. This abnormality on ECG, in the absence of clinical signs of cardiomyopathy, is not uncommon but requires monitoring. Pulmonary function will be evaluated as part of special tests.

Integumentary

The integumentary system is WNL. Some boys have been reported to show striae (stretch marks), especially on the abdomen, as a side effect of prednisone, but Sam was not noted to have striae.

Musculoskeletal

Musculoskeletal examination was unchanged from last year in terms of posture. Muscle performance and ROM will be examined in detail.

Neuromuscular

Neuromuscular examination is WNL in terms of motor control, sensory integrity, and tone. Specific functional activities documented previously will be examined in detail.

Cognition and Communication

Sam communicates at an age-appropriate level and follows instructions well.

Tests and Measures

Items include the same tests that were performed last year: muscle performance, ROM, timed motor function tests, and FVC (see Table 22.1).

> ### EVALUATION, DIAGNOSIS, AND PROGNOSIS (INCLUDING PLAN OF CARE)

Evaluation

Compared with his examination 1 year ago, Sam shows improvement. This is not unexpected; the randomized controlled trials of prednisone have shown that during the first 6 months there is an increase in muscle mass and muscle strength and an improvement in timed function tests and functional abilities. In the randomized controlled trials, this improvement lasted for 18 months or more, and even though the disease progresses thereafter, the progression is slower. With these tests and measures, physical therapists can assist the medical team in monitoring the effects of medications on muscle performance and functional abilities.

Diagnosis

Sam's physical therapy diagnoses continue to be impaired posture, ROM, and muscle performance.

Prognosis

Sam's prognosis, in general, remains poor because of the progressive nature of his condition, but because of his being on prednisone, it is difficult to make specific prognostic statements regarding his muscle performance and functional abilities in the short term.

Goals

Long-term goals include maintaining ROM, strength, and functional abilities. To facilitate Sam's assuming responsibility for his personal health care needs, short-term goals for this visit include teaching Sam techniques for self-stretching and incorporating these into his daily routine.

1. Sam will correctly perform self-stretching of gastrocnemius muscle.
2. Sam will demonstrate the appropriate prone position that he has been instructed to lie in for 30 minutes twice daily.
3. Sam will ride his bike around the neighborhood for up to 30 minutes daily during his summer vacation.

INTERVENTION

Coordination, Communication, and Documentation

During the past year, the school physical therapist continued to monitor Sam and to work with the classroom teacher and the physical education teacher to modify plans based on his recent improvements and current abilities. We will communicate with the school therapist in the fall and coordinate care for the new school year.

Patient/Client-Related Instruction

Sam's parents were encouraged to continue with the program of stretching, positioning, and swimming to maximize and build on the gains provided by the medical therapy. Sam was instructed in self-stretching exercises for the gastrocsoleus. We also reviewed the positioning for prevention of tightness at the hip by lying prone. Sam was encouraged to watch his after-school television programs in this

position. Parents were advised not to restrict Sam's activities unless he complained specifically of being tired after a good night's sleep or complained of cramps in specific muscles. The parents were also encouraged to increase the frequency of swimming over the summer, if at all feasible with their other family obligations.

EPISODE OF PHYSICAL THERAPY PREVENTION

Sam will continue to be followed at 6-month intervals in the progressive neuromuscular disorder clinic. Physical therapy services in this clinic visit include examination, instruction, and education. Sam and his family were independent in performing the home program of exercises and seemed to appreciate the importance of regular physical activity. The family was advised to contact the clinic if they had any questions or concerns before the next clinic visit.

EXAMINATION: AGE 10 YEARS

History

Sam has been healthy since his last visit to the clinic. He continues on prednisone and has developed cushingoid facies, a typical side effect of corticosteroid use. Sam has maintained the gains he had made when he started on medication and seems to be showing a very minimal decline. Both Sam and his parents are extremely pleased with the maintenance of his physical capabilities. Sam attended the 1-week summer camp sponsored by the MDA last month and is already looking forward to going next year.

Systems Review

Growth and Development

Sam is short for his age (20th percentile), and his parents are a little concerned about this because he will be starting middle school this fall. Sam and his parents are aware that growth retardation is the other major side effect of prednisone, besides weight gain, that has been documented in the previous clinical trials.

DUCHENNE MUSCULAR DYSTROPHY

Cardiovascular and Pulmonary

Sam's ECG done earlier today showed signs of cardiomyopathy. Sam will be referred to a cardiologist for long-term management of the cardiomyopathy. In terms of activities, no restrictions have been advised secondary to this new observation. Pulmonary function tests will be done to monitor his FVC.

Integumentary

The integumentary system is WNL.

Musculoskeletal

Sam's posture is a little more "lordotic." He stands with just a slightly wider base of support. ROM and muscle performance will be examined in detail.

Neuromuscular

Neuromuscular examination is WNL in terms of motor control, sensory integrity, and tone. Specific functional activities documented previously will be examined in detail.

Communication and Cognition

Sam communicates at an age-appropriate level and remains outgoing and curious. In school, he is interested in history and geography and is performing well. Unlike some boys with DMD, he is doing well intellectually and does not exhibit any problems with learning.

Tests and Measures

Results of the examination of ROM, muscle performance, timed functional activities, and FVC are presented in Table 22.1.

EVALUATION, DIAGNOSIS, AND PROGNOSIS

Evaluation

Results of Sam's examination support the observations made by Sam and his parents. Even though there are some declines compared with previous results, Sam continues to perform well above expectations from the natural history studies. He uses Gowers' maneuver again when getting up from the floor. When walking, he tends to go up on his toes more. Even though he is able to climb stairs without the railing, he prefers using the railing because it feels "safer." Sam's FVC continues to show an increase and is almost close to normal. Based on the natural history studies of pulmonary function in boys with DMD, we know that FVC continues to increase until about age 10 to 12 years, then plateaus for a couple of years, and then begins to decline.

Prognosis

Sam has done extremely well given the natural history of DMD. Reports of the effect of corticosteroids beyond a decade are currently unavailable; therefore it is difficult to predict the long-term future. Sam and his parents are aware of this and appreciate that we are learning from Sam's follow-up visits. In the short term, decreasing muscle performance, ROM, and functional abilities continue to be the main concern.

Goals

Long-term goals continue to be the maximizing of Sam's functional abilities within the limitations of a progressive disorder.

Short-term goals include maintaining ROM and strength through daily stretching exercises and participation in an adaptive gym program and/or a community pool program.

INTERVENTION

Coordination, Communication, and Documentation

The middle school that Sam will be attending has planned to accommodate him by ensuring that all his classes will be on the same level and he does not have to climb stairs. An assistance plan is already in place in case of emergencies and fire drills. Sam and his parents are concerned that Sam may not be able to participate to the same extent in physical education. A program of regular and adaptive physical education will be worked out with the physical education teacher and school physical therapist. It is important to let Sam have the opportunity to participate in team sports in some capacity, such as scorekeeper or timekeeper, especially for the social components. It is also important that Sam have an opportunity to meet his health and well-being needs as part of the physical education program. Because the school he will be attending has a pool, the option of swimming as part of physical education will be explored for Sam.

Patient/Client-Related Instruction

Sam and his father described the routine they have worked out. Sam does self-stretching for the heel cords and ITB/TFL as part of his physical education routine at school, and follows the positioning instructions when he comes home and watches television. His father does the stretches for the heel cord and ITB/TFL at bedtime. Sam also understands the importance of standing and weight-bearing and spends 3 to 4 hours a day on his feet.

SYNOPSIS OF VISIT AT AGE 15 YEARS

History

Sam has been healthy over the past year. He continues on prednisone, although at a reduced dose of 0.5 mg/kg/day because of his weight gain. He has also developed punctate cataracts in both eyes. These cataracts do not affect his vision or require surgery at this time. Sam will require annual checkups with an ophthalmologist. The cataracts are a long-term side effect of steroid use. The orthopedist obtained a baseline spine radiograph today to start monitoring Sam for development of scoliosis. Sam enjoys school and continues to do well in class. He is interested in history and computer sciences. He is already beginning to explore options regarding college. He is having greater difficulty walking long distances. Sam chose to use a wheelchair during the family's recent trip to Disney World. His parents are planning on getting a manual chair from MDA's "loan" closet for occasional family trips this summer. Sam is also having greater difficulty with stairs, and the family is exploring the option of either adding or converting space in their house on the first floor into a

bedroom and an accessible bathroom for Sam. They will be adding a ramp to the side door that comes in from the garage.

Systems Review

Growth and Development

Sam's growth has definitely slowed down since he started on prednisone. He continues to manage his weight well with his diet.

Cardiovascular and Pulmonary

Vital signs are WNL. Sam does not show any symptoms related to cardiac or pulmonary systems. He continues to be monitored yearly by the cardiologist. He also continues to have formal pulmonary function evaluations. Results of the FVC are noted in Table 22.1.

Integumentary

The integumentary system is WNL.

Musculoskeletal

Sam is up on his toes a lot more, his posture is very lordotic, and his gait is very much more wide based as he tries to maintain stability. He is getting tighter at all joints.

Neuromuscular

Sam is definitely weaker and had increasing difficulty with the timed tests. Even though he managed to get up from supine on the floor independently, at home he rarely gets down on the floor, and he tends to get up with the help of furniture. He is unable to climb stairs without a railing. At home, he comes down in the morning and does not go up to his room until the evening. He literally has to pull himself on the railing to make it up. He is unable to run and walked as fast as he could within safety for the timed test.

Tests and Measures

Results of the ROM, muscle performance tests, timed function tests, and FVC are detailed in Table 22.1.

INTERVENTION

Coordination, Communication, and Documentation

The high school has accommodated Sam by clustering his classes in one wing of the building. A manual wheelchair is also available for him for emergency evacuations, and if he needs to use it to get to the cafeteria or library. Currently, Sam has chosen to continue to walk even though it takes him longer. He gets out of classes earlier to change rooms, so he does not have to worry about being jostled in the crowds. Safety is a concern because he could easily fall because of his weakness. Sam works out in the training room with his peers. The school physical therapist and the physical education teacher have worked out a plan of exercises for the upper extremities using mild to moderate resistance. Sam is also doing pulmonary exercises daily with an incentive spirometer.

Patient/Client-Related Instruction

Sam is having difficulty continuing his self-stretching for the ankles. Stretching exercises for the heel cords, ITB/TFL, and hamstrings were reviewed with his father. Sam continues to spend 45 to 60 minutes prone daily when watching television. We also discussed the option of using night splints to maintain his ankle ROM. We do not routinely provide them because most children do not tolerate them all night. Also, they do not go above the knee and therefore provide only a partial stretch. Sam was willing to give them a try. We also discussed at length the options of motorized mobility, either a scooter or a motorized wheelchair. The pros and cons of each option in terms of cost, ease of transportation, need for a van, and so on were discussed at length. Sam and his family decided they would discuss the issue and talk to the school personnel, other families who had made these decisions, and the MDA services coordinator. They would also check with their insurance company to see how much of the costs would be covered and what out-of-pocket expenses would be incurred.

SYNOPSIS OF VISIT AT AGE 18 YEARS

History

Sam graduated from high school this May. He will be going to a college that is located about 4 hours away from home.

The college is well known for its services and environmental adaptations to meet the special needs of students with disabilities. Sam is excited about living on campus. He will receive aide service for 1 hour in the morning and at bedtime. Besides helping Sam with his activities of daily living needs, the aide will also continue with the stretching program that Sam's father used to follow. Sam will also have the opportunity to continue working out in the pool 2 to 3 times a week based on his schedule. The pool is completely accessible. The same aide will help Sam in the changing rooms at the pool and help him get in and out of the pool. In preparation for the move to college, Sam obtained a motorized chair this spring. The family has bought a van and equipped it with a lift so that they can transport Sam and his chair back and forth from college. At some point during the next 2 years, Sam hopes to have the van adapted to his needs and get driver training himself so that he can be completely independent.

Examination

Sam is unable to get up from the floor or climb stairs. He continues to be able to walk around the house, but tends to use the furniture and walls for occasional support. He needs assistance with some self-care activities but otherwise is fairly independent given the adaptations in the bathroom (a shower seat, raised toilet seat, grab bars) and bedroom (railings on the side of his bed). Sam has difficulty with overhead activities such as shampooing his hair and getting a shirt over his head. He is still able to feed himself, use his computer keyboard, and write. The shoulder girdle muscles are in the 3− range. The elbow flexors and extensors are 4−, and the distal hand muscles are in the 4 range. His grip is fair. Results of specific tests and measures are detailed in Table 22.1.

Coordination

Sam and his family are very knowledgeable about Sam's condition and the various treatment and management options. They have attended seminars and support groups offered by MDA and the Parent Project Muscular Dystrophy (PPMD). Sam has attended MDA camp every summer for the past 7 years and met other children with inherited neuromuscular disorders and therefore is very aware of the progression that occurs in these disorders. The whole family has been very proactive regarding Sam's care and management. Because Sam is going to college, we again reviewed the (1) plan for continuing visits with the multidisciplinary team at least once a year, (2) importance of a pulmonary workout to maintain respiratory function, (3) need to immediately seek care in case of even minor respiratory involvements, and (4) emergency plan in case of a fall when Sam is by himself.

DISCUSSION

This case report of a child with DMD illustrates the knowledge and processes necessary to create and implement evidence-based plans of care for children with inherited disorders. When preparing to see a child with a medical diagnosis that is uncommon or unfamiliar, it is important to collect information about the etiology, pathophysiology, resulting impairments in body structures and functions, and restrictions in activities and participation related to the medical diagnosis. It is also important to have information about the natural history or the prognosis of the condition, secondary complications, and current medical, surgical, and rehabilitative management. The *Guide* (APTA, 2001) provides information on specific tests and measures and the practice patterns related to the "physical therapy diagnoses." Review available literature regarding physical therapy interventions that have been shown to be effective and have been used based on empirical information. An evidence-based plan of care can be developed for any child with an inherited disorder using information regarding the elements listed above, as has been illustrated using the case of a child with DMD.

Having an understanding of the etiology, pathophysiology, and natural history of a disorder allows us to better define and describe the role physical therapy and physical therapists can play in intervention. The role of physical therapy and the physical therapist in the intervention of children with progressive disorders is different from that for a child with a condition from which complete recovery is expected (e.g., fracture) or a child with a nonprogressive neuromuscular disorder (e.g., cerebral palsy), who is expected to show some improvements. Even though all of these children may have "impaired muscle function" as one of their physical therapy diagnoses, the medical prognosis and natural history may determine the goals and interventions appropriate for the condition. In the case of a child with an inherited neuromuscular disorder with a progressive natural history, the goals are not necessarily to "normalize" strength and function but to prevent and/or delay losses and to maximize function and improve quality of life within the imposed limitations. This is an extremely important concept that needs to be understood and appreciated.

SUMMARY

Sam's case documents the changing natural history and prognosis for children with DMD attributable to advances in therapeutic options. Even though specific medications are not currently available for the other pediatric inherited neuromuscular disorders, the aggressive preventive care, surgical options for management of scoliosis, and the noninvasive options of pulmonary support have had a major impact on prognosis and life span. With the increasing life span and improved functional abilities, activities, and participation, these children are now graduating from high school, completing college, and looking forward to living independently, being employed, and living as productive members of society. As health-care providers, we need to make sure that our practices meet the changing needs of these children. As citizens, we also need to advocate on behalf of children, to make sure that societal barriers do not prevent them from achieving their full potential.

Campbell has summarized the issues faced by adults with cerebral palsy and myelodysplasia (1997). Some of the issues she emphasizes are also applicable in the management of children with inherited progressive neuromuscular disorders. These include (1) prevention of secondary disabilities by preparing children and adolescents to take personal responsibility for their health and wellness, (2) preparing these children educationally and vocationally so that they can be productive members of society,, and (3) enabling them to live independently by advocating for the appropriate services. She has also made recommendations for adapting our practices so that we take a more long-term view and develop programs for children so that they last a lifetime. In so doing, we may need to consider our role more as consultants, coordinators, and educators rather than primarily as direct care providers.

DISCUSSION QUESTIONS

1. Discuss the difficulty in developing and writing appropriate objectives for a child whose ability to function is expected to deteriorate over time.

2. What are some activities of daily living aids that might commonly be used to help the child with DMD?

3. What are some obstacles you would look for when evaluating a high school for a student with DMD who uses a power wheelchair?

RECOMMENDED READINGS

Florence, J. M. (1998). Neuromuscular disorders in childhood and physical therapy intervention. In J.S. Tecklin (Ed.), *Pediatric physical therapy* (3rd ed., pp. 223–246). Philadelphia: J.B. Lippincott.

Harris, S.E., & Cherry, D.B. (1974). Childhood progressive muscular dystrophy and the role of physical therapy. *Physical Therapy, 54* (1), 4–12. (*Even though published 30 years ago, this article is still pertinent today in terms of physical therapy examination, intervention, and management. It is a classic!*)

Pandya, S. (1993). Evaluation and management of patients with neuromuscular diseases. *Neurology Report 17* (3), 15–19.

Stuberg, W. A. (2000). Muscular dystrophy and spinal muscular atrophy. In S.K. Campbell, D.W. Vander Linden, & R.J. Palisano (Eds.), *Physical therapy for children* (2nd ed., pp. 338–369). Philadelphia: W.B. Saunders.

The following Worldwide Websites are recommended for up-to-date information regarding the latest research findings, clinical management, support groups, and advocacy initiatives.

National Institute of Neurological Disorders and Stroke: *http://www.ninds.nih.gov*

National Institute of Child Health: *www. Nichd.nih.gov*

Muscular Dystrophy Association: *http://www.mdausa.org*

Parent Project Muscular Dystrophy:*www.parentprojectmd.org*

REFERENCES

American Physical Therapy Association (APTA) (2001). *Guide to physical therapist practice* (2nd ed.). *Physical Therapy, 81,* 6–746.

Angelini, C., Pergoraro, E., Turella, E., Intino, M.T., Pini, A., & Costa, C. (1994). Deflazacort in Duchenne dystrophy: Study of long term effect. *Muscle and Nerve, 17,* 386–391.

Backman, E., & Henriksson, K.G. (1995). Low dose prednisone treatment in Duchenne and Becker muscular dystrophy. *Neuromuscular Disorders, 5,* 233–241.

Biggar, W.D., Gingras, M., Feblings, D.L., Harris, V.A., & Steele, C.A. (2001). Deflazacort treatment of Duchenne muscular dystrophy. *Journal of Pediatrics, 138,* 45–50.

Brooke, M.H., Fenichel, G., Griggs, R., Mendell, J.R., Moxley, R., Miller, J.P., et al. (1983). Clinical investigations in Duchenne dystrophy. Part 2. Determination of the "power" of therapeutic trials based on the natural history. *Muscle Nerve, 6,* 91–103.

Brooke, M.H., Fenichel, G., Griggs, R., Mendell, J.R., Moxley, R., Miller, J.P., et al. (1989). Duchenne muscular dystrophy: Patterns of clinical progression and effects of supportive therapy. *Neurology, 39,* 475–481.

Campbell, S.K. (1997). Therapy programs for children that last a lifetime. *Physical and Occupational Therapy in Pediatrics, 1,* 1–15.

De Lateur, B.J., & Giaconi, R.M. (1979). Effect on maximal strength of submaximal exercise in Duchenne muscular dystrophy. *American Journal of Physical Medicine, 58,* 26–36.

DeSilva, S., Drachman, D.B., Mellits, D., & Kunel, R.W. (1987). Prednisone treatment in Duchenne muscular dystrophy: Long term benefit. *Archives of Neurology, 44,* 818–822.

Dubowitz, V. (1995). *Muscle disorders in childhood* (2nd ed.). London: W.B. Saunders.

Duchenne, G.B. (1868). Recherches sur la paralysie musculaire pseudohypertrophique ou paralysie myosclérosique. *Archives Générales de Médecine (11)*5, 179, 305.

Eagle, M., Baudouin, S.V., Chandler, C., Giddings, D.R., Bullock, R., & Bushby, K. (2002). Survival in Duchenne muscular dystrophy: Improvements in life expectancy since 1967 and the impact of home nocturnal ventilation. *Neuromuscular Disorders, 12*(10), 926–930.

Emery, A.E.H. (1991). Population frequencies of inherited neuromuscular diseases: A world survey. *Neuromuscular Disorders, 1,* 19–29.

Emery, A.E.H. (2003). *Duchenne muscular dystrophy* (2nd ed.). Oxford: Oxford University Press.

Fenichel, G.M., Florence, J.M., Pestronk, A., Mendell, R.T., Griggs, R.C., Miller, J.P., et al. (1991). Long term benefit from prednisone in Duchenne muscular dystrophy. *Neurology, 41,* 1874–1877.

Florence, J.M., Pandya, S., King, W.M., Robinson, J.D., Signore, L.C., Wentzell, M., Province, M.A., & The CIDD Group (1984). Clinical trials in Duchenne muscular dystrophy: Standardization and reliability of evaluation procedures. *Physical Therapy, 64*(1), 41–45.

Florence, J.M., Pandya, S., King, W.M., Robinson, J.D., Baty, J., Miller, J.P., Schierbecker, J., & Signore, L.C. (1992). Intrarater reliability of manual muscle test (Medical Research Council Scale) grades in Duchenne's muscular dystrophy. *Physical Therapy, 72*(2), 115–122.

Galasko, C.S., Delaney, C., & Morris, P. (1992). Spinal stabilisation in Duchenne muscular dystrophy. *The Journal of Bone and Joint Surgery (British), 74B,* 210–215.

Gowers, W.R. (1879). Clinical lecture on pseudohypertrophic muscular paralysis. *Lancet, 2,* 37, 73, 113.

Griggs, R.C., Moxley, R.T., Mendell, J.R., Fenichel, G.M., Brooke, M.H., Pestronk, A., et al. (1991). Prednisone in Duchenne dystrophy. A randomized controlled trial defining the time course and dose response. *Archives of Neurology, 48,* 383–388.

Griggs, R.C., Moxley, R.T., Mendell, J.R., Fenichel, G.M., Brooke, M.H., Pestronk, A., et al. (1993). Duchenne dystrophy: Randomized controlled trial of prednisone (18 months) and azathioprine (12 months). *Neurology, 43,* 520–527.

Harris, S.E., & Cherry, D.B. (1974). Childhood progressive muscular dystrophy and the role of physical therapy. *Physical Therapy, 54*(1), 4–12.

Heckmatt, J.Z., Dubowitz, V., & Hyde, S.A. (1985). Prolongation of walking in Duchenne muscular dystrophy with lightweight orthoses: Review of 57 cases. *Developmental Medicine and Child Neurology, 27,* 149–154.

Hislop, H.J., & Montgomery, J. (2002). Techniques of manual examination. In *Daniels and Worthingham's muscle testing* (7th ed.). Philadelphia: W.B. Saunders.

Hoffman, E.P., Brown, R.H., & Kunkel, L.M. (1987). Dystrophin: The protein product of the Duchenne muscular dystrophy locus. *Cell, 51*, 919–928.

Kunkel, L.M., Monaco, A.P., Middlesworth, W., Ochs, S.D., & Latt, S.A. (1985). Specific cloning of DNA fragments absent from the DNA of a male patient with an X chromosome deletion. *Proceedings of the National Academy of Science USA, 82*, 4778–4782.

Luque, E.R. (1982). Segmental spinal stabilization for the correction of scoliosis. *Clinical Orthopedics 163*, 192–198.

Manzur, A.Y., Kuntzer, T., Pike, M., & Swan, A. (2004). Glucocorticoid corticosteroids for Duchenne muscular dystrophy (Cochrane Review). In: *The Cochrane Library*, Issue 3. Chichester, UK: John Wiley & Sons, Ltd.

Mendell, J.R., Moxley, R.T., Griggs, R.C., Brooke, M.H., Fenichel, G.M., Miller, J.P., et al. (1989). Randomized double blind six month trial of prednisone in Duchenne's muscular dystrophy. *New England Journal of Medicine, 320*, 1592–1597.

Mesa, L.E., Dubrovsky, A.L., Corderi, J., Maarco, P., & Flores, D. (1991). Steroids in Duchenne muscular dystrophy: Deflazacort trial. *Neuromuscular Disorders, 1*, 261–266.

Miller, F., Moseley, C.F., & Koreska, J. (1992). Spinal fusion in Duchenne muscular dystrophy. *Developmental Medicine and Child Neurology, 34*, 775–786.

Pandya, S., Florence, J.M., King, W.M., Robinson, V.D.,

Wentzell, M., Province, M.A., & The CIDD Group (1985). Reliability of goniometric measurements in patients with Duchenne muscular dystrophy. *Physical Therapy, 65*, 1339–1342.

Pandya, S., & Moxley, R.T. (2002). Long term prednisone therapy delays loss of ambulation and decline in pulmonary function (abstract). *Journal of Neurological Science, 199*, S120.

Rideau, Y., Jankowski, L.W., & Grellet, J. (1981). Respiratory function in the muscular dystrophies. *Muscle Nerve, 4*, 155–164.

Schara, U., Mortier, J., & Mortier, W. (2001). Long term steroid therapy in Duchenne muscular dystrophy: Positive results versus side effects. *Journal of Clinical Neuromuscular Disease, 2*, 179–183.

Scott, O.M., Hyde, S.A., Goddard, C., & Dubowitz, V. (1981). Prevention of deformity in Duchenne muscular dystrophy: A prospective study of passive stretching and splintage. *Physiotherapy, 67*, 177–180.

Scott, O.M., Hyde, S.A., & Goddard, E. (1982). Quantification of muscle function in children: A prospective study in Duchenne muscular dystrophy. *Muscle and Nerve, 5*, 291–301.

Vignos, P.J., Wagner, M.B., Karlinchak, B., & Katirji, B. (1996). Evaluation of a program for long-term treatment of Duchenne muscular dystrophy. Experience at the University Hospitals of Cleveland. *The Journal of Bone and Joint Surgery (British), 78*, 1844–1852.

Wong, B.L., & Christopher, C. (2002). Corticosteroids in Duchenne muscular dystrophy: A reappraisal. *Journal of Child Neurology, 17*, 183–190.

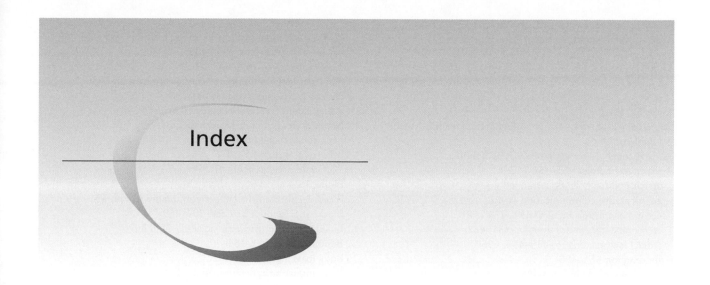

Index

Note: Page numbers followed by f indicate figures; page numbers followed by t indicate tables; and page numbers followed by b refer to boxed material.

A

AAC (augmentative and alternative communication) devices, 475–478, 477f

ABILITIES Index, 98

Abuse and neglect, of children, 35, 36b

Abuse of drugs, during childhood or adolescence, 402, 406
during pregnancy, teratogenic effects of, 52

Achondroplasia, 48t

Acquired nonprogressive disorders, of central nervous system, 192–201

Action, vs. movement, 254

Active alertness, in newborn, 436t

Active cycle-of-breathing techniques, in airway clearance, 314f, 314–315

Active movement, by newborn, 436, 439

Activities of daily living, assistive technology facilitating, 481, 483f

Activity-based instruction, in early intervention, 365, 370

Activity restrictions, in heat-stress environment, 408t
in presence of integumentary impairment, 355

Acute-care pediatric hospital, 419–429

Acute head trauma, 197–201, 420–422

Acute leukemia, 532t. See also Leukemia.

Adams forward bend test, 143–144, 144f

Adolescent(s), 77
development of, 77, 80t, 81
injury types specific to, 399
scoliosis in, 178
steroid use by, 406

Adult vs. pediatric cardiopulmonary physiology, 286t, 308, 308t, 309, 309t

Afference copy, 218

Affordances, 263

Age-equivalent score, expression of test result(s) as, 18

Agenesis, pulmonary, 293t

Ages & Stages Questionnaire (2nd ed.), 98

Agility, athletic fitness correlated with, 402t, 403t

Aided communication systems, 476–478

Airway, clearance of secretions from, 310–316
in management of cystic fibrosis, 428t–429t

Alberta Infant Motor Scale and Motor Assessment of Developing Infant, 98

Alcohol, teratogenic effects of, 51–52, 52f

Alertness, of newborn, 436t

Alginate dressings, 351

Allis test, 142–143, 143f

Alternative and augmentative communication (AAC) devices, 475–478, 477f

Alveolar-capillary membrane, 305f

American Sign Language, 485

Amorphous hydrogels, as wound dressings, 351

Anemia, sickle cell, 306t

Angelman syndrome, 48t

Ankle strategy, in postural control, 214, 214f

Anomalous pulmonary venous return, 301t

Antetorsion, 136

Aorta, coarctation of, 300f, 302t

Aortic valve, stenosis of, 302t

Apgar scoring, 430, 431t

Arena assessment, 17, 117, 368

Arm supports, for child in seating system, 467

Arnold-Chiari malformation, 296t